# Advances in Ceramic Biomaterials

## Related titles

Bioceramics and their clinical applications (ISBN 978-1-84569-204-9)

Bioactive glasses (ISBN 978-1-84569-768-6)

Non-metallic biomaterials for tooth repair and replacement (ISBN 978-0-85709-244-1)

Woodhead Publishing Series in Biomaterials

# Advances in Ceramic Biomaterials

## Materials, Devices and Challenges


*Edited by*

*Paola Palmero*

Politecnico di Torino, Torino, Italy

*Francis Cambier*

Belgium Ceramic Research Centre, Mons, Belgium

*Eamonn De Barra*

University of Limerick, Limerick, Ireland



ELSEVIER

WP WOODHEAD PUBLISHING

An imprint of Elsevier

Woodhead Publishing is an imprint of Elsevier
The Officers' Mess Business Centre, Royston Road, Duxford, CB22 4QH, United Kingdom
50 Hampshire Street, 5th Floor, Cambridge, MA 02139, United States
The Boulevard, Langford Lane, Kidlington, OX5 1GB, United Kingdom



**British Library Cataloguing-in-Publication Data**
A catalogue record for this book is available from the British Library

**Library of Congress Cataloging-in-Publication Data**
A catalog record for this book is available from the Library of Congress

ISBN: 978-0-08-100881-2 (print)
ISBN: 978-0-08-100882-9 (online)

For information on all Woodhead Publishing publications
visit our website at https://www.elsevier.com/books-and-journals



*Publisher:* Matthew Deans
*Acquisition Editor:* Laura Overend
*Editorial Project Manager:* Natasha Welford
*Production Project Manager:* Debasish Ghosh
*Cover Designer:* Miles Hitchen

Typeset by MPS Limited, Chennai, India

# Contents


**List of contributors** ix
**Preface** xiii
**Acknowledgments** xvii

## Part I An Overview of Biomedical Grade Ceramic Materials 1

**1 Materials for hard tissue applications: An overview** 3
*Laurent Gremillard and Solène Tadier*
1.1 Introduction: Hard tissues and how to replace them 3
1.2 Materials for hard tissue applications 4
1.3 Concluding remarks 16
References 16

**2 Types of ceramics: Material class** 21
*Christophe Drouet, Anne Leriche, Stuart Hampshire, Mitra Kashani, Artemis Stamboulis, Michele Iafisco and Anna Tampieri*
2.1 Active oxides 22
2.2 Inert oxides and composites 34
2.3 Nonoxide ceramics 40
2.4 Bioactive glasses 44
2.5 Glass ceramics and bioactive glass ceramics 49
2.6 Glass-ionomer cements 50
2.7 Magnetic ceramic materials in medicine 60
2.8 Conclusion 63
References 64
Further reading 82

**3 Assessment of mechanical properties of ceramic materials** 83
*Marc Anglada*
3.1 Introduction to mechanical properties 83
3.2 Bioactive glasses and glass ceramics 93
3.3 Calcium phosphates (CaP) and CaP composites 95
3.4 Calcium phosphate cements 100
3.5 Structural bioinert ceramics 102
3.6 Conclusions 105
References 106
Further reading 109

4 **Biological assessment of bioceramics** **111**
*Paola Torricelli, Nicolò Nicoli Aldini and Milena Fini*
4.1 Introduction 111
4.2 Regulations and international standard organization rules 112
4.3 In vitro and in vivo tests 113
4.4 Conclusions 122
References 123

**Part II Bioceramics on the Market: Issues and Perspectives 127**

5 **Ceramics for joint replacement: Design and application of commercial bearings** **129**
*Corrado Piconi*
Abbreviations 129
5.1 Introduction 130
5.2 Development of ceramics for joint replacements 132
5.3 Requirements of ceramics in joint replacements 145
5.4 Ceramic coatings in joint replacements 159
5.5 Commercial ceramics for joint replacements bearings 161
5.6 Conclusions 167
References 169

6 **Ceramics for dentistry: Commercial devices and their clinical analysis** **181**
*Loredana Cerroni*
Abbreviations 181
6.1 Introduction 182
6.2 Dental applications of load-bearing ceramics 182
6.3 Commercial load-bearing ceramics: a comparative analysis 217
6.4 Conclusions 232
References 232
Further reading 248

7 **Ceramics for bone replacement: Commercial products and clinical use** **249**
*Francesco Baino*
7.1 Introduction 249
7.2 Bone substitutes of human and animal origin 250
7.3 Bone substitutes of nonanimal biological origin: Ceramics from corals 252
7.4 Calcium orthophosphates of synthetic origin 254
7.5 Bioactive glasses and glass ceramics 256
7.6 Composites 262
7.7 Moldable and injectable ceramic-based cements 264
7.8 Conclusions and outlook 269
References 271

**8 Ceramic devices for bone regeneration: Mechanical and clinical issues and new perspectives 279**

*David Marchat and Eric Champion*

8.1 Introduction 279
8.2 The origins of failure 280
8.3 Rationale for the development of implant-based tissue engineering strategies 288
8.4 Concluding remarks 298
References 298
Further reading 311

**9 Clinical issues of ceramic devices used in total hip arthroplasty 313**

*Jonathan S. De Mattia, Emanuela Castiello and Saverio Affatato*

Abbreviations 313
9.1 Introduction 314
9.2 Ceramics as orthopedic medical devices: Advantages and disadvantages 317
9.3 Technical issues and surgical aspects 320
9.4 In vitro performance and in vivo failure analysis 321
9.5 Challenges and future trends 323
9.6 Conclusions 324
Acknowledgments 324
References 324
Further reading 328

## Part III Engineering and Challenges of New Ceramics for Medical Devices 329

**10 Design of ceramic materials for orthopedic devices 331**

*Frank Kern, Anke Bernstein and Andreas Killinger*

10.1 Bulk ceramics 331
10.2 Coatings 341
10.3 Conclusions and perspectives 346
References 348

**11 Design and development of dental ceramics: Examples of current innovations and future concepts 355**

*Marta Fornabaio, Helen Reveron, Erik Adolfsson, Laura Montanaro, Jerome Chevalier and Paola Palmero*

11.1 Introduction 355
11.2 Requirements for dental ceramic materials 357
11.3 The use and key advantages of zirconia as a dental material 361
11.4 Design and development of strong, tough, and stable $ZrO_2$-based dental materials 365
11.5 Bio-inspired design of dental ceramics 374

11.6 Dental tissue regeneration: advanced materials and technologies 379
11.7 Conclusions 383
Acknowledgments 384
References 384
Further reading 389

**12 Patient-specific design of tissue engineering scaffolds, based on mathematical modeling 391**
*Stefan Scheiner and Christian Hellmich*
12.1 Introduction 391
12.2 Overview of mathematical models in bone tissue engineering 393
12.3 Utilization of mathematical models for patient-specific scaffold design 396
12.4 Conclusions and outlook 402
References 402

**13 Tissue engineering and biomimetics with bioceramics 407**
*Simone Sprio, Monica Sandri, Andrea Ruffini, Alessio Adamiano, Michele Iafisco, Massimiliano Dapporto, Silvia Panseri, Monica Montesi and Anna Tampieri*
13.1 Introduction 407
13.2 Multisubstituted apatites 408
13.3 Apatitic, self-setting bone cements 412
13.4 Multifunctional, biohybrid scaffold obtained by bioinspired assembling/mineralization process 416
13.5 Porous bioceramics with hierarchical structure obtained by biomorphic transformation of natural structures 419
13.6 Conclusions and future perspectives 424
Acknowledgments 425
References 425
Further reading 432

**14 Advanced processing techniques for customized ceramic medical devices 433**
*Eric Champion, Amandine Magnaudeix, Patricia Pascaud-Mathieu and Thierry Chartier*
14.1 Introduction 433
14.2 Additive manufacturing: towards automization of customized organ fabrication 434
14.3 Freeze-templating: towards biomimetic architectured ceramics 443
14.4 Bioreactors and 3D cell culture techniques 446
14.5 Concluding remarks 458
References 459

**Index 469**

# List of Contributors

**Alessio Adamiano** National Research Council, Faenza, Italy

**Erik Adolfsson** Swerea, IVF AB, Mölndal, Sweden

**Saverio Affatato** Rizzoli Orthopaedic Institute, Bologna, Italy

**Marc Anglada** Universitat Politècnica de Catalunya, Barcelona, Spain

**Francesco Baino** Politecnico di Torino, Torino, Italy

**Anke Bernstein** University of Freiburg, Freiburg, Germany

**Emanuela Castiello** Ospedale "S.M.della Scaletta" Imola, Bologna, Italy

**Loredana Cerroni** University of Rome "Tor Vergata", Rome, Italy

**Eric Champion** University of Limoges, Limoges, France

**Thierry Chartier** University of Limoges, Limoges, France

**Jerome Chevalier** Université de Lyon-INSA Lyon, Villeurbanne, France

**Massimiliano Dapporto** National Research Council, Faenza, Italy

**Jonathan S. De Mattia** Rizzoli Orthopaedic Institute, Bologna, Italy

**Christophe Drouet** University of Toulouse, Toulouse, France

**Milena Fini** Rizzoli Orthopaedic Institute, Bologna, Italy

**Marta Fornabaio** Politecnico di Torino, Turin, Italy; École Polytechnique Fédérale de Lausanne (EPFL), Lausanne, Switzerland

**Laurent Gremillard** University of Lyon, Lyon, France

**Stuart Hampshire** University of Limerick, Limerick, Ireland

**Christian Hellmich** Vienna University of Technology, Vienna, Austria

**Michele Iafisco** National Research Council, Faenza, Italy

**Mitra Kashani** University of Birmingham, Birmingham, United Kingdom

**Frank Kern** University of Stuttgart, Stuttgart, Germany

**Andreas Killinger** University of Stuttgart, Stuttgart, Germany

**Anne Leriche** University of Valenciennes and Hainaut-Cambrésis, Maubeuge, France

**Amandine Magnaudeix** University of Limoges, Limoges, France

**David Marchat** University of Lyon, Saint-Etienne, France

**Laura Montanaro** Politecnico di Torino, Turin, Italy

**Monica Montesi** National Research Council, Faenza, Italy

**Nicolò Nicoli Aldini** Rizzoli Orthopaedic Institute, Bologna, Italy

**Paola Palmero** Politecnico di Torino, Turin, Italy

**Silvia Panseri** National Research Council, Faenza, Italy

**Patricia Pascaud-Mathieu** University of Limoges, Limoges, France

**Corrado Piconi** Catholic University "Sacro Cuore", Rome, Italy

**Helen Reveron** Université de Lyon-INSA Lyon, Villeurbanne, France

**Andrea Ruffini** National Research Council, Faenza, Italy

**Monica Sandri** National Research Council, Faenza, Italy

**Stefan Scheiner** Vienna University of Technology, Vienna, Austria

**Simone Sprio** National Research Council, Faenza, Italy

**Artemis Stamboulis** University of Birmingham, Birmingham, United Kingdom

**Solène Tadier** University of Lyon, Lyon, France

**Anna Tampieri** National Research Council, Faenza, Italy

**Paola Torricelli** Rizzoli Orthopaedic Institute, Bologna, Italy

# Preface

The unique properties of ceramics have resulted in their deployment as medical device implant materials in an expanding range of forms and applications of the last 50 years. As with metals and polymers, ceramics were initially deployed in medicine as materials developed for other engineering applications. Over the intervening decades, the developments in the understanding of the relationships between composition, processing parameters, and resultant structure and properties, have yielded significant advances in the clinical performance of biomaterials in general, and ceramics in particular. There does, however, still persist a divide within the classes of ceramic biomaterials, as Larry Hench classified them many years ago, in terms of their performance as high-strength mechanically reliable materials on the one hand and bioactivity and capacity to integrate with living tissue on the other.

In this context, led by Dr. Francis Cambier of the Belgian Ceramic Research Centre, a COST Action network MP1301 "New Generation Biomimetic and Customized Implants for Bone Engineering" was developed to address this very dichotomy in ceramic biomaterial performance; i.e., could advances in ceramic biomaterials science, with improved processing, enhanced bioactivity, and/or tailored morphologies and interfaces provide enough structural integrity as well as bone integration/regeneration? This network, with 120 researchers from across Europe, contains leading academic, industrial, and clinical specialists involved in synthesis, characterization and use of all types of ceramic biomaterials, including those trying to improve strength and reliability of bioactive materials, and those trying to confer bioactivity on high-toughness reliable materials via novel surface morphology or functionalization, as well as those focused on development of more reliable in vitro assessment methods. In addition, the emerging technologies of additive manufacturing, which have already seen the clinical application of a variety of porous titanium orthopedic implants, are being developed as a means of making new forms of ceramic materials with the potential of combined morphological and bioactive tissue integration.

We felt that the developments, perspectives and challenges that are collectively addressed in the work of this network could usefully be collated in a book, which we would hope to be of benefit to those with a developmental commercial or clinical interest in the scope and challenges for successful deployment of ceramics in medical applications.

The book is divided into three parts. The first is a review of classes of ceramic materials, their synthesis and processing, as well as methods of property assessment. The second part contains a review of materials developed, clinical applications, and some of the lessons learned from decades of clinical use. The third part outlines the challenges to improve performance and the directions that novel approaches are taking to meet these challenges.

To elaborate further: the first part of the book provides an overview of materials used in hard tissue surgery, highlighting the characteristics of ceramics—in comparison with the other classes of biomaterials—and their current fields of application (see *Chapter 1: Materials for hard tissue applications: an overview*). *Chapter 2, Types of ceramics: material class*, is a comprehensive description of the various ceramic and glass materials used in biomedical applications: from active oxides, used for bone regeneration and drug-delivery systems, to bioinert oxides and related composites used in load-bearing applications like dental and orthopedic devices, and to the recent developments of new oxide compositions, nonoxide ceramics, magnetic bioceramics, and bioglasses. The mechanical performances of both active and inert ceramics are described in *Chapter 3, Assessment of mechanical properties of ceramic materials*, highlighting the common requirements of higher fracture toughness, reliability, and prolonged clinical lifetimes, which should be taken into account in the design and development of new products and implants, as described in the third part of the book. *Chapter 4, Biological assessment of bioceramics*, deals with the biological assessment of ceramics intended for medical applications, through preclinical evaluation of biocompatibility and bioactivity, in order to assess their safety and efficacy. In vitro and in vivo tests, carried out according to the International Standards for the biological evaluation of medical devices are described, as well as innovative in vitro models—based on the use of cell cocultures and on three-dimensional models—and in vivo tests based on the use of pathological models.

The second part of the book describes the state of the art of current commercial medical devices based on ceramic materials: *Chapter 5, Ceramics for joint replacement: design and application of commercial bearings*, focuses on the devices used in joint arthroplasty (hip, knee, shoulder, ankle, finger, spine) and coatings; *Chapter 6: Ceramics for dentistry: commercial devices and their clinical analysis*, on the commercial products for dentistry (implants, abutments, endodontic posts, etc.) including ceramics, glass ceramics, and polymer–ceramic composites; *Chapter 7, Ceramics for bone replacement: commercial products and clinical use*, is focused on the products clinically used as bone substitutes, including calcium phosphates and calcium sulfates, bioactive glasses, composites, and injectable cements. Requirements, properties, configurations, specific applications, and clinical outcomes for those commercial products are reviewed. Clinical issues and new perspectives of ceramics used in bone tissue regeneration and in total hip arthroplasty are elucidated in *Chapter 8, Ceramic devices for bone regeneration: mechanical and clinical issues and new perspectives* and *Chapter 9, Clinical issues of ceramic devices used in total hip arthroplasty*, respectively.

The third part of the book aims to provide some guidance for the design and development of the 21st-century medical ceramics and products, able to satisfy the previously mentioned clinical and commercial requirements and to further enhance the properties and reliability of materials and products, especially when advanced, nonconventional manufacturing techniques are employed. In this context, the design of innovative load-bearing ceramics for orthopedics and dentistry is discussed in *Chapter 10, Design of ceramic materials for orthopedic devices*, and *Chapter 11, Design and development of dental ceramics: examples of current innovations and future concepts*, respectively. In tissue engineering, a major contemporary goal is the realization of appropriate patient-specific design of materials and structures, meaning the scaffold should be tailored to the physical, mechanical, and biological environment pertaining to a specific anatomical site in a specific patient. Therefore, *Chapter 12, Patient-specific design of tissue engineering scaffolds, based on mathematical modeling*, aims at discussing the potential of the computational and mathematical-based models for actually approaching true patient specificity and for properly designing customized scaffolds. The development of biomimetic and nature-inspired scaffolds is described in *Chapter 13, Tissue engineering and biomimetics with bioceramics*, such innovative approaches having the potential to overcome some of the critical limitations in conventional manufacturing processes, particularly if the ideal scaffold ought to reproduce very complex characteristics of bone tissue, such as composition, porosity, and hierarchical organization. Finally, the challenges of additive manufacturing methods and freeze-templating techniques to shape customized ceramic implants and scaffolds for bone repair are described in *Chapter 14, Advanced processing techniques for customized ceramic medical devices*. Principle, advantages and current limitations of these techniques are discussed, as well as examples of current applications.

The Editors would like to acknowledge the support of the COST Association for funding the network to do its work and thus enabling the assembly of the group of contributors, and in turn to acknowledge our gratitude to those contributors. We also would like to thank Ms. Véronique Huart (Belgian Ceramic Research Centre, Belgium) for her efficiency and dedication in the management and execution of the COST Action MP1301. Special thanks to Prof. A. Leriche (Universite de Valenciennes et Hainaut Cambresis, France), to Prof. S. Hampshire (University of Limerick, Ireland), Prof. M. Almeida (University of Aveiro, Portugal), and Dr. S. Hocquet (Belgian Ceramic Research Centre, Belgium) for contributing to writing a successful proposal, as well as to all other participants with a leading role in the action: Dr. E. Adolffson (Swerea IVF AB, Sweden), Dr. C. Baudin (Instituto de Ceramica y Vidrio, Spain), Prof. J. Chevalier (INSA de Lyon, France), Prof. F. Monteiro (INEB- Instituto de Engenharia Biomedica, Portugal). COST is supported by the EU Framework Programme Horizon 2020.

COST
EUROPEAN COOPERATION
IN SCIENCE & TECHNOLOGY

**Eamonn de Barra[1], Francis Cambier[2] and Paola Palmero[3]**
[1]University of Limerick, Limerick, Ireland
[2]Belgium Ceramic Research Centre, Mons, Belgium
[3]Politecnico di Torino, Turno, Italy

# Acknowledgments

The Editors would like to acknowledge Prof. C. Esnouf (INSA de Lyon), Dr. E. Meurice, Mr. Shaan Chamary (both from Université de Valenciennes et du Hainaut-Cambrésis) and Dr. D. Hautcoeur (BCRC) for providing some of the pictures on the book cover, in the frame of the LONGLIFE project (EU FP7/ 2007–2013, grant agreement no. 280741) and COST Action MP1301 "NEWGEN" (2013–2017).

# Part I

# An Overview of Biomedical Grade Ceramic Materials

# Materials for hard tissue applications: An overview

# 1

*Laurent Gremillard and Solène Tadier*
University of Lyon, Lyon, France

**Chapter Outline**

**1.1 Introduction: Hard tissues and how to replace them 3**
**1.2 Materials for hard tissue applications 4**
1.2.1 Dental applications 4
1.2.2 Orthopedic applications 9
1.2.3 Ceramics for bone repair 12
**1.3 Concluding remarks 16**
**References 16**

## 1.1 Introduction: Hard tissues and how to replace them

Hard tissues are living, mineralized tissues that posess a high degree of hardness, and are found in organs such as bones and teeth (enamel, dentin, and cementum). The replacement of damaged hard tissues by artificial devices has a long history, since the first known artificial tooth—a piece of nacre found in a 4000-year-old Mayan skull (Bobbio, 1972). Teeth were the first to benefit from the regular use of ceramic materials, since the late 18th century when porcelain crowns were first implanted. The late 19th century saw their first applications in orthopedics with the use of plaster of Paris, or gypsum (calcium sulfate dihydrate) for bone filling (Dreesman, 1892). However, only during the 20th century did ceramic materials specifically designed for hard tissue replacement become available, concurrently with the progress of chemistry making possible the synthesis of finer and more pure ceramic powders.

Even if the authors do not entirely condone this classification, ceramic materials can be separated using the "three generations" classification. First-generation ceramic materials are bioinert ceramics (such as zirconia, alumina and their composites, silicon nitride, and some glasses and glass ceramics used in dentistry), that do not elicit any adverse reaction from the body and are "transparent" to the immune system. Second-generation ceramic materials are bioactive ceramics (such as most calcium phosphates, bioactive glasses, calcium sulfate, etc.), that trigger a positive reaction from the body (in the case of ceramics, it is mostly an acceleration of bone regrowth). Third-generation ceramic materials are bioceramics that are able to release specific signals in vivo to improve the body response (e.g., bioceramics functionalized by growth factors, adhesion peptides, or containing drug-releasing

**Advances in Ceramic Biomaterials.**
**DOI: http://dx.doi.org/10.1016/B978-0-08-100881-2.00001-4**

polymer capsules, etc.). The first-generation bioceramics are used for orthopedic and dental applications, while the second and third generations are used for bone healing (bone filling, bone replacement, etc.). These three applications call for very different specifications.

Orthopedic applications (e.g., total hip arthroplasty) require strong and tough materials, that are able to resist millions of cycles of friction and mechanical fatigue. Moreover, they must not elicit any reaction from the body: no rejection from the immune system, no integration in the body (that would prevent movements). Alumina, zirconia, their composites, and silicon nitride are the most (if not the only) ceramic materials used for these applications, thanks to their reasonably high mechanical properties and almost perfect chemical inertness vs body fluids.

Dental applications also require high strength and toughness, but they also require more specific mechanical properties (that will be discussed below). Integration with bone is also at stake, when one considers dental implants. Since dental implants are mostly made with strong and tough but intrinsically inert materials, this can be achieved through surface modifications. Finally, esthetics are rather important in the final appreciation of the patient: one likes to avoid implants showing through a thin gingiva, or a crown with an unnatural color; here the white color of ceramic implants and the specific optical properties of dental glass ceramics are great advantages.

At present, bone healing applications do not require important mechanical properties (when necessary, mechanical loading is sustained by a system of metallic plaques and screws in addition to the bioactive material). However, they do require a rapid integration with bone, they should be osteoconductive (allow and favor the colonization of the material by bone tissue), and they should even be replaced by new bone. The interaction between bioactive ceramic materials and the bone cells (essentially osteoclasts mediating resorption, osteoblasts acting for bone growth) is thus crucial. When one considers the filling of critical bone defects, osteoinductivity (the ability to promote bone formation in nonosseous site) and angiogenicity (the ability to favor the growth of blood vessels) are also necessary, and may be achieved thanks to specific molecular interactions (with ions naturally released from the biomaterials, or with the molecules loaded in the materials in the case of third-generation bioceramics). Although these materials can be found in various shapes (blocks, granules and even injectable cement pastes to help in minimally invasive surgery), their architecture plays a key role in their success.

This chapter aims to provide a quick description of the ceramic materials used in dental, orthopedic, and bone reconstruction fields, and will develop the concepts exposed in this introduction.

## 1.2 Materials for hard tissue applications

### *1.2.1 Dental applications*

Dental materials may have to serve different functions, depending on the part of the tooth they are meant to replace. Indeed, one can distinguish between numerous dental restoration devices. A dental implant replaces the root of a tooth, and is screwed into the jawbone. On top of it, an abutment is affixed. This part provides an interface between the implant and the crown constituting the visible part of the tooth. One can also find bridges (replacing one or several teeth with a single device glued to the neighboring teeth), and inlays and onlays, that replace only a part of a tooth. This diversity of functions explains the wide number of materials used for dental applications. Indeed, dental materials may be made of metals, ceramics, polymers, composites, glass and glass ceramics, etc.

#### *1.2.1.1 Materials for dental implants*

First described by Carter et al. in 1967 (Carter and Smith, 1967), titanium is the material of choice for dental implants, thanks to its biocompatibility, efficient osteointegration, and good mechanical properties. It is either used pure (unalloyed grade 4, ISO 5832-2) or as a TA6V4 alloy (containing 6% aluminum and 4% vanadium, ISO 5832-3). Both materials spontaneously form a thin (<30 nm) titanium oxide passivation layer that avoids direct contact of metal with tissues, and favors osteointegration. Pure titanium is highly biocompatible, but possesses lower mechanical properties than TA6V4 (see Table 1.1). Since TA6V4 exhibits a perfectly acceptable biocompatibility and osteointegration, it has become the reference material for the fabrication of dental implants.

However, titanium has been challenged by ceramic materials almost ever since its introduction in dentistry. Indeed, Sandhaus proposed the first alumina dental implant (called CBS for Crystalline Bone Screw) as early as 1967. Other systems based on alumina were proposed in the 1970s (Frialit 1, also called Tübingen implant (Friadent, Germany)), Sapphire implants, made of single crystal alumina (Bioceram, Kyocera, Japan, etc.). Zirconia was introduced in the 1990s by Sigma implants (Incermed, Switzerland), and a decade later in its current, stronger version (3Y-TZP with Hot Isostatic Pressing, Z-look implants (Z-systems, Germany)). There is now a large number of zirconia implants manufacturers (Nobel Biocare, Straumann, Axis Biodental, etc.).

Dental implants have to fulfill a few requirements of mechanical, biological, and esthetical natures. They must not break, either during implantation or during

**Table 1.1 Orders of magnitude of the mechanical properties of dental materials**

| Material | Young's modulus (GPa) | Fracture strength (MPa) | Vickers hardness (Hv) |
|---|---|---|---|
| Pure Ti (grade 4) | 110 | Up to 700 | 200 |
| TA6V4 | 120 | Up to 1300 | 420 |
| Alumina | 400 | Up to 600 | 2000 |
| Zirconia | 200 | Up to 1400 | 1200 |

Data are extracted from CES EduPack 2015, Granta design.

mastication. They must be able to be attached to a pillar or to a dental crown. They must bond with the jawbone, and remain integrated for as long as possible. And finally, they should make the artificial tooth look like a natural one.

Mechanically, TA6V4 has an advantage due to its high fracture strength and toughness. Esthetically, ceramic implants take the lead: titanium implants may be visible through thin gingiva as dark-grayish areas, whereas the white color of ceramic implants makes them invisible. Integration in the jawbone is a trickier problem: it requires an adequate surface chemistry, but can be significantly improved by surface modification. For example, titanium implants are most often sandblasted and etched in hydrofluoric acid: this treatment induces craters on the surface at both micrometer and nanometer scales that improve bone growth. Such treatments are also explored on zirconia implants, but are more difficult to optimize (since they can significantly affect the mechanical resistance by introducing surface defects). Coatings (with calcium phosphates mostly) may also enhance bone bonding. However, their use is mostly discontinued because of coatings delamination during the implantation surgery. It is also possible to improve bone bonding by modifying the surface chemistry. This is only in the research stage for ceramics implants (Schickle et al., 2012; Caravaca, in press). One idea is to silanize the surface to immobilize interesting functional groups (amine, carboxylic acids) or biomolecules (such as bone morphogenetic protein or RGD peptide). Such a silanization can also be performed to improve the bonding of the pillar or crown, glued on the implant (in that case it is conducted directly during the dental surgery).

### 1.2.1.2 Materials for crowns and structures

Crowns are the visible parts of dental restorations. They must look like natural teeth, be hard, tough and strong enough to resist mastication and thermal stresses but not too hard so as to preserve the opposite teeth, and be chemically inert with respect to the mouth environment. They can be bonded to a prepared tooth (the enamel being removed, the dentin is tapered to an angle of 3–6 degrees) using a dental cement, or affixed to a pillar or abutment or directly to an implant.

Numerous materials or systems have been used to fabricate crowns. Among them, glass and glass ceramics are probably the most common, and have been around since the 18th century (with the use of porcelain for crowns). In more recent years, two techniques have been competing for the fabrication of crowns: molding and machining. Molding (called "hot pressing" in the dental community) involves fabricating a negative mold of the tooth (or teeth) to replace, and investing it with a glass or glass ceramic ingot heated above its glass transition temperature. Leucite ($KAlSi_2O_6$) glass ceramics (in the $SiO_2$-$Al_2O_3$-$K_2O$ system) were first used in this application, but their modest mechanical properties (fracture strength lower than 180 MPa) restricted their use for inlays and crowns (Dong et al., 1992; Holand et al., 1995). Then lithium-disilicate-based glass ceramics ($SiO_2$-$Li_2O$ system) were introduced, their satisfactory fracture strength (up to 400 MPa) and toughness of $\sim 3.5\ \mathrm{MPa}\sqrt{\mathrm{m}}$ making them adequate for the fabrication of bridges (Guazzato et al., 2004; Frank et al., 1998).

Machining of dental crowns has been made possible thanks to the development of computer-assisted design—computer-assisted machining (CAD-CAM) methods. These involve the knowledge of a numerical model of the tooth to replace. The first glass ceramic used with CAD-CAM was mica-based (Grossman, 1991) (in the $SiO_2$-$Al_2O_3$-MgO-$K_2O$ system), since the easy cleavage of mica sheets makes this material easy to machine. However these materials are rather weak (strength up to 140 MPa), and now three glass ceramic materials dominate the market (Denry and Holloway, 2010), either based on leucite, feldspar, or lithium disilicate. The latter is interesting in that it allows machining in a precrystallized state (with only a few lithium meta-silicate ($Li_2SiO_3$) crystals in the glass matrix), the final material being obtained after a second thermal treatment that crystallizes lithium disilicate and removes the microcracks left by the machining steps, thus allowing high fracture strength (up to 260 MPa) (Cattell et al., 2002). Other techniques to remove surface defects left by machining involve a careful polishing, or the adjunction of a superficial layer (a cosmetic ceramic that will both improve the visual aspect and fill the microcracks).

Most of these materials are part of a system, comprising several materials (structures, cosmetics, etc.) and the necessary processing and shaping tools (CAD-CAM systems, molding systems, dental furnaces, etc.).

Crowns and bridges, or even larger structures, can also be fabricated from zirconia blocks, using CAD-CAM techniques. These blocks (called "blanks") are most often machined in a presintered state, and sintered after machining. They can finally be coated by a veneer (see next section) to adjust their color. Many variations around zirconia are now coming onto the market. Tinted zirconia ceramics are more and more common, and allow the fabrication of natural-looking restoration without veneering. Blanks with a shade gradient (Katana Zirconium Multilayer, Kuraray Noritake) offer even more natural esthetics, with a deeper color close to the gingiva and a lighter one on the cutting edge of the restoration. Producers also increase the proportion of cubic phase, in cubic-tetragonal zirconia ((5—7)Y-TZP) to propose more translucent materials (Zfx BionX).

In parallel to monolithic ceramics, glass-infiltrated ceramics were still in use a few years ago (see, e.g., Vita In-Cera system). They consist of a partially sintered core (alumina, zirconia, or spinel) infiltrated with a glass phase (usually a lanthanum—alumina-silicate glass driven inside the porous core by capillary forces) (Narasimha Raghavan, 2012). These materials have been discontinued. Zirconia CAD-CAM materials became more important, mainly because the shorter production times of zirconia CAD-CAM dental restorations make them cheaper than glass-infiltrated ceramic devices.

Polymer-infiltrated-ceramic-network materials (PICNs, such as Vita Enamic) are new and interesting materials (Coldea et al., 2013). For example, Vita Enamic is composed of 75 vol.% aluminum-doped feldspar ceramic infiltrated by a methacrylate polymer phase (urethane dimetacrylate (UDMA)/triethyleneglycoldimetacrylate

(TEGMA)). It presents sufficient mechanical properties (up to 160 MPa fracture strength) to allow the fabrication of crowns and inlays (Vita Zahnfabrik, 2015), and a certain plasticity. Overall it presents a mechanical behavior rather similar to that of enamel.

Metals are still largely used for these applications. Cobalt—chromium alloys and titanium alloys (TA6V4) are machined, and then veneered by esthetic ceramics before implantation. Gold alloys are molded and often used without further color change.

### *1.2.1.3 Materials for esthetics*

Dental restorations must reproduce the aspect of the natural teeth of the patient. Thus, ideally their shade, fluorescence (Fluorescence: photonic emission after atomic excitation by one or two photons of usually different wavelengths. In a dental implant, fluorescence results in a shade changing with the ambient light), opalescence (Opalescence: the ability to show a yellowish—brownish shade in transmitted light, and a whitish—bluish shade in reflected light), and translucency should be adjustable. Among the materials presented above, lithium-disilicate-based glass ceramics meet this requirement (thanks to the reasonably low refractive index of the phases (Buchner et al., 2012): from 1.4 for the glass to 1.55 for $Li_2Si_2O_5$ and 1.62 for $Li_2SiO_3$). Zirconia ceramics may also be used without further adjustment, as discussed previously.

However, most often a "porcelain" (or "veneer") is used to coat the structures (glass ceramic, ceramic and metal structures) in order to optimize the aspect of the restoration. This layer is the outer layer of the restoration, thus must present other specific properties: abrasion resistance high enough to resist chewing but not so high as to wear the antagonist tooth (Holand and Beall, 2012), resistance to thermal stresses and mouth biochemical environment. It is sometimes an enamel (possibly tinted), highly transparent, that gives a smooth and glossy aspect to the restoration, and decreases the accumulation of dental plaque. Apatitic glass ceramics ($SiO_2$-$Al_2O_3$-$CaO$-$Na_2O$-$K_2O$-$P_2O_5$-F system) also give pleasing results. Depending on the exact composition and thermal treatment, small needles of fluorapatite ($Ca_5(PO_4)_3F$ with morphology similar to natural hydroxyapatite found in teeth) can be crystallized without the apparition of leucite, leading to optical properties rather close to those of teeth. In the same range of composition, one can also obtain opalescent glass ceramics containing both leucite and apatite.

### *1.2.1.4 Materials for caries filling*

The filling of caries probably necessitates materials that can be press-fit in the cavity, and harden in situ. Besides the well-known mercury-containing amalgams and photo-polymerizable composites, a special class of ceramic materials can also be used. Indeed, glass-ionomer cements (GICs) are mostly used for temporary dental filling. These cements are made of two constituents (Kovarik et al., 2005; Nicholson, 1998): the solid phase is composed of calcium-fluoroalumino-silicate glass particles, the liquid phase of polyacrylic acids solution. When mixed with the liquid phase, the glass is partially dissolved, releasing calcium and aluminum ions that form calcium- then aluminum-polyacrylate gels and provoke the setting of the cement. The whole process initiates in a few minutes, but the cement keeps on consolidating for a year or so. The claimed advantages of GICs are their strong adhesion to teeth tissue, their adequate wear rate, their low cost, the possibility to obtain them in different colors matching the teeth natural colors, and their ability to slowly release fluorine ions for long duration, thus improving the health of the neighboring teeth and the prevention of caries. However the latter gain is not statistically relevant as compared to classical composite teeth fillers (Mickenautsch and Yengopal, 2016). The cements can also be modified by reinforcing mineral particles (ex: zinc oxide for the ChemFil GIC (Dentsply)), and used with a coating that protects them at the early stages of setting. Classical cements are sold by such companies as Voco (IonoStar Molar), GC (Equia Fil), Dentsply (ChemFil).

### 1.2.2 Orthopedic applications

The most important orthopedic applications (in terms of number of surgeries worldwide) are total hip replacements and knee replacements. Both applications rely on the same concepts and materials: to replace the cartilage and damaged bone by synthetic devices affixed in the healthy bone (acetabulum and femur for the hip, femur and tibia for the knee). The materials used for these applications are not numerous. Articulating surfaces, submitted to high friction, are made of ultra-high-molecular-weight polyethylene (sometimes cross-linked), cobalt–chromium alloys, stainless steel, alumina, zirconia or alumina–zirconia composites. The nonarticulating surfaces, which ensure a bonding of articulating surfaces with bone, are exclusively made of metals (stainless steel, titanium alloy (TA6V4) or cobalt–chromium alloys). Only ceramic materials will be presented briefly here. Due to their high degree of hardness, but intrinsically brittle nature, the main concern for ceramic components in orthopedics is their fracture. However, the in vivo fracture rate of ceramic devices remains low: less than 0.3% of the patients may suffer from the fracture of a ceramic component during their lifetime, and only 2.5% of revision surgeries are conducted because of implant fracture (55% because of aseptic loosening) (Sadoghi et al., 2014).

#### 1.2.2.1 Alumina

Alumina was the first ceramic material introduced as bearing surfaces in hip prostheses. The first alumina hip heads were implanted in the early 1970s by Boutin (1972). Since then, almost 4 million alumina components have been implanted, with a good success rate (the failure rate is nowadays claimed to be below 0.01% (Willmann, 2000), but might be higher according to national arthroplasty registers (Sadoghi et al., 2014)). Alumina has evolved much since its first implantations, towards purer materials and finer microstructures that have enabled improvements in its mechanical properties, mostly its fracture strength (which went from

~400 MPa in the 1970s (Rieger, 2001) to ~600 MPa today (Früh and Willmann, 1998; Ben Nissan et al., 2008; Kyocera, 2014)). However even the strongest alumina ceramics are limited to "classical designs" of hip heads: the most loaded devices (22.2 mm heads, heads with extra-long necks, etc.) are forbidden to alumina. In contrast, alumina–alumina bearings are particularly well suited to young, active patients (D'Antonio et al., 2012), because of their low production of wear debris that is less likely to trigger osteolysis than, e.g., a metallic head wearing against a polyethylene cup.

#### *1.2.2.2 Zirconia (3Y-TZP)*

The need for more loaded orthopedic devices (smaller components, long-necked heads, knee prostheses, etc.) led to the search for a material that is both stronger and tougher than alumina. Zirconia (mostly 3Y-TZP, standing for 3 mol.% $Y_2O_3$–stabilized Tetragonal Zirconia Polycrystal) was first introduced in orthopedics in the early 1990s. Its mechanical properties are higher than alumina ones (toughness around 6 $MPa\sqrt{m}$, strength up to 1500 MPa), and the failure rate of zirconia components was equivalent to that of alumina. However, it suffers from two drawbacks as compared to alumina: its moderate stability in humid atmosphere, and its worse tribological behavior. Indeed, zirconia is sensitive to hydrothermal aging, a transformation of its surface from a metastable tetragonal polymorph to the stable monoclinic one, in the presence of water. This crystallographic transformation is accompanied by a volume increase of the transformed zones, thus an increase in roughness (hence the worse tribological properties) and microcracking (Chevalier et al., 2007). Nevertheless, around 600,000 zirconia hip heads were implanted, until 2001 when Prozyr heads from two defective batches were recalled by the FDA because of a high risk of fracture due to a change in the manufacturing process. Since this episode, 3Y-TZP orthopedic devices are no more available on the European and American markets. However, zirconia hip and knee components are still distributed in China and Japan (Kyocera, 2015a,b).

#### *1.2.2.3 Composites*

The problems met by zirconia and the limited mechanical properties of alumina allowed room for a third material. Zirconia–alumina composites seem to be the perfect candidate, presenting higher toughness (up to 8 $Mpa\sqrt{m}$) and strength (up to 1400 MPa) than alumina, and much better resistance to hydrothermal aging than zirconia (or even no sensitivity to it). The main zirconia–alumina composite materials are presented in Table 1.2. Two classes of composites are now in use: zirconia-toughened alumina (ZTA) in which alumina is the major phase, and alumina-toughened zirconia (ATZ) in which zirconia is the major phase. ATZ may present better mechanical properties than ZTA, but it is still sensitive to aging (although less so than 3Y-TZP) and softer than ZTA. Both ATZ and ZTA present excellent in vivo performance. Due to their high mechanical properties, fractures of components are very scarce. They are almost insensitive to wear,

**Table 1.2 Materials for orthopedics (toughness values might not be comparable, because the methods used to measure them are different from one reference to another)**

| Material | $K_{IC}$ MPa$\sqrt{m}$ | Strength (MPa) | Vickers hardness (GPa) |
|---|---|---|---|
| Alumina | 4 | 630 | 20 |
| 3Y-TZP | 6 | 1500 | 12 |
| Biolox Delta ZTA (Ceramtec, 2014) | 6.5 | 13844 pts bending | 19 |
| Bioceram AZ209 ZTA (Kyocera, 2014) | 4.5 | 1300 | 17 |
| Ceramys ATZ (Begand et al., 2005) | | 1150 Biaxial tests | |
| Bio Hip ATZ (Metoxit, 2016) | 8 | 20004 pts bending | 14 |
| $Si_3N_4$ (Bal et al., 2008) | 10 | 920 | 15 |
| MgPSZ Duracer (Signal_Medical_Corporation, 2014) | 10 | 620 | 10.7 |

decreasing the risk of aseptic loosening. Their behavior versus shock is also better than alumina (Perrichon et al., 2016). ZTA is nowadays the leading ceramic material in terms of number of implants, and represents 70%–80% of the market of ceramic heads and cups.

It is possible to associate ZTA or ATZ components with polyethylene or alumina counterparts. However (and this is also valid for alumina and zirconia components), they are never associated with metal counterparts: this would greatly accelerate the wear of the metallic part, with high risk of poisoning by metal ions.

### *1.2.2.4 Materials in development*

Magnesia partially stabilized zirconia (Mg-PSZ) materials are commonly used in many industries. They were foreseen as orthopedic materials as early as 1984. They have been sold as heads for hip prostheses since the end of the 1990s (Duracer, by Signal Medical Corporation). Duracer material presents mechanical strength equivalent to alumina (see Table 1.2), but a much higher toughness than even the best ZTA materials. Moreover, Mg-PSZ seems immune to hydrothermal aging. Explanted pieces show no degradation whatsoever after 5 years in vivo (Roy et al., 2007).

Silicon nitride is also widely used in industry, in particular for ceramic bearings, due to its better tribological behavior than oxide ceramics. It also offers a very limited sensitivity to slow crack propagation, and no hydrothermal aging. These properties make it an interesting candidate for the fabrication of heads for total hip arthroplasty. Indeed $Si_3N_4$ heads are currently tested by Amedica Corp. (Bal and Rahaman, 2012), with good success up until now.

### 1.2.3 Ceramics for bone repair

Resorbable ceramics are designed in order to make use of the bone remodeling process: they should act as a temporary graft, which will gradually be resorbed at a pace similar to bone growth rate and finally be replaced by a natural bone tissue.

Although the gold-standard autografts (bone harvested from the patient own's body), the allografts (from a donor), and xenografts (from animals, e.g., Bio-Oss, cerabone) remain the conventional techniques, they all face important limitations such as rationed availability of natural bone, morbidity of the donor site, risk of disease transmissions, and high refusal rates by the patients. This is why this section will focus on synthetic grafts only.

Bone is constituted of ~60 wt.% inorganic apatitic phase, ~30 wt.% organic tissue (collagen and bone cells) and ~10 wt.% water. Natural hydroxyapatite is polysubstituted and could be described with the chemical formula (Combes et al., 2016):

$Ca_{10-x}$ $(PO_4)_{6-x}$ ($HPO_4$ or $CO_3)_x$ (OH or ½ $CO_3)_{2-x}$ with $0<x<2$, where Ca could additionally be (slightly) substituted by K, Na, Sr, and OH by F (Wopenka and Pasteris, 2005). In spite of the huge presence of calcium phosphates in bone, the first attempted bone filling, in 1892, used calcium sulfate (Dreesman, 1892) (gypsum). Thirty years later, Albee et al. reported the first use of tricalcium phosphate suspension for the healing of bone fractures (Albee, 1920). These two historical steps already relied on injectable materials. However most of the synthetic bone grafts used during the following years were made of sintered calcium phosphates, either as rigid, porous pieces, or in the form of granules.

#### 1.2.3.1 Sintered calcium orthophosphates

Although many different phases of calcium orthophosphates exist, the two main compounds used in materials for bone healing are hydroxyapatite and β-tricalcium phosphate. Since the inorganic component of bone is made of carbonated hydroxyapatite, stoichiometric hydroxyapatite (usually abbreviated as HA or HAP, $Ca_{10}(PO_4)_6(OH)_2$) has been extensively studied and commercial products have been developed (for instance, Boneceram, ApaPore, etc.). HA ceramics can be of synthetic origin or obtained from natural sources (Barakat et al., 2008; Ivankovic et al., 2009; Lombardi et al., 2011). In all cases, hydroxyapatite suffers from a slow resorption rate that prevents its replacement by natural bone. For this reason, it is commonly used in combination with β-tricalcium phosphate (β-TCP, β-$Ca_3(PO_4)_2$) whose resorption is faster (Lu et al., 2002). HA-TCP composites are called "biphasic calcium phosphates" (BCPs) and are the basis of numerous commercial bone-substitution implants (Graftys, Medtronic, Biomatlante, e.g., are among the many companies that fabricate and sell these types of synthetic bone grafts). β-TCP has also been investigated alone (Antartik TCP, ChronOS, Cerasorb (Dorozhkin, 2013)), like more soluble phases, such as α-TCP (Biobase). Another route that has been studied is to form architectured scaffolds out of these phases, to favor the vascularization process and to increase the resorption rate. On this aspect, recent progress has been made concerning the use of so-called "rapid prototyping" manufacturing (or additive manufacturing) processes to thoroughly control the architectural features, such as macroporosity size, geometry, and interconnection (Lan Levengood et al., 2010; Habibovic et al., 2008).

### 1.2.3.2 Bone cements

Although polymer cements (such as poly (methyl-methacrylate) cements) are quite well used in dental and orthopedic fields (fixation of prosthetic implants, repair of vertebral fractures using minimally invasive techniques, etc.), this paragraph focuses on synthetic bone cements made of inorganic materials. The key point of these bone cements is their setting reaction, which is triggered by the mixing of one solid phase together with one liquid phase: starting from a viscous paste, the cement sets in vivo and hardens by crystal entanglements to form a monolithic ceramic.

First formulations of calcium phosphate cements (commonly referred to as CPCs) were developed and patented by Legeros et al. (1982) and Brown and Chow (1985) in the early 1980s. Since then, numerous other formulations have been developed and commercialized (Bohner, 2010). CPCs are classified in two groups, depending on the CaP phase precipitating during the setting reaction: apatite cements (made of a poorly crystallized, calcium-deficient HA; e.g.: Norian SRS, Bonesource) and brushite cements, made of dicalcium phosphate dihydrate (DCPD, $CaHPO_4.2H_2O$).

Compared to sintered ceramics obtained at high temperature, cements offer several benefits, summarized in Table 1.3. However, bone cements also suffer from their mechanical weakness, which restricts their use to nonload-bearing applications, and from too slow resorption kinetics. To address this last point, possible solutions are the use of cements mainly composed of more soluble compounds such as $CaCO_3$ (Combes et al., 2006; Fontaine et al., 2001) or $CaSO_4$ (Bohner, 2010; Devine, 1991) or the introduction of macroporosity in CPC (leaching of a pore former agent (Vandevelde et al., 2014), foaming, etc.) (Ginebra et al., 2010).

In addition to the specifications common to all materials for bone repair (low-cost production, good biological properties, resorption kinetics), bone cements also have to meet specifications relative to their distinct properties, to which are devoted a huge number of studies (Table 1.3). More recently, researchers and industries have paid more attention to easing the preparation procedure of their products: since the clinician has a limited time to prepare the paste just before implantation, it may be complicated and stressful to perform within a precise timeline a protocol composed of many steps, which must be done in a sterile environment. Therefore, ready-to use cements (for instance premixed calcium phosphate cements) have been developed (Takagi et al., 2003) and commercialized (Graftys QuickSet, VitalOs Cement). Their formulations are stable during storage in prefilled syringes, and hardened only after their delivery. This approach reduces the surgery time,

**Table 1.3 Advantages and requirements specific to a bone cement formulation**

| | |
|---|---|
| Advantages of CPCs compared to sintered CaPs | Injectability (minimally invasive surgery techniques can be used)<br>Moldability (can perfectly adapt to any geometry of the implanted site, allowing a good contact between the bone and the material)<br>In vivo self-setting<br>Setting reaction at body temperature:<br>1. leading to the formation of CaP phases, which are not obtained at high temperature (i.e. hydrated phases such as DCPD, or poorly crystallized apatite), have higher specific surface areas and are more reactive<br>2. enables the loading with temperature-sensitive molecules for drug-delivery (antibiotics, growth factors) or with cells (Chen et al., 2012) |
| Specifications relative to bone cements | Easy sterilization (not always the case when polymer additives are required to fulfill the other specifications) (Bohner, 2010)<br>Shelf-life (long-term stability during storage) (Bohner, 2010)<br>Easiness and robustness of routine preparation and handling (mixing, transfer into a delivery system, delivery)<br>Injectability without any filter-pressing phenomena (Bohner and Baroud, 2005; Dorozhkin, 2009);<br>Cohesion of the paste once injected (no "wash-out" or leaking in the surrounding tissues) (Dorozhkin, 2009; Bohner et al., 2006)<br>Radio-opacity (to trace the cement during and after injection)<br>Setting times suiting the surgical procedure (not too rapid to provide enough time for a clinician to perform the implantation, not too slow for the surgeon to be able to close the defect rapidly without delaying the operation) (Dorozhkin, 2009) |

*CPCs*, calcium phosphate cements; *DCPD*, dicalcium phosphate dihydrate.

increases the reproducibility of the cement preparation and therefore its performance (Ginebra et al., 2010; Dorozhkin, 2009).

#### *1.2.3.3 Bioactive glasses and glass ceramics*

First proposed by Larry Hench in 1969, bioactive glasses distinguish themselves by their ability to bond quickly with bone. The most known glass for such application is Bioglass (also called 45S5 or Hench's glass) (Hench, 1991, 1998), commercialized as granules by such companies as Novabone (PerioGlass) or Noraker (Activioss), or as cones (Endosseous Ridge Maintenance Implant, ERMI).

Immersed in biological fluid, bioactive glass undergoes a series of dissolution–reprecipitation steps (Hench et al., 1971) that lead to the formation of poorly crystalline, carbonated hydroxyapatite on which bone can strongly adhere and grow. Bioactive glasses have long found a use in dentistry. Indeed, a high quality of bone is necessary for good osteointegration of dental implants. Since the removal of a tooth leaves a cavity, a common practice in dentistry is to fill this cavity with osteoconductive materials that will favor the formation of new natural bone, in which the implant can be inserted (Karatzas et al., 1999). In addition to favoring bone–implant contact, 45S5 glass is thought to favor the differentiation of stem cells into osteoblasts (Bosetti and Cannas, 2005), to accelerate the bone growth kinetic through the activation of certain genes by the dissolution products (Xynos et al., 2001), and to promote angiogenesis (Day, 2004), three factors that favor bone growth. It gives excellent results in vivo (Stanley et al., 1997). However, these materials should be handled with care: indeed, their intrinsic basicity can make them toxic if their dissolution rate is too fast (either due to the composition of the glass or to a too-high specific surface area).

### 1.2.3.4 Ceramic-polymer composites

Although this is not the main focus of this chapter, it should be underlined that organic–inorganic composite materials using a biodegradable synthetic polymer have also been extensively studied (Yunos et al., 2008; Habraken et al., 2007). Two major reasons for this approach are the biomimetic strategy mimicking the bone composition and the already-mentioned limitations of the ceramics used for bone repair. For instance, polymer has been added to ceramic materials to improve their mechanical properties (toughness) (Martinez-Vazquez et al., 2014; Peroglio et al., 2007, 2010), to ease their delivery (nonsetting viscous polymer solution to deliver ceramic granules, see, e.g., Bio-Oss Collagen (Geistlich Pharma)), or to improve the rheological properties of bone cements. By the way, due to the recent development of the so-called additive manufacturing techniques, there has been a renewed interest, not only in self-setting CPC, but also in the design of composite slurries and paste, which can easily be extruded and shaped using three-dimensional printing technology. Some synthetic bone grafts based on this technology are already used clinically (OsteoFlux, from VIVOS-Dental AG).

Nonstructural properties of polymers are also exploited, such as the angiogenicity of chitosan (in chitosan/calcium phosphate composites (Di Martino et al., 2005; Zhang et al., 2003)), or the osteoconductivity of collagen (again in composites with calcium phosphate). But to the knowledge of the authors, no large clinical application has yet been made of these composites.

Conversely, polymer-based composites, reinforced by ceramic particles, have been extensively studied (Rezwan et al., 2006). This type of composite has only recently reached clinical application. For example, poly-(lactic acid)/bioactive glass composites are manufactured using classical polymer-processing techniques (extrusion, injection) into resorbable interference screws (attaching tendons to bones) (LockActiv, manufactured by Noraker).

## 1.3 Concluding remarks

This chapter aims to briefly present many ceramics that have found a path to clinical applications as hard tissue prosthetics, as well as the most promising candidates for these applications, from the point of view of the authors. However, many more have remained stuck in the laboratories, in spite of their potentially high interest for biological applications. Indeed, the requirements for a new material to be used in vivo are numerous, and sometimes unexpected for materials scientists. Among them, the necessity for sterilization has often put a stop to the development of new biomaterials. In particular many composites are difficult to sterilize without compromising their integrity. Also, scientists sometimes overlook the medical requisites of surgeons. Other difficulties arise from the high numbers of tests necessary for the acceptance of new medical devices by the health agencies, which make the introduction of completely new materials onto the market both costly and lengthy. Finally, the in vivo interactions between an implant, its surface and the surrounding tissues are very complicated to study and, therefore, still only partially understood. The reasons for this deficiency are of course ethical and financial, but there is also a lack of tools that could help to monitor the implanted material. Yet, understanding how a bioceramic and the host tissues influence each other is a crucial issue in improving the design of the materials currently used for hard tissues replacement.

## References

Albee, F.H., 1920. Studies in bone growth: triple calcium phosphate as a stimulus to osteogenesis. Ann. Surg. 71 (1), 32–39.

Bal, B.S., Rahaman, M.N., 2012. Orthopedic applications of silicon nitride ceramics. Acta. Biomater. 8 (8), 2889–2898.

Bal, B.S., Khandkar, A., Lakshminarayanan, R., Clarke, I., Hoffman, A.A., Rahaman, M.N., 2008. Testing of silicon nitride ceramic bearings for total hip arthroplasty. J. Biomed. Mater. Res. - Part B Appl. Biomater. 87 (2), 447–454.

Barakat, N.A.M., Khalil, K.A., Sheikh, F.A., Omran, A.M., Gaihre, B., Khil, S.M., et al., 2008. Physiochemical characterizations of hydroxyapatite extracted from bovine bones by three different methods: extraction of biologically desirable HAp. Mater. Sci. Eng. C. 28 (8), 1381–1387.

Begand, S., Oberbach, T., Glien, W., 2005. Investigations of the mechanical properties of an alumina toughened zirconia ceramic for an application in joint prostheses. Key Eng. Mater. 284-286, 1019–1022.

Ben Nissan, B., Choi, A.H., Cordingley, R., 2008. Alumina ceramics. In: Kokubo, T. (Ed.), Bioceramics and Their Clinical Applications. Woodhead Publishing, Cambridge, UK, pp. 223–242.

Bobbio, A., 1972. The first endosseous alloplastic implant in the history of man. Bull. Hist. Dent. 20 (1), 1–6.

Bohner, M., 2010. Design of ceramic-based cements and putties for bone graft substitution. Eur. Cell. Mater. 20, 1–12.

Bohner, M., Baroud, G., 2005. Injectability of calcium phosphate pastes. Biomaterials 26, 1553.

Bohner, M., Doebelin, N., Baroud, G., 2006. Theoretical and experimental approach to test the cohesion of calcium phosphate pastes. Eur. Cell. Mater. 12, 26.

Bosetti, M., Cannas, M., 2005. The effect of bioactive glasses on bone marrow stromal cells differentiation. Biomaterials 6 (26), 3873–3879.

Boutin, P., 1972. Arthroplastie total de la hanche par prothèse en alumine frittée. Total hip arthroplasty made of dense ceramics - frited alumina. Rev. Chir. Orthop. Reparatrice. Appar. Mot. 58 (3), 229.

Brown, W.E., Chow, L.C., inventors, 1985. Dental restorative cement pastes (US patent 4518430).

Buchner, S., Pereira, M.B., Balzaretti, N.M., 2012. Behavior of the refractive index of lithium disilicate glass ceramic processed at high pressure and high temperature. Opt Mater. 34 (5), 826–831.

Caravaca, C., Shi, L., Balvay, S., Rivory, P., Laurenceau, E., Chevolot, Y., et al. Direct silanization of zirconia for increased biointegration. Acta Biomater. in press:. http://dx.doi.org/10.1016/j.actbio.2016.09.034.

Carter, J.M., Smith, D.C., 1967. Studies of properties of titanium alloys for dental purposes. J. Dent. Res. 46 (1P1S), 115.

Cattell, M.J., Palumbo, R.P., Knowles, J.C., Clarke, R.L., Samarawickram, D.Y.D., 2002. The effect of veneering and heat treatment on the flexural strength of Empress® 2 ceramics. J. Dentistry 30, 161–169.

Ceramtec. BIOLOX®delta – Céramique nano-composite pour l'orthopédie. [cited 2014 27-08-2014]. Available from: http://www.ceramtec.com/files/mt_biolox_delta_fr.pdf.

Chen, W., Zhou, H., Weir, M.D., Bao, C., Xu, H.H.K., 2012. Umbilical cord stem cells released from alginate-fibrin microbeads inside macroporous and biofunctionalized calcium phosphate cement for bone regeneration. Acta. Biomater. 8, 2297.

Chevalier, J., Gremillard, L., Deville, S., 2007. Low-temperature degradation of Zirconia and implications for biomedical implants. Annu. Rev. Mater. Res. 37, 1–32.

Coldea, A., Swain, M.V., Thiel, N., 2013. Mechanical properties of polymer-infiltrated-ceramic-network materials. Dent. Mater. 29 (4), 419–426.

Combes, C., Miao, B., Bareille, R., Rey, C., 2006. Preparation, physical-chemical characterisation and cytocompatibility of calcium carbonate cements. Biomaterials 27, 1945.

Combes, C., Cazalbou, S., Rey, C., 2016. Apatite biominerals. Minerals 6 (2), 34.

D'Antonio, J.A., Capello, W.N., Naughton, M., 2012. Ceramic bearings for total hip arthroplasty have high survivorship at 10 years. Clin. Orthop. Relat. Res. 470 (2), 373–381.

Day, R.M., inventor, 2004. Bioactive material for use in stimulating vascularization patent WO2004071542 A8.

Denry, I., Holloway, J., 2010. Ceramics for dental applications: a review. Material 3 (1), 351–368.

Devine, T.K., inventor, 1991. Calcium sulfate hemihydrate composition having utility in the presence of blood.

Di Martino, A., Sittinger, M., Risbud, M.V., 2005. Chitosan: a versatile biopolymer for orthopaedic tissue-engineering. Biomaterial 26, 5983–5990.

Dong, J.K., Luthy, H., Wohlwend, A., Schärer, P., 1992. Heat-pressed ceramics: technology and strength. Int. J. Prosthodont. 5 (1), 9–16.

Dorozhkin, S.V., 2013. Calcium Orthophosphate-Based Bioceramics. Mater. Des. 6, 3840–3942.

Dorozhkin, S.V., 2009. Calcium orthophosphates cements and concretes. Material 2 (1), 221–291.

Dreesman, H., 1892. Uber Knochenplombierung. Beitr. Klin. Chir. 9, 804–810.
Fontaine, M.L., Combes, C., Mounic, S., Rey, C., inventors, 2001. Composition de ciment hydraulique à base de carbonates de calcium. (French patent FR2830249). France.
Frank, M., Schweiger, M., Rheinberger, V., Höland, W., 1998. High strength translucent sintered glass-ceramic for dental applications. Glastech. Ber Glass Sci. Technol. 71C, 345–348.
Früh, H.-J., Willmann, G., 1998. Tribological investigations of the wear couple alumina–CFRP for total hip replacement. Biomaterials. 19, 1145–1150.
Ginebra, M.P., Espanol, M., Montufar, E.B., Perez, R.A., Mestres, G., 2010. New processing approaches in calcium phosphate cements and their applications in regenerative medicine. Acta. Biomater. 6, 2863.
Grossman, D.G., 1991. Structure and physical properties of Dicor/MGC glass-ceramic. In: Mörmann, W.H. (Ed.), International Symposium on Computer Restoration. Quintessence Pub. Co, Chicago IL, pp. 103–115.
Guazzato, M., Albakry, M., Ringer, S.P., Swain, M.V., 2004. Strength, fracture toughness and microstructure of a selection of all-ceramic materials. Part II. Zirconia-based dental ceramics. Dental Mater. 20 (5), 449–456.
Habibovic, P., Gbureck, U., Doillon, C.J., Bassett, D.C., van Blitterswijk, C.A., Barralet, J.E., 2008. Osteoconduction and osteoinduction of low-temperature 3D printed bioceramic implants. Biomaterials 29 (7), 944–953.
Habraken, W.J.E.M., Wolke, J.G.C., Jansen, J.A., 2007. Ceramic composites as matrices and scaffolds for drug delivery in tissue engineering. Adv. Drug. Deliv. Rev. 59, 234.
Hench, L.L., Splinter, R.J., Allen, W.C., Greenlee, T.K., 1971. Bonding mechanisms at the interface of ceramic prosthetic materials. J. Biomed. Mater. Res. Symp. 5 (6), 117–141.
Hench, L.L., 1991. Bioceramics: from concept to clinic. J. Am. Ceram. Soc. 74 (7), 1487–1510.
Hench, L.L., 1998. Bioceramics. J. Am. Ceram. Soc. 81 (7), 1705–1728.
Holand, W., Beall, G.H., 2012. Glass Ceramic Technology. John Wiley & Sons, Hoboken, NJ.
Holand, W., Frank, M., Rheinberger, V., 1995. Surface crystallization of leucite in glasses. J. Non-Cryst Solids 180, 292–307.
Ivankovic, H., Gallego Ferrer, G., Tkalcec, E., Orlic, S., Ivankovic, M., 2009. Preparation of highly porous hydroxyapatite from cuttlefish bone. J. Mater. Sci. Mater. Med. 20 (5), 1039–1046.
Karatzas, S., Zavras, A., Greenspan, D., Amar, S., 1999. Histologic observations of periodontal wound healing after treatment with PerioGlas in nonhuman primates. Int. J. Periodontics Restor. Dent. 19 (5), 489–499.
Kovarik, R.E., Haubenreich, J.E., Gore, D., 2005. Glass ionomer cements: a review of composition, chemistry, and biocompatibility as a dental and medical implant material. J. Long. Term. Eff. Med. Implants 15 (6), 655–671.
Kyocera. Bioceram(r) AZ209. 2014 [cited 2014 22/08/2014]. Available from: http://kyocera-md.jp/bioceram/general/material.html.
Kyocera. Actiyas total knee system. 2015b [cited 2015 10/02/2015]. Available from: http://kyocera-md.jp/m_professional/yes/medical/pdf/actiyas_v1_0.pdf.
Kyocera. LFA total knee system. 2015a [cited 2015 10-02-2015]. Available from: http://kyocera-md.jp/m_professional/yes/medical/pdf/lfa_v6_2.pdf.
Lan Levengood, S.K., Polak, S.J., Wheeler, M.B., Maki, A.J., Clark, S.G., Jamison, R.D., et al., 2010. Multiscale osteointegration as a new paradigm for the design of calcium phosphate scaffolds for bone regeneration. Biomaterials 31 (13), 3552–3563.

Legeros, R.Z., Chohayeb, A., Shulman, A., 1982. Apatitic calcium phosphates: possible restorative materials. J. Dent. Res. 61S, 343.

Lombardi, M., Palmero, P., Haberko, K., Pyda, W., Montanaro, L., 2011. Processing of a natural hydroxyapatite powder: from powder optimization to porous bodies development. J. Eur. Ceram. Soc. 31 (14), 2513–2518.

Lu, J., Descamps, M., Dejou, J., Koubi, G., Hardouin, P., Lemaitre, J., et al., 2002. The biodegradation mechanism of calcium phosphate biomaterials in bone. J. Biomed. Mater. Res. 63 (4), 408–412.

Martinez-Vazquez, F.J., Pajares, A., Guiberteau, F., Miranda, P., 2014. Effect of polymer infiltration on the flexural behavior of β-tricalcium phosphate robocast scaffolds. Material 7, 4001.

Metoxit, 2016. Zirconia Ceramics. Available from: http://www.metoxit.com/english/downloads/mat_zr_e.pdf.

Mickenautsch, S., Yengopal, V., 2016. Caries-preventive effect of high-viscosity glass ionomer and resin-based fissure sealants on permanent teeth: a systematic review of clinical trials. PLoS One. 11 (1), e0146512.

Narasimha Raghavan, R., 2012. Ceramics in dentistry, sintering of ceramics – new emerging techniquesIn: Lakshmanan, A. (Ed.), InTech, Rijeka: Croatia, http:/dx.doi.org/10.5772/39090. Available from: https://www.intechopen.com/books/sintering-of-ceramics-new-emerging-techniques/ceramics-in-dentistry.

Nicholson, J.W., 1998. Chemistry of glass-ionomer cements: a review. Biomaterials 19, 485–494.

Peroglio, M., Gremillard, L., Chevalier, J., Chazeau, L., Gauthier, C., Hamaide, T., 2007. Toughening of bio-ceramics scaffolds by polymer coating. J. Eur. Ceram. Soc. 27 (7), 2679–2685.

Peroglio, M., Gremillard, L., Gauthier, C., Chazeau, L., Verrier, S., Alini, M., et al., 2010. Mechanical properties and cytocompatibility of poly(epsilon-caprolactone)-infiltrated biphasic calcium phosphate scaffolds with bimodal pore distribution. Acta. Biomater. 6 (11), 4369–4379.

Perrichon, A., Reynard, B., Gremillard, L., Chevalier, J., Farizon, F., Geringer, J., 2016. Effects of in vitro shocks and hydrothermal degradation on wear of ceramic hip joints: Towards better experimental simulation of in vivo ageing. Tribology International 100, 410–419.

Rezwan, K., Chen, Q.Z., Blaker, J.J., Boccaccini, A.R., 2006. Biodegradable and bioactive porous polymer/inorganic composite scaffolds for bone tissue engineering. Biomaterials 27 (18), 3413–3431.

Rieger, W., 2001. Ceramics in orthopedics - 30 years of evolution and experience. In: Rieker, C., Oberholzer, S., Wyss, U. (Eds.), World Tribology Forum on Arthroplasty. Hans Uber, Bern.

Roy, M.E., Whiteside, L.A., Katerberg, B.J., Steiger, J.A., Nayfeh, T., 2007. Not all zirconia femoral heads degrade in vivo. Clin. Orthop. Relat. Res. 465, 220–226.

Sadoghi, P., Pawelka, W., Liebensteiner, M.C., Williams, A., Leithner, A., Labek, G., 2014. The incidence of implant fractures after total hip arthroplasty. Int. Orthop. 38 (1), 39–46.

Schickle, K., Kaufmann, R., Duarte Campos, D.F., Weber, M., Fischer, H., 2012. Towards osseointegration of bioinert ceramics: introducing functional groups to alumina surface by tailored self assembled monolayer technique. J. Eur. Ceram. Soc. 32 (12), 3063–3071.

Signal_Medical_Corporation. DuraCer Ceramic Components, The Strong Choice In Ceramics. 2014 [cited 2014 28/08/2014]. Available from: http://www.signalmd.com/Hip_files/duracer-ceramic.pdf.

Stanley, H.R., Hall, M.B., Clark, A.E., King, C.J., Hench, L.L., Berte, J.J., 1997. Using 45S5 bioglass cones as endosseous ridge maintenance implants to prevent alveolar ridge resorption: a 5-year evaluation. Int. J. Oral Maxillofac Implants. [Article]. 12 (1), 95–105.

Takagi, S., Chow, L.C., Hirayama, S., Sugawara, A., 2003. Premixed calcium phosphate cement pastes. J. Biomed. Mater. Res. B. Appl. Biomater. 67, 689.

Vandevelde R, Bignon A, Cordier D, Meille S, Bouville F, Chevalier J, et al., inventors; Composition de substitut osseux (Bone substitute composition) (International Patent WO2014009674A1). France 2014 2014-01-16.

Vita Zahnfabrik. Vita Enamic®, Technical and scientific documentation 2015.

Willmann, G., 2000. Ceramic femoral head retrieval data. Clin. Orthop. Relat. Res. 379, 173–177.

Wopenka, B., Pasteris, J.D., 2005. A mineralogical perspective on the apatite in bone. Mater. Sci. Eng. C 25 (2), 131–143.

Xynos, I.D., Edgar, A.J., Buttery, L.D., Hench, L.L., Polak, J.M., 2001. Gene-expression profiling of human osteoblasts following treatment with the ionic products of Bioglass® 45S5 dissolution. J. Biomed. Mater. Rese. 55 (2), 151–157.

Yunos, D.M., Bretcanu, O., Boccaccini, A.R., 2008. Polymer-bioceramic composites for tissue engineering scaffolds. J. Mater. Sci. 43, 4433.

Zhang, Y., Ni, M., Zhang, M., Ratner, B., 2003. Calcium phosphate-chitosan composite scaffolds for bone tissue engineering. Tiss. Eng. 9 (2), 337–345.

# Types of ceramics: Material class

**2**

*Christophe Drouet*[1], *Anne Leriche*[2], *Stuart Hampshire*[3], *Mitra Kashani*[4], *Artemis Stamboulis*[4], *Michele Iafisco*[5] *and Anna Tampieri*[5]
[1]University of Toulouse, Toulouse, France, [2]University of Valenciennes and Hainaut-Cambrésis, Maubeuge, France, [3]University of Limerick, Limerick, Ireland, [4]University of Birmingham, Birmingham, United Kingdom, [5]National Research Council, Faenza, Italy

## Chapter Outline

**2.1 Active oxides 22**
- 2.1.1 Introduction 22
- 2.1.2 CaP-based systems 22
- 2.1.3 Other bioactive oxides 33
- 2.1.4 Conclusion 34

**2.2 Inert oxides and composites 34**
- 2.2.1 Introduction 34
- 2.2.2 Alumina ceramics 36
- 2.2.3 Zirconia ceramics 37
- 2.2.4 Alumina–zirconia composites 38
- 2.2.5 Further developments 39

**2.3 Nonoxide ceramics 40**
- 2.3.1 Silicon nitride: An introduction 40
- 2.3.2 Silicon carbide 43

**2.4 Bioactive glasses 44**

**2.5 Glass ceramics and bioactive glass ceramics 49**

**2.6 Glass-ionomer cements 50**
- 2.6.1 Introduction 50
- 2.6.2 The chemistry of GICs 52
- 2.6.3 Glass compositions to form GICs 54
- 2.6.4 Key factors affecting the properties of GICs 55
- 2.6.5 Fluoride release and recharge ability 58
- 2.6.6 Antimicrobial effectiveness 59

**2.7 Magnetic ceramic materials in medicine 60**

**2.8 Conclusion 63**

**References 64**

**Further reading 82**

**Advances in Ceramic Biomaterials.**
**DOI: http://dx.doi.org/10.1016/B978-0-08-100881-2.00002-6**

# 2.1 Active oxides

## 2.1.1 Introduction

Oxide materials are increasingly encountered in biomedical applications (Rey et al., 2011) such as tissue repair (e.g., bone regeneration), drug delivery, or medical diagnosis. Among these compounds, certain types of oxides not only play a "physical" role to fulfill a function (e.g., to fill bone defects and avoid invasion from surrounding soft tissues or to play an imaging role as in magnetic resonance imaging (MRI)), but can also take an active or "chemical" part in biological processes. Bioactivity, for example, consists of supplying constitutive building blocks (e.g., ions) for promoting tissue repair or of activating biological pathways (e.g., favoring or orienting cell activity). Such compounds are referred to as "bioactive oxides." This activity is directly related to features such as chemical composition (and related thermodynamic stability in body fluids), structure, morphology, degree of stoichiometry, crystal dimensions, surface state/reactivity, etc.

Among bioactive oxides, calcium phosphates (CaPs) represent by far the main group of compounds, used either as is or in combination with other compounds, and will be treated in the following. The family of active oxides, however, also encompasses other systems such as calcium carbonates and sulfates, which will also be briefly commented on at the end of this section.

## 2.1.2 CaP-based systems

CaPs are extensively developed in medicine and have become the most implanted bioactive ceramics. This interest is mainly linked to the chemical composition of these compounds, exhibiting similarities with vertebrates' hard tissues (bones and teeth) (LeGeros, 2008; Gomez-Morales et al., 2013). Also, from a practical point of view, their preparation is rather straightforward, low cost, and allows the preparation of synthetic bone substitute materials with a high similarity to bone mineral, in high quantity, and without the side effects of autografts (limitation of grating tissue, increased risks of infections, pain) or the possible spreading of infectious pathogens possibly associated with allografts. Plus, the bioactivity of these compounds is associated with significant bone regrowth efficacy due to osteoconductive and even sometimes osteoinductive properties.

CaP compounds are often classified on the basis of their Ca/P ratio, and Table 2.1 summarizes the main CaP phases.

Preparation methods of these CaPs have been widely treated in the literature (LeGeros, 2008; Elliott, 1994; Kurosawa et al., 1986), and CaP processing has also extensively been explored (e.g., Champion et al., 2013). Although some of these phases can be prepared at "low" temperature in solution, others can only be obtained by high-temperature dry-state reactions. Of particular relevance is the subgroup of apatite compounds, deriving from hydroxyapatite (HA), $Ca_{10}(PO_4)_6(OH)_2$. Indeed, bone and teeth biominerals crystallize in the apatite structure (hexagonal system, space group $P6_3/m$), and this structure is very accommodative for many

**Table 2.1 Classification of CaP compounds**

| CaP compound | Abbreviation | Chemical formula | Ca/P | Synthesis approach |
|---|---|---|---|---|
| **Monocalcium phosphate** | | | | |
| Anhydrous | MCPA | $Ca(H_2PO_4)_2$ | 0.5 | Low T |
| Monohydrate | MCPM | $Ca(H_2PO_4)_2 \cdot H_2O$ | 0.5 | Low T |
| **Dicalcium phosphate** | | | | |
| Anhydrous | DCPA/monetite | $CaHPO_4$ | 1 | Low T |
| Dihydrate | DCPD/brushite | $CaHPO_4 \cdot 2H_2O$ | 1 | Low T |
| Octocalcium phosphate (triclinic) | OCP | $Ca_8(PO_4)_4(HPO_4)_2 \cdot 5H_2O$ | 1.33 | Low T |
| **Tricalcium phosphate** | | | | |
| Amorphous | ACP (or $TCP_{am}$) | $Ca_3(PO_4)_2 \cdot nH_2O$ | 1.5 | Low T |
| Apatitic | ap-TCP | $Ca_9(PO_4)_5(HPO_4)(OH)$ | 1.5 | Low *or High T* |
| β | β-TCP | $Ca_3(PO_4)_2$ | 1.5 | *High T* |
| α | α-TCP | $Ca_3(PO_4)_2$ | 1.5 | *High T* |
| Nonstoichiometric apatites | | $Ca_{10-x}(PO_4)_{6-x}(HPO_4)_x(OH)_x$ | <1.67 | Low T |
| Stoichiometric hydroxyapatite | HA | $Ca_{10}(PO_4)_6(OH)_2$ | 1.67 | *High T (at least boiling, often calcined)* |
| Tetracalcium phosphate | TTCP | $Ca_4(PO_4)_2O$ | 2 | *High T* |

types of cations and anions, leading to a rich variety of substituted apatites with modulable properties.

For biomedical applications, CaPs can be used alone or in association with other mineral and/or organic (polymers) compounds with the view to adjoin new functionalities, to strengthen existing properties (e.g., mechanical), or to allow chemical reactions (as in bone cements for instance).

### *2.1.2.1 Pure and substituted HA and related apatite compounds*

Two types of apatite compounds have to be distinguished at this point: well-crystallized and nanocrystalline apatites.

#### Well-crystallized apatites

Well-crystallized apatites can be obtained either by solid state reaction at high temperature (e.g., 1000°C) (Suchanek and Yoshimura, 1998) or by heat treatment of precursors prepared by wet chemistry. The main compound encountered is stoichiometric HA, although well-crystallized nonstoichiometric apatites can also be produced, e.g., by hydrolysis of β-tricalcium phosphate (β-TCP) in hydrothermal conditions, then leading to the compound $Ca_9(PO_4)_5(HPO_4)(OH)$ also known as "apatitic tricalcium phosphate." HA is the most stable CaP phase in physiological conditions (Elliott, 1994). Due to its high thermodynamic stability, it exhibits a very low solubility in vivo and is thus characterized by a slow bioresorption (da Silva et al., 2007).

For the production of HA bioceramics, the sintering process is key, during which volatiles from synthesis (water, carbon dioxide, ammonia, nitrates, etc.) are eliminated and densification as well as grain coarsening occur. This sintering stage (generally involving temperatures around or above 1000°C) then leads to ceramics with increased mechanical strength (Khalil et al., 2007; Kobayashi et al., 2006; Raynaud et al., 2002). Stoichiometric HA is thermally rather stable and can be sintered up to ~1250°C without major alteration. Yet, under very low water-pressure conditions, HA may start to loose water from 850°C thus generating oxyapatite (Trombe and Montel, 1978); oxyapatite being known, however, to regenerate HA after immersion in aqueous medium. Care should be taken when calcining/sintering nonstoichiometric apatites often represented (Winand, 1961) by the formula $Ca_{10-x}(PO_4)_{6-x}(HPO_4)_x(OH)_{2-x}$): typically for samples with a Ca/P ratio between 1.5 and 1.67, they will ultimately decompose into a mixture of HA and β-TCP in relative proportions dependent on the initial Ca/P ratio. Note that a calcination at 1000°C for 15 hours has been proposed as a standard procedure (ISO 13779-3:2008) to validate the stoichiometry of an HA sample.

Despite a hardening phenomenon after sintering, HA ceramics are not suited to being applied alone in large load-bearing sites (Linhart et al., 2004). For instance, fracture toughness generally reaches $\sim 1.0\,MPa\sqrt{m}$ (to be compared with $2-12\,MPa\sqrt{m}$ for human bone), although HA mechanical properties can be improved by optimizing sintering/densification, e.g., via less conventional methods such as microwave sintering (Thuault et al., 2014). Mechanical limitations, however, limit bone-related applications of pure HA to mainly non-load-bearing sites, or for the coverage of tougher but less bioactive implants. HA can be processed in different forms such as powders, granules for bone filling, coatings (e.g., on metal implants), dense or porous scaffolds for orthopedic or dental surgeries.

Porous scaffolds (Sopyan et al., 2007; Meurice et al., 2012) are of particular interest as interconnected macropores (typically in the size range 300–500 μm) can favor cell migration (for osteoblasts but also endothelial cells to create neo-angiogenesis) and therefore promote osteointegration (Mastrogiacomo et al., 2006; Karageorgiou and Kaplan, 2005; Lu et al., 1999). Pore production can be created, for example, by incorporating either water-soluble porogens such as sodium chloride, or heat-sensitive compounds (e.g., glucose, paraffin, $CaCO_3$, etc.) that will be calcined during a subsequent heating process (Tancret et al., 2006; Walsh and Tanaka, 2001; Chevalier et al., 2008; Descamps et al., 2009). Other techniques can also be employed to obtain porous scaffolds such as freeze casting, stereolithography, the transformation of naturally porous biological calcium carbonates into CaP, etc. (e.g., Meurice et al., 2012; Gonzalez-McQuire et al., 2005; Liu, 1997; Walsh et al., 2005; Charriere et al., 2003).

Beside porous or dense scaffolds and pieces, coatings are another major form in which HA is nowadays commercially available, especially using the plasma spraying technology (Sun et al., 2001), regularly employed since the mid-1980s for the coverage of prosthetic devices (e.g., femoral tail of hip implants) in view of increasing their osteointegration and surface bioactivity (Buser et al., 1991; Jarcho, 1986). An important aspect for high-temperature coating processes as in plasma spray is linked to HA thermal decomposition due to transient exposure to temperatures of several thousands of degrees (e.g., 15,000°C). In such conditions, HA decomposes for reconstituting only partially after deposition on the substrate. With rapid cooling, this recovery is only incomplete and plasma-sprayed coatings are thus composed of, besides apatite, a mixture of other crystalline or amorphous phases such as amorphous calcium phosphate (ACP), CaO, and oxyapatite (Heimann, 2006). The presence of relatively soluble phases like ACP can, in particular, be seen as a potential coating-fracture pathway after implantation, due to preferential dissolution deteriorating the mechanical integrity of the interface and thus jeopardizing the long-term stability of HA-coated implants. The apatite structure is highly accommodative for numerous ionic species. Therefore, it is possible to tailor the properties of HA compounds by exploiting relevant ionic substitutions, e.g., for increasing thermal stability and/or modifying advantageously the powder thermal behavior in a plasma torch. In particular, the fluorination or chlorination of HA has been investigated. Indeed, on the one hand fluorohydroxyapatite (FHA) exhibits a greater stability than pure HA thus limiting its decomposition (Demnati et al., 2014; Gineste et al., 1999), and on the other hand chlorapatite (ClA) can melt at high temperature without decomposing (Demnati et al., 2015), thus allowing a better control of the coating.

The strategy to modulate the characteristics of HA-based systems by exploiting ion substitutions in the apatite lattice has also been employed for optimizing biological properties, although the underlying biological mechanisms are not always fully understood. For example, silicated HA was reported to improve biological properties of scaffolds in terms of bone regrowth (Qiu et al., 2013; Porter et al., 2004). Also, HA doped with cations (via substitutions for $Ca^{2+}$) known to exhibit antimicrobial capabilities such as $Ag^{+}$, $Cu^{2+}$, or $Zn^{2+}$, have been reported and shown to be active against bone-related pathogens (e.g., Kim et al., 1998; Stanić et al., 2010; Yang et al., 2007). Other cations like $Mg^{2+}$ or $Sr^{2+}$ are also regularly considered as potential doping ions with biological activity, typically for promoting osteoblastic activity (for both $Mg^{2+}$ and $Sr^{2+}$) or limiting osteoclastic resorption (for $Sr^{2+}$) (Marie et al., 2001). Modifying the chemical composition of HA by selected ionic substitutions also modulates its thermodynamic stability (Drouet, 2015), which can then be a way to tailor the solubility (and in vivo resorption) of apatite-based biomaterials.

## Nanocrystalline apatites

Well-crystallized stoichiometric HA represents, in a first approximation, a good model for human tooth enamel (Gomez-Morales et al., 2013; Eanes, 1979). However, it differs by several aspects from the apatite phase composing the mineral component of bone (as well as dentin) (Gomez-Morales et al., 2013). In the latter, the apatite phase exhibits a rather low degree of crystallinity due to the nanosized dimensions of their constitutive crystals and to a crystal disorder essentially linked to nonstoichiometry (calcium and hydroxide vacancies) (Legros et al., 1987). This nonstoichiometric character also involves the protonation of some phosphate ions in the form of $HPO_4^{2-}$ ions and some degree of carbonation ($CO_3^{2-}$ ions). The presence of these divalent anions replacing trivalent $PO_4^{3-}$ (thus attracting $Ca^{2+}$ ions with less energy) associated to the existence of ionic vacancies in Ca and OH sites leads to a significantly lower thermodynamic stability when compared to well-crystallized HA (Rollin-Martinet et al., 2013). This in turn leads to significantly more soluble apatite compounds than HA. Also, bone nanocrystals are composed of an "apatitic core" (often nonstoichiometric but consisting of ions localized in apatitic crystallographic sites) covered by an ionic but "nonapatitic" hydrated layer with ions located in distinct chemical environments (Eichert et al., 2007; Rey et al., 1990, 2007). The presence of this amorphous-like surface layer is at the origin of the high surface reactivity of bone crystals, playing a role in biological processes like homeostasis.

It is possible to prepare synthetic analogs to bone mineral, the so-called "biomimetic nanocrystalline apatite," by several soft-chemistry approaches such as double decomposition, hydrolysis of precursor unstable phases, etc. (Gomez-Morales et al., 2013; Markovic et al., 2011). These analogs (provided that they were produced by soft chemical routes without the use of elevated temperatures) then also exhibit the same characteristics as their biological counterparts presented above, and represent appropriate candidates for the setup of bioactive ceramics due to their high similarity to bone apatite nanocrystals and their high surface reactivity. The latter allows in particular two types of surface reactions: surface ion exchange (e.g., Drouet et al., 2008; Cazalbou et al., 2005) and molecular adsorption (Cazalbou et al., 2005; Ouizat et al., 1999).

Surface ion exchanges between ions contained in the surrounding fluid and ions composing the hydrated layer on apatite nanocrystals have been shown to be rapid (few minutes) and mostly reversible (Drouet et al., 2008). They allow the modification of surface composition to convey additional functionalities. This is related to the labile character of surface ions (Cazalbou et al., 2005). It is also possible to exploit ionic substitution within the whole nanocrystals, as for well-crystallized apatites (see previous section), by precipitating apatite in the presence of foreign biologically active ions (e.g., $Cu^{2+}$, $Ag^{+}$, $Zn^{2+}$, $Sr^{2+}$, etc.).

Adsorptive capabilities of apatite nanocrystals have also been widely explored, allowing surface functionalization with a large variety of (bio)molecules and drugs (e.g., antimicrobials, antitumor drug, growth factors, hemostatic agents, cell-targeting moieties, etc.) (e.g., Cazalbou et al., 2015; Grunenwald et al., 2014; Weber et al., 2014; Pascaud et al., 2014; Bosco et al., 2013; Iafisco et al., 2012a, 2013; Palazzo et al., 2007; Tabata et al., 2003; Guicheux et al., 1997; Schierano et al., 2010).

The physicochemical characteristics (degree of nonstoichiometry, crystal dimensions, extent of hydrated surface layer), surface reactivity, and thermodynamic metastability can be modulated by selecting appropriately synthesis and posttreatment conditions (Rollin-Martinet et al., 2013; Vandecandelaere et al., 2012; Iafisco et al., 2012b). In particular, one important aspect is the maturation state of the apatite crystals, which can be directly tailored by playing on experimental conditions (duration of aging in precipitating medium prior to drying, temperature and pH of maturation stage, relative concentrations of precursors, eventual presence of foreign ions/molecules in the medium, etc.). It is then possible to mimic immature or more mature bone mineral by choosing adequately these parameters: immature apatite nanocrystals exhibit a large proportion of surface layer thus leading to more reactive and resorbable material, whereas more mature crystals will dissolve at a slower rate and will exhibit a lower reactivity. Care should be taken when posttreatments are envisioned (Vandecandelaere et al., 2012) on nanocrystalline apatites as the compound characteristics may be altered by heating or inadequate chemical posttreatments. Considerations like sterilization pathway have thus to be selected accordingly.

Nanocrystalline apatites can be obtained not only as gels/suspensions and powders (after a (freeze)drying step), but can also be processed as genuine bioceramic materials by using soft chemical routes (typically using temperatures not greater than ~150°C), so as to preserve their hydrated character (directly linked to their surface reactivity) and nanosized dimensions of constitutive crystals. This often necessitates adapting production lines and protocols to the specific synthesis of such highly reactive compounds. Processing routes include, for example, flash sintering processes (e.g., spark plasma sintering (SPS) processing up to 150°C) (Grossin et al., 2010) or low-temperature gel consolidation (Sarda et al., 1999), limiting crystal dehydration and coarsening effects. The ion mobility from ions of the hydrated layer allows direct crystal–crystal (or crystal–substrate) bonding; and this facilitated ion diffusion explains the possibility of obtaining ceramic-like materials without significant thermally activated diffusion processes, in much a similar way to the "crystal fusion" mechanism proposed in the literature for dental apatite (Daculsi et al., 1984). Mechanical properties reported after consolidation of nanocrystalline apatites proved to be suitable for use in orthopedic or dental domains, e.g., with a Young's modulus in the range 12–37 GPa depending on the maturation state of the apatite, close to the range observed in cortical bone (7–30 GPa), thus lower than for well-crystallized dense HA (80–110 GPa) (Kokubo et al., 2003; Hench et al., 1971; Rho et al., 1998; Hench, 1991). Coatings of nanocrystalline apatites on metal or ceramic implants have also been explored, via several approaches such as dip coating in apatite gels/suspensions or electrodeposition (Chai and Ben-Nissan, 1999; Abe et al., 1990; Autefage et al., 2009; Blackwood and Seah, 2009). Again, the use of limited temperatures is key to preserving the interesting characteristics of biomimetic apatites.

Biomaterials based on nanocrystalline apatite have shown significant improvements on bone growth (osteoconduction like HA), but they were also recently shown to be osteoinductive (Autefage, 2009). Also, the possibility to functionalize them with high amounts of drugs opens the way to enhance local drug delivery capacities compared to high-temperature CaP ceramics.

The modularity of nanocrystalline apatite may thus be exploited for bone repair, but also in other biomedical domains as in nanomedicine (Iafisco et al., 2012a; Drouet et al., 2012, 2015; Welzel et al., 2004) for the setup of apatite nanoparticles for intracellular drug delivery (e.g., in oncology), as reported in Section 2.1.2.4, gene transfection, or else medical imaging (e.g., after $Eu^{3+}$ or $Tb^{3+}$ ionic substitutions), and new applications are regularly developed. In all cases, however, care should be taken in the fine characterization of these systems all along their production line, following adapted complementary techniques (Drouet, 2013). Process development is in progress in view of industrializing nanocrystalline apatite-based systems on a wide scale, as this requires adaptations of production lines or the setup of dedicated process pathways.

### *2.1.2.2 Associations with other inorganic compounds*

Bioactive oxides may be used alone as described above, but also in combination with other mineral compounds for modulating the overall biomaterial properties (as in the example of biphasic HA/β-TCP mixtures) or for allowing reactive pathways with phase transformations (example of inorganic bone cement formulations).

#### Biphasic HA/β-TCP and related mixtures

As mentioned above, stoichiometric CaP compounds such as HA are nowadays largely used in orthopedic and dental domains. One limitation of HA is however its very low solubility, which is appropriate for the setup of nonresorbable ceramic scaffolds but not when the biomaterial is expected to progressively disappear to give way to newly formed bone matter. In contrast, nanocrystalline apatites are resorbable but exhibit a lower mechanical resistance and have not yet reached wide industrial development, which is still in progress. Another way to increase (artificially) the resorption of HA-based systems is by associating HA to another, more soluble compound, such as typically β-TCP (Daculsi and Legeros, 2008; Descamps et al., 2013). Although β-TCP is theoretically not soluble in physiological conditions (as body fluids are supersaturated vs this phase) (Rey et al., 2008), β-TCP can nevertheless resorb upon cell activity. In this context, CaP mixtures HA/β-TCP (often referred to as biphasic calcium phosphates, BCPs) are widely used as bone-related biomaterials (Daculsi et al., 2003), for instance in the form of granules, porous, or dense scaffolds. Their resorbability will then be directly dependent on the β-TCP proportion (Daculsi et al., 2003; Yamada et al., 1997). Typically, the β-TCP content varies between 20 and 60 wt% in commercial products. The presence of HA as opposed to pure β-TCP limits the resorption but also facilitates biological apatite nucleation in body fluids. However, note that β-TCP alone can also be used as such for bone applications (Descamps et al., 2008).

Combinations of HA with CaP phases other than β-TCP can also be envisioned, for example, with even more soluble compounds, keeping in mind the general resorption order (Bohner, 2000) TTCP ≈ α-TCP > DCPD > DCPA > OCP > β-TCP > HA.

## Inorganic cement formulations

Another case where combinations of mineral compounds are used is for inorganic cements. This type of approach can be particularly appealing for filling complex shapes of bone defects via a mini-invasive surgical procedure using injectable formulations. With bone cements, CaP formulations are especially appealing due to excellent biocompatibility and bioactivity, and have been extensively developed in the last decade. Several kinds of CaP cements can be distinguished based on the type of setting process, and in particular "acid–base" and "hydrolyzable" formulations (Rey et al., 2008; Bohner et al., 2005). While the former involve an acid/base reaction such as by mixing α-TCP, $CaCO_3$, and MCPM (Constantz et al., 1995), the latter are based on the hydrolysis of one compound such as α-TCP (Ginebra et al., 1997) (known to progressively hydrolyze into apatite) or a multicomponent system (e.g., ACP + DCPD); the final product being usually bone-like nanocrystalline apatite. In hydrolyzable cements, the hydrolysis of the active phase determines the setting reaction. Passive phases on the other hand are used for their nucleating ability or as sources of calcium and phosphate ions (e.g., βTCP in DCPD-based cements). Acid–base reactions involved in CaP cement are exothermic, but the heat released is lower than for polymer-based cement formulations such as using polymethylmethacrylate (PMMA) (Baroud et al., 2006).

In practice, the cement paste is prepared by the surgeon at the time of use by mixing the solid phase with a predetermined amount of liquid phase (aqueous solution). After inclusion in the bone defect to be filled, the paste will then progressively harden. The hardening phenomenon is linked to the growth of interlaced crystals and, when nanocrystalline apatite crystals are involved, to strong interactions between adjacent nanocrystals.

Most of the commercial cements are microporous (~50% porosity) and with pore size smaller than a few micrometers, not allowing direct cell colonization. Despite a hardening process, the mechanical properties of such cements remain rather low (e.g., compressive strength of TCP-based cements in the range

3–80 MPa) (Rey et al., 2008), and they may also vary from characteristics provided by manufacturers due to difference of testing conditions in vitro and in vivo. Applications of such bone cements are thus more focused for non-load-bearing sites.

Mixed calcium carbonate–CaP cements have recently been reported (Combes et al., 2006) with the view to modulate their resorption rate. Cement formulations can also be associated with active (bio)molecules/drugs, for example, for conveying antimicrobial properties.

### *2.1.2.3 Organic/inorganic composites*

The association, via liquid/solid or solid/solid mixing (Zhang and Zhang, 2001; Kikuchi et al., 2004; Aunoble et al., 2006; Matsuno et al., 2006; Van Den Vreken et al., 2006), of an organic compound (e.g., synthetic or natural polymer) and bioactive oxides such as CaPs can be a way of modulating the biomaterials properties (Vallet-Regí et al., 1997), for example for improving mechanical specifications (Sanginario et al., 2006). This type of organic/inorganic combination is indeed exploited by Nature itself in bone tissue, where close interactions between apatite nanocrystals and collagen fibrils (protein) come into play. By tailoring preparation conditions and composite scaffold characteristics, mechanical properties close to those of bone can be obtained (Mathieu et al., 2006).

The possibility to consolidate synthetic nanocrystalline apatite in the presence of organic fibers (cellulose) has been recently reported (Brouillet et al., 2015), based on SPS treatment. Various trials have also been made to elaborate bone-like composite material for bone regeneration starting from apatite/collagen associations (e.g., Itoh et al., 2001; Tampieri et al., 2003; Kikuchi et al., 2004b; Kim et al., 2005). In vivo evaluation of apatite/collagen composites in weight-bearing sites, possibly in association with growth factors such as BMP-2, was e.g., reported to promote new bone formation (Itoh et al., 2002).

Generally speaking, several composite materials have been studied in the field of bone repair, although few of them have been commercialized such as Duosorb (60% β-TCP, 40% polylactic acid (PLA)) and MBCP gel (combination of BCP granules and silanized-hydroxypropylmethyl-cellulose) (Daculsi et al., 2003). Composites associating α-TCP and PLA- or PGA-ε-caprolactone copolymers have been prepared, relative contents of the inorganic/organic counterparts being found to modulate the crystallinity of the apatite formed (Van Den Vreken et al., 2006). β-TCP/collagen and β-TCP/chitosan and apatite/chitosan composites have also been prepared (Zhang and Zhang, 2001; Matsuno et al., 2006; Kong et al., 2005; Rusu et al., 2005), as in Calciresorb-collagen. Organic/inorganic cement formulations have also been reported, e.g., associating β-TCP and methacrylate monomers (Goto et al., 2006) or polysaccharides (Jacquart et al., 2013).

As presented above for purely inorganic scaffolds, macroporous composite pieces can also be produced, e.g., via porogen leaching (Tadic et al., 2004), freeze drying, or supercritical $CO_2$ foaming (Mathieu et al., 2006) processes, with the view to lead to interconnected macroporosity allowing cell colonization and increasing the surface of contact with surrounding body fluids.

In such composite materials, a faster degradation of the polymer can however be at the origin of a modification of the surface roughness and overall porosity with time. The resorption rate of the organic matrix can be in part modulated by its chemical composition, e.g., polylactic/glycolic-acid polymers will resorb faster for larger proportions of glycolic groups as opposed to lactic.

#### *2.1.2.4 CaPs for drug delivery systems*

The main driving force behind the use of CaPs as materials for healthcare is their chemical similarity to the mineral component of bones and teeth, as previously stated. CaPs are nontoxic, biocompatible and, most importantly, exhibit a bioactive behavior and may integrate into living tissues by the same processes as the ones that are active in remodeling healthy bone. Moreover, CaPs are well reported to strongly bind a wide variety of molecules (i.e., they are nowadays applied for separation of various proteins/molecules in a high-performance liquid chromatography system and as materials for wastewater remediation (Mavropoulos et al., 2002; Benmoussa et al., 1996)), therefore in the last decades they were largely explored as materials for drug delivery (Bose and Tarafder, 2012; Gómez-Morales et al., 2013; Roveri et al., 2008). CaPs, and in particular HA possess on their surface both positive and negative groups (i.e., calcium, phosphates, or hydroxyl groups) that can be exploited for their reactivity by specific electrostatic interactions with some charged/polarized end groups of biomolecules (Gómez-Morales et al., 2013). Negatively charged molecules are considered to bind to calcium sites and positively charged ones to phosphate sites. The interaction (i.e., adsorption and release) of biomolecules and CaP surfaces depends on the nature of the molecules as well as the chemical and structural characteristics of the substrates. Carboxyl-containing molecules are good binders of calcium sites, in fact, it has been published that, in the case of antibiotics, those containing carboxylic groups like cephalothin interacted better with HA (Stigter et al., 2004). Commonly, the adsorption equilibrium of biomolecules strongly interacting with an apatitic surface can be satisfactorily described by a Langmuir isotherm (Errassif et al., 2010; Ouizat et al., 1999; Iafisco et al., 2008, 2010, 2011, 2012a; Autefage et al., 2009). Conversely, a covalent functionalization of CaPs with bioactive molecules can be obtained using the reaction of surface hydroxyl groups with substituted alkoxysilanes (Russo et al., 2014). Silanol groups from hydrolyzed silicon alkoxides are able to condense with the hydroxyl groups of the CaPs, while the alkyl chain bears the functional group that can be exploited for further functionalization (Russo et al., 2014). Usually, the biomolecules release is mainly triggered by dissolution of the CaPs that occurs faster at acidic pH values.

Numerous bioactive molecules can indeed be associated with CaPs, including proteins, amino acids, antibiotics, growth factors, anticancer, and antiosteoporosis drugs, that make them able to interact selectively in the biological environment. This represents a big innovation for the development of novel bone substitute materials, in fact, functionalized CaPs will not only guarantee, for instance, either osteointegration or osteoinduction properties, but they will also perform functions at the molecular level by stimulating specific cellular responses (Bose and Tarafder, 2012;

Autefage et al., 2009; Iafisco and Margiotta, 2012). For example, some papers have investigated the use of HA as a smart bone filler delivery system, acting both as bone substitutes and as platinum drug releasing agents with the final goal of locally inhibiting the tumor regrowth and reducing the systemic toxicity (Iafisco and Margiotta, 2012; Palazzo et al., 2007; Iafisco et al., 2009, 2012b). Another interesting example is the functionalization of CaPs-coated titanium implants with antibiotics (Stigter et al., 2004) or antiosteoporotic drugs (i.e., bisphosphonates) (Bosco et al., 2015). In this way, a local release system of antibiotics could be used to prevent postsurgical infections favoring early osteointegration of prosthesis (Stigter et al., 2004), while the functionalization of HA with bisphosphonates and subsequent deposition of this material as a coating onto bone implants represents an approach for improving bone implant fixation and survival in patients suffering from osteoporosis (Bosco et al., 2015). The deposition of HA functionalized with bisphosphonate might have a dual effect during bone implant integration, and may offer a simultaneous targeting of peri-implant bone anabolic/catabolic processes (Alghamdi et al., 2014).

Due to their ability to be easily functionalized, crystalline or amorphous CaPs having nanodimensions were recently proposed as drug carriers in nanomedicine, thus for biomedical applications not strictly connected to bone. In fact, the recent advancements in the nanotechnology have prompted a rapid progress in the preparation of CaPs with tailored surface characteristics, nanometric dimensions, and colloidal stability opening new perspectives in their use in nanomedicine (Bouladjine et al., 2009; Uskoković and Uskoković, 2011). In comparison to other inorganic nanoparticles (silica, quantum dots, carbon nanotubes, and magnetic particles), CaPs show the following advantages: favorable biodegradability and biocompatibility, lower toxicity, low production costs and pH-dependent dissolution. In particular, they dissolve at low pH, e.g., in lysosomes, after cellular uptake or in the acidic environment of several solid tumors or inflammation sites, thereby releasing the incorporated drugs or ions or any other biologically active molecule (Rodríguez-Ruiz et al., 2013; Tabaković et al., 2012; Morgan et al., 2008; Kester et al., 2008). In recent years, a plethora of synthetic CaPs have been developed leading to a huge variety of nanoparticles differing in composition (i.e., Ca/P ratio, anionic or cationic substituents), hydration level, crystalline phase, crystallinity degree, dimension, morphology, aspect ratio, polydispersity index, aggregation degree, surface area, surface charge (total charge and charges present in surface), and colloidal stability (Sadat-Shojai et al., 2013; Lin et al., 2014). Overall, CaPs are versatile materials because all the cited parameters can be tuned for different specific requirements representing an important step toward the development of personalized medicine where CaP nanosystems can be customized based on the condition of the patient. A huge number of therapeutic agents has been loaded on CaP nanoparticles. Commonly, the therapeutic agent is a molecule adsorbed or encapsulated in the nanoparticles that when released explicates its pharmacological activity, i.e., activates or deactivates a receptor, enhances or suppresses a gene's expression, induces cell proliferation or apoptosis, etc. Some of the most employed drugs/molecules attached to CaPs are bisphosphonates and doxorubicin (DOX) (Victor et al., 2014; Iafisco et al., 2013a, 2016; Hirabayashi and Fujisaki, 2003). Bisphosphonates are used as drugs for the treatment of skeletal disorders (Nancollas et al., 2006) and also as a binding moiety (Hirabayashi and Fujisaki, 2003; Farbod et al., 2016): in fact, they strongly bind to synthetic as well as biological HA nanoparticles surfaces. DOX is commonly used in chemotherapies due to its therapeutic potential against solid tumors (Rodríguez-Ruiz et al., 2013). Moreover, DOX has strong visible absorption and fluorescence emission, and therefore is one of the best molecules to monitor the uptake and release from different CaPs (Iafisco et al., 2016). CaP nanoparticles have been also loaded with several advanced therapeutics for gene regulation, for instance, polypeptides, proteins, lipids, DNA, RNA, siRNA, and microRNAs (Mostaghaci et al., 2016; Xie et al., 2013; Di Mauro et al., 2016).

### 2.1.3 Other bioactive oxides

The preceding section dealt with the use of CaPs—a major class of bioactive oxides—pure or in association with other inorganic or organic compounds. Other active oxides can also be mentioned, such as calcium carbonate and calcium sulfate systems in particular.

#### 2.1.3.1 Calcium carbonates

Calcium carbonates arising from natural origins (e.g., from marine organisms such as coral and seashells) are regularly used as bone substitute materials (Arnaud et al., 1999; Atlan et al., 1999; Begley et al., 1995; Braye et al., 1996; Macha et al., 2015) and can be found as commercial products. Prior to use, these natural compounds are subjected to physical/chemical treatments for purification and control of physicochemical features. Carbonated apatites can also be prepared by hydrothermal conversion of coral in the presence of phosphate (Damien and Revell, 2004). The three-dimensional (3D) organization with interconnected porosity of coral is similar to that of trabecular bone, and may allow good osteointegration with cell colonization ability.

Body fluids are supersaturated relatively to calcium carbonates and the latter should thus not dissolve spontaneously, but enzymatic processes can degrade them; also in the presence of phosphate ions apatite remains the most stable phase which explains $CaCO_3$ transformation into (carbonated) apatite. The use of highly carbonated systems can thus be an appealing way to obtain highly resorbable scaffolds.

#### 2.1.3.2 Calcium sulfates

Another class of bioactive oxides lies in calcium sulfates (Ricci et al., 2008). Plaster of Paris (based on the hemihydrate form $CaSO_4 \cdot 0.5\ H_2O$) has been used for thousands of years by ancient civilizations. It is used to set up cement formulations as well as granules and resorbable composites (Thomas and Puleo, 2009; Mamidwar et al., 2007; Rosenblum et al., 1993). It derives from gypsum, the dehydrated form $CaSO_4 \cdot 2\ H_2O$, after heat treatment (typically 160°C), and the setting reaction of calcium sulfate cement lies in the rehydration process leading to interlaced gypsum crystals. The hemihydrate exists in two allotropic forms, $\alpha$ and $\beta$. The $\alpha$-form leads to denser materials than the β-form, and is preferable, e.g., in dental applications. The setting reaction can be accelerated by additives like $K_2SO_4$. Body fluids are undersaturated relatively to calcium sulfates, thus these compounds will resorb rapidly in vivo (typically within 4–7 weeks) (Ricci et al., 2008), which may limit use as bone substitutes to small defects. The use of preset calcium sulfate granulates and more efficiently a combination with an organic matrix (e.g., PLA) may allow the slowing down of the dissolution kinetics (Mamidwar et al., 2007). Calcium sulfate bioactivity can be related to the release of calcium ions inducing apatite formation (Ricci et al., 2008). As for CaP compounds, calcium sulfates can also be associated with active molecules/drugs for local delivery (Rosenblum et al., 1993; Beardmore et al., 2005).

### 2.1.4 Conclusion

Bioactive oxides represent central candidates for the setup of efficient and sometimes multifunctional biomaterials and medical devices dedicated to a variety of biomedical applications. In particular, the group of CaPs (including in (hydroxy) apatites, β-TCP, and related phases) is a major class of compounds, used alone or in combination with other inorganic or organic components, which are now used on a daily basis, e.g., in orthopedic and dental surgeries, but for which appealing novel applications are also under investigation as in nanomedicine. The possibility to synthesize them via several approaches, to tailor their physicochemical (and thermodynamic) characteristics in view of the targeted applications, to process them in various forms (granules, micro/nanoparticles, 3D scaffolds, injectable cements, coatings, etc.), and to modulate their activity via ion substitutions/surface ion exchanges and molecular adsorptions allows us to envision a large diversity of biomedical usages, some of which have still to be explored.

## 2.2 Inert oxides and composites

### 2.2.1 Introduction

Contrary to the previous chapter, this chapter is devoted to the description of load-bearing bioinert oxide ceramics meaning that no direct bone–ceramic interface is formed and that the ceramic part replaces permanently the bone for orthopedic or dental applications. Ceramics used for applications such as total hip and knee replacements, dental implants, dental crowns, etc., need to present sufficient high mechanical properties as compressive and tensile strengths, hardness, toughness, low wear and good corrosion resistance against biological medium. Alumina or alumina-based composites are the most used ceramics for joint replacement and are often preferred to metals due to their better compatibility with human cells without cation relaxing and their lower wear in friction stress conditions (McEntire et al., 2015). For dental applications, most commercial products are today alumina-stabilized–zirconia-based composites. The characteristics of inert oxide ceramics and some commercial parts used as medical devices are listed in Table 2.2.

**Table 2.2 Characteristics of bioinert oxide ceramics and composites**

| Properties | Unit | $Al_2O_3$ (McEntire et al., 2015) | 3Y-TZP (McEntire et al., 2015) | 12Ce-TZP (McEntire et al., 2015) | ZPTA (Kuntz et al., 2005) | ATZ (McEntire et al., 2015; Sequiera et al.,2017; Kern, 2014) | Ce-TZP/ $Al_2O_3$ (Benzaid et al., 2008) | Ce-TZP/ Spinel (Apel et al., 2012) |
|---|---|---|---|---|---|---|---|---|
| Theoretical density | $g/cm^3$ | 3.98 | 6.1 | | 4.40 | 5.51 | | |
| Thermal expansion | $10^{-6}/°C$ | 9.8 | 10.5 | | 8.1 | | | |
| Thermal conductivity (298 K) | W/mK | 36 | 2.9 | | 17 | | | |
| Grain size | μm | 1.7 | 0.3–0.5 | 0.1–0.6 | 0.6 $Al_2O_3$ | 0.4 | | 0.5 $ZrO_2$ 0.2 Spinel |
| Flexural strength | MPa | 630 | 900–1200 | 700 | 1380 | 755–1163 | 900 | 900 |
| Young's modulus | GPa | 407 | 210 | 223 | 360 | 240–250 | | |
| Fracture toughness ($K_{IC}$) | $MPa\sqrt{m}$ | 3.2 | 7–9 | 7.8–20 | 5.6 | 8–12 | 8.8–11.8 | >15 |
| Hardness | GPa | 20 | 12.5 | 11 | 17.8 | 14 | 13 | |
| Fracture threshold ($K_{I0}$) | $MPa\sqrt{m}$ | 2.4 | 3.5 | 5.1 | | | 4.6 | |
| Commercial grade | | BIOLOX® *forte* | | | BIOLOX® *delta* | Bio Hip | | |

ATZ, alumina-toughened zirconia; TZP, tetragonal zirconia polycrystals; ZPTA, zirconia-platelets-toughened alumina.

### 2.2.2 Alumina ceramics

The first oxide material developed for medical devices is the α-crystallographic phase of aluminum oxide owing to its good mechanical properties such as high hardness (superior to 20 GPa), high wear and corrosion resistance, and to its relatively good inertia to biological liquids. The excellent properties of α-$Al_2O_3$ are linked to its close-packed hexagonal crystal structure with strong ionic and covalent bonds between atoms. This induces a high melting temperature and consequently a fabrication of parts by sintering at relatively high temperatures (1500–1600°C). In order to limit grain growth during the densification and conserve high-strength values, a few hundred ppm of MgO is often added in the raw powder to induce grain boundary segregation slackening grain boundary mobility. The hardness decrease induced by MgO introduction is compensated for by the addition of small amounts of $Cr_2O_3$, responsible for the colorizing effect. Before thermal treatment, the green powder compacts are shaped by cold-isostatic pressing followed by computer-aided design/computer-aided manufacturing (CAD/CAM) machining, slip casting, or injection molding, depending on the final shape and size of the part. In the 1970s, it was suggested that alumina could be exploited to provide better implants for orthopedic applications such as total hip and knee replacements compared with metal plus ultrahigh-molecular-weight polyethylene devices (Banche at al., 2014). Post-hoc isostatic treatments are commonly used to fully eliminate intergranular porosity and by consequence increase flexural strength from 400 up to 650 MPa. Despite its brightness, owing to process improvement, the in vivo failure rate has considerably decreased; from 0.026 (first generation BIOLOX® alumina CERAMTEC) down to 0.0004% (BIOLOX® forte alumina (CERAMTEC) (Willmann, 2000; Piconi et al., 2003). In dental applications, besides mechanical performance, esthetic properties such as color and translucency are required. Owing to the development of CAD/CAM technology, from the 1990s, alumina veneered with feldspathic translucent porcelain (VITAVM9) was used to replace Cr–Co alloys as the crown framework (Denry and Holloway, 2010). Two kinds of alumina were commercially proposed: (1) In-Ceram ALUMINA and in-Ceram SPINELL (VITA) for spinel, which were fabricated from a porous ceramic crown framework processed by CAD/CAM and impregnated under vacuum by lanthanum-silicate-based glass. These products are no longer available because of their poor mechanical properties and the long fabrication duration due to the two steps heat treatment. (2) In-CeramAL (VITA) in dense alumina which are processed by CAD/CAM subtractive method from dense blocks and sintering and PROCERA which are processed by CAD/CAM subtractive method from dry pressed green compact and sintering. The fabrication of these products was also abandoned in 2014 because of a nonprofitable market.

The disadvantage of dense alumina ceramics is mainly its brittleness illustrated by a low toughness value (especially in the case of fine microstructure necessary to minimize the critical defect size and increase the strength) and by its low resistance to subcritical crack propagation occurring in a corrosive environment such as physiological medium (Fig. 2.1). Therefore, to counteract this property lack, zirconia-based ceramics were developed for 30 years.

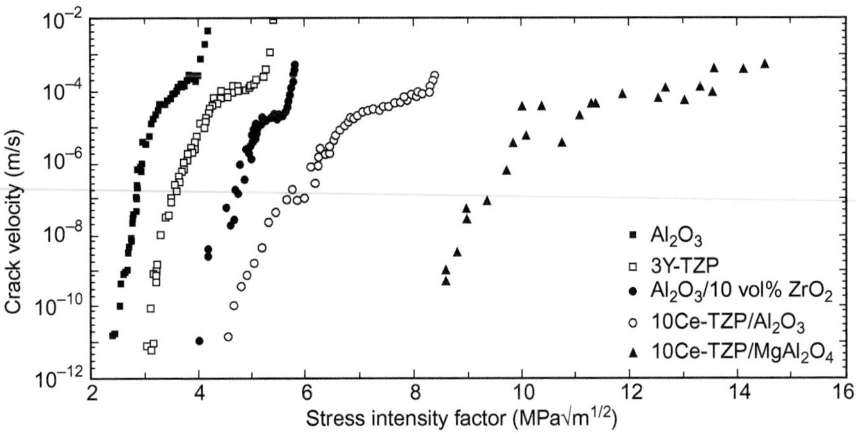


**Figure 2.1** $V-K_I$ curve of the 10Ce-TZP–magnesium aluminate spinel composite, compared to alumina, 3Y-TZP, alumina–10 vol% zirconia and Ce-TZP–alumina nanocomposite (Apel et al., 2012).

### 2.2.3 Zirconia ceramics

In order to understand the origin of the highest mechanical properties of zirconium oxide (zirconia) compared to other oxides (see Table 2.2), it is necessary to describe its atomic structure. At atmospheric pressure, zirconia exists in three different crystallographic forms depending on temperature: monoclinic (*m*) at room temperature, tetragonal (*t*) above 1170°C and cubic above 2370°C. The martensitic monoclinic and tetragonal phase transformation occurs following a hysteresis cycle with 4 vol% change of atom cell: a contraction on heating and an expansion on cooling. As the sintering temperature is ~1400–1450°C, the zirconia sample fabrication is affected by this reversible $m \leftrightarrow t$ phase transformation. Until the 1980s, it was impossible to fabricate sintered parts without them breaking into pieces on cooling. The discovery of the possibility to stabilize the tetragonal high-temperature zirconia phase by adding in the cell structure a few mole percent of cubic oxides ($Y_2O_3$, MgO, $CeO_2$, etc.) has allowed the processing of dense ceramics. Moreover, the presence of partially stabilized tetragonal particles inside zirconia or other matrices induces two toughening mechanisms, linked to the $t \rightarrow m$ phase transition occurrence. The first is the "microcracking phenomenon", which occurs in the parts cooling process for grains coarser than a critical size and slackens the further propagation of the main crack by increasing the multiple small cracks size located around the transformed zirconia grain. The second is the "stress-induced transformation phenomenon" which occurs during the material use by transformation of tetragonal grains induced by stress relaxation under crack propagation by compressive stresses development at the front of the main crack. Further details on the toughening mechanisms can be found elsewhere (Hannink et al., 2000). By the occurrence of these toughening mechanisms, high mechanical performances have been achieved. The most famous composition is the 3Y-TZP ceramic, a tetragonal zirconia polycrystal (TZP) partially stabilized by 3 mol% of $Y_2O_3$ which exhibits the highest strength (1000–1200 MPa) and toughness (9 MPa$\sqrt{m}$) and also a better subcritical crack propagation resistance than alumina, as presented in Fig. 2.1. Owing to its very low friction coefficient and higher strength, zirconia was used as the hip head instead of alumina. This application was abandoned due to some failure cases in the 1990s (Chevalier, 2006). Indeed, Y-TZP presents unfortunately a destabilization in vivo condition known as low-temperature hydrothermal degradation (LTD) which strongly compromises its use in such biomedical applications. So, today the main applications of Y-TZP are restricted to medical devices like orthodontic brackets, dental implants, or dental restoration.

Some research studies have been devoted to zirconia stabilized by 12 mol% of $CeO_2$ (Ce-TZP) which does not present this deleterious destabilization phenomenon (LTD) and is characterized by higher toughness values (up to 20 MPa$\sqrt{m}$) but lower flexural strength due to larger grain size (Chevalier and Gremillard, 2009). Thus, composite components have been developed in order to refine the microstructure.

### 2.2.4 Alumina–zirconia composites

Since 2000, new ceramics constituted by mixtures of alumina and zirconia have been developed to overcome the water destabilization problem occurring in Y-TZP and the modest strength of alumina or 12Ce-TZP. The zirconia-toughened alumina (ZTA) is a fully dense ceramic consisting of between 7 and 25 wt% of unstabilized or Y-stabilized zirconia and the alumina-toughened zirconia (ATZ), also fully dense but composed of 80/20 wt% of zirconia/alumina (McEntire et al., 2015). These composites, developed in 1980s (Orange et al., 1992; Claussen, 1997), and presenting both a strong increase in toughness (10 MPa$\sqrt{m}$) and strength (>1 GPa) compared to alumina and 12Ce-TZP, and a better subcritical crack propagation resistance than Y-TZP, were considered as good candidates for biomedical devices (Chevalier and Gremillard, 2009). Higher values of toughness and flexural strength are commonly reported for ATZ composites while ZTA composites present higher hardness and better aging (Sequeira et al., 2017) (see Table 2.2). Alternative ZTA or ATZ ceramics have also been developed using ceria as zirconia stabilizer or $La_2O_3$-doped Y-TZP in order to reduce the LTD phenomenon of Y-TZP (Zhang et al., 2017). Many ATZ products are today commonly used in orthopedics (Bio-Hip Metoxit) and dentistry such as glass-infiltrated porous alumina-Ce-TZP matrix (InCeram-Zirconia system Vita, Bad Sackingen, Germany), or ATZ composed of 76 wt% $ZrO_2$, 4 wt% $Y_2O_3$, and 20 wt% $Al_2O_3$ (Ziraldent Metoxit, Thayngen, Switzerland). ZTA (12Ce-TZP–$Al_2O_3$) produced by slip casting, sintering, and infiltration with lanthanum-based glass, was introduced in the 1990s for dental restorations (Guazzato et al., 2003).

Another strategy consisting of adding elongated aluminate second-phase grains ($BaAl_{12}O_{19}$, $CeAl_{11}O_{18}$,$CeMnAl_{11}O_{19}$, $LaAl_{11}O_{18}$, and $SrAl_{12}O_{19}$) to increase the fracture toughness by crack bridging and deflection mechanisms was tested by various authors (Cutler et al., 1991; Reveron et al., 2017; Kern, 2014). It was shown that toughening depends on the type of hexaluminate platelets. The German company CeramTec has produced higher hardness zirconia-platelet-toughened alumina (ZPTA) ceramic (named BIOLOX® *delta*) constituted in 17 vol% of dispersed Y-TZP particles in an alumina matrix with nucleation during the sintering of strontium aluminate platelets for orthopedic devices (Kuntz et al., 2005). Due to opacity of the material, this kind of product is not used in dentistry.

The last generation is alumina–zirconia nanocomposites constituted by homogeneous repartition either of submicronic zirconia inside coarser alumina grains or juxtaposition of submicronic both phases grains. This type of microstructure was initially developed by Niihara and consisted of 100-nm-sized silicon carbide particles dispersed in alumina matrix leading to a large increase in the flexural strength and largely improved wear, corrosion, and temperature resistances (Niihara, 1991). This concept was applied by Nawa et al. (1998) to perform a novel interpenetrated intragranular microstructure in which 200-nm-sized alumina particles or 30- to 50-nm-sized zirconia were trapped within de $ZrO_2$ or $Al_2O_3$ grains, respectively. This type of ceramic is now commercialized on the dental market for dental crown framework fabricated by CAD/CAM and veneered by feldspathic glass with the trade name of NANOZR (Panasonic Electric Works, Osaka, Japan). It is constituted by 12 mol% Ce-TZP matrix containing 30 vol% of alumina and 0.3 mol% of $TiO_2$ added as tetragonal zirconia stabilizer and grain growth enhancer. Its coloration, due to the presence of cerium, offers the advantage of masking the metallic pillars but impedes its use as a full crown part. The other reason not to use it to produce crowns is the higher hardness value than natural teeth, which would provoke the failure of opposite natural teeth in bruxism cases. By replacing alumina with $MgAl_2O_4$ in zirconia matrix, Apel et al. (2012) obtained impressive mechanical properties with fracture toughness up to 15 $MPa\sqrt{m}$ and flexural strength of 900 MPa with submicronic grain equiaxed morphology. The various alumina-based nanocomposites (Apel et al., 2012; Benzaid et al., 2008) present a slower crack growth compared to alumina, zirconia, or conventional ZTA, as shown in Fig. 2.1.

The tendency nowadays is to combine both strengthening and toughening effects by developing nanostructured matrix reinforced by dispersed equiaxed nanosized particles and elongated microsized particles (Palmero et al., 2015) or to study new zirconia dopant like germanium oxide (Matsui et al., 2014) or some cermet compositions (Y-TZP with Ta, Ti, or Nb) (Fernandez-Garcia et al., 2015). Lastly, the use of a nonoxide such as silicon nitride which presents no LTD (Bal et al., 2009) and displays the required strength and toughness is under investigation.

### 2.2.5 Further developments

Besides the perfecting of new ceramic composites, the novelties will mainly concern the new additive or subtractive manufacturing techniques in order to save consumables and reduce the part fabrication duration. Indeed, these advanced technologies, newly applied to ceramics, offer feasibility of customized complex shape. For instance, dental crowns can today be fabricated by ultraviolet-stereolithography of ceramic-powder-loaded polymeric resins with mechanical properties close to classical ceramic part machining (Fig. 2.2) (Dehurtevent et al., 2017) or by hybrid machining technology (Petit et al., 2015).

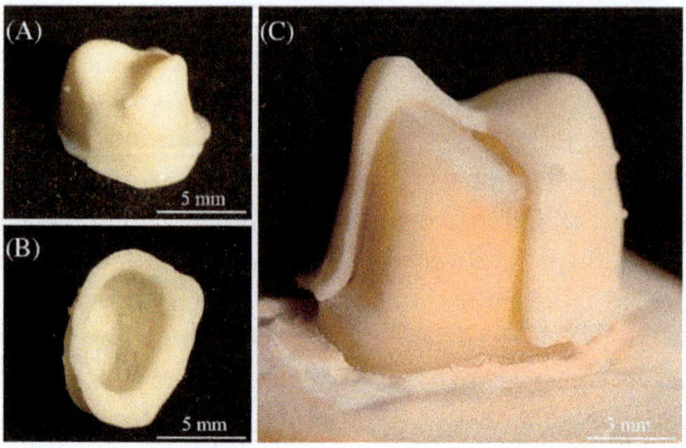


**Figure 2.2** Alumina crown processed by ultraviolet-stereolithography (Dehurtevent et al., 2017). Photographs of an alumina dental crown framework processed by ultraviolet-stereolithography: external ( A) and internal (B) views. Crown framework in place on an all-ceramic crown (C).
With thanks to Dr. Marion Dehurtevent (Lille dentistry faculty) and Dr. Norbert Schneider (Ceramtec).

## 2.3 Nonoxide ceramics

### 2.3.1 Silicon nitride: an introduction

Silicon nitride (Riley, 2000; Hampshire, 2016) is one of the major structural ceramics that has been developed for use in wear-resistant and high-temperature applications such as bearings, cutting tools, turbine blades, and glow plugs.

The ceramic form of silicon nitride ($Si_3N_4$) was first produced in 1955 (Collins and Gerby, 1955) for use as thermocouple tubes, molten metal crucibles, and also rocket nozzles. This type of material was formed by nitriding silicon powder compacts and was later termed “reaction-bonded silicon nitride” (RBSN) (Parr et al., 1960). Considerable internal rearrangement occurs as silicon nitride crystals grow within the preexisting pores of the silicon powder compact as it is heated in nitrogen at 1200–1400°C. However, the original dimensions of the component remain almost unchanged (linear shrinkage <0.1%) during nitriding allowing complex shapes to be machined to final size either before nitriding in the “green” state or after partial nitriding at 1000–1200°C to provide strength. The final silicon nitride product contains 20%–30% microporosity which limits its mechanical strength (<200 MPa) for certain engineering applications. Thus, subsequent developments to produce higher-strength material involved sintering of silicon nitride powder to form a dense ceramic.

Dense silicon nitride exhibits high flexural strength, high fracture resistance, good creep resistance, high hardness, and excellent resistance to erosion. These properties arise from the processing of the ceramic by liquid-phase sintering. Oxide additives ($Al_2O_3 + Y_2O_3$ or $RE_2O_3$) are mixed with silicon nitride powder and react at sintering temperatures of 1750–1900°C with silica present on the surface of the silicon nitride particles and some of the nitride itself to form an oxynitride liquid which promotes liquid-phase sintering and densification by solution precipitation (Riley, 2000; Hampshire, 2016). The $\alpha$-$Si_3N_4$ dissolves in the liquid and is precipitated as $\beta$-$Si_3N_4$ which grows in the longitudinal direction as prismatic hexagonal rod-like crystals that eventually impinge on each other forming an interlocked microstructure, consisting of high-aspect-ratio grains and intergranular glass films (Becher et al., 1998; Sun et al., 1998; Hampshire and Pomeroy, 2012), which leads to excellent fracture toughness and high strength. Fig. 2.3 is a scanning electron micrograph of silicon nitride densified with $Al_2O_3 + Y_2O_3$ and shows hexagonal $\beta$-$Si_3N_4$ grains, some with high length to diameter ratios, surrounded by a Y–Si–Al–O–N glass phase.

### 2.3.1.1 Emergence of silicon nitride as a biomedical material

The special combination of properties exhibited by silicon nitride led investigators to speculate that this structural ceramic might also have applicability in biomedical fields. In the late 1980s, it was already established that silicon nitride is biocompatible (Howlett et al., 1989). Following an initial in vitro study, an in vivo pilot investigation was carried out. Three femoral segmental $Si_3N_4$ endoprostheses were implanted in three adult rabbits, and the osseous reactions were monitored during their natural life. Each implant was enclosed by a stable cuff of bone within 4 months of implantation and remained unchanged during the rest of the animal's life. Autopsies confirmed the radiographic observations, and tissue adjacent to each prosthesis was morphologically normal (Howlett et al., 1989). A later study (Kue et al., 1999) gave further evidence that RBSN has a nontoxic, biocompatible ceramic surface for the propagation of functional human bone cells in vitro.

During the same period, 30 patients in Australia with long-term spinal degeneration problems underwent anterior interbody fusion of the lower spine using RBSN intervertebral spacers (Sorrell et al., 2004). A control population of 10 underwent the same procedure using autologous bone. After 5 years, there were no significant

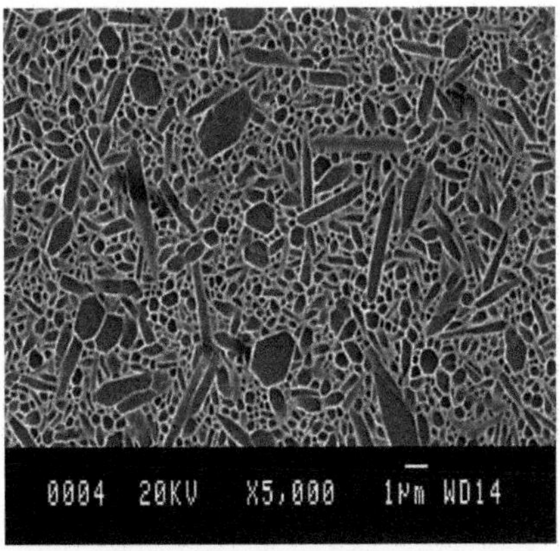


**Figure 2.3** Scanning electron micrograph of silicon nitride densified with 6 wt% yttria and 2 wt% alumina.

differences in patient satisfaction or rates of union between the autologous bone grafts and ceramic implants, but there was a significant reduction in interspace collapse with the silicon nitride implants. After 10 years, progressive degeneration was observed in 13 of 16 cases assessed which were thought likely to be the result of stress shielding due to elastic modulus mismatch.

Given the excellent combination of mechanical and tribological properties of silicon nitride, investigations of other properties critical in biomedical environments were subsequently examined (Neumann et al., 2004; Bodišová et al., 2013; Bal and Rahaman, 2012; Olofsson et al., 2012; Mazzocchi and Bellosi, 2008; Mazzocchi et al., 2008) such as cytotoxicity, wetting behavior, chemical stability in aqueous media (including simulated body fluid, SBF), and wear rates in physiological solutions with a view to developing silicon nitride components for orthopedic applications (Bal and Rahaman, 2012). $Si_3N_4$ sliding against itself showed low wear rates both in bovine serum and phosphate-buffered saline (PBS) compared with the other tested wear couples (Olofsson et al., 2012). Tribofilms were built up on the $Si_3N_4$ surfaces both in PBS and in bovine serum, controlling the friction and wear characteristics. Not only was silicon nitride nontoxic, but the material encouraged cell adhesion, normal proliferation, and differentiation. Cell growth, viability, and morphology on silicon nitride were comparable with Ti, and polished $Si_3N_4$ surfaces appeared to promote cell growth (Bal and Rahaman, 2012).

Prosthetic hip- and knee-replacement bearings require biomaterials with low wear rates and favorable frictional coefficients that remain stable in vivo for their service life. $Si_3N_4$ articulating against itself seems to satisfy this requirement (Bal and Rahaman, 2012; Olofsson et al., 2012), since under test conditions, the contact surface of $Si_3N_4$ becomes ultrasmooth as a result of tribochemical polishing, and the friction becomes very low at increasing sliding distances. In one study (Mazzocchi and Bellosi, 2008; Mazzocchi et al., 2008), a range of different materials were tested: (1) 90.0 vol% $Si_3N_4$ + 10.0 vol% bioglass, (2) 91.3 vol% $Si_3N_4$ + 8.7 vol% MgO, and (3) a $Si_3N_4$/TiN composite with 65.0 vol% matrix (93 wt% $Si_3N_4$ + 2 wt% $Al_2O_3$ + 5 wt% $Y_2O_3$) + 35.0 vol% TiN. For the latter composite material, some oxidation of TiN affected the friction coefficient, but for the monolithic silicon nitrides friction coefficients were found to be lower than results reported in the literature and the wear resistance is an order of magnitude higher than those reported for other ceramics used for hip joints (Mazzocchi et al., 2008). The results indicated that silicon nitride was a suitable biomaterial for bone substitution in load-bearing prostheses.

Silicon nitride components for orthopedic applications are now being manufactured by Amedica Corporation (Salt lake City, UT) and American Food and Drug Administration (FDA) certification has been approved for some of its products, including ceramic interbody vertebrae fusion devices for cervical and thoracic spine surgery (Fig. 2.4) (Taylor et al., 2010). The company is also working on the development of new joint replacements in silicon nitride. The silicon nitride is densified using 6 wt% $Y_2O_3$ and 4 wt% $Al_2O_3$ as additives and is sintered in nitrogen at $>$1700°C for $\sim$3 hours, followed by hot-isostatic pressing $>$1650°C under a nitrogen pressure of $>$200 MPa for $\sim$2 hours.

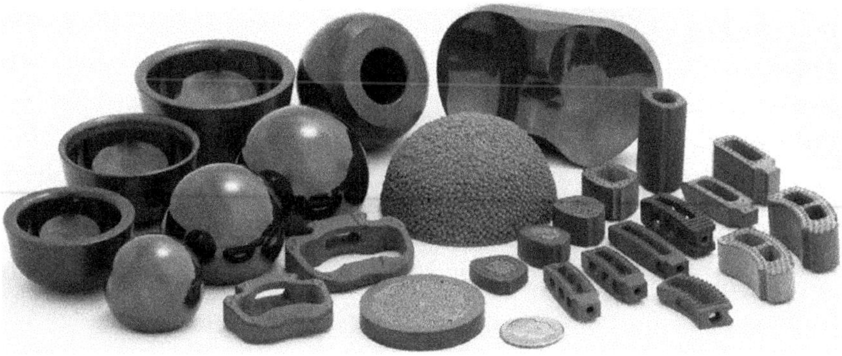

**Figure 2.4** Silicon nitride bioceramic components for joint and spinal reconstruction (Amedica Corp., Salt Lake City, UT, United States).

The surface texture and chemistry of silicon nitride in these materials has been tailored by applying thermal, chemical, and mechanical treatments, to yield ultra-smooth or highly fibrous surface structures that lead to enhanced osseointegration and bacterial resistance without compromising bulk mechanical properties (Bock et al., 2015). Chemical modification of $Si_3N_4$ surfaces results in stable formation of a balance of positively and negatively charged off-stoichiometric sites (Pezzotti et al., 2016a) such as N vacancies and N−N bonds (+ve) and silanol groups (SiO−), leading to enhanced in vitro cell adhesion and apatite formation. Altering the surface chemistry of $Si_3N_4$ by either chemical etching or thermal oxidation influences peroxynitrite formation and preventing bacterial growth in different ways (Pezzotti et al., 2016b). Thus, modification of the stoichiometry of silicon nitride surfaces enhances cell metabolism, affects bacteria metabolism and opens up the possibility of promoting faster healing in bone repair devices.

Silicon nitride has been shown to have very interesting and unique properties that would allow their use in orthopedic applications, but to date this has not been realized commercially. This is due partly to the long and costly process of approval by various regulatory authorities. It should also be noted that silicon nitride requires a different and, again, more costly process for manufacture, i.e., sintering at higher temperatures than oxides and under a nitrogen atmosphere and, with higher hardness, it is more difficult to machine. However, the development of silicon nitride devices in orthopedics should be realized in the near future.

### 2.3.2 Silicon carbide

SiC exists in many polymorphic forms called polytypes where the coordination between Si and C is always tetrahedral and the structures differ only in the sequence of identical layers of Si atoms coordinated to four C atoms (Pandey and Krishna, 1975). β-SiC adopts the cubic zinc blende structure whereas the other common polymorphs have a hexagonal structure, related to the Wurtzite crystal structure and, for historical reasons, are collectively referred to as α-SiC. Silicon carbide has been developed as an engineering ceramic with excellent high-temperature strength, good oxidation and thermal shock resistance, high hardness, and low specific weight. Because of its strong covalent bonding character, as with silicon nitride, SiC requires the use of sintering additives and external pressure to enable densification.

Both α- and β-SiC powders can be densified at temperatures of 1850–2000°C with the addition of $Al_2O_3$ and $Y_2O_3$ which involves liquid-phase sintering (Lee and Kim, 1994). With α-SiC, the microstructure consisted of equiaxed SiC grains, whereas with β-SiC, a platelike grain structure resulted from the grain growth associated with the β → α-SiC phase transformation during sintering. As grain size increased for the sintered SiC from α-SiC powder, fracture toughness increased slightly whereas for the sintered SiC from β-SiC powder, fracture toughness increased significantly, which was attributed to crack bridging and crack deflection by the platelike β-SiC grains.

Silicon carbide ceramics have been considered as potential materials for biomedical applications (Rade et al., 2013). SiC showed good wetting properties but bioactivity, estimated on the basis of HA formation in SBF, was only achieved by surface modification. Much of the literature is concerned with property assessments of SiC rather than biomedical aspects.

Biomorphic SiC can be fabricated by molten-Si infiltration of carbon templates obtained by controlled pyrolysis of wood. Through this process, the microstructure of the final SiC product mimics that of the starting material with porosity ranging from 30% to 70% and resembles the cellular microstructure and mechanical characteristics of bone (González et al., 2003). It can be coated with bioglass for potential implant applications. No further developments have been reported.

SiC has also been developed as coatings and in sensors for biomedical applications. Its use as a bone replacement may be well in the future.

## 2.4 Bioactive glasses

Common soda–lime–silica ($Na_2O$–$CaO$–$SiO_2$) glass, used for containers and windows, is a brittle material and would appear to be an unlikely candidate to replace metals and polymers as a biomedical implant material. Larry L. Hench (1938–2015) invented Bioglass in 1969 following his efforts to find a material that would bond to living bone (Hench, 1991, 2006, 2013; Jones, 2013). At that time, metals and polymers used as implants were "inert" within the human body and elicited a fibrous capsular response at the implant–tissue interface rather than forming a stable interface or bond. Hench (1991, 2006) discovered that Bioglass 45S5 of composition (in mol%): 46.1% $SiO_2$, 24.4% $Na_2O$, 26.9% $CaO$ and 2.6% $P_2O_5$, bonded with bone rapidly, did not form any interfacial scar tissue isolating it from the host femoral bone, and also stimulated bone growth away from the bone–implant interface. Instead, the glass formed a bond so strong that it could not be removed from the implant site (Hench et al., 1971). 45S5 signifies that the glass contains 45 wt% $SiO_2$ and has a Ca:P ratio of 5 which is significantly higher than in the mineral found in bone, HA, $Ca_5(PO_4)_3(OH)$ (Ca:P = 1.67).

Bioglass is known to bond to bone in the body through a sequence of surface reactions (Hench, 2013; Hench et al., 1971; Hren et al., 1976; Kim et al., 1989) with initial rapid release of soluble ionic species ($Na^+$, $Ca^{2+}$) from the glass into the interfacial solution. A high-surface-area hydrated silica gel and polycrystalline hydroxyl-carbonate apatite (HCA) bilayer is formed on the glass surface within hours. The reaction layers enhance subsequent adsorption and desorption of growth factors and greatly decrease the length of time macrophages need to prepare the implant site for tissue repair. The HCA layer is similar to the mineral content of bone and the final stage of the process consists of crystallization of the HCA which interacts with collagen fibrils thus integrating with the host bone. The osteogenic properties (often termed osteoinduction) of the glass are thought to be due to the dissolution products of the glass, i.e., soluble silica and calcium ions, that stimulate osteogenic cells to produce bone matrix. Fig. 2.5 shows a schematic of the overall process of bone bonding from implantation.

Application of Bioglass 45S5 particles to bone defects results in new bone growth during the first few weeks after surgery (Oonishi et al., 2000). It has been used in more than a million patients to repair bone defects in the jaw and in orthopedics (Hench, 2011).

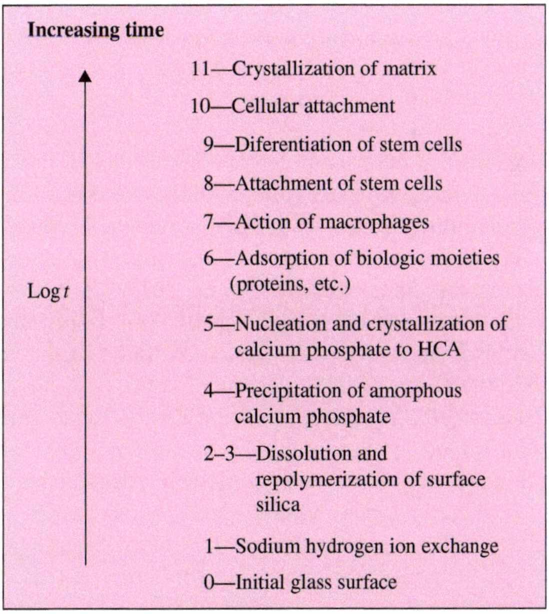


**Figure 2.5** Sequence of interfacial reactions involved in forming bond between bone and Bioglass
*Source*: After Hench, L.L., 1991. Bioceramics: from concept to clinic. J. Am. Ceram. Soc. 74 (7), 1487–1510.

The first Bioglass 45S5 clinical product in 1984 was used to replace two of the three bones of the middle ear in a previously deaf patient so that sound was transmitted from the eardrum to the cochlea, restoring hearing (Rust et al., 1996). Previous materials used, metals and plastics, failed because fibrous tissue formed around them after implantation. The Bioglass 45S5 middle-ear prosthesis was cast into shape from the melt to fit each patient's indication. Follow-up studies after 10 years found that four out of 21 had failed due to fracture, but the others continued to function. Custom design of each implant was not commercially viable, so the device was remodeled to cone shapes of three sizes (Douek-MED) for optimal mechanical properties.

The second commercial Bioglass 45S5 device (Stanley et al., 1997) was the Endosseous Ridge Maintenance Implant (ERMI) in 1988, which was also a simple cone of Bioglass 45S5. The devices were inserted into fresh tooth extraction sites to repair tooth roots and to provide a stable ridge for dentures. They proved to be extremely stable and a study after 5 years showed significant improvements over HA tooth root implants.

None of these products is in widespread clinical use, as surgeons need to be able to cut the implant to shape rather than be limited to cones of fixed size. Monolithic Bioglass 45S5 is more suited to implants that are custom made for the patient. Clinical trials were carried out on 30 trauma patients with orbital floors that were badly damaged causing blurred vision. Using computed axial tomography (CAT) scans of the defect site, rapid prototyping (or "additive manufacturing") equipment was used to produce molds for casting Bioglass 45S5 implants, which were then sutured into place (Thompson, 2011). After 5 years, patients regained full movement of their eyes and both their vision and the cosmetic appearance of the face were much improved.

Orthopedic surgeons and dentists prefer to use particles or granules which can be pressed easily into a defect and, thus, commercially based products consist of particles rather than monolithic shapes. The first particulate Bioglass 45S5 product in 1993 was PerioGlas which was a synthetic bone graft for repair of defects in the jaw that result from periodontal disease (Jones, 2013). It is now sold in over 35 countries. PerioGlas has a particle size range of 90–710 μm and can be used to regenerate bone around the root of a healthy tooth or to repair bone in the jaw so that it may anchor titanium implants. Because of these successes in dental bone regeneration, a Bioglass 45S5 particulate for orthopedic bone grafting of non-load-bearing sites named NovaBone was brought to market in 1999 (Jones, 2013).

While Bioglass 45S5 may have been limited, in terms of bone regeneration, to non-load-bearing applications, one major commercial success is as an active repair agent in toothpaste, under the name NovaMin (GlaxoSmithKline, UK). Clinical studies show that the dentifrice can mineralize tiny holes in dentine, reducing tooth sensitivity (Jones, 2013).

Since the first investigations on Bioglass, other bioactive glasses within a certain compositional range containing $SiO_2$, $Na_2O$, CaO, and $P_2O_5$ were also found that could be used as materials to repair, replace, or augment parts of the skeletal system promoting beneficial tissue response, encouraging new tissue formation and

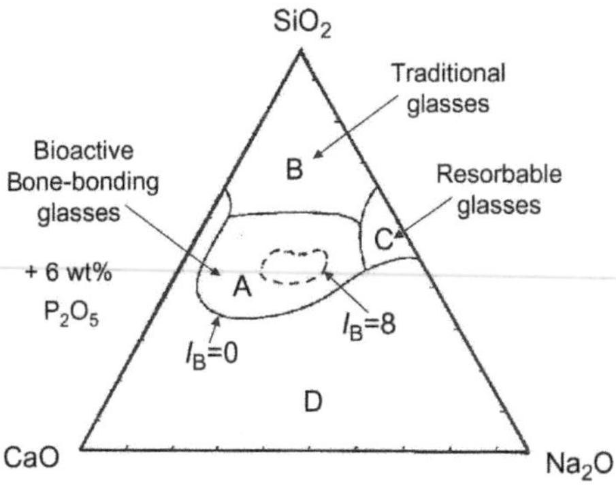


**Figure 2.6** The $Na_2O-CaO-SiO_2$ ternary system (+6 wt% $P_2O_5$) showing the range of bone bonding compositions.
*Source*: Adapted from Hench, L.L., 1991. Bioceramics: from concept to clinic. J. Am. Ceram. Soc. 74 (7), 1487–1510.

involving interactions of cells with the materials (Jones, 2013). The rate of bone bonding depends on the composition of the material (Hench, 2006, 2013; Jones, 2013). Fig. 2.6 shows the range of potential bone bonding compositions (in wt%) in the $Na_2O-CaO-SiO_2$ ternary system; all compositions also have 6 wt% added $P_2O_5$ (Hench, 1991). Compositions in region A in Fig. 2.6 form a bond with bone and therefore the boundary of region A is termed the "bioactive-bone-bonding boundary." Glasses in region B are high in $SiO_2$; with no added $P_2O_5$ these glasses would be used for windows or containers. They behave as almost inert materials and elicit a fibrous capsule at the implant–tissue interface. Glasses in region C are resorbable and disappear within 10–30 days of implantation as new bone growth occurs. Glasses in region D are not technically practical and so have not been tested as implants.

The bioactive glasses of region A have three key compositional features that distinguish them from traditional $Na_2O-CaO-SiO_2$ glasses (Hench, 1991); they have: (1) <60 mol% $SiO_2$, (2) high $Na_2O$ and CaO contents, and (3) high $CaO:P_2O_5$ ratio. These features make the surface highly reactive when exposed to an aqueous medium. Glass compositions with the fastest rates of bone bonding also bond to soft tissues (Wilson et al., 1981).

The level of bioactivity, or bioactivity index (Hench, 1988), $I_B$, of a specific material can be related to the time for more than 50% of the interface to be bonded, $t_{0.5bb}$ (days$^{-1}$), where $I_B = 100/t_{0.5bb}$. $I_B = 0$ at the bone bonding boundary of region A whereas glasses at the center of the region (within the dotted line) have $I_B \geq 8$. The collagenous constituent of soft tissues can strongly adhere to the bioactive glasses within this compositional range.

A significant bioactive glass research program at Abo Akademi, Turku, Finland (Kinnunen et al., 2000) led to the development of glasses of composition S53P4 (53.8 mol% $SiO_2$, 21.8 mol% CaO, 22.7 mol% $Na_2O$, 1.7 mol% $P_2O_5$) and initial trials were carried out in maxillofacial reconstruction with similar success to

Bioglass although S53P4 has a higher silica content than Bioglass and a lower bioactivity index. This material is now marketed as BonAlive (BonAlive Biomaterials, Turku, Finland) and received European approval for orthopedic use as a bone graft substitute in 2006 (Jones, 2013).

An ideal synthetic bone graft is a porous material that can act as a temporary template (scaffold) for bone growth in three dimensions. In order to produce porous scaffolds from bioactive glasses, melt-derived glass particles must be sintered, often around a template or foam or after solid freeform fabrication (also termed "additive manufacturing"). Sintering involves heating the particles above their glass transition temperature, Tg, which causes local flow of the glass, fusing the particles at their points of contact. However, to maintain the amorphous glass structure and properties, the temperature must not be raised above the onset of the crystallization temperature, $Tc_{onset}$. The temperature difference between Tg and $Tc_{onset}$ is termed the "sintering window." The size of the sintering window is dependent on the structure of the glass and therefore on its composition.

The commercially available bioactive glass particulates that have regulatory approval are compositions such as Bioglass 45S5 and BonAlive S53P4 both of which have sintering windows that are too small, so they cannot be sintered without crystallization which results in formation of a glass ceramic (Chen et al., 2006, 2011). Glass ceramic scaffolds have been produced from 45S5 particles with 90% porosity and open pores (Chen et al., 2011). However, full crystallization reduces bioactivity whereas partial crystallization can lead to instability, as the residual amorphous regions degrade preferentially (Hench, 2006, 2013; Jones, 2013). This was found for Ceravital, a glass ceramic synthesized by crystallizing glass of the 45S5 composition containing also small additions of $K_2O$ and MgO. Although Ceravital bonded successfully to bone, implants failed due to long-term instability of crystal phase boundaries (Hench, 2006).

One of the first compositions designed not to crystallize on sintering was **13–93** glass (54.6 mol% $SiO_2$, 22.1 mol% CaO, 6.0 mol% $Na_2O$, 1.7 mol% $P_2O_5$, 7.9 mol% $K_2O$, 7.7 mol% MgO) (Brink, 1997) with a particle size range of 0.5–1 mm and has shown improved bone repair in terms of quantity and quality, compared with synthetic HA (Jones, 2013). Bone growth is faster for BonAlive than for **13–93**, which is probably a result of the Mg content of **13–93** which reduces its bioactivity. It takes 7 days to form an HCA layer on **13–93** in SBF tests, whereas Bioglass 45S5 particles of similar size formed the layer within 8 hours.

A much broader compositional range for bioactivity is possible using a sol-gel chemistry-based synthesis route, where a solution containing the compositional precursors undergoes polymer-type reactions at room temperature to form a gel (Li et al., 1991). The gel is a hydrated inorganic network of covalently bonded silica, which can then be dried and heated to $\sim 600°C$ to form a glass with a high surface area due to inherent nanoporosity which can result in improved cellular response. Typical bioactive compositions are based on $CaO-SiO_2$ combinations: 70S30C (70 mol% $SiO_2$, 30 mol% CaO), 58 S (60 mol% $SiO_2$, 36 mol% CaO, 4 mol% $P_2O_5$), and 77 S (80 mol% $SiO_2$, 16 mol% CaO, 4 mol% $P_2O_5$). The high surface area of sol-gel glasses results in high dissolution rates in body fluids and, while $Na_2O$

increases bioactivity in melt-quenched bioactive glasses, it is not required in sol-gel glasses as its primary role is to lower the melting point, improving processability.

Sol-gel processing also makes it possible to produce bioactive sol-gel glass foams and other structures with highly controlled hierarchical porosity for scaffolds, a requirement for viable tissue repair situations (Sepulveda et al., 2002). Inorganic sol-gel solutions have been designed that can be electrospun into a cotton-wool-like 3D bioactive 70S30C glass scaffold (Poologasundarampillai et al., 2014). This flexible 3D fibrous structure is ideal for packing into complex defects. It also has large interfiber spaces to promote vascularization, penetration of cells, and transport of nutrients throughout the scaffold.

For phosphate-free bioactive $Na_2O-CaO-SiO_2$ glass particles, bone in-growth also occurs in a similar way to the glasses already described (Fujibayashi et al., 2003). Other studies of the effects of composition of glasses in the P-free $Na_2O-CaO-SiO_2$ system on bioactivity have shown that potential bioactive glasses have compositions in the range (mol%): **42–55% $SiO_2$ : 13.5–48% CaO : 10–35% $Na_2O$** (Duée et al., 2009). At the lower contents of silica, bioactivity is not too dissimilar to that for Bioglass 45S5 with HCA forming after 24 hours whereas, as silica content increases up to 55 mol%, apatite formation occurs after a much longer time (a few days), confirming again that bioactivity is closely related to composition.

## 2.5 Glass ceramics and bioactive glass ceramics

Bioactive glass ceramics are formed by controlled crystallization of preformed glasses in order to tailor the mechanical properties for particular applications. Heat treatment is carried out in two stages at two different temperatures to promote nucleation and growth of crystal phases(s).

Bioactive commercial products include (Zanotto, 2010): Cerabone A-W (apatite–wollastonite), Ceravital (apatite–devitrite), Bioverit I (mica–apatite), Bioverit II (mica), and Ilmaplant L1 and AP40. They have been used as granular fillers, artificial vertebrae, scaffolds, iliac spacers, spinous spacers, intervertebral spacers, middle-ear implants, and as other types of small-bone replacements. Some properties are listed in Table 2.3.

Cerabone, developed by Kokubo (Kokubo, 1991) and produced by Nippon Electric Glass, is probably the most widely used bioactive glass ceramic for bone replacement. Heat treatment of an $MgO-CaO-CaF_2-SiO_2-P_2O_5$ glass gave a glass ceramic containing crystalline apatite ($Ca_{10}(PO_4)_6[O,F]_2$) and β-wollastonite ($CaO{\bullet}SiO_2$) in an $MgO-CaO-SiO_2$ glassy matrix. It showed bioactivity and a reasonable mechanical strength which decreased only slowly with time, even under load-bearing conditions in the body. The bioactivity of this glass ceramic was attributed to apatite formation on its surface in the body as with bioactive glasses. Numerous clinical trials have shown intergrowth between this glass ceramic and

**Table 2.3 Properties of bioactive glass ceramics**

| Property | Cerabone | Bioverit I | Highly bioactive glass ceramic | Bioglass 45S5 |
|---|---|---|---|---|
| Bioactivity class | B | B | A | A |
| Machinability | Low | Good | Fair | Low |
| Density ($g/cm^3$) | 3.1 | 2.8 | 2.6 | 2.66 |
| Three-point flexural strength (MPa) | 215 | 140–180 | 210 | 42 |
| Young's modulus (GPa) | 120 | 70–90 | 70 | 35 |
| Vickers hardness (HV) | 680 | 500 | 600 | 460 |
| Fracture toughness ($MPa\sqrt{m}$) | 2.0 | 1.2–2.1 | 0.95 | – |

human bone. It was reported (Zanotto, 2010) in 2009 that ~50,000 successful implants had been made using Cerabone.

Bioverits I and II are glass ceramics containing mica as a crystal phase that allows them to be machined easily so that they can be modified in shape during clinical procedures.

A low-density highly bioactive glass ceramic in the Na–Ca–Si–P–O system that has a Young's modulus closer to that of cortical bone is 30%–50% crystalline, and its main phase is $Na_2O \cdot 2CaO \cdot 3SiO_2$ (Peitl et al., 2001). The first clinical trials for middle-ear bone replacements in 30 patients yielded very positive results. Table 2.3 summarizes the main properties of some bioactive glass ceramics and compares them with Bioglass 45S5.

A wide range of potential properties of glass ceramics is possible because of the ability to design their composition, thermal treatment, and resulting microstructure, and some of these may lend themselves for use as porous scaffolds.

## 2.6 Glass-ionomer cements

### 2.6.1 Introduction

Glass-ionomer cements (GICs), widely used as restorative materials, are formed from an acidic polymer solution and a basic glass powder. When these two components are mixed together, they undergo an acid–base reaction. The resulting material is a cement, which consists of glass filler particles embedded in a metal polyacrylate matrix (Wilson and Kent, 1971). Variation in the particle size and powder to liquid ratio can lead to several physico-mechanical properties and corresponding clinical applications, as reported later on.

GICs have several advantages: minimal exothermic reaction during setting, controlled setting properties, no shrinkage upon polymerization, excellent optical translucency, and very good surface adhesion. Radiopacity, which depends on the glass composition, is also an advantage. The main drawback of GICs is their lower mechanical properties compared with composite resin materials, which pushed research to develop specific compositions with increased mechanical performance.

In 1972 Wilson and Kent (1972) produced the first commercially available GIC, with the trade name aluminosilicate polyacrylate-I (ASPA-I). However, this cement showed two major drawbacks: it required 20 minutes to harden and it did not satisfy the esthetical specifications (it was opaque, due to the high fluoride content). For this reason, in 1972 Wilson and Mclean (1988) provided a new formulation by adding tartaric acid (TA) accelerators and by changing aluminum oxide to silicon dioxide in the silicate glass. The addition of TA, a stabilizer able to control the reaction, allowed the extension of the substance's working time (by complexing with $Al^{3+}$ and $Ca^{2+}$ cations to form tartaric aluminum and tartaric calcium), enabling the use of reduced fluoride content and further strengthening the cement. This product was named ASPA-II (Crisp et al., 1976; Wilson et al., 1976).

Conventional GICs (C-GIC) are provided as fine glass particles and a polyacid solution. If the polyacid is provided as a suspension, the viscosity could increase with time due to an increase in intermolecular hydrogen bonding (Garg and Garg, 2013; McLean and Wilson, 1977). As a consequence, the cement paste is more difficult to process. A small amount of methanol was added to the polyacrylic acid (PAA) in order to stop the flexible PAA chains forming intermolecular hydrogen bonds. This improved cement was called ASPA-III (Walls, 1986; Nagaraja and Kishore, 2005; Mount, 2002).

From 1979 to 1980, new dental cements, also called water-mixed or water-hardened cements, were distinguished from previous products by their improved shelf lives and mechanical properties (McLean et al., 1984). The trend was toward using PAA not in solution but in powder form. The PAA was mixed with either $H_2O$ or TA. This was the key to reducing the high viscosity in the early stages of mixing (Walls, 1986; Wilson and Kent, 1972; Mount, 2002).

The improved GIC was successfully used in low-stress-bearing areas. However, the fact that GICs had poor mechanical properties remained a concern (Naasan and Watson, 1998). Low tensile strength of 7–14 MPa made GICs virtually impossible to use in molar areas, where high stress is present. To increase the mechanical properties, an amalgam alloy was mixed with zinc phosphate cement (Massler et al., 1957; Mahler and Armen, 1962). In 1987 ESPE launched in the market a new cermet (ceramic + metal) under the tradename of Ketac-Silver (McLean and Gasser, 1985). The aluminosilicate glass particles were coated with silver, which resulted in a lower coefficient of friction due to abrasion resistance. Ketac-Silver uses pure Ag powder which, unfortunately, after a period of time, forms $Ag_2O$, inducing the discoloration of the tooth (Mandras et al., 2013). Cermet-ionomer cements have higher flexural strength as compared to C-GICs, but still not sufficient to replace amalgam alloys (Al-Badry and Kamel, 1994).

In 1988 Antonucci et al. (1988) introduced the first light-cured resin-modified glass-ionomer cement (RM-GIC). This material combines the best properties of composite resins and glass ionomers; it has a cariostatic property because of its fluoride-release, low thermal expansion, and the hydrophilic qualities of GICs.

The RM-GICs have improved fracture toughness, are wear resistant, and easier to polish in comparison to the original GICs (Garg and Garg, 2013). The first commercial light-cured GIC, Vitrebond, was developed by Mitra in 1989. This modified cement has two setting mechanisms: a light initiated polymerization reaction and a glass-ionomer acid–base reaction. In 1991 a modified resin was developed by Mitra (1991), which was able to polymerize without light. RM-GICs possess the advantages of both GIC and resin composites, though disadvantages remain such as setting shrinkage and limited depth of curing (Garg and Garg, 2013).

Furthermore, GICs were developed in order to enhance their ease of handling in practice. GICs with adequate powder:liquid ratios were launched to ensure a higher degree of dosing consistency and the corresponding consistent mechanical properties (Albers, 2002; 3M ESPE). Around the 1990s, Dentspy released a new restorative dental product, compomer (Dyract) (Hse et al., 1999). Compomers are fluoride-containing resin composites, also known as polyacid-modified resin composites. Compomers became popular because of their esthetic characteristics, which resemble resin composites. In compomers, fluoride is present in the reactive glass filler and becomes available for release following reaction of this glass with the acid functional groups, triggered by moisture uptake.

## 2.6.2 The chemistry of GICs

GICs are produced by a neutralization reaction (acid–base) involving the alkali, finely powdered fluoro-aluminosilicate glass particles, and an aqueous acrylic acid or copolymers (Garg and Garg, 2013; Crisp and Wilson, 1974a,b, 1976).

The acid–base setting reaction shown in Fig. 2.7, starts once the acrylic acid groups of PAA $(C_3H_4O_2)_n$ (which dissociate to form acrylic anions $COOH^-$ and hydron $H^+$) are mixed with the ion leachable glass powder. The hydrons ($H^+$) attack the surface of the inorganic glass structure, causing disintegration of the glass structure. The continuous attack on the ion leachable glass structure causes the release of $Ca^{2+}$, $Al^{3+}$, $Mg^{2+}$, and $F^-$, among others, depending on the glass composition. These ions enter the aqueous phase of the cement and form complexes with the anions of the carboxylates ($COO^-$) to form metal polysalts cross-linking the polyacid chains, resulting in the development of silica hydrogel (Si-OH) on the exterior of the glass particles linking the cement matrix and the glass particles. The general reaction may be simplified as:

$$MO \quad + H_2A \quad \rightarrow MA \quad + H_2O$$

$$\text{basic oxide} + \text{acidic liquid} \rightarrow \text{salt hydrogel} + \text{water}$$

The outer layer of the basic glass powder is attacked by the carboxylic acid, contrary to the glass core, which remains as filler in the GIC matrix (Nicholson, 1998). The two main cations, which are released from the alkali glass (which have an important role in both the polysalt matrix formation and the correspondent resulting mechanical properties of GIC) are $Ca^{2+}$ and $Al^{3+}$ ions. The degree to which the formation of the polysalt matrix is achieved is determined by the vulnerability of

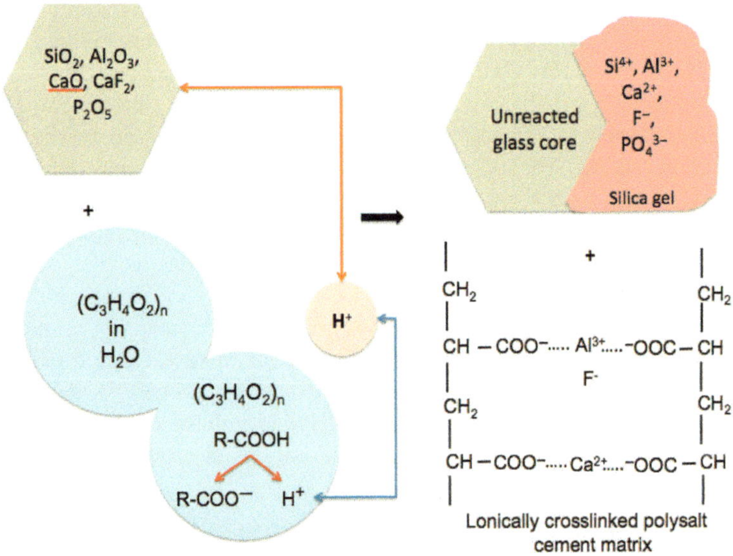


**Figure 2.7** Schematic representation of the setting reaction of the GICs.
*Source*: Information from Culbertson, B.M., 2001. Glass-ionomer dental restoratives. Prog. Polym. Sci. 26, 577–604.

the glass structure and the composition of the inorganic glass (Crisp and Wilson, 1974a,b, 1976; Pires et al., 2008).

The incorporation of the bivalent $Ca^{2+}$ ions and trivalent $Al^{3+}$ ions into the preformed matrix with additional $PO_4^{3-}$ and $F^-$ anions forms a hard, cross-linked, ceramic-like cement and results in the formation of a 3D water-insoluble calcium- and aluminum-carboxylate gel (Pires et al., 2008; Wasson and Nicholson, 1991).

Hatton and Brook (1992) demonstrated that in the polysalt matrix, ions such as $Na^+$, $PO_4^{3-}$, and $Si^{4+}$ are available throughout the cement structure. Wasson and Nicholson (1991, 1993) investigated the inorganic network based on $PO_4^{3-}$ and $Si^{4+}$ and its water solubility, suggesting a role in increasing the materials compressive strength. Sullivan and Hill (2000); Griffin and Hill (1998) reported that the molecular weight of the polymer defines the strength of the resulting GIC. It was also reported that the addition of $F^-$ ions can increase the compressive strength of a 1-day cement of up to 200 MPa (as a comparison to a fluoride-free GIC that has a strength of just 100 MPa (Wasson and Nicholson, 1991). $F^-$ ions are not involved in the polysalt matrix, and react with other ions to form $F^-$ complexes, which delay the reaction of the cations and help to create metal carboxylates. This increases the ability to react, retards the gelation, and extends the working time (Griffin and Hill, 2000a).

As mentioned above, GICs are composed of two essential elements: the ion leachable glass powder, which is based on a calcium fluoro-aluminosilicate glass composition, and the acidic polymer solution, which is made out of a water-soluble polymer (Wilson and Kent, 1971) such as PAA.

PAA is widely used to form cements, due to its very low toxicity, appropriate physical properties, and ability to adhere to the tooth substrate (Wall and Drenan, 1951). Initially, PAA was used as a 50% aqueous solution to form cement, but these cements required a lengthy period (10–30 minutes) to set. Furthermore, the aqueous solution started to increase in viscosity (gelation) after 10 weeks of storage (Wilson et al., 1976). Therefore, copolymers of acrylic acid, itaconic acid, maleic acid, and fumaric acid were introduced to enhance its storage life. The higher degree of carboxyl groups (–COOH) in these copolymers enhances the reactivity of the acidic polymer. Generally, increasing the molecular weight (Mw) (Cifford et al., 2001) or the concentration (ASTM C162—052010 C162-05, 2010) of PAA enhances the mechanical properties of the resulting GIC. Handling properties, however are compromised (Crisp et al., 1977). In order to ensure appropriate resulting mechanical properties without neglecting the handling properties, it is possible to either use higher powder content to constant liquid volume or incorporate vacuum- or freeze-dried PAA powder in anhydrous glass-ionomer or water-hardened cements (McLean et al., 1984).

### 2.6.3 Glass compositions to form GICs

Various glasses have been investigated as cement developers. Three main glasses have emerged.

#### 2.6.3.1 Aluminosilicate glasses

Oxide ($SiO_2-Al_2O_3-CaO$) and fluoride ($SiO_2-Al_2O_3-CaF_2$) glasses were investigated by Wilson and Kent (1970, 1972) Oxide glasses exhibited a typical random glass network structure composed of $AlO_4$ and $SiO_4$ bridges. Introducing $Al^{3+}$ as a network former into the glass structure resulted in fourfold coordination $[AlO^{4-}]$ with a surplus of negative charge, which was balanced by network modifiers (Hill and Wood, 1995). In fluoride glasses, calcium oxide (CaO) was substituted for calcium fluoride ($CaF_2$), resulting in nonbridging fluorines instead of nonbridging oxygens (NBOs). These fluoride glasses were observed to be stronger and characterized by a shorter setting time (Rey et al., 2008). Additional components such as NaF, $P_2O_5$, $K_2O$, were added to the original oxide and/or fluoride glasses (Hill et al., 2006; Greene et al., 2003). Presently, the glass component to form GICs is mainly aluminosilicate glass, whereas the addition of other compositional ingredients can vary (McLean and Wilson, 1977).

The ability of these glasses to form cements was observed to be dependent on the $Al_2O_3/SiO_2$ ratio ($Al^{3+}:Si^{4+} > 1.2:1$ mass ratio; equivalent to 1:1 by mole ratio (Drouet et al., 2012)), on the sodium content (Yamada et al., 1997), and the glass network connectivity (BO to NBO ratio) (Descamps et al., 2008), as reported in the following.

### 2.6.3.2 Aluminoborate glasses

Aluminoborate glasses have the general composition $Al_2O_3-B_2O_3-ZnO-ZnF_2$. Neve et al. (1992a,b) suggested that aluminoborate glasses absorb more water than aluminosilicate glasses. Generally, water-hardening cements, when in contact with moisture, absorb water which acts as a plasticizer (Prosser et al., 1984). Neve et al. investigated the mechanical properties and storage time as well as the powder:liquid ratio in aluminoborate-glass-based cements. They reported that the compressive strength (<ca. 60 MPa at 1 hour, with further reduction with aging time) of aluminoborate cements was poor and may have been related to the slow development of ionic cross-linking in the cement matrix. However, the tensile strength (5–8 MPa at 1 hour) exhibited more representative values. Furthermore, aluminoborate-glass-based cements were significantly affected by their powder content. An increase in strength was observed if powder content was increased by constant liquid volume. Increased $B_2O_3$ content in the glass powder raised the dissolution rate of the aluminoborate glasses (Neve et al., 1992b).

### 2.6.3.3 Zinc silicate glasses

Zinc silicate glasses with the composition of $CaO-ZnO-SiO_2$ and/or $Al_2O_3-ZnO-SiO_2$ contain $Zn^{2+}$ which is an intermediate and serves as both network modifier and network former (Likitvanichkal, 1995). In zinc silicate glasses which do not contain aluminum, the cement-forming ability of the glass is not dependent on the Si/Al ratio. In these glasses, low Si mole fraction and high ZnO provide the ability to form cements. The addition of $Zn^{2+}$ has several biological advantages: it enhances the bone formation and mineralization (Masayoshi, 1998) and it is recognized as an antibacterial agent (Cho et al., 2002). However, cements made of zinc silicate glass components exhibit poor mechanical properties in comparison with those containing aluminosilicate glass (Prosser et al., 1984).

## 2.6.4 Key factors affecting the properties of GICs

### 2.6.4.1 $Al_2O_3/SiO_2$ ratio in the glass

The $Al_2O_3/SiO_2$ ratio determines the reactivity of the glass in an acidic solution and the extent of leaching of the ions from the glass structure (Wilson et al., 1980). Setting rate and vulnerability of the glass toward acid attack are dependent on this ratio. Resistance to acid attack decreases if $Si^{4+}$ is substituted with $Al^{3+}$, which results in a higher polarizability of Al–O–Si bridges in the glass structure when attacked by $H^+$. Furthermore, Wilson et al. (1980) concluded that the BO to NBO ratio is as important as the Al/Si ratio in determining the cement formation abilities. Introducing $Al^{3+}$ in the glass structure as network formers may lead to the susceptibility of the glass toward acid attack by creating a higher degree of NBOs (Wood and Hill, 1990).

### 2.6.4.2 Phosphorus content in the glass

$PO_4^{3-}$ ions in the aqueous phase might interfere with the setting reaction by complexing with other cations ($Al^{3+}$ or $Ca^{2+}$), affecting the setting time and properties of the resulting cement (Griffin and Hill, 2000b). High amounts of phosphorus in the glass prevent the development of the metal salt ionic cross-linking, which is responsible for the strength of the resulting cement (Griffin and Hill, 2000b). Griffin and Hill (investigated the role of $PO_4^{3-}$ in the glass composition $(4.5 - 2_x)SiO_2{-}3.0Al_2O_3{-}(3.0 - x)CaO{-}(1.5 + x)P_2O_5{-}2.0CaF_2$, where $P_2O_5$ was substituted for CaO and $SiO_2$. The Al/P ratio in these glasses was kept at >1. The compressive strength of the resulting cement over a 1-month period was observed and for low-formulation cements ($x = 0$), a maximum strength of $121.8 \pm 4.5$ MPa was found. They also reported that the incorporation of $PO_4^{3-}$ in the glass structure lead to a high degree of plasticity before failure in the resulting cement. The plasticity of the cement decreased, while the strength increased with aging. A high amount of phosphorus in the glass component reduces the compressive strength and the elastic modulus of the resulting cement. The reduction in the mechanical strength could have been caused by phosphate stabilizing the aluminum in the network through the formation of Al–O–P bonds, making the network hydrolysis and release of $Al^{3+}$ ions slower. Conversely, adding a low amount of phosphorus in the glass component can extend the setting and working time, resulting in improved strength of the resulting cement. Ray (1978) reported that the solubility of phosphate glasses is dependent on the double bonded oxygen connected to phosphorus. Generally, the Al/P ratio is kept at <1, to avoid the double-bonded oxygen–phosphorus complexes resulting in hydrolysis.

### 2.6.4.3 $F^-$ content in the glass

The role of fluoride in GICs has been investigated by (De Barra and Hill, 2000) and Stamboulis et al. (2006). Fluoride and phosphates were incorporated into the calcium aluminosilicate glass, to investigate the effect on the setting and mechanical properties of the GIC. Fluoride, originally added to the glass mixture to decrease the melting temperature, was found to disrupt the glass network by forming Al–F–Ca($n$) and F–Ca($n$) species (Stamboulis et al., 2006). In glasses with high fluoride content, additional Si–F–Ca($n$) species are formed. The incorporation of calcium into these species results in a reduction in the number of available cations to charge balance NBOs. This made the glass more reactive which improved the mechanical properties of the GIC. De Barra and Hill (2000) investigated the influence of $CaF_2$ ($Ca^{2+}$ and $F^-$ ions) on the glass composition $1.5SiO_2{-}0.5P_2O_5{-}Al_2O_3{-}CaO{-}XCaF_2$ and observed a weakened glass network associated with the inclusion of $F^-$ in the glass structure and a reduction in the Tg. The cement setting time showed a reduction due to glass structure disturbance coupled with increased cement viscosity. Thus, an increase in glass reactivity in the form of higher cation diffusion in the aqueous phase and higher degree of polysalt ionic cross-linking was observed to be associated with increased $CaF_2$ content, corresponding to an increase in compressive strength and elastic modulus.

In current GICs, $F^-$ ions provide several important characteristics: they reduce the index of refraction of the glass, making it translucent and provide a cariostatic effect, when released in the oral environment (Griffin et al., 1992; Maltz and Emilson, 1982).

### 2.6.4.4 *$Na^+$ content in the glass*

By investigating the decomposition of single-component glass powder containing $Na^+$ as the main cation, Crisp and Wilson (1974a,b) found that $Na^+$ was mobile and replaced $H^+$ from the carboxylate group $(RCOO)_n$ when the powder was under acid attack. Kent et al. (1979) investigating the $Na^+$ and $Ca^{2+}$ effect in multicomponent glasses, stated that the higher the $Na^+$ content, the greater the susceptibility of the glass toward the acid attack, resulting in a faster setting time in comparison with $Ca^{2+}$. Furthermore, they reported that a high content of $Na^+$ in the glass would result in the solubility of the glass surface in an aqueous state. De Barra and Hill (1998) investigated the substitution of $Na^+$ for $Ca^{2+}$ in two series of glass compositions based on the generic composition $PSiO_2{-}QAl_2O_3{-}0.75P_2O_5{-}(1-z)$ $CaO{-}xCaF_2{-}ZNa_2O$ with a high $F^-$ ion content ($x = 0.75$) and a low $F^-$ ion content ($x = 0.5$) and monitored the effect on the resulting properties of the cement. The presence of $Na^+$ in the high $F^-$ ion content glass had minimal effect on the resulting cement properties, compared with the dominant influence exerted by the high $F^-$ ion content. In contrast, in the low $F^-$ ion content glass, $Na^+$ had greater influence on the resulting mechanical properties of the cement with a significant decrease in the elastic modulus, fracture strength, and toughness consistent with $Na^+$ ions complexing with the carboxylate anions and disturbing the ionic cross-linking in the resulting cement matrix.

### 2.6.4.5 *Glass reactivity*

Heat treatment and acid washing are the two main processes employed to control glass reactivity and diffusion of ions into the cement matrix.

#### Heat treatment

Preheating the glass powder—before mixing with other constituents—improves both the handling properties and the strength of the resultant cement. Brune (1982) investigated the effect of preheating (at 100°C) aluminosilicate glass powder on the properties of the cement, and reported a 10% enhancement of the compressive strength compared to the traditional procedure. A reduction of the glass reactivity with heat treatment of the glass at 300°C was also reported by Neve et al. (1993).

### Acid washing

This process, carried out on the glass component of the GIC before the addition of acidic solution, can delay the leaching of ions from the glass structure into the cement matrix resulting in a delay of cation diffusion from the glass structure into the aqueous phase and therefore an increase in the setting and working time of the cement (Crowley et al., 2007).

### 2.6.4.6 Particle size

The glass particle size can influence the speed of reaction. The smaller the size of the glass powder, the larger the surface area, leading to an increase in the chemical kinetics, thus an increase in the speed of reaction (Croll and Nicholson, 2008). Furthermore, if higher amounts of glass particle are available, which is the source of ions, a higher amount of ions can diffuse from the glass structure into the aqueous phase to cross-link with carboxylate anions (Prosser et al., 1986). The combination of reduced glass particles size with a high amount of glass powder content results in a decreased working time. Generally, the glass particle size and the distribution of glass powder content have a considerable influence on the resulting properties of the cement. An improvement in compressive strength with a decrease in particle size was observed (Prentice et al., 2005) and, at low powder:liquid ratio, the working time was extended, due to the ions diffusing out of the glass matrix into the aqueous phase to form ionic cross-linking. In this case, the acid–base reaction was dominant. At a higher powder:liquid ratio, the handling of the paste was better than the rate of reaction, although there was a decrease in the working time. In this case, the acid–base reaction was in the background and the paste viscosity was in the foreground (Karantakis et al., 2000).

## 2.6.5 Fluoride release and recharge ability

One of the major characteristics of $F^-$ ions is their anticariogenic action. A number of studies reported the $F^-$ ion release from restorative dental materials, such as GICs (Brune, 1982; Rothwell et al., 1998; Damen et al., 1996; Karantakis et al., 2000; Marks et al., 2000; Wiegand et al., 2007; Verbeeck et al., 1998; Guida et al., 2002; Williams et al., 2001; Creanor et al., 1994; Moshaverinia et al., 2011). While it is believed that the release of $F^-$ ions in the oral environment has a beneficial cariostatic effect (Brune, 1982; Fross and Seppa, 1990), to date the precise amount of $F^-$ ions required to inhibit caries remains unknown (Marks et al., 2000).

The $F^-$ ion release of GICs can be divided into two stages (Creanor et al., 1994). First, is the short-term (up to 24 hours) discharge of $F^-$ ions on the surface of the restorative material into the oral environment, followed by a long-term release, via a diffusion process from the inner cement (Creanor et al., 1994). Several authors have reported that the maximum release of $F^-$ ions occurs in the first 48 hours, followed by a rapid decline to a modest, residual level, which endures up to a few years (Williams et al., 2001; Fross and Seppa, 1990).

Generally, several factors can influence the $F^-$ ion release into the oral environment: storage media (such as deionized/distilled water and artificial saliva (AS) (Dhondt et al., 2001), plaque formation (Svanberg et al., 1990a), pH (Crisp et al., 1980), and the $F^-$ ion source (glass component of the GIC) (Williams et al., 2003). In vitro experiments demonstrated that the $F^-$ release in AS was not as high as in deionized or distilled water. This was related to similar ion distribution, as between AS, saliva, and GIC, which caused a low diffusion gradient (Bell et al., 1999). Plaque formation can hinder the $F^-$ ion release, or even the formation of saliva set down on the tooth structure can hinder or delay the $F^-$ ion release. A reduction of pH in the oral environment can cause dissolution of the restorative material, resulting in a higher $F^-$ ion release (Dhondt et al., 2001).

Furthermore, GICs possess the ability to recharge $F^-$ ions. This recharge ability of the restorative material is dependent on permeability and frequent exposure to the $F^-$ ion source (Preston et al., 1999).

The recharge ability of the restorative materials if exposed to an $F^-$ ion source is believed to be superficial, since the recharge occurs rapidly (Diaz-Arnold et al., 1995). The ionic cross-linking of the cement structure affects the material permeability and plays a major role on the recharge ability. Air voids and cracks facilitate the diffusion process, but might decrease the strength of the restorative material (Svanberg et al., 1990a).

## 2.6.6 Antimicrobial effectiveness

Fluoride not only has an effect on the de- and re-mineralization of the tooth structure, but also affects the physiology of microbial cells, including streptococci (Koo, 2008; Marquis, 1995). Hydrogen fluoride is formed easily under acidic conditions, which could permeate the bacterial cell easily. The presence of intracellular $F^-$ ions inhibits glycolytic enzymes, resulting in a decrease in acid production and acid tolerance of *Streptococcus mutans* (*S. mutans*) (Nouri and Titley, 2003). The presence of $F^-$ ions also inhibits the plasma membrane $H^+$-ATPase's ($H^+$ is one of the substrates as well as one of the products), hence excreted $H^+$ are brought back into the bacteria cell, causing a decrease of the $H^+$ excretion from the bacteria cell (Nouri and Titley, 2003; Marquis et al., 2003; Nakajo et al., 2009).

*S. mutans* are Gram-positive, anaerobic, spherical bacteria, and are the major cause of tooth decay. Of all the oral streptococci, *S. mutans* are thought to develop and promote the most caries (Fejerskov and Kidd, 2008). Mainly *Streptococcus* genus nourish on food debris in the oral cavity (Banche et al., 2010). *S. mutans* are acidogenic; they attach to the enamel and metabolize sucrose to lactic acid that is released into the resultant meshwork (Rose and Turner, 1998). The tooth pellicle is generally colonized by early colonizers. Co-aggregation contributes to sequential binding and colonization (including *Streptococcus mitis*, *Streptococcus gordonii*, and *Streptococcus sanguinis*). The acidic environment favors the demineralization of teeth. The dental substance is composed of 98% HA crystals ($Ca_5(PO_4)_3OH$). After digesting sucrose, the microorganisms secrete a sticky polymer of sucrose that cannot be removed solely by saliva. The acidic environment makes the hard and highly mineralized enamel susceptible to caries. The acid in the plaque causes demineralization of the outer mineral structure and progresses into the inner dental substance (dentin), finally resulting in decaying of the tooth structure and the formation of a cavity (Tabaković et al., 2012).

In vitro and in vivo studies established the inhibitory effect of fluoride on bacterial growth (Bell et al., 1999; Herrera et al., 2000; Koch and Hatibović-Kofman, 1990; Svanberg et al., 1990b). Because of the porous matrix of the tooth, $F^-$ ions may become incorporated in the HA matrix. This makes the tooth matrix become more resistant to the acidic environment (formation of FHA). $F^-$ ions with an ionic radius of 1.36 nm replace $OH^-$ ions (ionic radius of 1.40 nm) of the HA matrix, resulting in the formation of the more resistant fluorapatite. The acidic environment causes a reduction in pH and release of $Ca^{2+}$ and $PO_4^{3-}$ ions into the oral cavity. During the demineralization, $F^-$ ions complex to $CaF_2$ crystals, which position themselves on and penetrate into the tooth structure during remineralization (Rolla and Saxegaard, 1990). However, the precise level of fluoride concentration that is needed to have an antimicrobial effect is still unclear (Williams et al., 2001).

## 2.7 Magnetic ceramic materials in medicine

One of the most innovative and promising topics in material science is the development of bioceramics endowed with magnetic features. The first class of magnetic bioceramics were conceived as thermo-seeds for the local treatment of bone cancer by hyperthermia (Ohura et al., 1991). Magnetically induced hyperthermia consists of heat generation by means of materials with ferromagnetic, ferromagnetic, or superparamagnetic properties subjected to alternate external magnetic fields (Bañobre-López et al., 2013). The mechanism by which materials heat depends on the chemical composition, magnetic structure, and size. Bone metastases are treated by internal fixation after curettage of the tumor, followed by postoperative radiation or chemotherapy. However, these latter procedures are not always sufficient and the tumor often recurs. Ideally, biocompatible magnetic ceramics can be implanted after tumor resection replacing the damaged site and allowing adhesion, proliferation, and differentiation of healthy cells on their surface, and at the same time generating heat in situ in the range of 43–47°C. Within this interval of temperature, the malignant cells are selectively destroyed whereas the healthy ones only undergo small and/or reversible damage (Overgaard, 1977). However the optimal heating temperature depends on the materials properties, magnetic field parameters (intensity, frequency), and tissue characteristics (i.e., blood flow, tissue density, cancer cells, etc.).

In the last decades, magnetic mesoporous silica glass ceramics (bioglass) incorporating ferrimagnetic, ferromagnetic, and superparamagnetic phases have been extensively studied as hyperthermia-biocompatible mediators for the treatment of bone cancer (Bretcanu et al., 2017; Arcos et al., 2003; Singh and Srinivasan, 2011). For the same aim, a few kinds of injectable CaP cements mixed with iron oxide magnetic nanoparticles have also been developed (C-h et al., 2009; Xu et al., 2015; Matsumine et al., 2007). CaPs are to accommodate in their crystal lattice a huge variety of doping ions in order to improve and widen their performance, while maintaining their intrinsic biocompatibility (Boanini et al., 2010). According to this approach, superparamagnetic HA obtained by doping with ~10 wt% $Fe^{2+}/Fe^{3+}$ was hailed as a far less toxic alternative to magnetite when used as a heating material for hyperthermia-based bone cancer therapies (Tampieri et al., 2012).

Remaining in the field of bone cancer therapy, an innovative approach involves the use of external stimuli (i.e., magnetic fields) to activate the release in situ of anticancer drugs previously loaded on the magnetic implanted matrices (Manzano and Vallet-Regí, 2012; Vallet-Regí et al., 2007). At present, it has been reported that only polymeric porous scaffolds doped with magnetic nanoparticles, the so-called ferrogels are endowed with magnetically modulated drug-release features (Zhao et al., 2011), therefore the preparation of bioceramics scaffolds with the same characteristic is a novel scientific and technological challenge. In the optic of the theranostic approach that aims at exploiting materials having a therapeutic action and at the same time delivers diagnostic information through an imaging technique, magnetic bioceramics doped with iron ions or containing iron oxide phases can be visualized by magnetic resonance allowing a noninvasive in vivo monitoring of the scaffold efficacy (Bock et al., 2010).

More recently the use of magnetic-ceramic-biocompatible and bioresorbable scaffolds to promote bone healing triggering cell adhesion and proliferation under the stimulus of magnetic field is emerging (Bock et al., 2010; Panseri et al., 2012a; Xu and Gu, 2014). In this way bioceramics scaffolds were not conceived to kill cells by hyperthermia or to release cytotoxic molecules but to promote proliferation and differentiation. In fact, under magnetic fields, these scaffolds could provide on-demand release of drugs or biomolecules (i.e., growth factors) inducing osteogenesis and angiogenesis and at the same time magneto-mechanical stimulation on bone cells favoring proliferation, differentiation, and bone healing. The influence of magnetic fields in the cell stimulation has been recently reported including magneto-mechanical stimulation of cell constructs (Markaki and Clyne, 2004), mechano-sensitive ion channels (Hughes et al., 2008), magnetic cell seeding, and controlled cell proliferation and differentiation (Kanczler et al., 2010). Therefore, the association of magneto-mechanical stimulation and suitable biochemical agents could lead to more efficient treatments for the regeneration of extended bone regions (Xu and Gu, 2014; Kotani et al., 2002). It was demonstrated that iron oxide magnetic nanoparticles embedded in ceramic scaffolds have a positive effect on the osteoinduction with and without application of external magnetic force. In particular, it was reported that the introduction of magnetic nanoparticles into CaP bioceramics promoted bone formation and growth in vitro and in vivo (Xu and Gu, 2014; Yao et al., 2010). In this view, magnetic scaffolds might offer great potential in bone regenerative medicine particularly if biocompatible and biodegradable magnetic phases such as iron-doped CaPs (Panseri et al., 2012b; Iafisco et al., 2013b) can completely replace magnetite and the other iron oxide phases (maghemite, etc.).

In fact, the long-term cytotoxic effects of the iron oxides in the human body are not yet completely assessed and nowadays their use is becoming a critical issue due to their accumulation in soft tissues and organs such as liver and kidney (Almeida et al., 2011; Mahmoudi et al., 2012).

With the advent of nanomedicine, which is the application of nanotechnology, to address healthcare problems, the use of individual nanosystems/nanoparticles as drug carriers has been widely explored in the last 20 years to precisely administer therapeutic molecules in specific parts of the body to improve their efficacy and to reduce side effects (Peer et al., 2007). In this domain, the use of magnetic nanoparticles as injectable drug nanocarriers has strongly emerged because they could be manipulated upon application of magnetic fields (Reddy et al., 2012). In particular, the drug attached to the nanoparticles could be efficiently remotely controlled and targeted in desired areas of the body using external magnetic fields (Arruebo et al., 2007). Moreover, magnetic nanoparticles can also be employed for several other biomedical applications, such as cell labeling and separation (Wilhelm and Gazeau, 2008), immunoassay (Ranzoni et al., 2012), and MRI contrast agents (Lee et al., 2014). For biomedical applications, a required property of magnetic nanoparticles is the superparamagnetism, which is the ability to be strongly magnetized (i.e., the alignment of all magnetic moments of atoms in parallel along the direction of magnetic fields) when they are exposed to low-intensity magnetic fields, without having a remnant or residual magnetization when the magnetic fields are removed (Neuberger et al., 2005). This feature is strictly necessary to avoid coagulation and agglomeration of nanoparticles causing possible embolization of capillary vessels when they are used in vivo (Xu and Sun, 2013). So far, ceramic magnetic nanoparticles employed for biomedical applications are mainly based on superparamagnetic iron oxide nanoparticles (SPIONs), consisting of mixtures of magnetite, maghemite, and hematite, which have been demonstrated successfully both in vitro and in vivo (Xu and Sun, 2013). SPIONs can be synthesized with different morphologies, chemical compositions, and magnetic properties, but some limitations still exist including a low magnetic moment and low cargo capacity (Kievit and Zhang, 2011). In addition, although the FDA approve SPIONs for human use, several concerns about their cytotoxicity have emerged. In fact, their chronic administration can lead to the accumulation of a high quantity of iron in soft tissues and organs, causing an imbalance in their homeostasis and even cytotoxic and inflammatory effects (Huang et al., 2010).

To overcome the limitations of SPIONs, new forms of ceramic superparamagnetic nanoparticles with a good magnetic moment, high drug-loading capability, and low iron content are strongly required. For this purpose, iron-doped nano-HAs have been reported to be a competitive substitute for SPIONs (Iafisco et al., 2016). These particles have been proven to be excellent MRI contrast agents while having a minor long-time toxicity compared to SPIONs, and it has also been reported that the if loaded with drugs, application of low pulsed alternate magnetic field could trigger the drug release (i.e., DOX), because it induces the mechanical shaking of superparamagnetic nanoparticles breaking the bonding with the drug and allowing detachment of the drug from the surface (Iafisco et al., 2016).

## 2.8 Conclusion

In this chapter, the state of the art in composition and processing techniques of bioceramics and bioglasses was highlighted for scaffolds and prosthesis applications. Pure and substituted CaP ceramics and related composites are today largely used for bone regeneration applications. These materials offer a large variety of items according to the stoichiometry, the substitution elements nature and content, the crystallinity and the crystal size with, as a consequence, different osteoconduction or osteoinduction properties. They are commercially available in different shapes as granules, scaffolds, coatings, and injectable cements. Bioglasses were also commercialized as bone substitutes for a long time after their discovery by Hench in 1969 and the recent developments are mainly devoted to sol-gel processing allowing achievement of a larger composition range at lower temperature treatment and to the performance of coatings on various substrates. The subsequent development of bioactive glass ceramics was carried out to enhance the mechanical properties of bioglasses and led to satisfactory commercial products for small-bone replacements.

The bioinert ceramics are used as permanent load-bearing parts and include inert oxides like alumina, stabilized zirconia, spinel and related micro- or nanocomposites, and more recently silicon nitride and carbide. Many different products based from alumina, zirconia, and composites are successfully applied for dental restoration and orthopedic devices. The main innovations in progress concern two different aspects: the material and the process techniques. Concerning the material, researches are focused on the development of particular microstructure favorable to better mechanical properties, the use of new stabilizer ions for tetragonal zirconia and cermet compositions. For the fabrication methods, the novelties concern the additive and substractive manufacturing techniques recently applied to ceramics materials and promising time consumption reduction.

The GICs constituted of glass filler particles embedded in a metal polyacrylate matrix are widely used as dental restorative materials. The main improvement in this material was made on the acidic polymer solution and the basic glass powder mixing conditions set up to obtain viscosity and hardening time compatible to the manipulation, on the control of the leaching of the ions from the glass structure in the acidic solution affecting the setting reaction, and on the influence of the glass composition on the biological properties. For instance, the presence of zinc or fluorine elements in the glass has been shown to have an inhibitory effect on bacterial growth.

The development of magnetic bioceramics constituted of a ferrimagnetic, ferromagnetic, or superparamagnetic phase incorporated inside any bioceramics is probably the most innovative and promising topic as it offers several application fields such as cancer-curing action by hyperthermia or bone substitution favoring the osteoinduction phenomenon under (or not under) magnetic field application. Individual nanosystems/nanoparticles can also be used as drug carriers targeted in desired areas of the body using external magnetic fields.

In all the fields examined, a tendency to nanoscale for particles or grains is observed to induce higher bioreactivity or mechanical properties or more localized drug delivery devices.

# References


3M ESPE. Ketac™Molar Easymix Glass-Ionomer Filling Material. <http://multimedia.mmm.com/mws/mediawebserver.dyn?6666660Zjcf6lVs6EVs66S3IzCOrrrQ->. 30.09.2010.

Abe, Y., Kokubo, T., Yamamuro, T., 1990. Apatite coating on ceramics, metals and polymers utilizing a biological process. J. Mater. Sci. Mater. Med. 1 (4), 233–238.

Abo-Naf, S.M., El Batal, F.H., Azooz, M.A., 2003. Characterisation of some glasses in the system $SiO_2$ $Na_2O \cdot RO$ by infrared spectroscopy. Mater. Chem. Phys. 77, 846–852.

Al-Badry, I.A., Kamel, F.M., 1994. Clinical use of glass-ionomer cement: a literature review. Saudi Dent. J. 6 (2), 107–116.

Albers, H.F., 2002. Tooth-Colored Restoratives: Principles and Techniques. 9th ed. BC Beckers Inc, ON, p. 44.

Alghamdi, H.S., Bosco, R., Both, S.K., Iafisco, M., Leeuwenburgh, S.C.G., Jansen, J.A., et al., 2014. Synergistic effects of bisphosphonate and calcium phosphate nanoparticles on peri-implant bone responses in osteoporotic rats. Biomaterials 35, 5482–5490.

Almeida, J.P.M., Chen, A.L., Foster, A., Drezek, R., 2011. In vivo biodistribution of nanoparticles. Nanomedicine 6, 815–835.

Antonucci J.M., McKinney, J.E., Stansbury, J.W., 1988. Resin-modified glass-ionomer cement. US Patent Application 160:856.

Apel, E., Ritzberger, C., Courtois, N., Reveron, H., Chevalier, J., Scweiger, M., et al., 2012. Introduction to a tough, strong and stable Ce-TZP/$MgAl_2O_4$ composite for biomedical applications. J. Eur. Ceram. Soc. 32, 2697–2703.

Arcos, D., del Real, R.P., Vallet-Regí, M., 2003. Biphasic materials for bone grafting and hyperthermia treatment of cancer. J. Biomed. Mater. Res. A. 65A, 71–78.

Arnaud, E., De Pollak, C., Meunier, A., Sedel, L., Damien, C., Petite, H., 1999. Osteogenesis with coral is increased by BMP and BMC in a rat cranioplasty. Biomaterials 20 (20), 1909–1918.

Arruebo, M., Fernández-Pacheco, R., Ibarra, M.R., Santamaría, J., 2007. Magnetic nanoparticles for drug delivery. Nano Today 2, 22–32.

ASTM C162—05(2010) C162-05, 2010. Standard Terminology of Glass and Glass Products.

Atlan, G., Delattre, O., Berland, S., LeFaou, A., Nabias, G., Cot, D., et al., 1999. Interface between bone and nacre implants in sheep. Biomaterials 20 (11), 1017–1022.

Aunoble, S., Clement, D., Frayssinet, P., Harmand, M.F., Le Huec, J.C., 2006. Biological performance of a new beta-TCP/PLLA composite material for applications in spine surgery: in vitro and in vivo studies. J. Biomed. Mater. Res. A. 78 (2), 416–422.

Autefage H., , 2009. PhD Thesis. Rôle ostéoinducteur d'un revêtement d'apatite carbonatée nanocristalline sur des céramiques de phosphate de calcium biphasique—INP Toulouse, 171 pp.

Autefage, H., Briand-Mesange, F., Cazalbou, S., Drouet, C., Fourmy, D., Goncalves, S., et al., 2009. Adsorption and release of BMP-2 on nanocrystalline apatite-coated and uncoated hydroxyapatite/beta-tricalcium phosphate porous ceramics. J. Biomed. Mater. Res. B Appl. Biomater. 91B (2), 706–715.

Bal, B.S., Rahaman, M.N., 2012. Orthopedic applications of silicon nitride ceramics. Acta Biomater. 8 (8), 2889–2898.

Bal, B.S., Khandkar, A., Lakshminarayanan, R., Clarke, I., Hofmann, A.A., Rahaman, M.N., 2009. Fabrication and testing of silicon nitride bearings in total hip arthroplasty. J. Arthroplast. 24, 110–116.

Banche, G., Tullio, V., Allizond, V., Mandras, N., Roana, J., Scalas, D., et al., 2010. Synergistic effect of erythromycin on polymorphonuclear cell antibacterial activity against erythromycin-resistant phenotypes of *Streptococcus pyogenes*. Int. J. Antimicrob. Agents. 36, 319–323.

Banche, G., Allizond, V., Bracco, P., Bistolfi, A., Boffano, M., Cimino, A., et al., 2014. Interplay between surface properties of standard, vitamin E blended and oxidised ultra high molecular weight polyethylene used in total joint replacement and adhesion of *Staphylococcus aureus* and *Escherichia coli*. Bone Joint J. 96 B (4), 497–501.

Bañobre-López, M., Teijeiro, A., Rivas, J., 2013. Magnetic nanoparticle-based hyperthermia for cancer treatment. Rep. Pract. Oncol. Radiother. 18, 397–400.

Baroud, G., Swanson, T., Steffen, T., 2006. Setting properties of four acrylic and two calcium-phosphate cements used in vertebroplasty. J. Long Term Eff. Med. Implants. 16 (1), 51–59.

Beardmore, A.A., Brooks, D.E., Wenke, J.C., Thomas, D.B., 2005. Effectiveness of local antibiotic delivery with an osteoinductive and osteoconductive bone-graft substitute. J. Bone Joint Surg. Am. 87A (1), 107–112.

Becher, P.F., Sun, E.Y., Plucknett, K.P., Alexander, K.B., Hsueh, C.-H., Lin, H.T., et al., 1998. Microstructural design of silicon nitride with improved fracture toughness: I. Effects of grain size and shape. J. Am. Ceram. Soc. 81 (11), 2821–2830.

Begley, C.T., Jo Doherty, M., Mollan, R.A.B., Wilson, D.J., 1995. Comparative study of the osteoinductive properties of bioceramic, coral and processed bone graft substitutes. Biomaterials 16 (15), 1181–1185.

Bell, A., Creanor, S.L., Foye, R.H., Saunders, W.P., 1999. The effect of saliva on fluoride release by a glass-ionomer filling material. J. Oral Rehab. 26, 407–412.

Benmoussa, A., Lacout, J.L., Loiseau, P.R., Mikou, M., 1996. Calcium phosphate hydroxyapatite and lead phosphate hydroxyapatite for separation by liquid chromatography. Chromatographia 42, 177–180.

Benzaid, R., Chevalier, J., Saadaoui, M., Fantozzi, G., Nawa, M., Diaz, L.A., 2008. Fracture toughness, strength and slow crack growth in a ceria stabilized zirconia–alumina nanocomposites for medical applications. Biomaterials 29, 3636–3641.

Blackwood, D.J., Seah, K.H.W., 2009. Electrochemical cathodic deposition of hydroxyapatite: improvements in adhesion and crystallinity. Mater. Sci. Eng. C. 29 (4), 1233–1238.

Boanini, E., Gazzano, M., Bigi, A., 2010. Ionic substitutions in calcium phosphates synthesized at low temperature. Acta Biomater. 6, 1882–1894.

Bock, N., Riminucci, A., Dionigi, C., Russo, A., Tampieri, A., Landi, E., et al., 2010. A novel route in bone tissue engineering: magnetic biomimetic scaffolds. Acta Biomater. 6, 786–796.

Bock, R.M., McEntire, B.J., Bal, B.S., Rahaman, M.N., Boffelli, M., Pezzotti, G., 2015. Surface modulation of silicon nitride ceramics for orthopaedic applications. Acta Biomater. 26, 318–330.

Bodišová, K., Kašiarová, M., Domanická, M., Hnatko, M., Lenčéš, Z., Nováková, Z.V., et al., 2013. Porous silicon nitride ceramics designed for bone substitute applications. Ceram. Int. 39, 8355–8362.

Bohner, M., 2000. Calcium orthophosphates in medicine: from ceramics to calcium phosphate cements. Injury 31, D37–D47.

Bohner, M., Gbureck, U., Barralet, J.E., 2005. Technological issues for the development of more efficient calcium phosphate bone cements: a critical assessment. Biomaterials 26 (33), 6423–6429.

Bosco, R., Iafisco, M., van den Beucken, J., Leeuwenburgh, S., Jansen, J., 2013. Adsorption of alendronate onto biomimetic apatite nanocrystals to develop drug carrier coating for bone implants. Bioceramics. 24 (529–530), 475–479.

Bosco, R., Iafisco, M., Tampieri, A., Jansen, J.A., Leeuwenburgh, S.C.G., van den Beucken, J.J.J.P., 2015. Hydroxyapatite nanocrystals functionalized with alendronate as bioactive components for bone implant coatings to decrease osteoclastic activity. Appl. Surf. Sci. 328, 516–524.

Bose, S., Tarafder, S., 2012. Calcium phosphate ceramic systems in growth factor and drug delivery for bone tissue engineering: a review. Acta Biomater. 8, 1401–1421.

Bouladjine, A., Al-Kattan, A., Dufour, P., Drouet, C., 2009. New advances in nanocrystalline apatite colloids intended for cellular drug delivery. Langmuir. 25, 12256–12265.

Braye, F., Irigaray, J.L., Jallot, E., Oudadesse, H., Weber, G., Deschamps, N., et al., 1996. Resorption kinetics of osseous substitute: natural coral and synthetic hydroxyapatite. Biomaterials 17 (13), 1345–1350.

Bretcanu, O., Miola, M., Bianchi, C.L., Marangi, I., Carbone, R., Corazzari, I., et al., 2017. In vitro biocompatibility of a ferrimagnetic glass-ceramic for hyperthermia application. Mater. Sci. Eng. C. 73, 778–787.

Brink, M., 1997. The influence of alkali and alkaline earths on the working range for bioactive glasses. J. Biomed. Mater. Res. 36, 109–117.

Brouillet, F., Laurencin, D., Grossin, D., Drouet, C., Estournes, C., Chevallier, G., et al., 2015. Biomimetic apatite-based composite materials obtained by spark plasma sintering (SPS): physicochemical and mechanical characterizations. J. Mater. Sci. Mater. Med. 26 (8), 5553.

Brune, D.A.G., 1982. Heat treatment of glass ionomer, silicate, zinc phosphate and zinc polycarboxylate cements. Eur. J. Oral Sci. 90 (5), 409–412.

Buser, D., Schenk, R.K., Steinemann, S., Fiorellini, J.P., Fox, C.H., Stich, H., 1991. Influence of surface characteristics on bone integration of titanium implants. A histomorphometric study in miniature pigs. J. Biomed. Mater. Res. 25 (7), 889–902.

Cazalbou, S., Eichert, D., Ranz, X., et al., 2005. Ion exchanges in apatites for biomedical application. J. Mater. Sci. Mater. Med. 16 (5), 405–409.

Cazalbou, S., Bertrand, G., Drouet, C., 2015. Tetracycline-loaded biomimetic apatite: An adsorption study. J. Phys. Chem. B. 119, 3014–3024.

Chai, C.S., Ben-Nissan, B., 1999. Bioactive nanocrystalline sol-gel hydroxyapatite coatings. J. Mater. Sci. Mater. Med. 10 (8), 465–469.

Champion, E., Damia, C., Viana, M., Beaubrun-Giry, K., Drouet, C., Grossin, D., 2013. Processing of calcium phosphate bioceramics. MATEC Web Conf. 7, 04010/1–04010/4.

Charriere, E., Lemaitre, J., Zysset, P., 2003. Hydroxyapatite cement scaffolds with controlled macroporosity: fabrication protocol and mechanical properties. Biomaterials 24 (5), 809–817.

Chen, Q.Z., Thompson, I.D., Boccaccini, A.R., 2006. 45S5 Bioglass®-derived glass-ceramic scaffolds for bone tissue engineering. Biomaterials 27, 2414–2425.

Chen, Q.Z., Mohn, D., Stark, W.J., 2011. Optimization of Bioglass® scaffold fabrication process. J. Am. Ceram. Soc. 94, 4184–4190.

Chevalier, E., Chulia, D., Pouget, C., Viana, M., 2008. Fabrication of porous substrates: a review of processes using pore forming agents in the biomaterial field. J. Pharm. Sci. 97 (3), 1135–1154.

Chevalier, J., 2006. What future for zirconia as a biomaterial? Biomaterials 27, 535–543.

Chevalier, J., Gremillard, L., 2009. Ceramics for medical applications: a picture for the next 20 years. JECS 29, 1245–1255.

Cho, Y.-H., Lee, S.-J., Lee, J.Y., Kim, S.W., Lee, C.B., Lee, W.Y., et al., 2002. Antibacterial effect of intraprostatic zinc injection in a rat model of chronic bacterial prostatis. Int. J. Antimicrob. Agents 19, 576–582.

Cifford, A., Rafferty, A., Hill, R., Mooney, P., Wood, D., Samuneva, B., et al., 2001. The influence of calcium to phosphate ratio on the nucleation and crystallization of apatite glass-ceramics. J. Mater. Sci. Mater. Med. 12, 461–469.

Claussen, N., 1997. Fracture toughness of $Al_2O_3$ with an unstabilized $ZrO_2$ dispersed phase. J. Am. Ceram. Soc. 59, 1–7.

Collins, J.F., Gerby, R.W., 1955. New refractory uses for silicon nitride reported. J. Metals 7, 612–615.

Combes, C., Bareille, R., Rey, C., 2006. Calcium carbonate–calcium phosphate mixed cement compositions for bone reconstruction. J. Biomed. Mater. Res. A. 79 (2), 318–328.

Constantz, B.R., Ison, I.C., Fulmer, M.T., Poser, R.D., Smith, S.T., VanWagoner, M., et al., 1995. Skeletal repair by in situ formation of the mineral phase of bone. Science 267 (5205), 1796–1799.

Cook, W.D., 1983. Dental polyelectrolyte cements. II Effect of powder/liquid ratio on their rheology. Biomaterials 4, 21–24.

Creanor, S.L., Carruthers, L.M., Saunders, W.P., Strang, R., Foye, R.H., 1994. Fluoride uptake and release characteristics of glass ionomer cements. Caries Res. 28, 322–328.

Crisp, S., Wilson, A.D., 1974a. Reactions in glass ionomer cements. III The precipitation reaction. J. Dent. Res. 53, 1420–1424.

Crisp, S., Wilson, A.D., 1974b. Reactions in glass ionomer cements. I Decomposition of the powder. J. Dent. Res. 53, 1408–1413.

Crisp, S., Wilson, A.D., 1976. Reactions in glass ionomer cements. V Effect of incorporating tartaric acid in the cement liquid. J. Dent. Res. 55, 1023–1031.

Crisp, S., Lewis, B.G., Wilson, A.D., 1976. Characterization of glass-ionomer cements 1. Long term hardness and compressive strength. J. Dent. 4 (4), 162–166.

Crisp, S., Lewis, B.G., Wilson, A.D., 1977. Characterization of glass-ionomer cements: 3: Effect of polyacid concentration on the physical properties. J. Dent. Res. 5, 51–56.

Crisp, S., Lewis, B.G., Wilson, A.D., 1980. Characterization of glass-ionomer cements. 6. A study of erosion and water absorption in both neutral and acidic media. J. Dent. Res. 8, 68–74.

Croll, T.P., Nicholson, J.W., 2008. Glass-ionomer cements: history and current status. Inside Dent. 4 (3), 7–14.

Crowley, C.M., Doyle, J., Towler, M.R., Rushe, N., Hampshire, S., 2007. Influence of acid washing on the surface morphology of ionomer glasses and handling properties of glass ionomer cements. J. Mater. Sci. Mater. Med. 18, 1497–1506.

Culbertson, B.M., 2001. Glass-ionomer dental restoratives. Prog. Polym. Sci. 26, 577–604.

Cutler, A.C., Mayhew, R.J., Prettymann, K.M., Virkar, A.V., 1991. High toughness CeTZP/Al2O3 ceramics with improved hardness and strength. J. Am. Ceram. Soc. 74 (1), 179–186.

Daculsi, G., Legeros, R., 2008. 17—Tricalcium Phosphate/Hydroxyapatite Biphasic Ceramics A2—Kokubo, Tadashi, Bioceramics and their Clinical Applications. Woodhead Publishing, Cambridge, pp. 395–423.

Daculsi, G., Menanteau, J., Kerebel, L.M., Mitre, D., 1984. Length and shape of enamel crystals. Calcified Tiss. Int. 36 (5), 550–555.

Daculsi, G., Laboux, O., Malard, O., Weiss, P., 2003. Current state of the art of biphasic calcium phosphate bioceramics. J. Mater. Sci. Mater. Med. 14 (3), 195–200.

Damen, J.J.M., Buijs, M.J., Ten Cate, J.M., 1996. Uptake and release of fluoride by saliva-coated glass ionomer cement. Caries Res. 30 (6), 454–457.

Damien, E., Revell,, P.A., 2004. Coralline hydroxyapatite bone graft substitute: a review of experimental studies and biomedical applications. J. Appl. Biomat. Biomech. 2 (4), 65.

da Silva, R.V., Bertran, C.A., Kawachi, E.Y., Camilli, J.A., 2007. Repair of cranial bone defects with calcium phosphate ceramic implant or autogenous bone graft. J. Cran. Surg. 18 (2), 281–286.

De Barra, E., Hill, R.G., 1998. Influence of alkali metal ions on the fracture properties of glass polyalkenoate (ionomer) cements. Biomaterials 19, 495–502.

De Barra, E., Hill, R.G., 2000. Influence of glass composition on the properties of glass polyalkenoate cements. Part III: Influence of fluorite content. Biomaterials 21, 563–569.

Dehurtevent, M., Robberecht, L., Hornez, J.C., Thuault, A., Devaux, E., Dehin, P., 2017. Stereolithography: a new method for processing dental ceramics by additive computer aided manufacturing. Dent. Mater. <http://dx.doi.org/10.1016/j.dental.2017.01.018>.

Demnati, I., Grossin, D., Errassifi, F., Combes, C., Rey, C., Le Bolay, N., 2014. Synthesis of fluor-hydroxyapatite powder for plasma sprayed biomedical coatings: characterization and improvement of the powder properties. Powder Technol. 255, 23–28.

Demnati, I., Grossin, D., Marsan, O., Bertrand, G., Collonges, G., Combes, C., et al., 2015. Comparison of physical–chemical and mechanical properties of chlorapatite and hydroxyapatite plasma sprayed coatings. Open Biomed. Eng. J. 9, 42–55.

Denry, I., Holloway, J.A., 2010. Ceramics for dental applications: a review. Materials 3, 351–368. Available from: http://dx.doi.org/10.3390/ma3010351.

Descamps, M., Duhoo, T., Monchau, F., Lu, J., Hardouin, P., Hornez, J.C., et al., 2008. Manufacture of macroporous β-tricalcium phosphate bioceramics. J. Eur. Ceram. Soc. 28 (1), 149–157.

Descamps, M., Hornez, J.C., Leriche, A., 2009. Manufacture of hydroxyapatite beads for medical applications. J. Eur. Ceram. Soc. 29 (3), 369–375.

Descamps, M., Boilet, L., Moreau, G., Tricoteaux, A., Lu, J., Leriche, A., et al., 2013. Processing and properties of biphasic calcium phosphates bioceramics obtained by pressureless sintering and hot isostatic pressing. J. Eur. Ceram. Soc. 33 (7), 1263–1270.

Dhondt, C.L., De Maeyer, E.A.P., Verbeeck, R.M.H., 2001. Fluoride release from glass ionomer activated with fluoride solutions. J. Dent. Res. 80 (5), 1402–1406.

Diaz-Arnold, A.M., Holmes, D.C., Wistrom, D.W., Swift, E.J., 1995. Short-term fluoride release/uptake of glass ionomer restoratives. Dent. Mater. 11, 96–101.

Di Mauro, V., Iafisco, M., Salvarani, N., Vacchiano, M., Carullo, P., Ramírez-Rodríguez, G. B., et al., 2016. Bioinspired negatively charged calcium phosphate nanocarriers for cardiac delivery of microRNAs. Nanomedicine 11, 891–906.

Drouet, C., 2013. Apatite formation: why it may not work as planned, and how to conclusively identify apatite compounds. Biomed. Res. Int.12, Article ID 490946.

Drouet, C., 2015. A comprehensive guide to experimental and predicted thermodynamic properties of phosphate apatite minerals in view of applicative purposes. J. Chem. Thermodyn. 81, 143–159.

Drouet, C., Carayon, M.-T., Combes, C., Rey, C., 2008. Surface enrichment of biomimetic apatites with biologically-active ions $Mg2+$ and $Sr2+$: a preamble to the activation of bone repair materials. Mater. Sci. Eng. C. 28 (8), 1544–1550.

Drouet C., J. Gomez-Morales, M. Iafisco, S. Sarda, 2012. Calcium phosphate surface tailoring technologies for drug delivering and tissue engineering. In: Rimondini, L., Bianchi, C.L., Vernè, E. (Eds.), Surface Tailoring of Inorganic Materials for Biomedical Applications, Bentham Science, e-book, pp. 43–111.

Drouet, C., Al-Kattan, A., Choimet, M., Tourrette, A., Santran, V., Dexpert-Ghys, J., et al., 2015. Biomimetic apatite-based functional nanoparticles as promising newcomers in nanomedicine: overview of 10 years of initiatory research. HSOA J. Gen. Pract. Med. Diagn. 1 (1), 1–9.

Duée, C., Desanglois, F., Lebecq, I., Moreau, G., Leriche, A., Follet-Houttemane, C., 2009. Mixture designs applied to glass bioactivity evaluation in the Si–Ca–Na system. J. Non-Cryst. Sol. 355, 943–950.

Eanes, E.D., 1979. Enamel apatite: chemistry, structure and properties. J. Dent. Res. 58 (Spec Issue B), 829–836.

Eichert, D., Drouet, C., Sfihi, H., Rey, C., Combes, C., 2007. Nanocrystalline apatite-based biomaterials: synthesis, processing and characterization. In: Kendall, J.B. (Ed.), Biomaterials Research Advances. Nova Science Publishers, pp. 93–143.

Elliott, J.C., 1994. Structure and Chemistry of the Apatites and Other Calcium Orthophosphates. Elsevier Science, Amsterdam.

Errassif, F., Menbaoui, A., Autefage, H., Benaziz, L., Ouizat, S., Santran, V., et al., 2010. Adsorption on apatitic calcium phosphates: applications to drug delivery. In: Narayan, R., Singh, M., McKittrick, J. (Eds.), Advances in Bioceramics and Biotechnologies. Wiley-VCH Verlag GmbH & Co. KGaA.

Farbod, K., Curci, A., Diba, M., Zinkevich, T., Kentgens, A.P.M., Iafisco, M., et al., 2016. Dual-functionalisation of gelatine nanoparticles with an anticancer platinum(ii)-bisphosphonate complex and mineral-binding alendronate. RSC Adv. 6, 113025–113037.

Fejerskov, O., Kidd, E., 2008. Dental Caries. The Disease and its Clinical Management. second ed. Blackwell Munksgaard, Oxford, p. 8.

Fernandez-Garcia, E., Guillem-Marti, J., Gutierrez-Gonzalez, C.F., Fernandez, A., Ginabra, M.P., Lopez-Esteban, S., 2015. Osteoblastic cell response to spark plasma-sintered zirconia/titanium cermets. J. Biomater. Appl. 29:, 813–823.

Fross, H., Seppa, L., 1990. Prevention of enamel demineralization adjacent to glass ionomer filling materials. Scand. J. Dent. Res. 98 (2), 173–178.

Fujibayashi, S., Neo, M., Kim, H.M., Kokubo, T., Nakamura, T., 2003. A comparative study between in vivo bone ingrowth and in vitro apatite formation on $Na_2O$–$CaO$–$SiO_2$ glasses. Biomaterials 24, 1349–1356.

Garg, N., Garg, A., 2013. Textbook of Operative Dentistry. second ed. Jaypee Brothers Medical Publishers (P) Ltd, New Delhi, p. 428.

Ginebra, M.P., Fernandez, E., De Maeyer, E.A., Verbeeck, R.M., Boltong, M.G., Ginebra, J., et al., 1997. Setting reaction and hardening of an apatitic calcium phosphate cement. J. Dent. Res. 76 (4), 905–912.

Gineste, L., Gineste, M., Ranz, X., Ellefterion, A., Guilhem, A., Rouquet, N., et al., 1999. Degradation of hydroxylapatite, fluorapatite, and fluorhydroxyapatite coatings of dental implants in dogs. J. Biomed. Mater. Res. 48 (3), 224–234.

Gomez-Morales, J., Iafisco, M., Delgado-Lopez, J.M., Sarda, S., Drouet, C., 2013. Progress on the preparation of nanocrystalline apatites and surface characterization: overview of fundamental and applied aspects. Progr. Cryst. Growth Character. Mater. 59 (1), 1–46.

González, P., Serra, J., Liste, S., Chiussi, S., León, B., Pérez-Amor, M., et al., 2003. New biomorphic SiC ceramics coated with bioactive glass for biomedical applications. Biomaterials 24 (26), 4827–4832.

Gonzalez-McQuire, R., Green, D., Walsh, D., Hall, S., Chane-Ching, J.Y., Oreffo, R.O., et al., 2005. Fabrication of hydroxyapatite sponges by dextran sulphate/amino acid templating. Biomaterials 26 (33), 6652–6656.

Goto, K., Shinzato, S., Fujibayashi, S., Tamura, J., Kawanabe, K., Hasegawa, S., et al., 2006. The biocompatibility and osteoconductivity of a cement containing β-TCP for use in vertebroplasty. J. Biomed. Mater. Res. A. 78A (3), 629–637.

Greene, K., Pomeroy, M.J., Hampshire, S., Hill, R.G., 2003. Effect of composition on the properties of glasses in the $K_2O-BaO-MgO-SiO_2-Al_2O_3-B_2O_3-MgF_2$ system. J. Non-Crystall. Solids 325, 193–205.
Griffin, E., Donly, K.J., Erickson, R., 1992. Caries inhibition by fluoride releasing liners. Am. J. Dent. 5, 293–295.
Griffin, S.G., Hill, R.G., 1998. Influence of poly(acrylic acid) molar mass on the fracture properties of glass polyalkenoate cements. J. Mater. Sci. 33, 5383–5396.
Griffin, S.G., Hill, R.G., 2000a. Influence of glass composition on the properties of glass polyalkenoate cements. Part IV: Influence of fluorine content. Biomaterials 21, 693–698.
Griffin, S.G., Hill, R.G., 2000b. Influence of glass composition on the properties of glass polyalkenoate cements. Part II: Influence of phosphate content. Biomaterials 21, 399–403.
Grossin, D., Rollin-Martinet, S., Estournes, C., Rossignol, F., Champion, E., Combes, C., et al., 2010. Biomimetic apatite sintered at very low temperature by spark plasma sintering: physico-chemistry and microstructure aspects. Acta Biomater. 6 (2), 577–585.
Grunenwald, A., Keyser, C., Sautereau, A.M., Crubezy, E., Ludes, B., Drouet, C., 2014. Adsorption of DNA on biomimetic apatites: toward the understanding of the role of bone and tooth mineral on the preservation of ancient DNA. Appl. Surf. Sci. 292, 867–875.
Guazzato M., M. Albakry, M.V. Swain, S.P., 2003. Ringer Microstructure of alumina and alumina/zirconia-glass infiltrated dental ceramics. Bioceramics, 240–242, 875–882.
Guicheux, J., Grimandi, G., Trecant, M., Faivre, A., Takahashi, S., Daculsi, G., 1997. Apatite as carrier for growth hormone: in vitro characterization of loading and release. J. Biomed. Mater. Res. 34 (2), 165–170.
Guida, A., Hill, R.G., Towler, M.R., Eramo, S., 2002. Fluoride release from model glass ionomer cements. J. Mater. Sci. Mater. Med. 13, 645–649.
Hampshire, S., 2016. Silicon nitride ceramics. In: Ohji, T., Singh, M. (Eds.), Engineered Ceramics: Current Status and Future Prospects. John Wiley & Sons, Hoboken, NJ, pp, 79–97. ISBN-978-1-119-10040-9.
Hampshire, S., Pomeroy, M.J., 2012. Grain boundary glasses in silicon nitride: a review of chemistry, properties and crystallisation. J. Eur. Ceram. Soc. 32, 1925–1932.
Hannink, R.J., Kelly, P.M., Muddle, B.C., 2000. Transformation toughening in zirconia containing ceramics. J. Am. Ceram. Soc. 83 (3), 461–487.
Hatton, P.V., Brook, I.M., 1992. Characterisation of the ultrastructure of glass-ionomer (poly-alkenoate) cement. Br. Dent. J. 173, 275–277.
Heimann, R.B., 2006. Thermal spraying of biomaterials. Surf. Coat. Technol. 201 (5), 2012–2019.
Hench, L.L., 1988. Bioactive ceramics. In: Ducheyne, P., Lemons, J. (Eds.), Bioceramics: Materials Characteristics Versus In Vivo Behavior, Vol. 523. Annals of New York Academy of Sciences, New York, NY, p. 54.
Hench, L.L., 1991. Bioceramics: from concept to clinic. J. Am. Ceram. Soc. 74 (7), 1487–1510.
Hench, L.L., 2006. The story of bioglass. J. Mater. Sci. Mater. Med. 17, 967–978.
Hench, L.L., 2011. Bioactive materials for gene control. In: Hench, L.L., Jones, J.R., Fenn, M.B. (Eds.), New Materials and Technologies for Healthcare. World Scientific, Singapore, pp. 25–48.
Hench, L.L., 2013. Chronology of bioactive glass development and clinical applications. New J. Glass Ceram. 3, 67–73.
Hench, L.L., Splinter, R.J., Allen, W.C., Greenlee Jr., T.K., 1971. Bonding mechanisms at the interface of ceramic prosthetic materials. J. Biomed. Mater. Res. 5 (6), 117–141.

Herrera, M., Castillo, A., Bravo, M., Liébana, J., Carrión, P., 2000. Antibacterial activity of resin adhesives, glass ionomer and resin-modified glass ionomer cements and a compomer in contact with dentin caries samples. Oper. Dent. 25 (4), 265–269.

Hill, R.G., Wood, D., 1995. Apatite-mullite glass-ceramics. J. Mater. Sci. Mater. Med. 6, 311–318.

Hill, R.G., Stamboulis, A., Law, R.V., 2006. Characterisation of fluorine containing glasses by 19F, 27Al, 29Si and 31P MAS-NMR spectroscopy. J. Dent. 34, 525–532.

Hirabayashi, H., Fujisaki, J., 2003. Bone-specific drug delivery systems. Clin. Pharmacokinet. 42, 1319–1330.

Hou, C.-h, Chen, C.-w, Hou, S.-m, Li, Y.-t, Lin, F.-h, 2009. The fabrication and characterization of dicalcium phosphate dihydrate-modified magnetic nanoparticles and their performance in hyperthermia processes in vitro. Biomaterials 30, 4700–4707.

Howlett, C.R., McCartney, E., Ching, W., 1989. The effect of silicon nitride ceramic on rabbit skeletal cells and tissue. An in vitro and in vivo investigation. Clin. Orthopaed. Relat. Res. 244, 293–304.

Hren, J.J., Johnson, P.F., Bates, S.R., Hench, L.L., 1976. STEM/EDX analysis of bone–bioglass interface. In: Bailey, G.W. (Ed.), Proceedings of the Electron Microscopy Society of America: 34th Annual Meeting. Claitor's Publishing, Baton Rouge, LA, pp. 290–291.

Hse, K.M.Y., Leung, S.K., Wei, S.H.Y., 1999. Resin-ionomer restorative materials for children: a review. Austr. Dent. J. 44 (1), 1–11.

Huang, J., Bu, L., Xie, J., Chen, K., Cheng, Z., Li, X., et al., 2010. Effects of nanoparticle size on cellular uptake and liver MRI with polyvinylpyrrolidone-coated iron oxide nanoparticles. ACS Nano. 4, 7151–7160.

Hughes, S., McBain, S., Dobson, J., El Haj, A.J., 2008. Selective activation of mechanosensitive ion channels using magnetic particles. J. Royal Soc. Interf. 5, 855–863.

Iafisco, M., Margiotta, N., 2012. Silica xerogels and hydroxyapatite nanocrystals for the local delivery of platinum–bisphosphonate complexes in the treatment of bone tumors: a mini-review. J. Inorgan. Biochem. 117, 237–247.

Iafisco, M., Palazzo, B., Falini, G., Foggia, M.D., Bonora, S., Nicolis, S., et al., 2008. Adsorption and conformational change of myoglobin on biomimetic hydroxyapatite nanocrystals functionalized with alendronate. Langmuir 24, 4924–4930.

Iafisco, M., Palazzo, B., Marchetti, M., Margiotta, N., Ostuni, R., Natile, G., et al., 2009. Smart delivery of antitumoral platinum complexes from biomimetic hydroxyapatite nanocrystals. J. Mater. Chem. 19, 8385–8392.

Iafisco, M., Sabatino, P., Lesci, I.G., Prat, M., Rimondini, L., Roveri, N., 2010. Conformational modifications of serum albumins adsorbed on different kinds of biomimetic hydroxyapatite nanocrystals. Colloids Surf. B Biointerf. 81, 274–284.

Iafisco, M., Foggia, M.D., Bonora, S., Prat, M., Roveri, N., 2011. Adsorption and spectroscopic characterization of lactoferrin on hydroxyapatite nanocrystals. Dalton Transact. 40, 820–827.

Iafisco, M., Varoni, E., Di Foggia, M., Pietronave, S., Fini, M., Roveri, N., et al., 2012a. Conjugation of hydroxyapatite nanocrystals with human immunoglobulin G for nanomedical applications. Colloids Surf. B Biointerf. 90, 1–7.

Iafisco, M., Palazzo, B., Martra, G., Margiotta, N., Piccinonna, S., Natile, G., et al., 2012b. Nanocrystalline carbonate-apatites: role of Ca/P ratio on the upload and release of anticancer platinum bisphosphonates. Nanoscale 4 (1), 206–217.

Iafisco, M., Manuel Delgado-Lopez, J., Varoni, E.M., Tampieri, A., Rimondini, L., Gomez-Morales, J., et al., 2013a. Cell surface receptor targeted biomimetic apatite nanocrystals for cancer therapy. Small 9 (22), 3834–3844.

Iafisco, M., Sandri, M., Panseri, S., Delgado-López, J.M., Gómez-Morales, J., Tampieri, A., 2013b. Magnetic bioactive and biodegradable hollow Fe-doped hydroxyapatite coated poly(L-lactic) acid micro-nanospheres. Chem. Mater. 25, 2610–2617.

Iafisco, M., Drouet, C., Adamiano, A., Pascaud, P., Montesi, M., Panseri, S., et al., 2016. Superparamagnetic iron-doped nanocrystalline apatite as a delivery system for doxorubicin. J. Mater. Chem. B. 4, 57–70.

Itoh, S., Kikuchi, M., Takakuda, K., Koyama, Y., Matsumoto, H.N., Ichinose, S., et al., 2001. The biocompatibility and osteoconductive activity of a novel hydroxyapatite/collagen composite biomaterial, and its function as a carrier of rhBMP-2. J. Biomed. Mater. Res. 54 (3), 445–453.

Itoh, S., Kikuchi, M., Takakuda, K., Nagaoka, K., Koyama, Y., Tanaka, J., et al., 2002. Implantation study of a novel hydroxyapatite/collagen (HAp/col) composite into weight-bearing sites of dogs. J. Biomed. Mater. Res. 63 (5), 507–515.

Jacquart, S., Belime, A., Pigasse, C., Siadous, R., Fatnassi, M., Tadier, S., et al., 2013. Development of an injectable composite for bone regeneration. IRBM. 34 (2), 176–179.

Jarcho, M., 1986. Biomaterial aspects of calcium phosphates. Properties and applications. Dent. Clin. North Am. 30 (1), 25–47.

Jones, J.R., 2013. Review of bioactive glass: From Hench to hybrids. Acta Biomater. 9, 4457–4486.

Kanczler, J.M., Sura, H.S., Magnay, J., Green, D., Oreffo, R.O.C., Dobson, J.P., et al., 2010. Controlled differentiation of human bone marrow stromal cells using magnetic nanoparticle technology. Tissue Eng. A. 16, 3241–3250.

Karageorgiou, V., Kaplan, D., 2005. Porosity of 3D biomaterial scaffolds and osteogenesis. Biomaterials 26 (27), 5474–5491.

Karantakis, P., Helvatjoglou-Antoniades, M., Theodoridou-Pahini, S., Papadogiannis, Y., 2000. Fluoride release from three glass ionomers, a compomer, and a composite resin in water, artificial saliva, and lactic acid. Oper. Dent. 25 (1), 20–25.

Kent, B.E., Lewis, B.G., Wilson, A.D., 1979. Glass ionomer cement formulations: I. The preparation of novel fluoroaluminosilicate glasses high in fluorine. J. Dent. Res. 58, 1607–1619.

Kern, F., 2014. A comparison of microstructure and mechanical properties of 12Ce-TZP reinforced with alumina and in-situ formed strontium or lanthanum hexaaluminate precipitates. J. Eur. Ceram. Soc. 34, 413–423.

Kester, M., Heakal, Y., Fox, T., Sharma, A., Robertson, G.P., Morgan, T.T., et al., 2008. Calcium phosphate nanocomposite particles for in vitro imaging and encapsulated chemotherapeutic drug delivery to cancer cells. Nano Lett. 8, 4116–4121.

Khalil, K.A., Kim, H.Y., Kim, S.W., Kim, K.W., 2007. Observation of toughness improvement of the hydroxyapatite bioceramics densified using high-frequency induction heat sintering. Int. J. Appl. Ceram. Technol. 4 (1), 30–37.

Kievit, F.M., Zhang, M., 2011. Surface engineering of iron oxide nanoparticles for targeted cancer therapy. Accounts Chem. Res. 44, 853–862.

Kikuchi, M., Koyama, Y., Yamada, T., Imamura, Y., Okada, T., Shirahama, N., et al., 2004a. Development of guided bone regeneration membrane composed of beta-tricalcium phosphate and poly (L-lactide-co-glycolide-co-epsilon-caprolactone) composites. Biomaterials 25 (28), 5979–5986.

Kikuchi, M., Ikoma, T., Itoh, S., Matsumoto, H.N., Koyama, Y., Takakuda, K., et al., 2004b. Biomimetic synthesis of bone-like nanocomposites using the self-organization mechanism of hydroxyapatite and collagen. Comp. Sci. Technol. 64 (6), 819–825.

Kim, C.Y., Clark, A.E., Hench, L.L., 1989. Early stages of calcium-phosphate layer formation in bioglass. J. Non-Cryst. Sol. 113 (2-3), 195–202.

Kim, H.W., Knowles, J.C., Kim, H.E., 2005. Porous scaffolds of gelatin–hydroxyapatite nanocomposites obtained by biomimetic approach: characterization and antibiotic drug release. J. Biomed. Mater. Res. B Appl. Biomater. 74 (2), 686–698.

Kim, T.N., Feng, Q.L., Kim, J.O., Wu, J., Wang, H., Chen, G.C., et al., 1998. Antimicrobial effects of metal ions ($Ag^+$, $Cu^{2+}$, $Zn^{2+}$) in hydroxyapatite. J. Mater. Sci. Mater. Med. 9 (3), 129–134.

Kinnunen, I., Aitasalo, K., Pollonen, M., Varpula, M., 2000. Reconstruction of orbital floor fractures using bioactive glass. J. Craniofac. Maxillofac. Surg. 28, 229–234.

Kobayashi, S., Kawai, W., Wakayama, S., 2006. The effect of pressure during sintering on the strength and the fracture toughness of hydroxyapatite ceramics. J. Mater. Sci. Mater. Med. 17 (11), 1089–1093.

Koch, G., Hatibović-Kofman, S., 1990. Glass ionomer cements as a fluoride release system in vivo. Swedish Dent. J. 14 (6), 267–273.

Kokubo, T., 1991. Bioactive glass ceramics: properties and applications. Biomaterials 12 (2), 155–163.

Kokubo, T., Kim, H.-M., Kawashita, M., 2003. Novel bioactive materials with different mechanical properties. Biomaterials 24 (13), 2161–2175.

Kong, L., Gao, Y., Cao, W., Gong, Y., Zhao, N., Zhang, X., 2005. Preparation and characterization of nano-hydroxyapatite/chitosan composite scaffolds. J. Biomed. Mater. Res. A. 75 (2), 275–282.

Koo, H., 2008. Strategies to enhance the biological effects of fluoride on dental biofilms. Adv. Dent. Res. 20, 17–21.

Kotani, H., Kawaguchi, H., Shimoaka, T., Iwasaka, M., Ueno, S., Ozawa, H., et al., 2002. Strong static magnetic field stimulates bone formation to a definite orientation in vitro and in vivo. J. Bone Miner. Res. 17, 1814–1821.

Kue, R., Sohrabi, A., Nagle, D., Frondoza, C., Hungerford, D., 1999. Enhanced proliferation and osteocalcin production by human osteoblast-like MG63 cells on silicon nitride ceramic discs. Biomaterials 20, 1195–1201.

Kuntz, M., Schneider, N., Heros, R., 2005. Controlled zirconia phase transformation in BIOLOX® delta? A feature of safety. Bioceram. Altern. Bear. Jt. Arthroplast. Steinkopff, New York, pp. 79–84.

Kurosawa, H., Aoki, H., Akao, M., 1986. Tissue reactions to calcined bone graft. Biomaterials 7 (2), 132–136.

Lee, S.H., Kim, B.H., Na, H.B., Hyeon, T., 2014. Paramagnetic inorganic nanoparticles as T1MRI contrast agents. Wiley Interdisciplin. Rev. Nanomed. Nanobiotechnol. 6, 196–209.

Lee, S.K., Kim, C.H., 1994. Effects of α-SiC *vs.* β-SiC starting powders on microstructure and fracture toughness of SiC sintered with $Al_2O_3$–$Y_2O_3$ additives. J. Am. Ceram. Soc. 77, 1655–1658.

LeGeros, R.Z., 2008. Calcium phosphate-based osteoinductive materials. Chem. Rev. 108 (11), 4742–4753.

Legros, R., Balmain, N., Bonel, G., 1987. Age-related changes in mineral of rat and bovine cortical bone. Calcified Tissue Int. 41 (3), 137–144.

Li, R., Clark, A.E., Hench, L.L., 1991. An investigation of bioactive glass powders by sol-gel processing. J. Appl. Biomater. 2 (4), 231–239.

Likitvanichkal, S., Lacourse, W.C., 1995. The effect of fluorine content on the crystallisation of canasite, glass-ceramics. J. Mater. Sci. 3 (30), 6151–6155.

Lin, K., Wu, C., Chang, J., 2014. Advances in synthesis of calcium phosphate crystals with controlled size and shape. Acta Biomater. 10, 4071–4102.
Linhart, W., Briem, D., Amling, M., Rueger, J.M., Windolf, J., 2004. Mechanisches Versagen einer porösen Hydroxylapatitkeramik 7,5 Jahre nach Implantation an der proximalen Tibia. Der Unfallchirurg. 107 (2), 154–157.
Liu, D.-M., 1997. Fabrication of hydroxyapatite ceramic with controlled porosity. J. Mater. Sci. Mater. Med. 8 (4), 227–232.
Lu, J.X., Flautre, B., Anselme, K., Hardouin, P., Gallur, A., Descamps, M., et al., 1999. Role of interconnections in porous bioceramics on bone recolonization in vitro and in vivo. J. Mater. Sci. Mater. Med. 10 (2), 111–120.
Macha, I.J., Cazalbou, S., Ben-Nissan, B., Harvey, K.L., Milthorpe, B., 2015. Marine structure derived calcium phosphate–polymer biocomposites for local antibiotic delivery. Mar. Drug. 13 (1), 666–680.
Mahler, Armen, G.K., 1962. Addition of amalgam alloy to zinc phosphate cement. J. Prosthet. Dent. 12, 157–164.
Mahmoudi, M., Hofmann, H., Rothen-Rutishauser, B., Petri-Fink, A., 2012. Assessing the in vitro and in vivo toxicity of superparamagnetic iron oxide nanoparticles. Chem. Rev. 112, 2323–2338.
Maltz, M., Emilson, C.G., 1982. Susceptibility of oral bacteria to various fluoride salts. J. Dent. Res. 61, 786–790.
Mamidwar, S.S., Arena, C., Kelly, S., Alexander, H., Ricci, J., 2007. In vitro characterization of a calcium sulfate/PLLA composite for use as a bone graft material. J. Biomed. Mater. Res. B Appl. Biomater. 81B (1), 57–65.
Mandras, N., Roana, J., Allizond, V., Pasqualini, D., Crosasso, P., Burlando, M., et al., 2013. Antibacterial efficacy and drug-induced tooth discolouration of antibiotic combinations for endodontic regenerative procedures. Int. J. Immunopathol. Pharmacol. 26 (2), 557–563.
Manzano, M., Vallet-Regí, M., 2012. Revisiting bioceramics: bone regenerative and local drug delivery systems. Prog. Solid State Chem. 40, 17–30.
Marie, P.J., Ammann, P., Boivin, G., Rey, C., 2001. Mechanisms of action and therapeutic potential of strontium in bone. Calcif. Tissue Int. 69 (3), 121–129.
Markaki, A.E., Clyne, T.W., 2004. Magneto-mechanical stimulation of bone growth in a bonded array of ferromagnetic fibres. Biomaterials 25, 4805–4815.
Markovic, S., Veselinovic, L., Lukic, M.J., Karanovic, L., Bracko, I., Ignjatovic, N., et al., 2011. Synthetical bone-like and biological hydroxyapatites: a comparative study of crystal structure and morphology. Biomed. Mater. 6 (4), .
Marks, L.A., Verbeeck, R.M., De Maeyer, E.A., Martens, L.C., 2000. Effect of a neutral citrate solution on the fluoride release of resin-modified glass ionomer and polyacid-modified composite resin cements. Biomaterials 21 (19), 2011–2016.
Marquis, R.E., 1995. Antimicrobial actions of fluoride for oral bacteria. Can. J. Microbiol. 41 (11), 955–964.
Marquis, R.E., Clock, S.A., Mota-Meira, M., 2003. Fluoride and organic weak acids as modulators of microbial physiology. FEMS Microbiol. Rev. 26 (5), 493–510.
Masayoshi, Y., 1998. Role of zinc in bone formation and bone resorption. J. Trace Elem. Exp. Med. 11, 119–135.
Massler, M., Berman, D.S., James, V.E., 1957. Pulp capping and pulp amputation. Dent. Clin. North Am. 797.
Mastrogiacomo, M., Scaglione, S., Martinetti, R., Dolcini, L., Beltrame, F., Cancedda, R., et al., 2006. Role of scaffold internal structure on in vivo bone formation in macroporous calcium phosphate bioceramics. Biomaterials 27 (17), 3230–3237.

Mathieu, L.M., Mueller, T.L., Bourban, P.-E., Pioletti, D.P., Müller, R., Månson, J.-A.E., 2006. Architecture and properties of anisotropic polymer composite scaffolds for bone tissue engineering. Biomaterials 27 (6), 905–916.

Matsui, K., Yoshida, H., Ikuhara, Y., 2014. Nanocrystalline, ultra-degradation-resistant zirconia: its grain boundary nanostructure and nanochemistry. Sci. Rep. 4, 4758.

Matsumine, A., Kusuzaki, K., Matsubara, T., Shintani, K., Satonaka, H., Wakabayashi, T., et al., 2007. Novel hyperthermia for metastatic bone tumors with magnetic materials by generating an alternating electromagnetic field. Clin. Exp. Metastasis 24, 191–200.

Matsuno, T., Nakamura, T., Kuremoto, K., Notazawa, S., Nakahara, T., Hashimoto, Y., et al., 2006. Development of beta-tricalcium phosphate/collagen sponge composite for bone regeneration. Dent. Mater. J. 25 (1), 138–144.

Mavropoulos, E., Rossi, A.M., Costa, A.M., Perez, C.A.C., Moreira, J.C., Saldanha, M., 2002. Studies on the mechanisms of lead immobilization by hydroxyapatite. Environ. Sci. Technol. 36, 1625–1629.

Mazzocchi, M., Bellosi, A., 2008. On the possibility of silicon nitride as a ceramic for structural orthopaedic implants. Part I: Processing, microstructure, mechanical properties, cytotoxicity. J. Mater. Sci. Mater. Med. 19, 2881–2887.

Mazzocchi, M., Gardini, D., Traverso, P.L., Faga, M.G., Bellosi, A., 2008. On the possibility of silicon nitride as a ceramic for structural orthopaedic implants. Part II: Chemical stability and wear resistance in body environment. J. Mater. Sci. Mater. Med. 19, 2889–2896.

McEntire, B.J., Bal, B.S., Rahaman, M.N., Chevalier, J., Pezzotti, G., 2015. Ceramics and ceramic coatings in orthopaedics. J. Eur. Ceram. Soc. 35, 4327–4369.

McLean, J.W., Gasser, O., 1985. Glass-cermet cements. Quintessence Int. 16 (5), 333–343.

McLean, J.W., Wilson, A.D., 1977. The clinical development of glass ionomer cements: I Formulations and properties. Austral. Dent. J. 22, 33–36.

McLean, J.W., Wilson, A.D., Prosser, M.J., 1984. Development and use of water-hardening glass ionomer luting cements. J. Prosthet. Dent. 52, 175–181.

Meurice, E., Leriche, A., Hornez, J.-C., Bouchart, F., Rguiti, E., Boilet, L., et al., 2012. Functionalisation of porous hydroxyapatite for bone substitutes. J. Eur. Ceram. Soc. 32 (11), 2673–2678.

Mitra S.B., 1989. Photocurable ionomer cement systems. European Patent Application 0 323 120 A2.

Mitra, S.B., 1991. Adhesion to dentin and physical properties of a light-cured glass-ionomer liner/base. J. Dent. Res. 70 (1), 72–74.

Morgan, T.T., Muddana, H.S., Altinoglu, E.I., Rouse, S.M., Tabakovic, A., Tabouillot, T., et al., 2008. Encapsulation of organic molecules in calcium phosphate nanocomposite particles for intracellular imaging and drug delivery. Nano Lett. 8, 4108–4115.

Moshaverinia, A., Ansari, S., Roohpour, N., Reshad, M., Schricker, S.R., Chee, W.L., 2011. Effects of *N*-vinylcaprolactam containing polyelectrolytes on hardness, fluoride release and water sorption of conventional glass ionomers. J. Prosthet. Dent. 105 (5), 323–331.

Mostaghaci, B., Loretz, B., Lehr, C.M., 2016. Calcium phosphate system for gene delivery: historical background and emerging opportunities. Curr. Pharm. Design. 22, 1529–1533.

Mount, G.J., 2002. An Atlas of Glass-Ionomer Cements: A Clinician's Guide. third ed. Thieme, New York, NY, pp. p1–p6.

Naasan, M.A., Watson, T.F., 1998. Conventional glass-ionomers as posterior restorations: a status report for the American Journal of Dentistry. Am. J. Dent. 11, 36–45.

Nagaraja, P.U., Kishore, G., 2005. Glass-ionomer cement—the different generations. Trends Biomater. Artif. Organs. 18 (2), 158–165.

Nakajo, K., Imazato, S., Takahashi, Y., Kiba, W., Ebisu, S., Takahashi, N., 2009. Fluoride released from glass-ionomer cement is responsible to inhibit the acid production of caries-related oral streptococci. Dent. Mater. 25 (6), 703–708.

Nancollas, G.H., Tang, R., Phipps, R.J., Henneman, Z., Gulde, S., Wu, W., et al., 2006. Novel insights into actions of bisphosphonates on bone: differences in interactions with hydroxyapatite. Bone 38, 617–627.

Nawa, M., Bamba, N., Sekino, T., Niihara, K., 1998. The effect of $TiO_2$ addition on strengthening and toughening in intragranular type of 12Ce-TZP/$Al_2O_3$ nanocomposites. J. Eur. Ceram. Soc. 18, 2–219.

Neuberger, T., Schopf, B., Hofmann, H., Hofmann, M., von Rechenberg, B., 2005. Superparamagnetic nanoparticles for biomedical applications: possibilities and limitations of a new drug delivery system. J. Magn. Magn. Mater. 293, 483–496.

Neumann, A., Reske, T., Held, M., Jahnke, K., Ragoss, C., Maier, H.R., 2004. Comparative investigation of the biocompatibility of various silicon nitride ceramic qualities in vitro. J. Mater. Sci. Mater. Med. 15, 1135–1140.

Neve, A.D., Piddock, V., Combe, E.C., 1992a. Development of novel dental cements. I. Formulation of aluminoborate glasses. Clin. Mater. 9, 7–12.

Neve, A.D., Piddock, V., Combe, E.C., 1992b. Development of novel dental cements. II. Cement properties. Clin. Mater. 9, 13–20.

Neve, D., Piddock, V., Combe, E.C., 1993. The effect of glass heat treatment on the properties of a novel polyalkenoate cement. Clin. Mater. 12, 113–115.

Nicholson, J.W., 1998. Chemistry of glass-ionomer cements: a review. Biomaterials 19, 485–494.

Niihara, K., 1991. New design concept of structural ceramics—ceramic nanocomposites. J. Ceram. Soc. Jpn. 99, 974–982.

Nouri, M.R., Titley, K.C., 2003. Paediatrics: a review of the antibacterial effect of fluoride. Oralhealthgroup 1–7.

Ohura, K., Ikenaga, M., Nakamura, T., Yamamuro, T., Ebisawa, Y., Kokubo, T., et al., 1991. A heat-generating bioactive glass-ceramic for hyperthermia. J. Appl. Biomater. 2, 153–159.

Olofsson, J., Grehk, T.M., Berlind, T., Persson, C., Jacobson, S., Engqvist, H., 2012. Evaluation of silicon nitride as a wear resistant and resorbable alternative for total hip joint replacement. Biomatter. 2 (2), 94–102.

Oonishi, H., Hench, L.L., Wilson, J., Sugihara, F., Tsuji, E., Matsuura, M., 2000. Quantitative comparison of bone growth behavior in granules of Bioglass®, a-W glass-ceramic, and hydroxyapatite. J. Biomed. Mater. Res. 51, 37–46.

Orange, G., Fantozzi, G., Homerin, P., Thevenot, F., Leriche, A., Cambier, F., 1992. Preparation and characterization of a dispersion toughened ceramic for thermomechanical uses (ZTA). Part II: Thermomechanical characterization. Effect of microstructure and temperature on toughening mechanisms. J. Eur. Ceram. Soc. 9, 177–185.

Ouizat, S., Barroug, A., Legrouri, A., Rey, C., 1999. Adsorption of bovine serum albumin on poorly crystalline apatite: influence of maturation. Mater. Res. Bull. 34 (14–15), 2279–2289.

Overgaard, J., 1977. Effect of hyperthermia on malignant cells in vivo: a review and a hypothesis. Cancer 39, 2637–2646.

Palazzo, B., Iafisco, M., Laforgia, M., Margiotta, N., Natile, G., Bianchi, C.L., et al., 2007. Biomimetic hydroxyapatite-drug nanocrystals as potential bone substitutes with antitumor drug delivery properties. Adv. Funct. Mater. 17 (13), 2180–2188.

Palmero, P., Fornabaio, M., Montanaro, L., Reveron, H., Esnouf, C., Chevalier, J., 2015. Towards long lasting zirconia-based composites for dental implants. Part I: Innovative synthesis, microstructural characterization and in vitro stability. Biomaterials 50, 38–46.

Pandey, D., Krishna, P., 1975. Influence of stacking faults on the growth of polytype structures. II. Silicon carbide polytypes. Philosoph. Mag. 31 (5), 1133–1148.

Panseri, S., Cunha, C., D'Alessandro, T., Sandri, M., Russo, A., Giavaresi, G., et al., 2012a. Magnetic hydroxyapatite bone substitutes to enhance tissue regeneration: evaluation in vitro using osteoblast-like cells and in vivo in a bone defect. PLoS ONE. 7, e38710.

Panseri, S., Cunha, C., D'Alessandro, T., Sandri, M., Giavaresi, G., Marcacci, M., et al., 2012b. Intrinsically superparamagnetic Fe-hydroxyapatite nanoparticles positively influence osteoblast-like cell behaviour. J. Nanobiotechnol. 10, 32.

Parr, N.L., Martin, G.F., May, E.R.W., 1960. Preparation, microstructure and mechanical properties of silicon nitride. In: Popper, P. (Ed.), Special Ceramics 1. Heywood, London, pp. 102–135.

Pascaud, P., Errassifi, F., Brouillet, F., Sarda, S., Barroug, A., Legrouri, A., et al., 2014. Adsorption on apatitic calcium phosphates for drug delivery: interaction with bisphosphonate molecules. J. Mater. Sci. Mater. Med. 25 (10), 2373–2381.

Peer, D., Karp, J.M., Hong, S., Farokhzad, O.C., Margalit, R., Langer, R., 2007. Nanocarriers as an emerging platform for cancer therapy. Nat. Nano. 2, 751–760.

Peitl, O., Zanotto, E.D., Hench, L.L., 2001. Highly bioactive $P_2O_5$–$Na_2O$–CaO–$SiO_2$ glass-ceramics. J. Non-Cryst. Solids. 292, 115–126.

Petit F., Lardot, V., Ott, C., Juste, E., Cambier, F., 2015. Ceramic particle mixture and method for manufacturing ceramic parts from such a mixture. US Patent 9,115,034 B2.

Pezzotti, G., McEntire, B.J., Bock, R.M., Boffelli, M., Zhu, W.L., Vitale, E., et al., 2016a. Silicon nitride: a synthetic mineral for vertebrate biology. Sci. Rep. 6, 31717.

Pezzotti, G., Bock, R.M., McEntire, B.J., Jones, E., Boffelli, M., Zhu, W., et al., 2016b. Silicon nitride bioceramics induce chemically driven lysis in *Porphyromonas gingivalis*. Langmuir 32 (12), 3024–3035.

Piconi, C., Maccauro, G., Muratori, F., Brach del Prever, E., 2003. Alumina and zirconia ceramics in joint replacements. J. Appl. Biomater. Biomech. 1, 19–32.

Pires, R.A., Nunes, T.G., Abrahams, I., Hawkes, G.E., 2008. The role of aluminium and silicon in the setting chemistry of glass ionomer cements. J. Mater. Sci. Mater. Med. 19, 1687–1692.

Poologasundarampillai, G., Wang, D., Li, S., Nakamura, J., Bradley, R., Lee, P.D., et al., 2014. Cotton-wool-like bioactive glasses for bone regeneration. Acta Biomater. 10, 3733–3746.

Porter, A.E., Best, S.M., Bonfield, W., 2004. Ultrastructural comparison of hydroxyapatite and silicon-substituted hydroxyapatite for biomedical applications. J. Biomed. Mater. Res. A. 68A (1), 133–141.

Prentice, H.L., Tyas, M.J., Burrow, M.F., 2005. The effect of particle size distribution on an experimental glass-ionomer cement. Dent. Mater. 21, 505–510.

Preston, A.J., Higham, S.M., Agalamanyi, E.A., Mair, L.H., 1999. Fluoride recharge of aesthetic dental materials. J. Oral Rehab. 26, 936–940.

Prosser, H.J., Powis, D.R., Brant, P., Wilson, A.D., 1984. Characterisation of glass ionomer cements 7. The physical properties of current materials. J. Dent. Res. 12, 231–240.

Prosser, H.J., Powis, D.R., Wilson, A.D., 1986. Glass-ionomer cements of improved flexural strength. J. Dent. Res. 65 (2), 146–148.

Qiu, Z.-Y., Noh, I.-S., Zhang, S.-M., 2013. Silicate-doped hydroxyapatite and its promotive effect on bone mineralization. Front. Mater. Sci. 7 (1), 40–50.

Rade, K., Martinčič, A., Novak, S., Kobe, S., 2013. Feasibility study of SiC-ceramics as a potential material for bone implants. J. Mater. Sci. 48, 5295–5301.
Ranzoni, A., Sabatte, G., van Ijzendoorn, L.J., Prins, M.W.J., 2012. One-step homogeneous magnetic nanoparticle immunoassay for biomarker detection directly in blood plasma. ACS Nano. 6, 3134–3141.
Ray, N.H., 1978. Inorganic Polymers. Academic Press, Inc, London, p. 16.
Raynaud, S., Champion, E., Bernache-Assollant, D., Thomas, P., 2002. Calcium phosphate apatites with variable Ca/P atomic ratio I. Synthesis, characterisation and thermal stability of powders. Biomaterials 23 (4), 1065–1072.
Reddy, L.H., Arias, J.L., Nicolas, J., Couvreur, P., 2012. Magnetic nanoparticles: design and characterization, toxicity and biocompatibility, pharmaceutical and biomedical applications. Chem. Rev. 112, 5818–5878.
Reveron, H., Fornabaio, M., Palmero, P., Furderer, T., Adolfsson, E., Lughi, V., et al., 2017. Towards long lasting zirconia-based composites for dental implants: transformation induced plasticity and its consequence on ceramic reliability. Acta Biomater. 48, 423–432.
Rey, C., Shimizu, M., Collins, B., Glimcher, M.J., 1990. Resolution-enhanced Fourier-transform infrared-spectroscopy study of the environment of phosphates ions in the early deposits of a solid-phase of calcium phosphate in bone and enamel and their evolution with age. 1. Investigations in the $V_4$ $PO_4$ domain. Calcified Tissue Int. 46 (6), 384–394.
Rey, C., Combes, C., Drouet, C., Sfihi, H., Barroug, A., 2007. Physico-chemical properties of nanocrystalline apatites: implications for biominerals and biomaterials. Mater. Sci. Eng. C. 27 (2), 198–205.
Rey, C., Combes, C., Drouet, C., et al., 2008. Tricalcium phosphate-based ceramics. In: Kokubo, T. (Ed.), Bioceramics and Their Clinical Applications. CRC/Woodhead, Boca Raton, FL, pp. 326–366.
Rey, C., Combes, C., Drouet, C., Grossin, D., 2011. Bioactive ceramics: physical chemistry. In: Ducheyne, P., Healy, K.E., Hutmacher, D.W., Grainger, D.W., Kirkpatrick, C.J. (Eds.), Comprehensive Biomaterials. Elsevier, pp. 187–221.
Rho, J.-Y., Kuhn-Spearing, L., Zioupos, P., 1998. Mechanical properties and the hierarchical structure of bone. Med. Eng. Phys. 20 (2), 92–102.
Ricci, J.L., Weiner, M.J., Mamidwar, S., Alexander, H., 2008. 14 - Calcium sulphate A2 - Kokubo, Tadashi,. Bioceramics and Their Clinical Applications. Woodhead Publishing, pp. 302–325.
Riley, F.L., 2000. Silicon nitride and related materials. J. Am. Ceram. Soc. 83 (2), 245–265.
Rodríguez-Ruiz, I., Delgado-López, J.M., Durán-Olivencia, M.A., Iafisco, M., Tampieri, A., Colangelo, D., et al., 2013. pH-responsive delivery of doxorubicin from citrate–apatite nanocrystals with tailored carbonate content. Langmuir. 29, 8213–8221.
Rolla, G., Saxegaard, E., 1990. Critical evaluation of the composition and use of topical fluorides with emphasis on the role of calcium fluoride in caries inhibition. J. Dent. Res. 69, 780–785.
Rollin-Martinet, S., Navrotsky, A., Champion, E., Grossin, D., Drouet, C., 2013. Thermodynamic basis for evolution of apatite in calcified tissues. Am. Mineral. 98, 2037–2045.
Rose, R.K., Turner, S.J., 1998. Fluoride-induced enhancement of diffusion in streptococcal model plaque biofilms. Caries Res. 32 (3), 227–232.
Rosenblum, S.F., Frenkel, S., Ricci, J.R., Alexander, H., 1993. Diffusion of fibroblast growth factor from a plaster of Paris carrier. J. Appl. Biomater. 4 (1), 67–72.
Rothwell, M., Anstice, H.M., Pearson, G.J., 1998. The uptake and release of fluoride by ion-leaching cements after exposure to toothpaste. J. Dent. 26, 591–597.

Roveri, N., Palazzo, B., Iafisco, M., 2008. The role of biomimetism in developing nanostructured inorganic matrices for drug delivery. Expert Opin. Drug Deliv. 5, 861–877.

Russo, L., Taraballi, F., Lupo, C., Poveda, A., Jiménez-Barbero, J., Sandri, M., et al., 2014. Carbonate hydroxyapatite functionalization: a comparative study towards (bio)molecules fixation. Interf. Focus. 4, 20130040.

Rust, K.R., Singleton, G.T., Wilson, J., Antonelli, P.J., 1996. Bioglass middle ear prosthesis: long-term results. Am. J. Otolaryngol. 17, 371–374.

Rusu, V.M., Ng, C.-H., Wilke, M., Tiersch, B., Fratzl, P., Peter, M.G., 2005. Size-controlled hydroxyapatite nanoparticles as self-organized organic–inorganic composite materials. Biomaterials. 26 (26), 5414–5426.

Sadat-Shojai, M., Khorasani, M.-T., Dinpanah-Khoshdargi, E., Jamshidi, A., 2013. Synthesis methods for nanosized hydroxyapatite with diverse structures. Acta Biomater. 9, 7591–7621.

Sanginario, V., Ginebra, M.P., Tanner, K.E., Planell, J.A., Ambrosio, L., 2006. Biodegradable and semi-biodegradable composite hydrogels as bone substitutes: morphology and mechanical characterization. J. Mater. Sci. Mater. Med. 17 (5), 447–454.

Sarda, S., Tofighi, A., Hobatho, M.C., Lee, D., Rey, C., 1999. Associations of low temperature apatite ceramics and proteins. Phosphorus Res. Bull. 10, 208–213.

Schierano, G., Pejrone, G., Roana, J., Scalas, D., Allizond, V., Martinasso, G., et al., 2010. A split-mouth study on microbiological profile in clinical healthy teeth and implants related to key inflammatory mediators. Int. J. Immunopathol. Pharmacol. 23 (1), 279–288.

Sepulveda, P., Jones, J.R., Hench, L.L., 2002. Bioactive sol-gel foams for tissue repair. J. Biomed. Mater. Res. 59 (2), 340–348.

Sequeira, S., Fernandes, M.H., Neves, N., Almeida, M.M., 2017. Development and characterization of zirconia–alumina composites for orthopedic implants. Ceram. Int. 43, 693–703.

Singh, R.K., Srinivasan, A., 2011. Magnetic properties of bioactive glass-ceramics containing nanocrystalline zinc ferrite. J. Magn. Magn. Mater. 323, 330–333.

Sopyan, I., Mel, M., Ramesh, S., Khalid, K.A., 2007. Porous hydroxyapatite for artificial bone applications. Sci. Technol. Adv. Mater. 8 (1–2), 116–123.

Sorrell, C.C., Hardcastle, P.H., Druitt, R.K., Howlett, C.R., McCartney, E., 2004. Results of 15-year clinical study of reaction-bonded silicon nitride intervertebral spacers. Proc. 7th World Biomater. Cong. 7, 1872.

Stamboulis, A., Matsuya, S., Hill, R.G., Law, R.V., Udoh, K., Nakagawa, M., et al., 2006. MAS-NMR spectroscopy studies in the setting reaction of glass ionomer cements. J. Dent. 34 (8), 574–581.

Stanić, V., Dimitrijević, S., Antić-Stanković, J., Mitrić, M., Jokić, B., Plećaš, I.B., et al., 2010. Synthesis, characterization and antimicrobial activity of copper and zinc-doped hydroxyapatite nanopowders. Appl. Surf. Sci. 256 (20), 6083–6089.

Stanley, H.R., Hall, M.B., Clark, A.E., King, C.J., Hench, L.L., Berte, J.J., 1997. Using 45S5 bioglass cones as endosseous ridge maintenance implants to prevent alveolar ridge resorption: a 5-year evaluation. Int. J. Oral Maxillofac. Implant. 12, 95–105.

Stigter, M., Bezemer, J., de Groot, K., Layrolle, P., 2004. Incorporation of different antibiotics into carbonated hydroxyapatite coatings on titanium implants, release and antibiotic efficacy. J. Contr. Release. 99, 127–137.

Suchanek, W., Yoshimura, M., 1998. Processing and properties of hydroxyapatite-based biomaterials for use as hard tissue replacement implants. J. Mater. Res. 13 (1), 94–117.

Sullivan, A., Hill, R.G., 2000. Influence of poly(acrylic acid) molar mass on the fracture properties of glass polyalkenoate cements based on waste gasifier slags. J. Mater. Sci. 35, 1125–1134.

Sun, E.Y., Becher, P.F., Plucknett, K.P., Hsueh, C.-H., Alexander, K.B., Waters, S.B., et al., 1998. Microstructural design of silicon nitride with improved fracture toughness: II. Effects of yttria and alumina additives. J. Am. Ceram. Soc. 81 (11), 2831–2840.

Sun, L., Berndt, C.C., Gross, K.A., Kucuk, A., 2001. Material fundamentals and clinical performance of plasma-sprayed hydroxyapatite coatings: a review. J. Biomed. Mater. Res. 58 (5), 570–592.

Svanberg, M., Krasse, B., Ornerfeldt, H.O., 1990a. Mutans streptococci in interproximal plaque from amalgam and glass ionomer restorations. Caries Res. 24 (2), 133–136.

Svanberg, M., Mjör, I.A., Ørstavik, D., 1990b. Mutans streptococci in plaque from margins of amalgam, composite, and glass-ionomer restorations. J. Dent. Res. 69 (3), 861–864.

Tabaković, A., Kester, M., Adair, J.H., 2012. Calcium phosphate-based composite nanoparticles in bioimaging and therapeutic delivery applications. Wiley Interdisc. Rev. Nanomed. Nanobiotechnol. 4, 96–112.

Tabata, M., Shimoda, T., Sugihara, K., Ogomi, D., Serizawa, T., Akashi, M., 2003. Osteoconductive and hemostatic properties of apatite formed on/in agarose gel as a bone-grafting material. J. Biomed. Mater. Res. B Appl. Biomater. 67B (2), 680–688.

Tadic, D., Beckmann, F., Schwarz, K., Epple, M., 2004. A novel method to produce hydroxyapatite objects with interconnecting porosity that avoids sintering. Biomaterials 25 (16), 3335–3340.

Tampieri, A., Celotti, G., Landi, E., Sandri, M., Roveri, N., Falini, G., 2003. Biologically inspired synthesis of bone-like composite: self-assembled collagen fibers/hydroxyapatite nanocrystals. J. Biomed. Mater. Res. A. 67 (2), 618–625.

Tampieri, A., D'Alessandro, T., Sandri, M., Sprio, S., Landi, E., Bertinetti, L., et al., 2012. Intrinsic magnetism and hyperthermia in bioactive Fe-doped hydroxyapatite. Acta Biomater. 8, 843–851.

Tancret, F., Bouler, J.M., Chamousset, J., Minois, L.M., 2006. Modelling the mechanical properties of microporous and macroporous biphasic calcium phosphate bioceramics. J. Eur. Ceram. Soc. 26 (16), 3647–3656.

Taylor, R.M., Bernero, J.P., Patel, A.A., Brodke, D.S., Khandkar, A.C., 2010. Silicon nitride—a new material for spinal implants. J. Bone Jt. Surg. Br. 92 (Suppl. 1), 133.

Thomas, M.V., Puleo, D.A., 2009. Calcium sulfate: properties and clinical applications. J. Biomed. Mater. Res. B Appl. Biomater. 88B (2), 597–610.

Thompson, I.D., 2011. Clinical applications of bioactive glasses for maxillofacial repair. In: Hench, L.L., Fenn, M.B., Jones, J.R. (Eds.), New Materials and Technologies for Healthcare. World Scientific, Singapore, pp. 77–96.

Thuault, A., Savary, E., Hornez, J.C., Moreau, G., Descamps, M., Marinel, S., et al., 2014. Improvement of the hydroxyapatite mechanical properties by direct microwave sintering in single mode cavity. J. Eur. Ceram. Soc. 34 (7), 1865–1871.

Trombe, J.C., Montel, G., 1978. Some features of the incorporation of oxygen in different oxidation states in the apatitic lattice—I On the existence of calcium and strontium oxyapatites. J. Inorgan. Nucl. Chem. 40 (1), 15–21.

Uskoković, V., Uskoković, D.P., 2011. Nanosized hydroxyapatite and other calcium phosphates: chemistry of formation and application as drug and gene delivery agents. J. Biomed. Mater. Res. B Appl. Biomater. 96B, 152–191.

Vallet-Regí, M., Gordo, M., Ragel, C.V., Cabañas, M.Y., Román, J.S., 1997. Synthesis of ceramic–polymer–drug biocomposites at room temperature. Solid State Ionics. 101, 887–892.

Vallet-Regí, M., Balas, F., Arcos, D., 2007. Mesoporous materials for drug delivery. Angewandte Chem. Int. Ed. 46, 7548–7558.

Van Den Vreken, N.M., Pieters, I.Y., De Maeyer, E.A., Jackers, G.J., Schacht, E.H., Verbeeck, R.M., 2006. Apatite formation in composites of alpha-TCP and degradable polyesters. J. Biomater. Sci. Polym. Ed. 17 (9), 953–967.

Vandecandelaere, N., Rey, C., Drouet, C., 2012. Biomimetic apatite-based biomaterials: on the critical impact of synthesis and post-synthesis parameters. J. Mater. Sci. Mater. Med. 23 (11), 2593–2606.

Verbeeck, R.M., De Maeyer, E.A., Marks, L.A., De Moor, R.J., De Witte, A.M., Trimpeneers, L.M., 1998. Fluoride release process of (resin-modified) glass-ionomer cements versus (polyacid-modified) composite resins. Biomaterials 19 (6), 509–519.

Victor, S.P., Paul, W., Jayabalan, M., Sharma, C.P., 2014. Supramolecular hydroxyapatite complexes as theranostic near-infrared luminescent drug carriers. Cryst. Eng. Comm. 16, 9033–9042.

Wall, F.T., Drenan, S.W., 1951. Gelation of polyacrylic acid by divalent cations. J. Polym. Sci. 1 (7), 83–90.

Walls, A.W.G., 1986. Glass polyalkenoate (glass-ionomer) cements: a review. J. Dent. 14, 231–246.

Walsh, D., Tanaka, J., 2001. Preparation of a bone-like apatite foam cement. J. Mater. Sci. Mater. Med. 12 (4), 339–343.

Walsh, D., Boanini, E., Tanaka, J., Mann, S., 2005. Synthesis of tri-calcium phosphate sponges by interfacial deposition and thermal transformation of self-supporting calcium phosphate films. J. Mater. Chem. 15 (10), 1043–1048.

Wasson, E.A., Nicholson, J.W., 1991. Studies on the setting chemistry of glass-ionomer cements. Clin. Mater. 7 (4), 289–293.

Wasson, E.A., Nicholson, J.W., 1993. New aspects of the setting chemistry of glass-ionomer cements. J. Dent. Res. 72, 481–483.

Weber, C.G., Mueller, M., Vandecandelaere, N., Trick, I., Burger-Kentischer, A., Maucher, T., et al., 2014. Enzyme-functionalized biomimetic apatites: concept and perspectives in view of innovative medical approaches. J. Mater. Sci. Mater. Med. 25 (3), 595–606.

Welzel, T., Radtke, I., Meyer-Zaika, W., Heumann, R., Epple, M., 2004. Transfection of cells with custom-made calcium phosphate nanoparticles coated with DNA. J. Mater. Chem. 14 (14), 2213–2217.

Wiegand, A., Buchalla, W., Attin, T., 2007. Review on fluoride-releasing restorative materials—fluoride release and uptake characteristics, antibacterial activity and influence on caries formation. Dent. Mater. 23, 343–362.

Wilhelm, C., Gazeau, F., 2008. Universal cell labelling with anionic magnetic nanoparticles. Biomaterials 29, 3161–3174.

Williams, J.A., Billington, R.W., Pearson, G.J., 2001. A long study of fluoride release from metal-containing conventional and resin-modified glass-ionomer cements. J. Oral Rehab. 28, 41–47.

Williams, J.A., Briggs, E., Billington, R.W., Pearson, G.J., 2003. The effects of adding fluoride compounds to a fluoride-free glass ionomer cement on subsequent fluoride and sodium release. Biomaterials 24, 1301–1308.

Willmann, G., 2000. Ceramic femoral head retrieval data. Clin. Orthoped. Relat. Res. 379, 22–28.

Wilson, A.D., Kent, B.E., 1970. Dental cements: dental silicate cements IX. Decomposition of the powder. J. Dent. Res. 49, 7–13.

Wilson, A.D., Kent, B.E., 1971. The glass-ionomer cement, a new translucent dental filling material. J. Appl. Chem. Biotechnol. 21 (11), 13.

Wilson, A.D., Kent, B.E., 1972. A new translucent cement for dentistry: the glass-ionomer cement. Br. Dent. J. 132 (4), 133–135.

Wilson, A.D., Mclean, J.W., 1988. Glass-Ionomer Cement. Quintessence, Chicago, IL, pp. 43–55.

Wilson, A.D., Crisp, S., Ferner, A.J., 1976. Reactions in glass ionomer cements, IV Effect of chelating comonomers on setting behaviour. J. Dent. Res. 55, 489–495.

Wilson, D., Crisp, S., Prosser, H.J., Lewis, B.G., Merson, S.A., 1980. Aluminosilicate glasses for polyelectrolyte cements. Ind. Eng. Chem. Prod. Res. Dev. 19, 263–270.

Wilson, J., Pigott, G.H., Schoen, F.J., Hench, L.L., 1981. Toxicology and biocompatibility of bioglass. J. Biomed. Mater. Res. 15 (6), 805–817.

Winand, L., 1961. Ann Chim (Paris), 13th series 6, pp. 951–967.

Wood, D., Hill, R.G., 1990. Glass ceramic approach to controlling the properties of a glass-ionomer bone cement. Biomaterials 12, 164–170.

Xie, Y., Chen, Y., Sun, M.J., Ping, Q.N., 2013. A mini review of biodegradable calcium phosphate nanoparticles for gene delivery. Curr. Pharm. Biotechnol. 14, 918–925.

Xu, C., Sun, S., 2013. New forms of superparamagnetic nanoparticles for biomedical applications. Adv. Drug. Deliver. Rev. 65, 732–743.

Xu, C.Y., Zheng, Y.Y., Gao, W., Xu, J.S., Zuo, G.Q., Chen, Y., et al., 2015. Magnetic hyperthermia ablation of tumors using injectable $Fe_3O_4$/calcium phosphate cement. ACS Appl. Mater. Interf. 7, 13866–13875.

Xu, H.-Y., Gu, N., 2014. Magnetic responsive scaffolds and magnetic fields in bone repair and regeneration. Front. Mater. Sci. 8, 20–31.

Yamada, S., Heymann, D., Bouler, J.M., Daculsi, G., 1997. Osteoclastic resorption of calcium phosphate ceramics with different hydroxyapatite/β-tricalcium phosphate ratios. Biomaterials 18 (15), 1037–1041.

Yang, L., Ning, X., Xiao, Q., Chen, K., Zhou, H., 2007. Development and characterization of porous silver-incorporated hydroxyapatite ceramic for separation and elimination of microorganisms. J. Biomed. Mater. Res. B Appl. Biomater. 81 (1), 50–56.

Yao, W., Wen, J., Xiantao, W., Bin, H., Xiaobo, Z., Gang, W., et al., 2010. A novel calcium phosphate ceramic–magnetic nanoparticle composite as a potential bone substitute. Biomed. Mater. 5, 015001.

Zanotto, E.D., 2010. A bright future for glass-ceramics. Bull. Am. Ceram. Soc. 89 (8), 19–27.

Zhang, F., Chevalier, J., Olagnon, C., Van Meerbeek, B., Vleugels, J., 2017. Slow crack growth and hydrothermal aging stability of an alumina-toughened zirconia composite made from $La_2O_3$-doped 2Y-TZP. J. Eur. Ceram. Soc. 37, 1865–1871.

Zhang, Y., Zhang, M., 2001. Synthesis and characterization of macroporous chitosan/calcium phosphate composite scaffolds for tissue engineering. J. Biomed. Mater. Res. 55 (3), 304–312.

Zhao, X., Kim, J., Cezar, C.A., Huebsch, N., Lee, K., Bouhadir, K., et al., 2011. Active scaffolds for on-demand drug and cell delivery. Proc. Natl. Acad. Sci. 108, 67–72.

## Further reading

Ventura, M., Sun, Y., Cremers, S., Borm, P., Birgani, Z.T., Habibovic, P., et al., 2014. A theranostic agent to enhance osteogenic and magnetic resonance imaging properties of calcium phosphate cements. Biomaterials 35, 2227–2233.

Singh, A., Sahoo, S.K., 2014. Magnetic nanoparticles: a novel platform for cancer theranostics. Drug Discov. Today 19, 474–481.

# Assessment of mechanical properties of ceramic materials

**3**

*Marc Anglada*
Universitat Politècnica de Catalunya, Barcelona, Spain

**Chapter Outline**

**3.1 Introduction to mechanical properties 83**
3.1.1 Bioceramics 83
3.1.2 Fracture of ceramics 84
3.1.3 Weibull statistics of the strength 85
3.1.4 Subcritical crack growth 88
3.1.5 $K_{IC}$ and curve *R*-behavior of ceramics 90
3.1.6 Mechanisms of increase in fracture toughness 90
**3.2 Bioactive glasses and glass ceramics 93**
**3.3 Calcium phosphates (CaP) and CaP composites 95**
**3.4 Calcium phosphate cements 100**
**3.5 Structural bioinert ceramics 102**
**3.6 Conclusions 105**
**References 106**
**Further reading 109**

## 3.1 Introduction to mechanical properties

### 3.1.1 Bioceramics

Bone is a natural composite, mainly composed of inorganic bone mineral and organic collagen matrix and it has a complex hierarchical structure on different scales. It performs many different functions in the body. One of them is structural, such that the microstructure and corresponding mechanical properties of the bone have changed through human evolution for optimizing this function. The mineral constituent is about 0.45 volume fraction of the bone and is formed of calcium phosphates similar to synthetic hydroxyapatite (HA) which has a stoichiometric chemical formula of $Ca_{10}(PO_4)_6(OH)_2$ and a Ca:P ratio of 1.67 (Hench, 1998).

Bioceramics are used for bone substitution in case of disease, for making medical devices like femoral heads and acetabular cups for total hip replacement, dental implants and restorations, as well as bone fillers and scaffolds for tissue engineering. They are commonly divided in two different types according to their interaction with the body of the host. Bioactive ceramics are those that chemically bond with bone or tissue of the host, while bioinert ceramics retain their structure after implantation and do not induce an immunologic response in the host. In spite of the

**Advances in Ceramic Biomaterials.**
**DOI: http://dx.doi.org/10.1016/B978-0-08-100881-2.00003-8**

different level of mechanical properties of bioinert and bioactive ceramics, all of them suffer from fragility to a higher or lower degree.

Most inert bioceramics are based on alumina, zirconia doped with yttria or ceria, and composites of alumina–zirconia. On the other hand, bioactive ceramics are based on calcium phosphates, glass, glass ceramics, bioactive organic–inorganic hybrids, and bioactive composites. Bioactive ceramics are considered in the field of tissue engineering, although the translation of engineering tissues to clinical applications has been limited. Bone tissue engineering aims to develop alternatives to allogenic and autologous bone grafts in order to address the needs of an increasingly older population. Scaffolds can be used to repair defects guiding bone regeneration or be combined with cells which are added to enhance bone regeneration. Basic characteristics of bone scaffolds are biocompatibility, osteoconductivity and interconnected porosity, biodegradability, permeability, and mechanical integrity. Regarding this last property, from the beginning of implantation through complete healing, the target mechanical properties that should be achieved are not usually established. As referred to in a recent review on calcium phosphates (Wagoner Johnson and Herschler, 2011), the target properties, such as strength and elastic modulus, that have been explicitly stated or implied in the literature, span several orders of magnitude and several different approaches have been taken with regard to the design for mechanical properties. Nevertheless, as is well known in the structural engineering ceramics community, the key limiting factor for ceramics in load-bearing applications lies in the inherent brittleness of this class of materials. In spite of that, there are few studies in the literature on bioactive ceramics where properties associated with the brittleness, such as fracture toughness, reliability (i.e., Weibull modulus), or energy to failure, are reported (Wagoner Johnson and Herschler, 2011).

### 3.1.2 Fracture of ceramics

Ceramic materials fail by brittle fracture that originates at flaws, which can be generated during processing or in service. They are of different sizes and shapes and are distributed all through the material. Elastic fracture mechanics can be used to predict the strength if flaws are considered as very sharp cracks embedded in an elastic continuous. Cracks can propagate if the elastic energy released when they extend is larger than the energy necessary to create the new crack surfaces. The reader is referred to Lawn (1993) for background elastic fracture mechanics focused on ceramic materials.

The condition for fracture under a tensile stress acting perpendicular to the crack surface, i.e., in mode $I$, can be also established in terms of the stress intensity factor, $K_I$, crack length $a$, and the fracture toughness of the material, $K_{Ic}$. $K_I$ describes the elastic stress field very near the crack tip and it depends on the tensile stress, $\sigma$, the crack length, and the geometry of the specimen. Very often it can be written in a simple form, such as:

$$K_I = \sigma Y \sqrt{\pi a} \tag{3.1}$$

In this expression, $Y$ is a geometrical factor which accounts for the loading mode, the geometry of the crack and of the specimen. Processing flaws in ceramic materials are generally very small in comparison to specimen dimensions, so that in this case $Y$ may be independent of the crack length. This is the case for a bulk small penny crack loaded in the direction perpendicular to the crack surface, where $Y$ is equal to $2/\pi$ all along the crack front. $K_{Ic}$ represents the critical value of $K_I$ for which fracture occurs and it is in principle a material property. Therefore the fracture strength, $\sigma_S$, can be written as:

$$\sigma_S = \frac{K_{Ic}}{Y\sqrt{\pi a}} \tag{3.2}$$

This expression indicates that the fracture strength depends linearly on $K_{Ic}$ and is inversely proportional to the square root of the crack length. It shows two possible strategies to increase the strength of ceramic materials, namely, increase the fracture toughness or decrease the defect size. From Eq. (3.2) it can be seen that the smallest strengths are associated with the largest flaws.

Although specimens often contain many defects of different sizes, the strength will be determined by the larger crack size. On the other hand, if we know the strength of a specimen we can determine the minimum crack length or critical crack size for fracture. From Eq. (3.2) we obtain:

$$a_c = \frac{K_{Ic}^2}{\pi Y^2 \sigma_S^2} \tag{3.3}$$

In elastic fracture mechanics the strain energy rate energy, $G$, is the energy available for unit of area of crack extension. Under plane strain in mode $I$ it is given by:

$$G_I = \frac{K_I^2}{E}\left(1 - \nu^2\right) \tag{3.4}$$

where $E$ is the Young's modulus and $\nu$ is the Poisson coefficient (see, e.g., Anderson, 1995). Crack extension takes place when $G$ reaches a critical value, $G_{Ic}$, which is the critical value for creating the unit surface of crack area. This is then related to the fracture toughness, $K_{Ic}$, by the above Eq. (3.4) when fracture occurs:

$$G_{IC} = \frac{K_{Ic}^2\left(1 - \nu^2\right)}{E} \tag{3.5}$$

The units of $G_I$ are energy per unit of area and are often expressed in kJ/m$^2$ while the units of $K_I$ are stress per square root of length and are often given in terms of MPa$\sqrt{\text{m}}$.

### 3.1.3 Weibull statistics of the strength

If we measure the strength of a large number of specimens, the result will be a distribution of the strength according to the distribution of the largest flaw present in each specimen. The Weibull distribution is usually considered the best choice for fracture strength analysis. His fundamental assumption is the weakest link hypothesis, i.e., the specimen fails if its weakest volume element fails. In its simplest form, for a uniaxial homogenous tensile stress $\sigma$ and volume $V$, the Weibull cumulative probability function can be written as (see, e.g., Danzer et al., 2008):

$$P_f = 1 - \exp\left[ -\frac{V}{V_0}\left(\frac{\sigma - \sigma_u}{\sigma_\theta}\right)^m \right] \tag{3.6}$$

This is known as the Weibull three-parameter strength distribution. The threshold stress parameter, $\sigma_u$, represents a minimum stress below which a test specimen will not break. Eq. (3.6) is reduced to the Weibull two-parameter strength distribution if $\sigma_u = 0$. The scale parameter or characteristic strength, $\sigma_\theta$, is dependent on the stress configuration and test specimen size. The distribution shape parameter, $m$, is the Weibull modulus and $V_0$ is the chosen normalizing volume. Generally, approximately 30 test specimens provide adequate Weibull strength distribution parameters, with more test specimens contributing little towards better uncertainty estimates (Quinn and Quinn, 2010). The coefficient of variation $C_V$ is a dimensionless measure of the dispersion of the data and is defined as the ratio of the standard deviation, $s$, and the average strength, $\overline{\sigma}$. It can be shown that it depends only on $m$ and an approximate form which is accurate to a few percent for $m \gtrsim 15$, as given by (Wachtman et al., 2009):

$$C_V = \frac{s}{\overline{\sigma}} \approx \frac{1.28}{m} \tag{3.7}$$

The Weibull modulus can be obtained by fitting with a straight line a plot of $\ln(\ln(1/(1 - P_f))$ versus $\ln\sigma_f$. Such plots are displayed in Fig. 3.1 for the strength of 3Y-TZP after aging, where it can be noticed that the increase in the slope with aging (higher $m$) does not necessarily imply an increase in $\overline{\sigma}$. The Weibull modulus is a measure for the scatter of strength data so that high values of $m$ mean low scatter in the strength.

Tension tests are rarely used in ceramics and glasses because of several important disadvantages in comparison with flexural tests, among them the high cost of specimen fabrication and the difficulty in gripping without introducing bending stresses and damaging contact stresses. Flexural tests on rectangular specimens involving three- and four-point bending are often used. Today the most common testing configuration in advanced ceramic materials is a 3-mm by 4-mm cross-section rectangular specimen on 20-mm by 40-mm span four-point flexure fixtures. Standard procedures are available for advanced technical and advanced ceramics (ENV-843-1 and ENV-843-5).

When testing specimen configurations in which the stress is not uniform, the substitution of the actual stressed volume of the specimen by the Weibull effective volume in Eq. (3.6) allows us to still use this equation. The equivalent volume represents the volume that is subjected to a uniform stress equal to the maximum

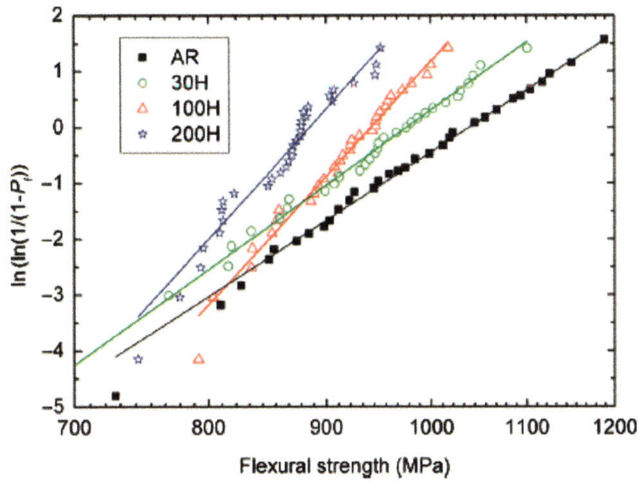


**Figure 3.1** Weibull representation of the strength data for 3Y-TZP rod specimens in four-point bending (diameter 8 mm, span 60 mm, and internal span 30 mm); before (AR) and after hydrothermal degradation in autoclave at 134°C for 30, 100, and 200 h (Marro et al., 2014).

stress in the actual specimen will give the same probability of failure. This allows the strength to be scaled from one loading configuration and specimen size to another. If the mean strength and the volume of specimens of type 1 are $\overline{\sigma}_1$ and $V_1$, and those of type 2 are $\overline{\sigma}_2$ and $V_2$, respectively, it can be shown that the ratio between average mean strengths is given by (see, e.g., Danzer et al., 2008):

$$\frac{\overline{\sigma}_1}{\overline{\sigma}_2} = \left(\frac{\overline{V}_2}{\overline{V}_1}\right)^{1/m} \tag{3.8}$$

where $\overline{V}_1$ and $\overline{V}_2$ are the effective volumes of specimens of types 1 and 2, respectively. Eq. (3.8) allows us to analyze the influence of volume and stress distribution on the strength. Thus, for the flexural strength of rectangular specimens of identical transversal dimensions subjected to the three-point bending (with external span $L_3$) and to four-point bending (with external and internal spans $L_4$ and $L_{4/2}$, respectively) the ratio of average strengths can be calculated with Eq. (3.8) (Quinn and Quinn, 2010):

$$\frac{\overline{\sigma}_3}{\overline{\sigma}_4} = \left(\frac{L_4}{L_3}\right)^{1/m}\left(\frac{m+2}{2}\right)^{1/m} \tag{3.9}$$

For example, if $m = 10$, and $L_4 = 10L_3$, $\overline{\sigma}_3$ is about 50% higher than $\overline{\sigma}_4$. As there is now a tendency to test miniature specimens, the influence of loading configuration and specimen size can convey significant higher values of strength than big macroscopic specimens used in conventional testing. This has to be taken especially into account when measuring the strength of bioceramics since testing of miniature specimens is often necessary because the amount of material available is limited and often $m$ is relatively small. Of course, if $m$ becomes very large, the difference becomes negligible, i.e., $\overline{\sigma}_3 \sim \overline{\sigma}_4$.

### 3.1.4 Subcritical crack growth

Ceramics can sustain static or cyclic loads without breaking immediately but they might fail after some time in service. This delayed fracture at room temperature is caused by subcritical crack growth (SCCG) as well as by cyclic fatigue. The crack velocity, $v$, in the range of low crack velocities of engineering interest, namely the range between $10^{-13}$ and $10^{-6}$ m/s, which is referred to as region $I$, can often be written in terms of the stress intensity factor, $K$, by using a power law (Munz and Fett, 1998; Danzer et al., 2008):

$$v = v_0 \left( \frac{K}{K_c} \right)^n \tag{3.10}$$

where $v_0$ and $n$ are constants. Fig. 3.2 shows SCCG for alumina where it can be seen that Eq. (3.10) is obeyed with an exponent equal to 33. There is also a threshold of $K$, $K_{th}$, below which SCCG does not occur. The value of $n$ is usually in the range 10–100 and $K_{th}$ may be around half the fracture toughness. Very often static or constant stress rate tests to fracture are used to study SCCG.

In constant stress tests the time to failure is measured, i.e., the time for incubation of an initial crack of length $a_i$ and its propagation to a critical length $a_f$ when failure takes place. If, for simplicity, it is assumed that: (1) the tensile stress in the specimen is uniform, (2) $K$ is given by Eq. (3.1) with $Y$ = constant, (3) the incubation time is negligible, and (4) $n$ is much larger than 1, then from integration of Eq. (3.10) we obtain the time of failure, $t_f$, in terms of the initial crack length and the applied stress, $\sigma_{stat}$, (Danzer et al., 2008).

$$t_f \propto a_i^{-(n-2)/2} \sigma_{stat}^{-n} \tag{3.11}$$

As $n$ is usually large, small changes in the stress and in the initial crack size induce very large changes in the time of failure under a static stress.

SCCG may also occur during loading in a strength test, so that the strength of ceramics and glasses will also depend on the loading rate. For a test under constant stress rate, $\dot{\sigma}$, the strength can be derived from Eqs. (3.1) and (3.10) and it can be written as (Wachtman et al., 2009; Munz and Fett, 1998):

$$\sigma_f \propto \dot{\sigma}^{1/(n+1)} \tag{3.12}$$

As can be seen in Fig. 3.3 for alumina the effect of stress rate is important at low stress rates while at very high stress rates the effect is negligible (Lathabai and Lawn, 1989).

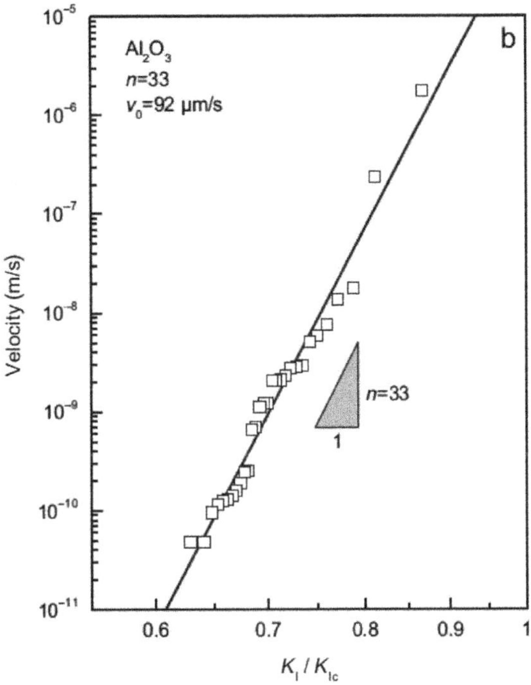


**Figure 3.2** Crack growth rate versus normalized stress intensity factor for alumina (Baierl, 1999).
Reproduced from Danzer, R., Lube, T., Supancic, P., Damani, R., 2008. Fracture of ceramics. Adv. Eng. Mater. 10(4), 275–298.

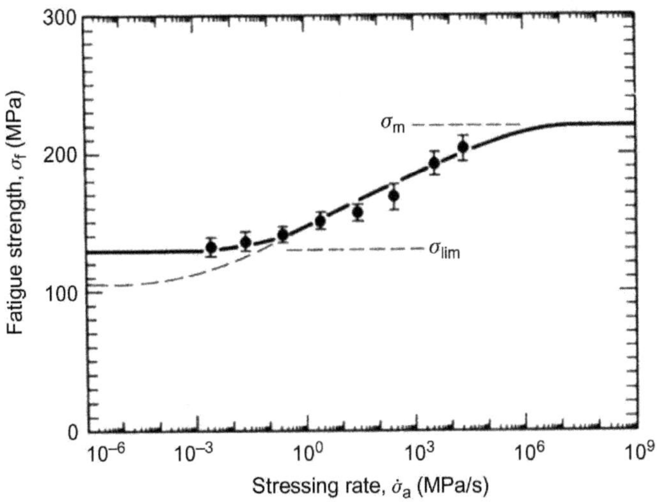


**Figure 3.3** Mean strength (fatigue strength) of alumina versus stress rate in water for constant stress rate bending tests in Vickers preindented specimens with a load of 30 N. $\sigma_m$ is the inert strength and $\sigma_{lim}$ corresponds to the fatigue threshold (Lathabai and Lawn, 1989).

Static and fatigue crack growth experiments were investigated by Alcalá and Anglada (1997) showing that SCCG is significant during the fatigue crack growth behavior in 3Y-TZP (see Fig. 3.4A and B). The threshold region is where true cyclic fatigue effects are more clearly detected as suggested by the strong effect of $R$ on the threshold for crack growth, but for $K_{max} > 2.6\ \mathrm{MPa}\sqrt{m}$, the effect of SCCG during cyclic loading fatigue crack growth is evidenced by the relative stronger influence of $K_{max}$ with respect to $\Delta K$ on crack velocity. The prediction of fatigue crack growth based on static crack growth results is shown in Fig 3.4B for $K_{max} > 3\ \mathrm{MPa}\sqrt{m}$.

### 3.1.5 $K_{IC}$ and curve R-behavior of ceramics

In the preceding paragraphs, $K_{Ic}$ has been assumed to be a material parameter. However, in many structural ceramics the value of $K_{Ic}$ depends on crack extension so that the fracture toughness cannot be considered to have a single value. In this case, the material is characterized by a crack resistance curve ("R-curve") which represents the stress intensity factor that has to be applied by an external load for the onset and maintenance of crack extension. The R-curve behavior can be caused by several intrinsic effects such as crack-face bridging, phase transformations, microcracking, etc. The effect of an increasing crack-resistance ("R-curve behavior") is commonly described by a function $K_R\ (\Delta a)$ in which $K_R$ is the stress intensity factor necessary for crack propagation by an amount of $\Delta a$ (Fig. 3.5) (Fett, 2012). The R-curve is commonly obtained by inducing a long sharp crack and observing its stable extension as the stress intensity factor is increased until unstable fracture takes place. The condition for unstable fracture is now given by (Munz and Fett, 1998):

$$K = K_R \tag{3.13}$$

$$\frac{dK}{da} = \frac{dK_R}{da} \tag{3.14}$$

This means that for unstable fracture the functions $K$ and $K_R$ must have a common point where the tangents to both curves have the same value. The strength of a ceramic with R-curve behavior will be determined by the initial crack length as well as by the details of how much and how fast $K_R$ increases with $\Delta a$.

### 3.1.6 Mechanisms of increase in fracture toughness

The critical stress intensity factor, $K_{Ic}$ (fracture toughness) of a ceramic that presents R-curve behavior is formally written as:

$$K_R = K_{Ic} = K_{I0} + \Delta K_c, \quad \Delta K_c > 0 \tag{3.15}$$

where $K_{I0}$ is the matrix toughness and $\Delta K_c$ the contribution from various crack-shielding mechanisms. In alumina with large grain size, the most important

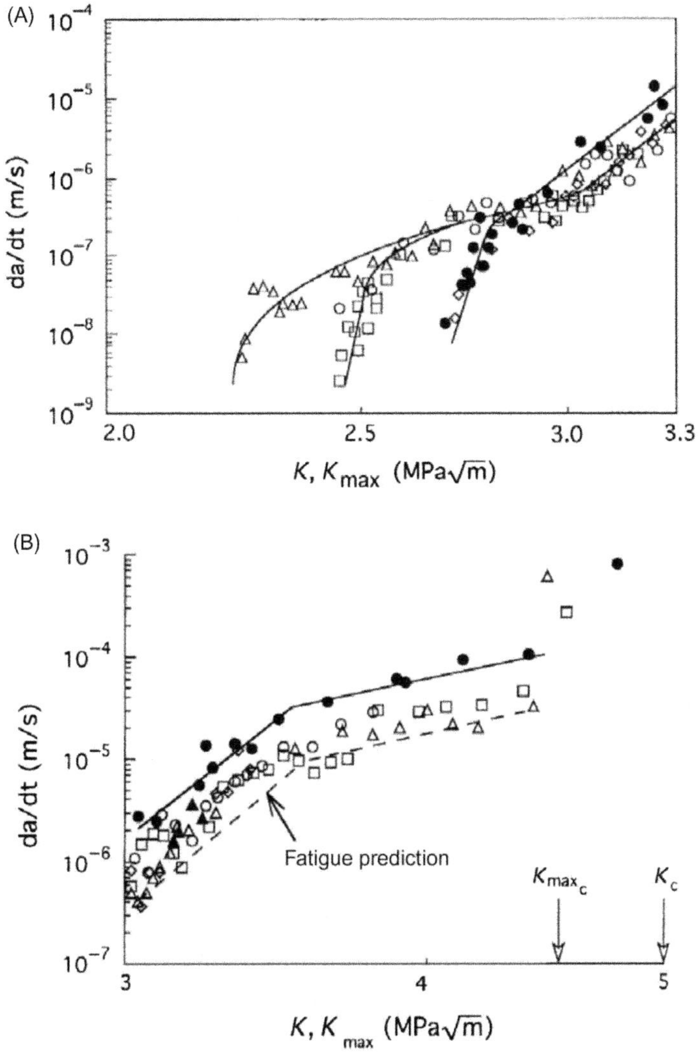


**Figure 3.4** Overall fatigue crack growth and static crack growth results determined with load-bridge-precracked specimens: (●) static crack growth; fatigue crack growth for $\nu = 2$ Hz and $R$ values of (Δ) 0.05, (□) 0.15, (○) 0.35, and (◇) 0.60). (A) Region close to the threshold and after initial crack growth discontinuities. (B) Comparison of the fatigue crack growth and static crack growth results for applied $K$ values of >3 MPa$\sqrt{m}$; the prediction of the fatigue crack growth behavior based on the static crack growth results also is included (Alcalá and Anglada, 1997).

contribution is that of grains bridging the crack faces near the crack tip, i.e., $\Delta K_c = |K_{br}|$ in Fig. 3.5 (Knehans and Steinbrech, 1982; Steinbrech et al., 1983; Swanson et al., 1987; Rödel, 1992; Bennison and Lawn, 1989). In the case of tetragonal zirconia, the main contribution is related to the stress activated $t$–$m$

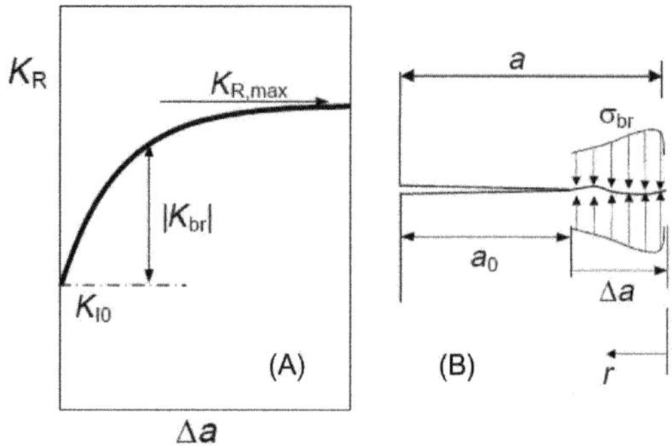


**Figure 3.5** (A) Schematic of an increasing crack growth resistance curve starting from the crack-tip toughness $K_{I0}$ and exhibiting a saturation value $K_{R,max}$. (B) A crack in a ceramic material exhibiting crack surface interactions described by bridging stresses $\sigma_{br}$ (Fett, 2012).

phase transformation in the crack tip process zone, which is accompanied by an increase in volume which in turn creates a compressive strain field which opposes crack extension. The contribution to the toughness resulting from stress activated transformation, $\Delta K_{cT}$, is commonly given by (see review by Hannink et al., 2000):

$$\Delta K_{cT} = \frac{\eta E^* e_T V_f h^{1/2}}{1-\nu} \tag{3.16}$$

where $\eta$ is a factor depending on the zone shape at the crack tip and the nature of the stress field in that zone, $E^*$ the effective modulus of the material, $e^T$ the dilatational strain, $V_f$ the transformed volume fraction of particles, $h$ the width of the transformation zone from the crack surface (i.e., the half-height of the zone), and $\nu$ the Poisson ratio. The matrix modulus $E^*$ plays an important role in determining the effectiveness of the dilatational strain. For example, a stiffer matrix, such as $Al_2O_3$ ($E^* = 380$ GPa, $\nu = 0.2$), constrains the transformation more than does $ZrO_2$ ($E^* = 210$ GPa, $\nu = 0.3$) decreasing the extent of the transformation zone $h$. The decreased $h$ is due to a decrease in $V_f$ that results from the high matrix $E^*$ value that opposes the transformation. For a review of transformation toughening of zirconia ceramics see (Hannink et al., 2000).

In principle, it is possible to predict accurately the strength from fracture mechanics if the critical natural flaw and the $K_R$ curve are precisely determined. The R-curve is usually known for long straight and artificial cracks of several millimeters or centimeters in length. However, fracture in advanced ceramics is caused by flaws with variable dimensions generally of only several tens of micrometers. If R-curves for macroscopic cracks are used to predict the strength of ceramics containing natural small defects, then by applying Eqs. (3.13) and (3.14) the common point of tangency between $K_{app}$ and $K_R$ may lie close to the intrinsic fracture toughness value so that the high increase in fracture toughness

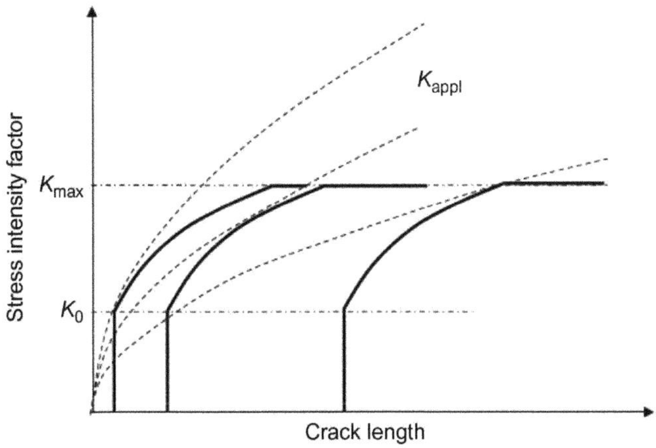


**Figure 3.6** $K_{app}$ and $K_R$ for three initial crack lengths (Munz, 2007).

corresponding to the plateau of the R-curve may never be reached. Fig. 3.6 is a schematic graphical representation of the condition of unstable fracture for different initial crack sizes where it can be seen that a small crack may not have any advantage of the existence of the R-curve as compared to a large crack for which the tangency point is practically at the plateau of the R-curve (Munz, 2007). This implies that a ceramic with large plateau toughness does not necessarily has a high strength.

This is the case when the R-curve increases sharply with crack extension, which is usually observed when a crack is growing only with partial crack-face separation. Remaining crack–surface interactions cause so-called "bridging stresses" which act against the externally applied load mainly very close behind the crack tip. The strength then depends very much on the details of how fast $K_R$ increases with initial crack growth rather than on the final plateau toughness. 3Y-TZP is also another ceramic that presents a small but very sharp increase in the R-curve at the beginning of crack extension (see Fig. 3.7, Casellas et al., 2001).

However, it is not clear whether R-curves for large cracks can be used to predict the strength from small cracks. In the few studies where the R-curve has been determined for small cracks, it has been shown that is different from that of macroscopic cracks lying always significantly below the R-curves for macrocracks (Munz, 2007; Marshall and Swain, 1988; Ramachandran et al., 1993; Yu and Shetty, 1990).

## 3.2 Bioactive glasses and glass ceramics

Bioactive glasses, similarly to soda lime glasses, have very low levels of $K_{Ic}$ and are very sensitive to SCCG. Fig. 3.8 shows experimental data of SCCG of a set of experimental bioactive glasses in the system Si–Na–K–Mg–Ca–P–O including

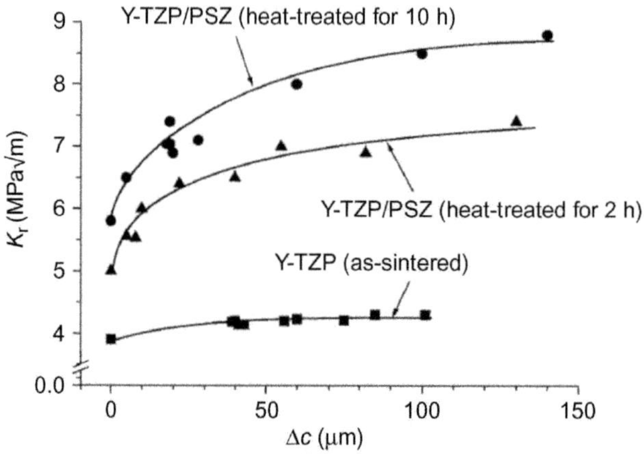


**Figure 3.7** R-curve behavior for 3Y-TZP as sintered and after different heat treatment at 1650°C (Casellas et al., 2001).

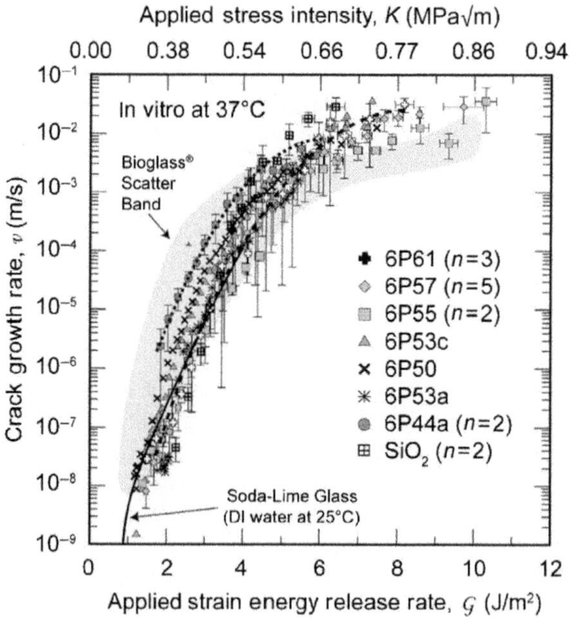


**Figure 3.8** The average SCCG data for glasses (*n* designates the number of samples in each population if greater than one).
The gray band describes data for Bioglass 45S5 taken from Barry and Nicholson (1988) and the solid line describes data for soda-lime glass taken from Michalske and Frechette (1980). All data except for soda-lime glass were taken in simulated body fluid (SBF) at 37°C (Bloyer et al., 2007).

Bioglass in simulated human physiological environment (Bloyer et al., 2007). The compositions of the glasses are related to that of the original Bioglasss developed by Hench (1998) but with silica contents ranging between 46 and 69 mol% and MgO and $K_2O$ partially substituted for CaO and $Na_2O$.

It can be seen that the threshold stress intensity factor for crack growth is roughly less than half the fracture toughness in SBF. It appears that the aqueous attack of the Si–O network of the glass is the dominant mechanism of SCCG in these bioactive/biocompatible glasses. In this study, a weak but measurable increase in crack growth rates with increasing bioactivity was detected in region *I*, i.e., where crack growth rates are largely controlled by the chemical reactivity (Bloyer et al., 2007).

The very low load-bearing capacity of bioglasses makes them unsuitable for medical devices in which strength and toughness are required. These characteristics restrict their use to only a few applications that do not demand these properties. However, they exhibit an early strong interfacial bonding with bone. Their bioactivity is attributed to the formation on their surface of a hydroxycarbonated apatite (HCA) layer similar to a large extent to the mineral part of bone.

One way to increase mechanical properties of bioglasses is by developing bioactive glass ceramics, i.e., various types of glasses that undergo the precipitation of suitable crystalline phases under heat treatment. For a recent review, the reader is referred to Montazerian and Zanotto (2016).

Examples of better known and commercially available bioactive glass ceramics are given in Table 3.1.

For example, the first development was that of Ceravital which has apatite ($CaO-P_2O_5$) precipitates in a $Na_2O-K_2O-MgO-CaO-SiO_2-P_2O_5$ glass matrix. Cerabone, developed later, is formed by apatite and wollastonite crystals in $MgO-CaO-SiO_2-P_2O_5$ glass, and is one of the commercial types with the higher mechanical properties, see Table 3.1. The fracture toughness of glass ceramics is generally in the range 1–2 $MPa\sqrt{m}$, which is much higher than the fracture toughness of their matrices, but only just reaches the lower end values of the fracture toughness of cortical bone.

## 3.3 Calcium phosphates (CaP) and CaP composites

The compositions that have received the most attention is hydroxyapaptite (HA) with the chemical composition $Ca_5(PO_4)_3OH$ and a calcium to phosphate ratio of 1.67, β-tricalcium phosphate (β-TCP), with the chemical composition $Ca_3(PO_4)_2$ and a calcium to phosphate ratio of 1.5, and biphasic calcium phosphate (BCP), which refers to composites of HA and β-TCP with no specific ratio. The main difference between the properties of HA and β-TCP is their relative degradation rates; HA is considered relatively nondegrading while TCPs degrade readily. Thus, the use of BCP with different HA to β-TCP ratios allows manipulation of the degradation rate as well as other properties.

**Table 3.1 Commercially available bioactive glass ceramics**

| Material | Main composition | Young's modulus (GPa) | Bending strength (MPa) | Fracture toughness (MPa$\sqrt{m}$) | Reference |
|---|---|---|---|---|---|
| Human bone | Mainly apatite and collagen | 6–20 | 160 | 2–12 | Kokubo (2008) |
| Parent glass | 100% glass | 30–50 | 70 | 0.8 | Kokubo (2008) |
| Ceravital© | CaO–$P_2$O5 (apatite) in $SiO_2$– | 100–150 | 90 | 1 | Brömer et al. (1977) |
| Cerabone© | 38% apatite + 34% wollastonite + 28% glass | 35–118 | 220 | 2 | Kokubo (2008) |
| Biovert I© | $Na_2O$–MgO–CaO–$Al_2O_3$–$SiO_2$–$P_2O_5$–F glass Mica + apatite + glass | 70–88 | 90–140 | 1.2–1.8 | Höland and Beall (2012) |
| Biovert II© | Mica + glass | 70 | 140–180 | 1.2–2.1 | Höland and Beall (2012) |
| Biosilicate© | $Na_2O$–CaO–$SiO_2$–$P_2O_5$ glass + ($Na_2$Ca-$Si_2O_6$) + ($NaCaPO_4$) | 80 | 200 | 1 | Peitl et al. (2001) |

CaPs have excellent properties for use in bone replacement, but one of the limiting factors in load-bearing applications often mentioned is the strength. The existence of porosity has a very strong effect on reducing the strength. Nevertheless, there is a range of porosities and architectures of CaPs for which they have strengths and stiffness that are similar to those of cortical and cancellous bone in some forms (Wagoner Johnson and Herschler, 2011). The real limiting factor for CaPs in load-bearing applications may be in the inherent brittleness of this class of materials. Unfortunately, few studies in the literature report properties such as fracture toughness, reliability (i.e., Weibull modulus), or energy to failure for CaP scaffolds. Cordell et al. (2009), found that the reliability of HA depends on deformation mode (bending or compression), along with pore size and pore size distribution; reliability was higher for smaller average pore sizes in bending, but lower for smaller pore sizes in compression.

Regarding SCCG, it was studied in HA by the double torsion technique and the crack velocity versus stress intensity factor, $K_I$, was obtained for different environments and processing conditions (Benaqqa et al., 2005). HA was found to be very sensitive to slow crack growth, with crack propagation beginning at $K_I$ as low as $0.4\ \mathrm{MPa}\sqrt{\mathrm{m}}$, which compromises its use in load-bearing applications. This was explained by a strong decrease in surface energy by water adsorption on the crack surface. The sintering temperature was shown to play a key role in $V-K_I$ laws. Fig. 3.9 shows the crack velocity in terms of $K_I$ for different environments (water, air, and oil). Values of n of about 60 were found for the stress exponent in stage *I*.

One effective strategy for increasing mechanical properties of CaP is to decrease the grain size from the micro- to the nano-scale. The result is a substantial increase in the compressive strength, making in this way the size of the grains closer to the size of natural HA which allows a better ionic exchange, producing larger protein adsorption and better cell response (Zhang et al., 2008). In this last study macroporous scaffolds were successfully fabricated from nanocrystalline β-TCP powders using the spark plasma sintering (SPS) technique with a degree of porosity

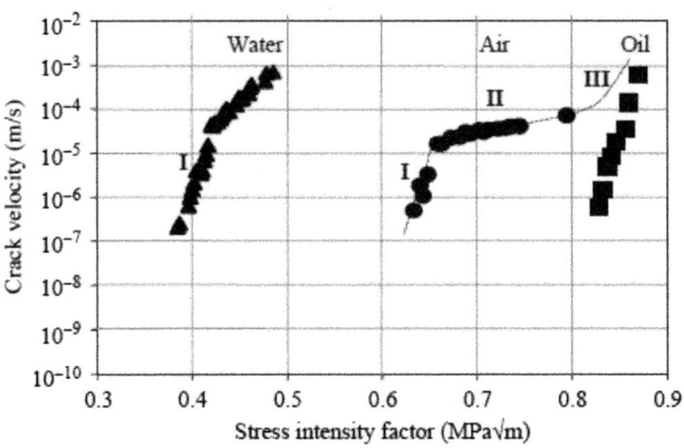


**Figure 3.9** SCCG of HA in three different media (Benaqqa et al., 2005).

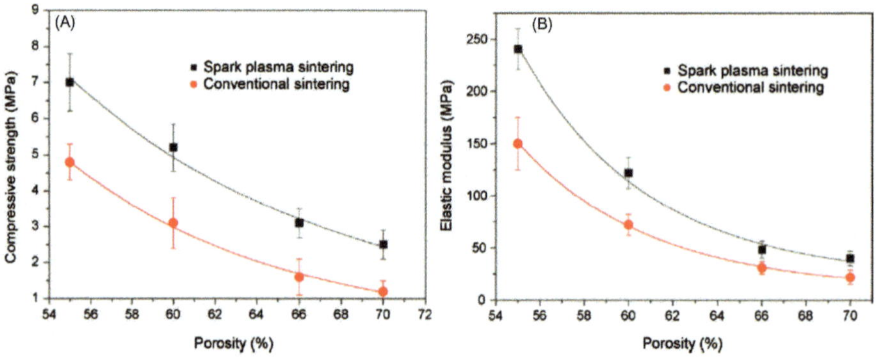


**Figure 3.10** Compressive strength (A) and elastic modulus (B) of the β–TCP scaffolds by SPS and conventional sintering (Zhang et al., 2008).

(55%–70%) and a macropore size (300–500 μm). Grain growth was inhibited, the density of the solid matrix increased and the elastic modulus and compressive strength increased between 50% and 100% with respect to the conventional one with micrometric microstructure (Zhang et al., 2008). However, only compressive strength was reported (Fig. 3.10).

Ceramic–polymer composites have been used to increase the fracture toughness of bioactive ceramics and to match the elastic modulus of bone. In general, if a *polymer matrix* is used and HA particles are incorporated into the matrix, the strength of the polymer decreases with increasing HA. In addition, with the presence of the polymer, bioactivity and osteoconductivity may decrease. Therefore, with this approach there is concern about decreasing properties such as bioactivity. Another limitation is the creep resistance and the low modulus of polymers.

The approach of polymer-bioactive glass has also been used. For instance, Niemelä et al. (2005) prepared composite rods of polymer matrix (high molecular weight poly-L, DL-lactide) containing up to 50 wt% of bioactive glass spheres which were drawn to a diameter of approximately 3 μm. The bioactive glass spheres were well dispersed and with the open pores formed on the composite surface during drawing. It was found that the addition of bioactive glass reduced the bending strength, bending modulus, shear strength, compression strength and torsion strength of the polymers (poly-L, DL-lactide). However, the strain at maximum bending load increased in the composites.

On the other hand, by preparing *ceramic matrix–polymer composites* better properties can be achieved. For instance, Martínez-Vázquez et al. (2010) studied by polymer infiltration of β-TCP scaffolds fabricated by robocasting. Porous structures consisting of a tetragonal three-dimensional mesh of interpenetrating rods were fabricated from concentrated TCP and biodegradable polymers (polylactic acid (PLA) and poly(e-aprolactone) (PCL)) which were infiltrated into selected scaffolds by immersion of the structure in a polymer melt. Infiltrating polymers into the porous ceramic structure was shown to considerably boost the strength and toughness of the material—threefold and more than sixfold increases in scaffold compressive

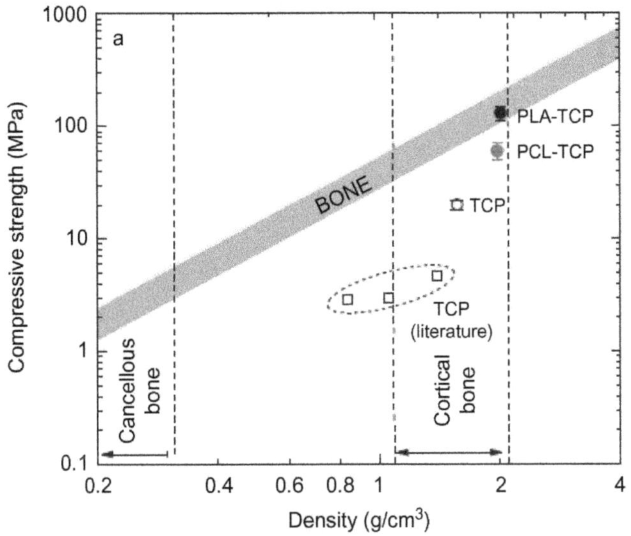


**Figure 3.11** Comparative plot of compressive strength for scaffolds fabricated by Martínez-Vázquez et al. (2010) (circles) in comparison with other literature reports (Sous et al., 1998; Gao et al., 1997; Ramay and Zhang, 2004), for conventional TCP scaffolds (squares); different literature sources are not distinguished. The results are plotted as a function of material density. The shaded band represents bone properties (including data dispersion) as a function of apparent bone dry density, estimated using an empirical power law model of Keller (1994) (Martínez-Vázquez et al., 2010).

strength were found with PCL and PLA infiltration, respectively. The PLA–TCP composite not only greatly exceeded the mechanical performance of other TCP scaffolds reported to date, but had strength values similar to those of cortical bone with the same density (Fig. 3.11).

A general view of the dependence of the compression strength in terms of porosity of CaPs and Ca/polymer composites for applications in bone replacement and repair is shown in Fig. 3.12 (Wagoner Johnson and Herschler, 2011). It can be seen that CaPs show definitive promise for the repair of bone load-bearing defects because the data show that most of the HA and BCP scaffolds overlap with cortical and cancellous bone in either strength, porosity, or both.

In hybrid organic–inorganic materials, the bioactive inorganic component chemically bonds to the polymer and is homogeneously distributed in this organic phase. Integration of organic and inorganic components in a very fine scale seems to have a much better cellular response and improved strain to failure. They can combine the bioactive properties of a glass with the toughness of a polymer. In addition, the mechanical properties may be better tailored to degradation rates (Valliant et al., 2013). The preparation of hybrids can be carried out from organo-silica polymers such as polydimethylsiloxane (Mahony et al., 2010), or from separate organic and inorganic starting materials. Through the sol-gel process, hybrids can be formed by incorporating a polymer into the sol, allowing a silica network to form around the polymer chains.

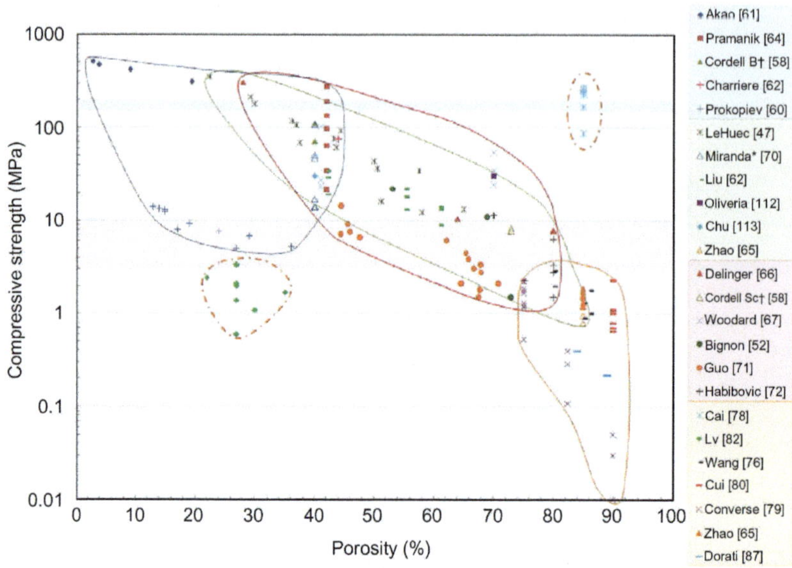


**Figure 3.12** Plot illustrating the dependence of compressive strength on total porosity for all references included in Wagoner Johnson and Herschler (2011). The data are grouped by material category using colored lines. Bulk HA and biphasic calcium phosphate (BCP), HA scaffolds, BCP scaffolds, HA/polymer and polymer scaffolds are represented by *blue*, *green*, *red*, and *orange* lines, respectively. One exception is Miranda et al. (2008) (denoted by *). These data are included in the BCP category, but are the only study in that category with β-tricalcium phosphate (β-TCP) and no HA. Two datasets from two different groups are considered "outliers" and are demarcated with dashed lines (Wagoner Johnson and Herschler, 2011).

The fine-scale integration of interpenetrating networks of silica and the polymer at the molecular level results in improved mechanical properties over bioactive glasses. Composite materials tend to fail at the interface between components. Thus, removing this interface and having covalent coupling between the components should lead to improved mechanical properties. As an example of mechanical properties achieved in hybrid materials with respect to glass, Fig. 3.13A shows the stress–strain curves for γCaPGA/silica hybrids. All stress–strain curves show strengths greater than 300 MPa and strains to failures reaching higher than 26%. Regarding the strain to failure of sol-gel glasses of less than 4% and strengths of 66 MPa, this is a significant improvement (Valliant et al., 2013).

## 3.4 Calcium phosphate cements

Calcium phosphate cements (CPCs) are well-established materials for the repair of bone defects with excellent biocompatibility and bioactivity, but their high

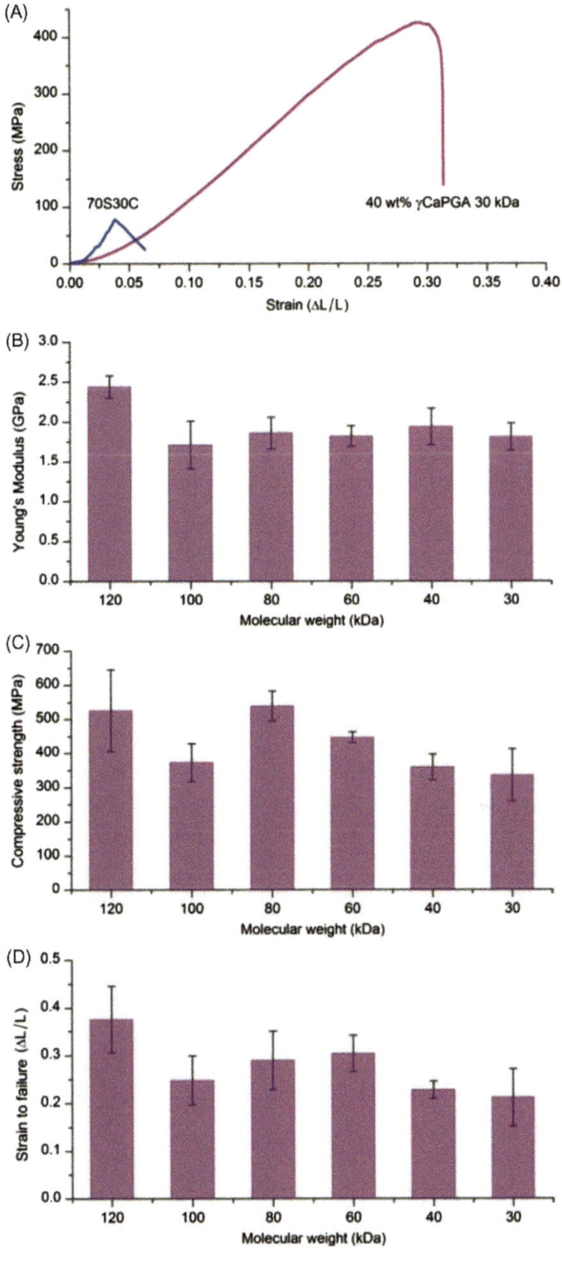


**Figure 3.13** Compression testing for hybrids of 40 wt% γCaPGA/silica hybrids of varying molecular weight. (A) Stress–strain curve for 30-kDa γPGA hybrid and stress–strain curve for a 70 mol%$SiO_2$, 30 mol% CaO glass (70S30C). (B) Young's modulus, (C) compressive strength, and (D) strain to failure (Valliant et al., 2013).

brittleness and low flexural/tensile strength limits their application to nonload-bearing areas. Efforts are made in order to reinforce CPCc with fibers (fiber-reinforced CPCs (FRCPCs)) in order to improve the fracture toughness and the strength. The addition of fibers to CPC matrix is shown to be an effective method to improve fracture toughness through crack-bridging and crack deflection toughening mechanisms (Zhang et al., 2014). Composition and mechanical properties of CPCs prepared with different processing parameters can be found in the review of Krûger and Groll (2012). FRCPCs bear a great potential for future development and optimization. Future research for load-bearing applications will have to focus on the selection of suitable fibers and matrix–fiber interfaces to optimize fracture toughness and strength and to tailor the degradation kinetics of fibers and matrix to retain strengthening and toughening over the entire the desired period (Zhang et al., 2014). According to this reference, although the mechanical strength of CPCs is generally low, it is not a critical issue for their application for bone repair—an observation not often realized by researchers and clinicians. The authors show that CPCs with compressive strengths comparable to those of cortical bones can be produced through densification and/or homogenization of the cement matrix, but the real limitation for CPCs appears to be their low fracture toughness and poor mechanical reliability (Weibull modulus) (Zhang et al., 2014).

## 3.5 Structural bioinert ceramics

Alumina, zirconia doped with yttria or ceria, and alumina–zirconia are the most used structural ceramics. One of the main applications of zirconia at present is in dental restorations using CAD/CAM technology. They are currently fabricated from presintered 3Y-TZP blanks by soft machining and sintering at temperatures around 1450°C. Their microstructure consists mainly of submicrometric tetragonal grains. Fracture toughness is mainly determined by transformation toughening and is in the range 4–6 MPa$\sqrt{m}$ depending on grain size, sintering temperature and exact yttria content. Regarding other mechanical properties, 3Y-TZP has high hardness and a flexural strength generally around 1000 MPa, but can easily be even higher.

The main limitation of zirconia is represented by low temperature degradation (LTD), also known as hydrothermal degradation or aging (Chevalier et al., 2007). It consists of the spontaneous transformation of the surface to the monoclinic phase in humid environments and moderate temperatures, including human body conditions. LTD is slow at room temperature and affects only a superficial layer of a few micrometers in well-densified 3Y-TZP, but it is accompanied by the formation of surface microcracks, surface roughening, and loss of cohesion, making the material unsuitable for joint replacement where surface stability is fundamental (Muñoz-Tabares et al., 2011). LTD is related to the diffusion of water radicals in zirconia with large numbers of oxygen vacancy sites induced by doping with trivalent yttrium as is the case with 3Y-TZP. If tetragonal Zirconia is doped with $Ce^{+4}$, as in 12Ce-TZP, the material is resistant to LTD. According to Schubert and Frey,

(Schubert and Frey, 2005) the penetration of water radicals leads to a lattice contraction, which results in the formation of tensile stresses in the surface grains that destabilize the tetragonal phase. The increase in volume associated with the tetragonal–monoclinic transformation induces tensile stresses in the neighboring grains, leading to transformation and microcracking. Detailed analysis is given in Chevalier et al. (2007). Powders of 3Y-TZP with small amounts of alumina are now used, which increase the resistance to LTD. It seems that the strength of the grain boundary is increased by the presence of a high concentration of $Al^{+3}$ on the grain boundaries (Samodurova et al., 2015).

Latest trends in dental restorative ceramics involve the development of full-contour 3Y-TZP ceramics which can avoid chipping of veneering porcelains. Among the challenges are the low translucency and the hydrothermal stability of 3Y-TZP ceramics. (Zhang et al. 2015, 2016) selected different trivalent oxides ($Sc_2O_3$, $Nd_2O_3$ and $La_2O_3$) to add in small concentrations to conventional $Al_2O_3$ doped 3Y-TZP. They showed that dopant segregation was a key factor to design hydrothermally stable and high-translucent 3Y-TZP ceramics and the cation dopant radius could be used as a controlling parameter. A large trivalent dopant, oversized as compared to $Zr^{4+}$, exhibiting strong segregation at the $ZrO_2$ grain boundary was preferred. The introduction of 0.2 mol% $La_2O_3$ in conventional 0.1–0.25 wt% $Al_2O_3$-doped 3Y-TZP resulted in an excellent combination of high translucency and superior hydrothermal stability, while retaining excellent mechanical properties.

In dental restorations with veneering porcelain, the 3Y-TZP is protected so that LTD is expected to be less significant as far as it is completely isolated from the aggressive oral environment by the veneering porcelain. However, in the porcelain-free full-contour 3Y-TZP ceramics directly in contact with the oral environment, the resistance to LTD must be kept in mind.

Zirconia toughened alumina ceramics combine the advantageous properties of monolithic alumina and zirconia: they exhibit high strength, high toughness, outstanding wear resistance, and excellent biocompatibility (Kurtz et al., 2014; Roualdes et al., 2010; Pezzotti et al., 2009). Thanks to these remarkable properties, in the last decade they have become the new gold standard in orthopedics for the fabrication of ceramic-bearing components. In particular, in the case of hip replacements, their superior mechanical properties as compared to alumina improve the reliability and enable the manufacture of smaller femoral heads and thinner liners, providing a larger range of motion in the joint (Piconi et al., 2005; Lee and Goodman, 2008). The stabilization of zirconia is achieved by the presence of the stiff alumina matrix so that the tetragonal structure may be stable even without any doping with yttria. This composite is now used in the fabrication of femoral heads (Biolox delta by Ceramtec) with additions of SrO and $Cr_2O_3$, with some grains of platelet-like morphology to deflect the cracks (see Fig. 3.14).

Ce-TZP shows extremely high toughness and a limited level of strength. Transformation zones are large and the stress to induce the beginning of transformation is significantly lower than in Y-TZP, and it may be even lower than the fracture stress of natural defects. This is shown in Fig. 3.15 for different ceramics (Hannink et al., 2000).

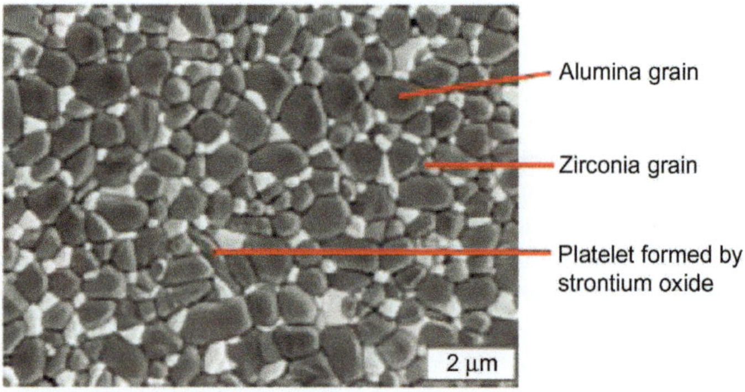


**Figure 3.14** Microstructure of Biolox delta.
Courtesy of Ceram Tec AG.

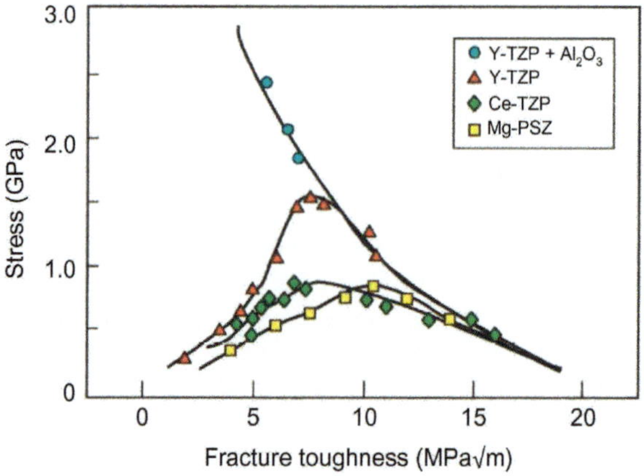


**Figure 3.15** Strength versus fracture toughness for a selection of $ZrO_2$-toughened engineering ceramics. Maximums in the curves indicate a transition from flaw-size control of strength to transformation-limited strength.
Reproduced in Hannink, R.H.J., Kelly, P.M., Muddle, B.C., 2000. Transformation toughening in zirconia-containing ceramics. J. Am. Ceram. Soc. 83, 461–487, Fig. 4, from Swain, M.V., 1985. Inelastic deformation of Mg-PSZ and its significance for strength–toughness relationship of zirconia-toughened ceramics. Acta Metall. 33(11), 2083–2091 (Swain, 1985).

Ce-TZP is often alloyed with alumina, and the composites are referred to as ATZ and show enhanced strength and high indentation fracture toughness. For example, in Ce-TZP–alumina, referred to under the commercial name Nanozir, both phases have submicrometric grain size and high toughness >10 MPa$\sqrt{m}$ and strength >900 MPa can be achieved (Benzaid et al., 2008).

Ce-TZP reinforced with several types of platelets made of hexaluminates as second phases has shown good compromise between high toughness and strength (Palmero et al., 2015; Reveron et al., 2017). For a review of these composites, we

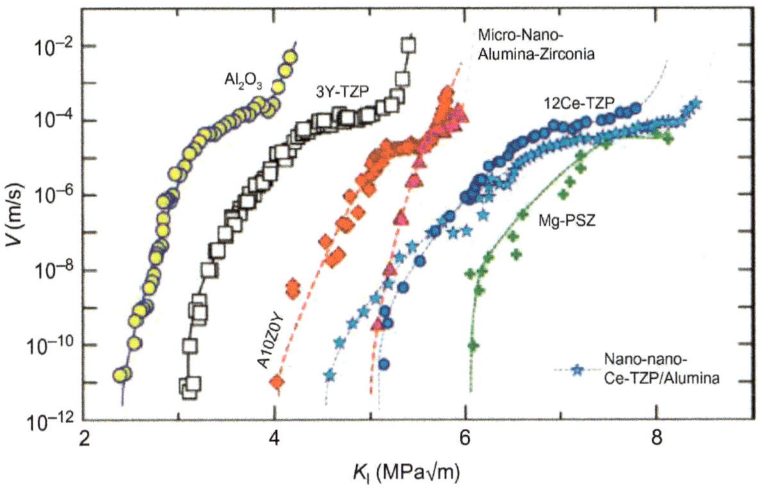


**Figure 3.16** Comparison of different $K_{Ic}$ and SCCG of bioinert ceramics: alumina, 3Y-TZP, 12Ce-TZP (El Attaoui, 2003), Mg-PSZ (Nagl et al., 1996), Al10Z0Y, micro-nano-alumina-zirconia composite (Chevalier et al., 2005), and nano-nano Ce-TZP-alumina composite (Chevalier and Gremillard, 2009).

suggest Kern (2014). This new class of composites offer the potential to overcome the disadvantages of Y-TZP.

With reference to SCCG resistance of bionert ceramics, Fig. 3.16 shows the crack velocity in terms of $K_I$ for alumina, zirconia doped with 3 mol% $Y_2O_3$ and composites of alumina reinforced with zirconia (Chevalier and Gremillard, 2009). One interesting point is to observe that all the materials displayed are sensitive to SCCG with $K_I$ threshold values which are generally around 60% of the fracture toughness. On the other hand, the fine microstructure of "micro-nano-alumina zirconia" has similar threshold to high toughness zirconia doped with 12 mol% ceria in spite of its lower fracture toughness. Reduction of grain size and more homogeneous distribution of zirconia increase the threshold for crack growth (De Aza et al., 2002).

For the design of implants for long life, these data on thresholds have to be taken into account in order to increase long-term reliability of devices which are subjected to static or dynamic stresses over long periods of time.

## 3.6 Conclusions

Mechanical properties of ceramics of interest in biomaterials applications, such as in bone substitution, making medical devices, and dental implants and restorations, depend in general on each application, but common requirements include the need for a higher fracture toughness and reliability, and prolonged clinical lifetimes. This is the major drawback of ceramics, since their low reliability, low fracture toughness, and the influence of the environment which could induce SCCG at levels much lower than the fracture toughness, are real limitations to their use in the biomedical field. In the development of bioceramics, these are the properties which need to be optimized and which, in general, are the most relevant from a mechanical viewpoint.

## References

Alcalá, J., Anglada, M., 1997. Fatigue and static crack propagation in yttria-stabilized tetragonal zirconia polycrystals: crack growth micromechanisms and precracking effects. J. Am. Ceram. Soc. 80 (11), 2759–2772.

Anderson, T.L., 1995. Fracture Mechanics, second ed. CRC Press, New York, NY.

Baierl, R.G.A., 1999. Langsames Rißwachstum in Aluminiumoxid. Diplomarbeit am Institut für Strukturund Funktionskeramik, Montanuniversität Leoben.

Barry, C., Nicholson, P.S., 1988. Stress corrosion cracking of a bioactive glass. Adv. Ceram. Mat. 3 (2), 127–130.

Benaqqa, C., Chevalier, J., Saädaoui, M., Fantozzi, F., 2005. Slow crack growth behaviour of hydroxyapatite ceramics. Biomaterials. 26, 6106–6112.

Bennison, S.J., Lawn, B.R., 1989. Role of interfacial grain-bridging sliding friction in the crack-resistance and strength properties of non transforming ceramics. Acta Metall. 37, 2659–2671.

Benzaid, R., Chevalier, J., Saâdaoui, M., Fantozzi, G., Nawa, M., Diaz, L.A., et al., 2008. Fracture toughness, strength and slow crack growth in a ceria stabilized zirconia-alumina nanocomposite for medical applications. Biomaterials. 29, 3636–3641.

Bloyer, R.D., James, M., McNaney, J.M., Cannon, R.M., Saiz, E., Tomsia, A.P., et al., 2007. Stress–corrosion crack growth of Si–Na–K–Mg–Ca–P–O bioactive glasses in simulated human physiological environment. Biomaterials. 28, 4901–4911.

Brömer, H., Deutscher, K., Blencke, B., Pfeil, E., Strunz, V., 1977. Properties of the bioactive implant material Ceravital®. Sci. Ceram. 9, 219.

Chevalier, J., et al., 2005. Nanostructured ceramic oxides with a slow crack growth resistance close to covalent materials. Nano Lett. 5 (7), 1297–1301.

Casellas, D., Alcalá, J., Llanes, L.M., Anglada, M., 2001. Fracture variability and R-curve behavior in yttria-stabilized zirconia ceramics. J. Mater. Sci. 36, 3011–3025.

Chevalier, J., Gremillard, L., 2009. Ceramics for medical applications: a picture for the next 20 years. J. Eur. Ceram. Soc. 29, 1245–1255.

Chevalier, J., Gremillard, L., Deville, S., 2007. Low-temperature degradation of zirconia and implications for biomedical implants. Annu. Rev. Mater. Res. 37, 1–32.

Cordell, J., Vogl, M., Johnson, A., 2009. The influence of micropore size on the mechanical properties of bulk hydroxyapatite and hydroxyapatite scaffolds. J. Mech. Behav. Biomed. Mater. 2, 560–570.

Danzer, R., Lube, T., Supancic, P., Damani, R., 2008. Fracture of ceramics. Adv. Eng. Mater. 10 (4), 275–298.

De Aza, A.H., Chevalier, J., Fantozzi, G., Schehl, M., Torrecillas, R., 2002. Crack growth resistance of alumina, zirconia and zirconia toughened alumina ceramics for joint prostheses. Biomaterials. 23, 937–945.

El Attaoui, H., 2003. Influence du renforcement sur le comportement en fatigue statique et cyclique des céramiques monolithiques de type alumine et zircone. PhD Thesis, INSA-Lyon, France.

Fett, T., 2012. New Contributions to R-Curves and Bridging Stresses—Applications of Weight Functions. Schriftenreihe des Instituts für Angewandte Materialien Band 3, KIT Scientific Publishing, Karlsruhe. Dedicated to Prof. Dr. Dietrich Munz on the occasion of his 75th Birthday.

Gao, T.J., et al., 1997. Morphological, biomechanical difference in healing in segmental tibial defects implanted with Biocoral(R) or tricalcium phosphate cylinders. Biomaterials. 18, 219–223.

Hannink, R.H.J., Kelly, P.M., Muddle, B.C., 2000. Transformation toughening in zirconia-containing ceramics. J. Am. Ceram. Soc. 83, 461–487.

Hench, L.L., 1998. , "Bioceramics. J. Am. Ceram. Soc. 81, 1705–1728.

Höland, W., Beall, G., 2012. Glass-Ceramic Technology, second ed. The American Ceramic Society & Wiley, USA.

Keller, T.S., 1994. Predicting the compressive mechanical-behavior of bone. J. Biomech. 27, 1159–1168.

Kern, F., 2014. A comparison of microstructure and mechanical properties of 12Ce-TZP reinforced with alumina and in situ formed strontium- or lanthanum hexaaluminate precipitates. J. Eur. Ceram. Soc. 34, 413–423.

Knehans, R., Steinbrech, R., 1982. Memory effects of crack resistance during slow crack growth in notched $Al_2O_3$ bend specimens, J. Mater. Sci., 1. 327–339.

Kokubo, T., 2008. Bioceramics and Their Clinical Applications. Woodhead Publishing Limited, USA.

Krüger, R., Groll, J., 2012. Fiber reinforced calcium phosphate cements–On the way to degradable load bearing bone substitutes? Biomaterials. 33, 5887–5900.

Kurtz, S.M., Kocagöz, S., Arnholt, C., Huet, R., Ueno, M., Walter, W.L., 2014. Advances in zirconia toughened alumina biomaterials for total joint replacement. J. Mech. Behav. Biomed. Mater. 31, 107–116.

Lathabai, S., Lawn, B.R., 1989. Fatigue limits in noncyclic loading of ceramics with crack-resistance curves. J. Mater. Sci. 24, 4298–4306.

Lawn, B., 1993. Fracture of Brittle Solids. second ed. Cambridge University Press, Cambridge, 1993. Cambridge Books Online. Web. 26 August 2016.

Lee, K., Goodman, S.B., 2008. Current state and future of joint replacements in the hip and knee. Expert Rev. Med. Devices. 5, 383–393.

Mahony, O., et al., 2010. Silica-gelatin hybrids with tailorable degradation and mechanical properties for tissue regeneration. Adv. Funct. Mater. 20, 3835–3845.

Marro, F.G., Mestra, A., Anglada, M., 2014. Weibull strength statistics of hydrothermally aged 3 mol% yttria-stabilised tetragonal zirconia. Ceram. Int. 40 (8, Part B), 12777–12782.

Marshall, D.B., Swain, M.V., 1988. Crack resistance curves in magnesia-partially-stabilized zirconia. J. Am. Ceram. Soc. 71, 399–404.

Martínez-Vázquez, F.J., Perera, F.H., Miranda, P., Pajares, A., Guiberteau, F., 2010. Improving the compressive strength of bioceramic robocast scaffolds by polymer infiltration. Acta Biomater. 6, 4361–4368.

Michalske, T.A., Frechette, V.D., 1980. Dynamic effects of liquids on crack growth leading to catastrophic failure in glass. J. Am. Ceram. Soc. 63 (11-12), 603–609.

Miranda, P., Pajares, A., Saiz, E., Tomsia, A.P., Guiberteau, F., 2008. Mechanical properties of calcium phosphate scaffolds fabricated by robocasting. J. Biomed. Mater. Res. A. 85, 218–227.

Montazerian, M., Zanotto, E.D., 2016. History and trends of bioactive glass-ceramics. J. Biomed. Mater. Res. Part A. 104A, 1231–1249.

Muñoz-Tabares, J.A., Jiménez-Piqué, E., Anglada, M., 2011. Subsurface evaluation of hydrothermal degradation of zircònia. Acta Mater. 59 (2), 473–484.

Munz, D., 2007. What can we learn from R-curve measurements?. J. Am. Ceram. Soc. 90 (1), 1–15.

Munz, D., Fett, T., 1998. Ceramics, Mechanical Properties, Failure Behaviour, Materials Selection. Springer, Berlin.

Nagl, M., Llanes, L., Fernandez, R., Anglada, M., 1996. The fatigue behaviour of Mg-PSZ and ZTA ceramics. In: Bradt, R.C., et al., (Eds.), Fracture Mechanics of Ceramics, 12. Plenum Press, New York, pp. 61–76.

Niemelä, T., Niiranen, H., Kellomäki, M., Törmälä, P., 2005. Self-reinforced composites of bioabsorbable polymer and bioactive glass with different bioactive glass contents. Part I. Initial mechanical properties and bioactivity. Acta Biomater. 1, 235–242.

Palmero, P., Fornabaio, M., Montanaro, L., Reveron, H., Esnouf, C., Chevalier, J., 2015. Towards long lasting zirconia-based composites for dental implants. Part I: innovative synthesis, microstructural characterization and in vitro stability. Biomaterials. 50, 38–46.

Peitl, O., Zanotto, E.D., Hench, L.L., 2001. Highly bioactive $P_2O_5$–$Na_2O$–CaO–$SiO_2$ glass-ceramics. J. Non-Cryst Solids. 292, 115–126.

Pezzotti, G., Yamada, K., Porporati, A.A., Kuntz, M., Yamamoto, K., 2009. Fracture toughness analysis of advanced ceramic composite for hip prosthesis. J. Am. Ceram. Soc. 92, np, 1817–1822.

Piconi, C., Maccauro, G., Muratori, F., 2005. Alumina matrix composites in arthroplasty. Key Eng. Mater. 284-286, 979–982. Available from: http://dx.doi.org/10.4028/www.scientific.net/KEM.284-286.979.

Quinn, J.B., Quinn, G.D., 2010. A practical and systematic review of Weibull statistics for reporting strengths of dental materials. Dent. Mater. 26, 135–147.

Ramachandran, N., Chao, L.-Y., Shetty, D.K., 1993. R-Curve behaviour and flaw insensitivity of Ce-TZP/Al2O3 composite. J. Am. Ceram. Soc. 76, 961–969.

Ramay, H.R.R., Zhang, M., 2004. Biphasic calcium phosphate nanocomposite porous scaffolds for load-bearing bone tissue Engineering. Biomaterials. 25, 5171–5180.

Reveron, H., Fornabaio, M., Palmero, P., Furderer, T., Adolfsson, E., Lughi, V., et al., 2017. Towards long lasting zirconia-based composites for dental implants: transformation induced plasticity and its consequence on ceramic reliability. Acta Biomater. 48, 424–432.

Rödel, J., 1992. Crack closure forces in ceramics: characterization and formation. J. Eur. Ceram. Soc. 9, 323–334.

Roualdes, O., Duclos, M.E., Gutknecht, D., Frappart, L., Chevalier, J., Hartmann, D.J., 2010. In vitro and in vivo evaluation of an alumina-zirconia composite for arthroplasty applications. Biomaterials. 31, 2043–2054.

Samodurova, A., Kocjan, A., Swain, M.V., Kosmac, T., 2015. The combined effect of alumina and silica co-doping on the ageing resistance of 3Y-TZP bioceramics. Acta Biomater. 11, 477–487.

Schubert, H., Frey, F., 2005. Stability of Y-TZP during hydrothermal treatment: neutron experiments and stability considerations. J. Eur. Ceram. Soc. 25, 1597–1602.

Sous, M., et al., 1998. Cellular biocompatibility and resistance to compression of macroporous β-tricalcium phosphate ceramics. Biomaterials. 19, 2147–2153.

Steinbrech, R.W., Knehans, R., Schaarwächter, W., 1983. Increase of crack resistance during slow crack growth in Al2O3 bend specimens. J. Mater. Sci. 18, 265–270.
Swain, M.V., 1985. Inelastic deformation of Mg-PSZ and its significance for strength–toughness relationship of zirconia-toughened ceramics. Acta Metall. 33 (11), 2083–2091.
Swanson, P.L., Fairbanks, C.J., Lawn, B.R., Mai, Y.-W., Hockey, B.J., 1987. Crack–interface grain bridging as a fracture resistance mechanism in ceramics: I experimental study on alumina. J. Am. Ceram. Soc. 70, 279.
Valliant, E.M., Romer, F., Wang, D., McPhail, D.S., Smith, M.E., Hanna, J.V., et al., 2013. Bioactivity in silica/poly(y-glutamic acid) sol-gel hybrids through calcium chelation. Acta Biomater. 9, 7662–7671.
Wachtman, J.B., Roger Cannon, W., Matthewson, M.J., 2009. Mechanical Properties of Ceramics, second ed. John Wiley & Sons, USA.
Wagoner Johnson, A.J., Herschler, B.A., 2011. Review of the mechanical behavior of CaP and CaP/polymer composites for applications in bone replacement and repair. Acta Biomater. 7, 16–30.
Yu, C.S., Shetty, D.K., 1990. Transformation yielding, plasticity and crack-growth-resistance (R-curve) behaviour of $CeO_2$-TZP. J. Mater. Sci. 25, 2025–2035.
Zhang, F., Lin, K., Chang, J., Lu, J., Ning, C., 2008. Spark Plasma Sintering of macro-porous calcium phosphate scaffolds from nano-crystalline powders. J. Eur. Ceram. Soc. 28 (3), 539–545.
Zhang, J., Liu, W., Schnitzler, V., Tancret, F., Bouler, J.M., 2014. Calcium phosphate cements for bone substitution: chemistry, handling and mechanical properties. Acta Biomater. 10, 1035–1049.
Zhang, F., et al., 2015. Highly-translucent, strong and aging-resistant 3YTZP ceramics for dental restoration by grain boundary segregation. Acta Biomater. 16, 215–222.
Zhang, F., et al., 2016. Effect of cation dopant radius on the hydrothermal stability of tetragonal zirconia: grain boundary segregation and oxygen vacancy annihilation. Acta Mater. 106, 48–58.

## Further reading

ENV-843-1, 1995. Advanced technical ceramics, monolithic ceramics, mechanical properties at room temperature. Part 1: determination of flexural strength.
ENV-843-5, 1996. Advanced technical ceramics, monolithic ceramics, mechanical properties at room temperature. Part 5: statistical analysis.
Juhasz, J.A., Best, S.M., 2012. Bioactive ceramics: processing, structures and properties. J. Mater. Sci. 47 (2), 610–624.
Kokubo, T., Ito, S., Sakka, S., Yamamuro, T., 1986. Formation of a high-strength bioactive glass-ceramic in the system MgO-CaO-SiO2-P2O5. J. Mater. Sci. 21 (2), 536–540.

# Biological assessment of bioceramics

**4**

*Paola Torricelli, Nicolò Nicoli Aldini and Milena Fini*
Rizzoli Orthopaedic Institute, Bologna, Italy

## Chapter Outline

**4.1 Introduction 111**
**4.2 Regulations and international standard organization rules 112**
**4.3 In vitro and in vivo tests 113**
4.3.1 In vitro tests 113
4.3.2 In vivo tests 115
4.3.3 In vivo evaluation of biocompatibility 116
4.3.4 Pathological models 119
4.3.5 Advanced preclinical in vitro models 120
**4.4 Conclusions 122**
**References 123**

## 4.1 Introduction

Biomaterials based on ceramics have been widely used over recent decades for dentistry and orthopedic applications (Baino et al., 2015). According to their behavior when implanted in the organism, bioceramics could be divided into bioinert (i.e., alumina, zirconia), resorbable and bioactive (i.e. hydroxyapatite and biological glasses), or able to stimulate specific cellular responses at the molecular level as scaffolds for tissue engineering (Navarro et al., 2008). All these type of bioceramics are reported to be biocompatible, but different bioactivity levels have been shown when investigating the property of interaction with the biological environment to improve the biological integration with tissues and the tissue/surface bonding. Therefore, bioactive ceramics can be used to improve strategies for the biological and biomechanical integration between the material and bone. The mechanism of bioactivity is related to the induction of biomineralization at the bone–biomaterial interface by bioceramics with specific composition and structure involving ionic, molecular and cellular mechanisms. Glass ceramics were the first biomaterials endowed with bioactivity, which means the direct chemical bonding with host tissues and stimulatory effects on bone cells (osteoinduction) (Han et al., 2007). Bioactivity performance may change as a result of the type of processing, the surface treatment and topography, the porosity of the construct, the addition of molecules, and the sterilization process (Zhang et al., 2014).

**Advances in Ceramic Biomaterials.**
**DOI: http://dx.doi.org/10.1016/B978-0-08-100881-2.00004-X**

Before the assessment of the clinical performance, the confirmation of safety and efficacy of any new formulation of ceramic-based material or development of existing biomaterials is a mandatory requirement. Safety and efficacy are defined in terms of a risk and a benefit, respectively. The evaluation of safety is obtained by tests, which try to measure the probability and severity of risks for the patients. Efficacy could be considered to be the probability of advantages due to the use of the medical device and is usually evaluated by means of preclinical "proof of concept" and "pivotal" studies.

The first step of a complex route to validate a material or a device proposed for clinical use is the performance of standardized regulatory tests *in vitro* and *in vivo* to license materials for use in humans, according to defined programs of biocompatibility and safety. Biocompatibility is related not only to chemical properties of ceramic composition, but also to ion release, degradation and corrosion. After having assessed the safety of the biomaterials, *in vitro* and *in vivo* tests to investigate the functional properties are required (Fini and Giardino, 2003).

## 4.2 Regulations and international standard organization rules

Different countries have adopted regulatory bodies to evaluate materials and devices intended for use in humans in order to establish biocompatibility and safety. Current regulations, in accordance with the US Food and Drug Administration (FDA), the International Organization for Standardization (ISO), or the Japanese Ministry of Health and Welfare (JMHW), require that manufacturers conduct adequate safety testing of their finished devices through preclinical and clinical phases as part of the regulatory clearance process.

Among the International Standards, the ISO 10993 "Biological evaluation of medical devices" refers to the fundamental principles governing the biological evaluation and testing within a risk-management process (UNI EN ISO 10993-1, 2010). ISO tests should be applied with interpretation and judgement by well-trained and experienced professionals and many factors relevant to the material, the expected applications, and the current knowledge provided by scientific literature, as previous clinical experience must be considered. The definition of categories of devices is mainly based on the nature and duration of the contact with the body, and the selection of appropriate tests is performed consequently. In particular, the biocompatibility tests must be performed on bioceramics-based materials and the final sterilized products taking into account the type, duration, and conditions of the exposure in the human body, the physical and chemical features of the product, the toxicological activity of the chemical elements or compounds, the presence of leachable materials. Biocompatibility tests investigate toxic, immunogenic, inflammatory, thrombogenic, and mutagenic effects on cells or tissues (Tables 4.1 and 4.2).

Table 4.1 **In vitro tests according to the ISO 10993**

| Test | Model | Evaluation at proper experimental times |
|---|---|---|
| Cytotoxicity ISO 10993-5 | Mammalian cell lines | Cell morphology, viability and proliferation |
| Genotoxicity, carcinogenicity ISO 10993-3 | Mammalian cells or bacteria transgenic model | Mutated cells or reverted colonies counting tumor development |
| Hemocompatibility ISO 10993-4 | Human blood | Thrombosis, coagulation, platelets, hematology, complement system |

Table 4.2 **In vivo tests according to the ISO 10993**

| Test | Model | Evaluation at proper experimental times |
|---|---|---|
| Irritation | Rabbit | Skin reaction: erythema and edema |
| Sensitization | Guinea pig | Skin reaction: erythema and edema |
| Systemic toxicity | Mouse (nonrodents: if required and appropriate) | Clinical signs, hematology, clinical chemistry, urinalysis, gross pathology, histopathology |
| Local effects after implantation (short- and long-term tests) | Mouse, rat, hamster, rabbit, sheep, goat, pig | Macroscopical and histopathological response at the implant site |

## 4.3 In vitro and in vivo tests

### *4.3.1 In vitro tests*

Test methods to assess the cytotoxicity of medical devices, according to the ISO10993-5 (UNI EN ISO 10993-5, 2009), are designed to evaluate the response of cultured mammalian cells in direct contact with the tested material or with a liquid extract test, using biological parameters. In general, established cell lines, well standardized and reproducible, are preferred to primary cultures, for both direct-contact tests, and liquid extract tests. Cytotoxic effects should be qualitatively and quantitatively evaluated after short periods of incubation by measuring cell proliferation and viability, release of enzymes in cell culture supernatant, and by examining cell morphology, membrane damage, cell lysis, and death.

Neutral Red dye is a suggested example to assess cell viability and morphology: the dye is actively incorporated by living cells, that appear red to light-microscope observation. Vacuolization, detachment, and lysis of cells can be evaluated and measured, according to a semiquantitative score (Fig. 4.1A, B).

(A) (B)

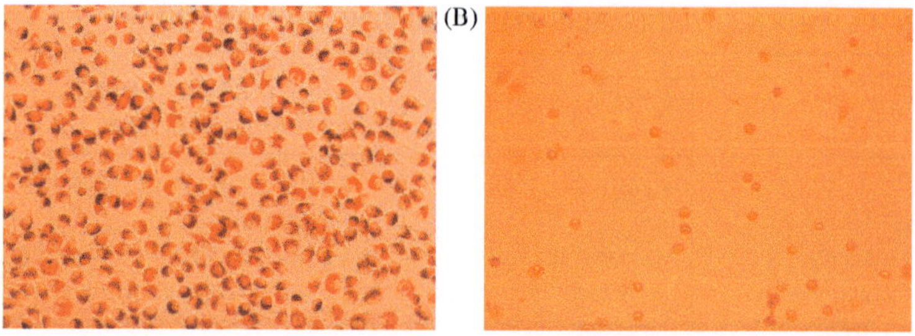

**Figure 4.1 Neutral Red staining.** Murine Fibroblasts L929 stained with Neutral Red. (A) Cells are well stained and display a normal morphology: fusiform shapes, and well-defined cell membrane margins can be observed. (B) Cell proliferation is markedly decreased and cells are not stained because they are dead, as suggested also by their rounded shape (original magnification ×4).

Genotoxicity results from alterations of the sequence of DNA and carcinogenicity describe damages of DNA that promote alteration in cell proliferation and generation of tumors. The possible risks of germ and somatic cell genetic changes by materials that will have a prolonged body contact may be investigated (ISO 10993-3) (UNI EN ISO 10993-3, 2015). The test can be performed both *in vitro* and *in vivo*. The simplest and sensitive *in vitro* assays are those involving gene mutation in bacteria and chromosomal damage in cultured mammalian cells. Only if justified on a scientific basis, and if the *in vitro* test results indicate potential genotoxicity, can the *in vivo* tests be performed (search of chromosomal aberration). The most common *in vitro* tests used are the AMES test and the micronucleus test.

#### *4.3.1.1 Ames test (OECD test Guideline 471)*

The Ames test uses different strains of *Salmonella typhimurium* that are have either frameshift or point mutations in the genes required to synthesize histidine (OECD test Guideline 471, 1997). The mutagenicity of a substance, added to the culture medium, causes a reversal (back mutation) and restores the bacteria's ability to synthesize histidine, and it is proportional to the number of colonies observed.

#### *4.3.1.2 Micronucleus assay (MN, OECD test Guideline 487)*

The guideline suggests the cell lines suitable for the *in vitro* micronucleus assay (MN) test (OECD Test Guideline 487, 2014). Micronuclei may originate from acentric chromosome fragments (i.e., lacking a centromere), or from whole chromosomes unable to migrate to the poles during the anaphase stage of cell division. A positive result is a dose-dependent significant increase in the number of cells containing MN in comparison with negative control cultures (Fig. 4.2).

In vitro test methods (ISO 10993-4) (UNI EN ISO 10993, 2002) to assess hemocompatibility include different categories (thrombosis, coagulation, platelets, hematology, and complement systems), depending on the type of device. The

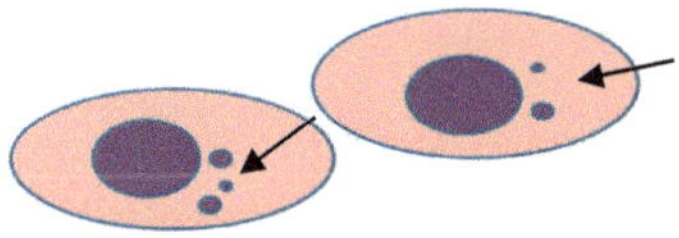

**Figure 4.2 MN test.** Scheme of Giemsa staining of TK6 cells: micronuclei are detected (*arrows*) near nuclei.

international Standard suggests a selection of the appropriate tests for the evaluation of different implant device categories and blood interaction is required for medical devices which contact circulating blood directly or indirectly. Because of species differences in blood reactivity, human blood is preferred.

## 4.3.2 *In vivo tests*

In vivo preclinical models still represent an essential step for the validation of any biomaterial with respect both to its efficacy and safety. One could say that they represent a bridge between *in vitro* studies and clinical applications (Giardino et al., 1998). In vivo studies require a thorough knowledge of and compliance with the ethical and legislative rules on laboratory animal experimentation. These regulations are accepted worldwide and are part of the International standards of material evaluation (Russell and Burch, 1959). The *Animal Welfare Act* was approved in the United States in 1966 and was followed by the *Public Health Service Policy on Human Care and Use of Laboratory Animals* and by the NIH *Guide for the care and Use of Laboratory Animals*. In the European Union the first Directive was the 86/609 – *Protection of Experimental Animals*, which indicated to the member states the guidelines to be applied in the regulation of animal research. This document was recently updated and replaced by the directive 2010/63 of 22 September 2010 on the protection of animals used for scientific purposes. As an example, in agreement with this directive, the Italian government approved the animal research Law by the Legislative Decree 26/2014 of March 29, 2014, that canceled the previous one (116/92).

Overall, the new provisions are based on the principle of the "three Rs" (Replacement, Reduction, and Refinement), an ethical guide suggesting and encouraging alternative methods to the animal models, following different strategies, from the reduction of the number of animals for each test to the complete substitution with *in vitro* tests (Smith et al., 1999). Consequently, procedures alternative to the use of animals may be adopted to minimize the number of animals involved; animal tests can be performed only if preliminary *in vitro* tests have been carried out that give suitable results. Animal experiments must be carried out in authorized laboratories, under veterinary control, with appropriate facilities for animal welfare. Surgical procedures must be performed under general anesthesia and in properly equipped operating rooms, under the control and responsibility of well-trained scientists and veterinarians. In every phase of the study, pain, suffering, and stress must be carefully monitored and avoided. A

Supervisory Board on Animal Welfare must be present where animal experiments are carried out.

The prerequisites to be accomplished when animal tests are to be performed are also pointed out in part 2 of ISO 10993 regarding the biological evaluation of medical devices entitled *Animal Welfare Requirements* (UNI EN ISO 10993, 2006). According to this guideline, the tests are justified only when the expected results are not otherwise available and are essential for the material characterization, when no other scientific validation method – not involving animals – could be used, and only after the acquisition of data obtained by *in vitro* evaluation. The strategies to minimize pain, suffering, distress, and lasting harm must be carefully considered, as well as the animal welfare, the anesthesia, and the procedures for euthanasia. The research protocol must describe in detail the scientific aims of the research, the features of the material to be investigated, the rationale for the use of animals, stating clearly that alternatives to *in vivo* experiments are not possible, and must include careful and complete study documentation. The protocol must also be approved by an Ethical Committee and submitted to the public authority, according to the regulations of each country.

Regarding the proper choice of the animal model, Einhorn emphasizes that "the appropriate use of animal models begins with careful considerations of the question asked" (Einhorn, 1999). During the *in vivo* validation of a material, the choice of more than one animal species, namely a small-/medium- and a large-sized animal could therefore be required. The use of small animals could be considered appropriate during the early stage of testing, but the tissue healing characteristics of large animals will better approximate those of humans during the last stages of research. In conclusion, the choice of an animal model must take into account regulatory requirements and assessments on ethics, availability of the animal, housing, ease of handling, costs, susceptibility to the disease, and must be supported by an appropriate background and literature data (Torricelli et al., 2004; Muschler et al., 2010; Pearce et al., 2007; O'Loughlin et al., 2008).

### 4.3.3 In vivo evaluation of biocompatibility

The irritation test (ISO 10993-10) assesses the potential of the material under test to produce dermal irritation in a relevant animal model (UNI EN ISO 10993, 2013). The test is generally performed in rabbit, using direct contact. Skin is observed for the evaluation of local effects (erythema and edema) to detect the changes. The potential for irritation is evaluated according to a suggested score grading for erythema and edema, in order to obtain the Primary Irritation Index (PII) that defines the category of response for the tested material, ranging from negligible to severe.

The maximization test (ISO 10993-10) assess the potential of a material under test to produce a cutaneous reaction mediated by the immune system. The sensitization test is performed in guinea pigs. The test is performed in three phases:

1. Intradermal induction: first contact of the material with the body by the injection of the extract material.

2. Topical induction: second contact by a topical application at the same site as intradermal induction.
3. Challenge: topical application at a different site.

Skin reaction for erythema and edema is observed and graded according to the Magnusson and Kligman grading: 0=no visible changes; 1=discrete erythema; 2=moderate erythema; 3 = intense erythema and/or swelling.

The *systemic toxicity* test evaluates the possible effects of the absorption, distribution, or metabolism of products that originate from a material or device, involving parts of the body or organs not in direct contact with them. The test will determine the systemic adverse effects that can be observed after the administration of a single dose or multiple doses of a test sample during a period of 24 hours (acute toxicity), or by exposures for a prolonged time (subacute, subchronic, and chronic systemic toxicity).

The test of *acute systemic toxicity* (ISO 10993-11) is performed in mouse by intramuscular injection of extract material. Animals are observed immediately after injection for up to 72 hours. If an animal shows severe symptoms of toxicity, further analyses are required, including gross appearance of main organs.

The test of *subchronic systemic toxicity* (ISO 10993-11) is performed in rodents, and the experimental time is usually 90 days (UNI EN ISO 10993, 2009a). The administration of a single dose or multiple doses will be established according to the characteristics of the tested material or depending on its use. If the clinical observation of animals shows severe symptoms of toxicity, further analyses are required and animals should be subjected to gross pathological examination of main organs, which should be preserved for possible future histopathological examination.

The evaluation of tissue reaction after the implantation of the material is predictive regarding the expected clinical behavior. Part 6 of the ISO 10993 considers the test to investigate the local effects after a material implant, in comparison with the effects caused by a clinically used control materials with well-assessed properties (UNI EN ISO 10993, 2009b). Surgical procedures in experimental animals are like those used in humans. Consequently, the same iatrogenic potential related to the procedure alone can be expected. An appropriate surgical technique is anyway a prerequisite for a correct *in vivo* evaluation of any device. Care must be taken to minimize tissue damage, or a possible displacement of the implant. The size and shape of the implant must be suitable for the site of the proposed implant and in agreement with the ISO 10093-6 rules. After an appropriate experimental time, several macroscopic and histologic parameters must be collected for evaluation, namely the presence of infection, inflammation, or fibrous reaction.

Bone implants are performed when the material is proposed mainly for orthopedic or maxillo-facial applications. When the evaluation concerns biomaterials intended for skeletal implants, some particular features of bone tissue must be keep in mind. Skeletal texture is in fact the combination of many components: bone, cartilage, connective, mesenchymal stromal tissue, vascular, and hemopoietic. Due to the differences in architecture, vascularization, mechanical stress, and the healing capacity of the site after the implant greatly affect both the osteointegration and the biodegradation of some biomaterials. The bone remodeling around an implant is a long-lasting process.

The sites of bone implants are usually the diaphysis (cortical bone), the epiphysis (cancellous bone) or both (Giavaresi et al., 2008b). The samples are designed according to their clinical use, and their size depends on the animal species in which the tests are performed, and of the skeletal segment in which the implant is placed.

Regarding preclinical "efficacy" tests, the capability of a material to improve bone regeneration in an *in vivo* model must be evaluated using critical size defects, namely the smallest bone defect that is incapable of spontaneous healing. The extents of these defects are related to the anatomical features of the bone, animal species and age. According to Lindsey et al. (2006), a bone defect could be considered "critical" when its length is about 2.5-times the external diameter of the same bone. As an example, in sheep metatarsus (cortical bone) the length is about 30 mm (Filardo et al., 2014), in rabbit radius diaphysis the critical defect has a length of about 10 mm, while in cancellous bone (rabbit femoral condyle), it is about 6 mm in diameter and 10 mm deep (Ambrosio et al., 2012). The histological evaluation, following the procedure used for the undecalcified or decalcified tissues, requires an accurate drawing of the samples. An adequate amount of tissue or bone surrounding the material must be withdrawn to evaluate the quality of the tissue around the implant. When hard materials are implanted in bone, the required procedure is the same as for undecalcified bone. After fixation in 4% buffered paraformaldehyde and dehydratation in graded series of alcohols, the samples are included in methyl-metacrilate. To obtain sections of appropriate thickness, the most useful procedure is obtained by a cutting-grinding system (Donath and Brenner, 1982) composed of a cutting device based on a diamond-saw and a rotable clamp on which the sample is held. The thick slices obtained thus are glued on a plexiglas slide, and are then thinned to the required thickness using a grinding system with a graded series of abrasive paper. Sections could be stained with Fast Green/Toluidine Blue/Acid Fucsin, or Stevenel's Blue.

Histology considers that the contact between bone tissue and the material at the bone/implant interface is matter of particular interest. Regarding this aspect, osteointegration is defined as the direct structural and functional connection between living bone and the surface of the implant (Mavrogenis et al., 2009).

To evaluate osteointegration, the histological observation of samples is usually performed to measure some morphological parameters. The histomorphometry measures should be obtained with image analysis systems with appropriate software. The most commonly evaluated parameters evaluated with histomorphometry are the *bone to implant contact* (e.g., the length of bone directly opposed to the implant/the total length of bone implant interface), the *bone ingrowth* (e.g., the area of the bone tissue grown into the screw thread/area between the screw threads) (Giavaresi et al., 2008a), and the *bone mirror area* which indicates the quality of the bone in the region closely contiguous to the implant (Tavares et al., 2007). The extent of fibrous tissue between the bone and the implant, if present, will also be evaluated.

The parameters related to the quality of cancellous bone in which the implant is placed are evaluated according to Parfitt (Parfitt et al., 1987; Parfitt, 1988): among them, the most significant are the trabecular bone volume (e.g., bone volume/tissue volume, BV/TV, %), the trabecular thickness (Tb.Th, μm), the trabecular number (Tb.N, /mm) and the trabecular separation (Tb.Sp, $\mu m^2$); these latter parameters are calculated from BV/TV and the perimeter of bone trabeculae using Parfitt formulae (Parfitt et al., 1987; Parfitt, 1988).

To evaluate tissue and/or inflammatory response, histomorphometric measures can be obtained with image analysis systems. These systems are composed by a microscope and a PC with appropriate software to perform interactive and automatic measurements, connected by a camera to capture images. Semi-quantitative grading scores are used to evaluate the amount of cellular infiltration, the presence of multinucleated giant cells, the vascularity, and the degree of connective tissue organization.

Considering bone implants, the rates of bone deposition and mineralization are evaluated by dynamic histomorphometry. To label the new bone deposition, fluorochromes (i.e., tetracycline, alizarin red, calcein blue, xylenol orange) are used, which are administered to the animal by injecting them at scheduled times. The fluorescence is evident on histological unstained sections at microscopic observation with appropriate filters and enhances the new deposition of bone (Jee, 2005).

Mechanical tests are also useful to evaluate the integration of the material with the bone and the bone quality. Implants in bone can be submitted to pull out and push out tests, and the whole bone to tests of three-point bending, torsion, compression (Borsari et al., 2009). Microhardness investigations, performed on the cutting surface of samples embedded in resin as for histology and carefully grounded and polished, are useful for evaluating the quality of the bone surrounding the implant (Bacchelli et al., 2009).

Besides these investigations, it is possible to perform computerized microtomography on the explanted samples; this is a nondestructive technique and the time required to capture the images is short; furthermore, the same sample can be used afterwards for the histology and histomorphometry. Microtomography gives quantitative information on the ceramic biomaterial microstructure before implantation and, after implantation, on re-adsorption rate, bone ingrowth, osteointegration, and colonization (Martini et al., 2012).

### 4.3.4 Pathological models

The use of healthy animal models for the *in vivo* validation of biomaterials is a well assessed procedure, but for a complete evaluation of materials or devices it is advisable to match as closely as possible the clinical situation in which the final product will be placed, which is often characterized by a morbid condition that may affect the outcome. This is particularly evident when the material, such as a bioceramic, is designed for use in bone. Preclinical models were therefore developed to obtain pathological conditions of clinical significance. One of the most frequent bone diseases is osteoporosis, which is related to age, postmenopausal status, or is secondary to systemic diseases or pharmacological therapies. Osteoporotic animal models are commonly used in the preclinical validation of biomaterials. Bilateral ovariectomy is the better procedure to reproduce the clinical situation of postmenopausal osteoporosis. The rat, rabbit, and sheep are the species most suitable for this purpose. In rats the osteoporotic state after ovariectomy is present from 8 to 16 weeks after ovariectomy, while in sheep the development of osteoporosis is recognizable 12 months after ovariectomy, and more evident after 24 months (Borsari et al., 2007).

The use of pathological bone-derived cell culture for *in vitro* tests (Torricelli et al., 2004), in association with pathological animal models, allows the evaluation of the different responses of bone to candidate orthopedic materials by comparing healthy and pathological conditions.

The sheep model is suitable for studies on long bones such as femur and tibia, and on the spine, were the decrease in bone mass is recognizable in the vertebral bodies (Fini et al., 2003; Nicoli Aldini et al., 2002). It must be emphasized that studies on small-sized animals like the rat are acceptable in the early stages of testing, but some differences between rat and human bone quality exist (Torricelli et al., 2003). Therefore, tests on large animals better approximate the behavior of humans, and are preferred during the last stages of research.

### 4.3.5 Advanced preclinical in vitro models

Bioceramics are mainly used for bone application, taking into account its chemical nature, typically hydroxyapatite (HA) and tricalcium phosphate (TCP), and their ability to closely bond with the host bone and to enhance bone matrix formation (Ebrahimi et al., 2017; Yunus Basha et al., 2015). HA is in fact the main inorganic component of bone tissue and its composites are considered as bone substitutes for their properties of biocompatibility, bioactivity, osteoconductivity, and osteointegration. It has been well established that HA implants or coatings show good performance in adhesion to the local tissue and in supporting bone repair processes.

In recent years, many new, complex materials based on HA have been proposed (Kuttappan et al., 2016; Deepthi et al., 2016; Khajuria et al., 2017) and their effectiveness has to be proven. To predict the *in vivo* behavior, *in vitro* tests are in general based on the study of osteoblasts, being the main cells involved in the interface with bioceramics material. Biological tests to assess osteoblast activity and differentiation, when cultured on bioceramics samples, are currently performed. Nevertheless, osteoblasts are not the only cells that interact with HA. Moreover, the microenvironment in which the biomaterials are implanted is often pathological, including inflammation, oxidative stress, and osteoporosis. Currently, research is geared toward advanced preclinical models simulating the microenvironment cell/tissue during the onset and progression of diseases. The simple and basic *in vitro* test, performed with osteoblast cell lines have, in recent years have been improved by more complex and smart *in vitro* models. These models allow better exploration of the bioactivity of new and more advanced materials, such as bulk or coatings, synthesized in the presence of various different molecules, such as antiosteoporotic agents, antibiotics, or antibacterial ions, to improve their effectiveness. These advanced models are also aimed at focusing the attention on the 3Rs principle (Russell and Burch, 1959).

#### *4.3.5.1 Co-culture in vitro models*

Co-culture models are suitable for testing biomaterials, such as bioceramics, that are able to interact with bone tissue. The system involves the interplay of different cell populations, participating in the process of bone remodeling and repair, by modulating each other's behavior.

These models require the definition of the precise settings of culture conditions, to allow proliferation and differentiation of all cell types used in the microenvironment of the model. These models may be set up using differentiated cell lines or starting from mesenchymal stem cells, whose differentiation is induced *in vitro*. Some examples are described below.

##### Osteoblasts/osteoclasts

This co-culture permits the exploration of the activity of cells that are strictly correlated in the maintenance of bone balance. It may be performed with cells in direct contact between them and with the biomaterials, or using inserts to separate different cells, but allowing the exchange of cellular products (Boanini et al., 2015).

##### Osteoblasts/osteoclasts/endothelial cells

Osteoblast and osteoclast cells are fundamental for bone turnover and angiogenetic processes that play a crucial role, as the formation of new capillaries supports osteogenesis during bone remodeling. The tri-culture model is suitable to investigate the interaction among the several cell types comprising the bone microenvironment, in which human osteoblasts are essential for bone deposition, osteoclasts for bone resorption, while endothelial cells are necessary to provide growth factors, nutrients, and oxygen in the mature tissue. Factors produced during the interaction between cells and biomaterials may be measured (Forte et al., 2016). The set-up of the tri-culture model is shown in Fig. 4.3.

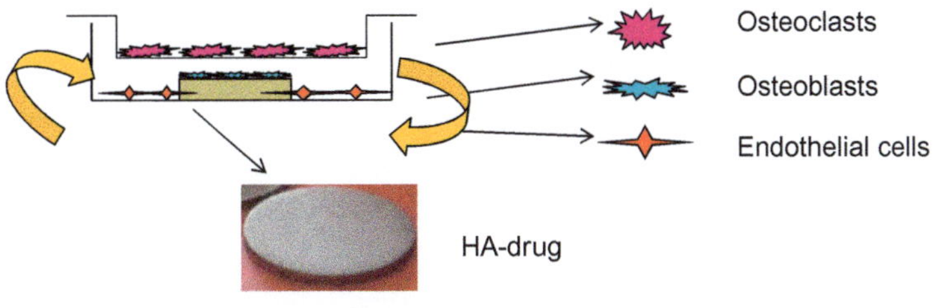


**Figure 4.3** Tri-culture model to evaluate hydroxyapatite (HA) functionalized with an antiosteoporotic agent.

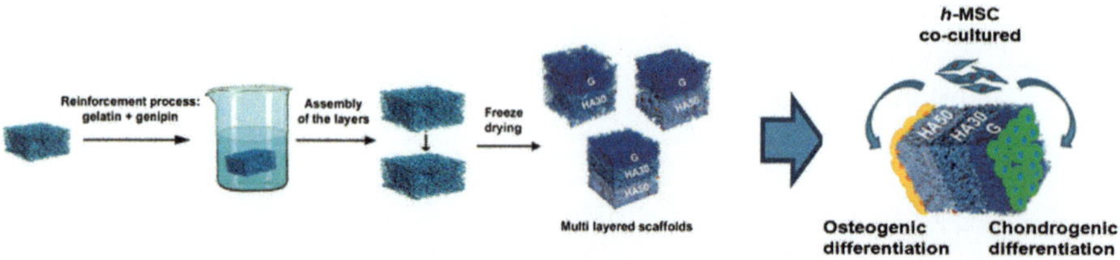


**Figure 4.4** Three-dimensional μ-CT representation of bi- and three-layered hydroxyapatite (HA) scaffolds cultured with MSCs.

### Osteoblasts/chondrocytes differentiated from mesenchymal stem cells

The model studies in which way a biomaterial or a scaffold may influence the differentiation of mesenchymal stem cells (MSCs) by means of a specific osteogenic and chondrogenic culture medium, to explore the osteochondral tissue regeneration (Amadori et al., 2015). In Fig. 4.4, a three-dimensional micro-computerized tomography (μ-CT) representation of bi- and three-layered HA scaffolds cultured with MSCs is shown. The development of multilayer, hybrid scaffolds composed of distinct but integrated layers able to mimic the different regions of cartilage and bone, is considered a promising strategy for osteochondral interface regeneration.

### *4.3.5.2 Three-dimensional models*

These models recreate *in vitro* osteochondral or bone lesions or defects and are aimed at testing biomaterials performance in a three-dimensional environment. These models allow investigation of osteointegration, microarchitecture of subchondral bone, quality of neoformed matrix, and the analyis of cell differentiation.

### Osteochondral model

An osteochondral defect is created in a biopsy of articular cartilage to simulate a lesion in the articular surface. The defect may be treated by a scaffold, cultured with cells, and also under biological or biophysical stimulation. At the end of the experimental time the model may be tested by the measure of cell products in the supernatant of culture and by histological and histomorphometric parameters.

### Bone fracture model

From a bone biopsy, a fracture is recreated *in vitro* and the regeneration of bone tissue may be simulated after the implant of a scaffold in the bone defect (Sundelacruz et al., 2013). The fracture artificial model can be evaluated over up to 6 weeks of culture by means of immunoenzymatic and histological measures.

## 4.4 Conclusions

Many and different experimental models may be adopted in order to study the safety and efficacy of ceramic materials. Many questions can be asked and the answers always require different experimental designs with the adoption of advanced evaluation techniques for both safety and efficacy. Ceramic biomaterials and scaffolds are more and more complex as far as microstructure, topography, and chemistry are concerned and, therefore, intelligent *in vitro* and *in vivo* testing strategies are mandatory.

## References


Amadori, S., Torricelli, P., Panzavolta, S., Parrilli, A., Fini, M., Bigi, A., 2015. Multi-layered scaffolds for osteochondral tissue engineering: in vitro response of co-cultured human mesenchymal stem Cells. Macromol. Biosci. 15 (11), 1535–1545.

Ambrosio, L., Guarino, V., Sanginario, V., Torricelli, P., Fini, M., Ginebra, M.P., et al., 2012. Injectable calcium-phosphate-based composites for skeletal bone treatments. Biomed. Mater. 7 (2), 024113.

Bacchelli, B., Giavaresi, G., Franchi, M., Martini, D., De Pasquale, V., Trirè, A., et al., 2009. Influence of a zirconia sandblasting treated surface on peri-implant bone healing: an experimental study in sheep. Acta Biomater. 5 (6), 2246–2257.

Baino, F., Novajra, G., Vitale-Brovarone, C., 2015. Bioceramics and scaffolds: a winning combination for tissue engineering. Front Bioeng. Biotechnol. 3, 202.

Boanini, E., Torricelli, P., Forte, L., Pagani, S., Mihailescu, N., Ristoscu, C., et al., 2015. Antiresorption implant coatings based on calcium alendronate and octacalcium phosphate deposited by matrix assisted pulsed laser evaporation. Colloids Surf. B. Biointerfaces. 136, 449–456.

Borsari, V., Fini, M., Giavaresi, G., Rimondini, L., Consolo, U., Chiusoli, L., et al., 2007. Osteointegration of titanium and hydroxyapatite rough surfaces in healthy and compromised cortical and trabecular bone: in vivo comparative study on young, aged, and estrogen-deficient sheep. J. Orthop. Res. 25 (9) September, 1250–1260

Borsari, V., Fini, M., Giavaresi, G., Tschon, M., Chiesa, R., Chiusoli, L., et al., 2009. Comparative in vivo evaluation of porous and dense duplex titanium and hydroxyapatite coating with high roughnesses in different implantation environments. J. Biomed. Mater. Res. A. 89 (2), 550–560.

Deepthi, S., Venkatesan, J., Kim, S.K., Bumgardner, J.D., Jayakumar, R., 2016. An overview of chitin or chitosan/nano ceramic composite scaffolds for bone tissue engineering. Int. J. Biol. Macromol. 93 (Pt B), 1338–1353.

Donath, K., Brenner, G., 1982. A method for the study of undecalcified bone and teeth with attached soft tissue. J. Oral Pathol. 11, 318.

Ebrahimi, M., Botelho, M.G., Dorozhkin, S.V., 2017. Biphasic calcium phosphates bioceramics (HA/TCP): Concept, physicochemical properties and the impact of standardization of study protocols in biomaterials research. Mater. Sci. Eng. C. Mater. Biol. Appl. 71, 1293–1312.

Einhorn, T.A., 1999. Clinically applied models of bone regeneration in tissue engineering research. Clin. Orthop. Relat. Res. 367 (Suppl), S59–S67.

Filardo, G., Kon, E., Tampieri, A., Cabezas-Rodríguez, R., Di Martino, A., Fini, M., et al., 2014. New bio-ceramization processes applied to vegetable hierarchical structures for bone regeneration: an experimental model in sheep. Tissue Eng. Part A. 20 (3–4), 763–773.

Fini, M., Giardino, R., 2003. In vitro and in vivo tests for the biological evaluation of candidate orthopedic materials:benefits and limits. J. Appl. Biomat. Biomech. 1, 155–163.

Fini, M., Giavaresi, G., Greggi, T., Martini, L., Nicoli Aldini, N., Parisini, P., et al., 2003. Biological assessment of the bone-screw interface after insertion of uncoated and hydroxyapatite-coated pedicular screws in the osteopenic sheep. J. Biomed. Mater. Res. A. 66 (1), 176–183.

Forte, L., Torricelli, P., Boanini, E., Gazzano, M., Rubini, K., Fini, M., et al., 2016. Antioxidant and bone repair properties of quercetin-functionalized hydroxyapatite: an *in vitro* osteoblast-osteoclast-endothelial cell co-culture study. Acta Biomater. 32, 298–308.

Giardino, R., Fini, M., Giavaresi, G., 1998. Experimental surgery in the research of artificial organs. Int. J. Artif. Organs. 21, 506–508.

Giavaresi, G., Chiesa, R., Fini, M., Sandrini, E., 2008a. Effect of a multiphasic anodic spark deposition coating on the improvement of implant osseointegration in the osteopenic trabecular bone of sheep. Int. J. Oral Maxillofac. Implants. 23 (4), 659–668.

Giavaresi, G., Fini, M., Chiesa, R., Giordano, C., Sandrini, E., Bianchi, A.E., et al., 2008b. A novel multiphase anodic spark deposition coating for the improvement oforthopedic implant osseointegration: an experimental study in cortical bone of sheep. J. Biomed. Mater. Res. A. 85 (4), 1022–1031.

Han, Y.J., Loo, S.C., Lee, J., Ma, J., 2007. Investigation of the bioactivity and biocompatibility of different glass interfaces with hydroxyapatite, fluorohydroxyapatite and 58S bioactive glass. Biofactors. 30 (4), 205–216.

Jee, W.S., 2005. The past, present, and future of bone morphometry: its contribution to an improved understanding of bone biology. J. Bone Miner. Metab. 23 (Suppl), 1–10, Review.

Khajuria, D.K., Vasireddi, R., Trebbin, M., Karasik, D., Razdan, R., 2017. Novel therapeutic intervention for osteoporosis prepared with strontiumhydroxyapatite and zoledronic acid: in vitro and pharmacodynamic evaluation. Mater. Sci. Eng. C. Mater. Biol. Appl. 71, 698–708.

Kuttappan, S., Mathew, D., Nair, M.B., 2016. Biomimetic composite scaffolds containing bioceramics and collagen/gelatin for bone tissue engineering – A mini review. Int. J. Biol. Macromol. 93 (Pt B), 1390–1401.

Lindsey, R.W., Gugala, Z., Milne, E., Sun, M., Gannon, F.H., Latta, L.L., 2006. The efficacy of cylindrical titanium mesh cage for the reconstruction of a critical-size canine segmental femoral diaphyseal defect. J. Orthop. Res. 24 (7), 1438–1453.

Martini, L., Staffa, G., Giavaresi, G., Salamanna, F., Parrilli, A., Serchi, E., et al., 2012. Long-term results following cranial hydroxyapatite prosthesis implantation in a large skull defect model. Plast Reconstr. Surg. 129 (4), 625e–635ee.

Mavrogenis, A.F., Dimitriou, R., Parvizi, J., Babis, G.C., 2009. Biology of implant osseointegration. J. Musculoskelet. Neuronal Interact. 9 (2), 61–71.

Muschler, G.F., Raut, V.P., Patterson, T.E., Wenke, J.C., Hollinger, J.O., 2010. The design and use of animal models for translational research in bone tissue engineering and regenerative medicine. Tissue Eng. Part B. Rev. 16 (1), 123–145.

Navarro, M., Michiardi, A., Castano, O., Planell, J.A., 2008. Biomaterials in orthopaedics. J. R. Soc. Interface. 5 (27), 1137–1158.

Nicoli Aldini, N., Fini, M., Giavaresi, G., Giardino, R., Greggi, T., Parisini, P., 2002. Pedicular fixation in the osteoporotic spine: a pilot in vivo study on long-term ovariectomized sheep. J. Orthop. Res. 20 (6), 1217–1224.

O'Loughlin, P.F., Morr, S., Bogunovic, L., Kim, A.D., Park, B., Lane, J.M., 2008. Selection and development of preclinical models in fracture-healing research. Bone Joint Surg. Am. 90 (Suppl 1), 79–84.

OECD Test Guideline 471, 1997. Bacterial reverse mutation test.

OECD Test Guideline 487, 2014. In vitro mammalian cell micronucleus test.

Parfitt, A.M., 1988. Bone histomorphometry proposed system for standardization of nomenclature, symbols and units. Calcif. Tissue Int. 42, 284–286.

Parfitt, A.M., Drezner, M.K., Glorieux, F.H., Kanis, J.A., Malluche, H., Meunier, P.J., et al., 1987. Bone histomorphomety: standardization of nomenclature, symbols and units; report of the ASBMR histomorphometry nomenclature committee. J. Bone Miner. Res. 2, 595–610.

Pearce, A.I., Richards, R.G., Milz, S., Schneider, E., Pearce, S.G., 2007. Animal models for implant biomaterial research in bone: a review. Eur. Cell Mater. 2 (13), 1–10.

Russell, W.M.S., Burch, R.L., 1959. The Principles of Humane Experimental Technique. Methuen, London.

Smith, A.C., Fasse, R.T., Swindle, M.M., 1999. Ethics and regulations for the care and use of laboratory animals. In: An, Y.H., Friedman, R.J. (Eds.), Animal models in orthopaedic research. CRC Press, Oxford.

Sundelacruz, S., Li, C., Jun Choi, Y., Levin, M., Kaplan, D.L., 2013. Bioelectric modulation of wound healing in a 3D in vitro model of tissue-engineered bone. Biomaterials. 34, 6695–6705.

Tavares, M.G., de Oliveira, P.T., Nanci, A., Hawthorne, A.C., Rosa, A.L., Xavier, S.P., 2007. Treatment of a commercial, machined surface titanium implant with H2SO4/H2O2 enhances contact osteogenesis. Clin. Oral Implants Res. 18 (4), 452–458.

Torricelli, P., Fini, M., Giavaresi, G., Borsari, V., Carpi, A., Nicolini, A., et al., 2003. Comparative interspecies investigation on osteoblast cultures: data on cell viability and synthetic activity. Biomed. Pharmacother. 57 (1), 57–62.

Torricelli, P., Fini, M., Giavaresi, G., Giardino, R., 2004. In vitro models to test orthopedic biomaterials in view of their clinical application in osteoporotic bone. Int. J. Artif. Organs. 27 (8), 658–663.

UNI EN ISO 10993, 2002. Biological evaluation of medical devices. Part 4 Selection of tests for interactions with blood.

UNI EN ISO 10993, 2006. Biological evaluation of medical devices. Part 2 Animal welfare requirements.

UNI EN ISO 10993, 2009a. Biological evaluation of medical devices. Part 11 Tests for systemic toxicity.

UNI EN ISO 10993, 2009b. Biological evaluation of medical devices. Part 6 Tests for local effects after implantation.

UNI EN ISO 10993, 2013. Biological evaluation of medical devices. Part 10 Tests for irritation and skin sensitization.

UNI EN ISO 10993-3, 2015. Biological evaluation of medical devices Part 3 Tests for genotoxicity, carcinogenicity and reproductive toxicity.

UNI EN ISO 10993-5, 2009. Biological evaluation of medical devices Part 5 Tests for in vitro cytotoxicity.

UNI EN ISO 10993-1, 2010. Biological evaluation of medical devices Part 1 Evaluation and testing with a risk management process.

Yunus Basha, R., Sampath Kumar, T.S., Doble, M., 2015. Design of biocomposite materials for bone tissue regeneration. Mater. Sci. Eng. C. Mater. Biol. Appl. 57, 452–463.

Zhang, B.G., Myers, D.E., Wallace, G.G., Brandt, M., Choong, P.F., 2014. Bioactive coatings for orthopaedic implants-recent trends in development of implant coatings. Int. J. Mol. Sci. 15 (7), 11878–11921.

# Part II

# Bioceramics on the Market: Issues and Perspectives

# Ceramics for joint replacement: Design and application of commercial bearings

**5**

*Corrado Piconi*
Catholic University "Sacro Cuore", Rome, Italy

**Chapter Outline**

**Abbreviations 129**
**5.1 Introduction 130**
**5.2 Development of ceramics for joint replacements 132**
5.2.1 Oxide biomaterials 132
5.2.2 Nonoxide bioceramics 143
**5.3 Requirements of ceramics in joint replacements 145**
5.3.1 Application of ceramics in hip replacements 145
5.3.2 Applications of ceramic in knee replacements 154
5.3.3 Application of load-bearing ceramics in other joints 157
**5.4 Ceramic coatings in joint replacements 159**
5.4.1 Nitride coatings 159
5.4.2 Zirconium dioxide coatings 160
5.4.3 Diamond-like carbon coatings 160
**5.5 Commercial ceramics for joint replacements bearings 161**
5.5.1 CeramTec 161
5.5.2 Mathys 162
5.5.3 Ceraver 165
5.5.4 Kyocera 165
5.5.5 CoorsTek medical 166
5.5.6 Amedica 166
5.5.7 Groupe Lépine 167
5.5.8 Morgan advanced ceramics 167
5.5.9 Signal medical corp 167
**5.6 Conclusions 167**
**References 169**

## Abbreviations

**ATZ** alumina-toughened zirconia
**CFR-PEEK** carbon fiber reinforced PEEK
**CoC** ceramic-on-ceramic
**CoP** ceramic-on-polyethylene
**DLC** diamond-like carbon

**Advances in Ceramic Biomaterials.**
**DOI: http://dx.doi.org/10.1016/B978-0-08-100881-2.00005-1**

**HIP** hot isostatic pressing
**LPS** liquid phase sintering
**Mg-PSZ** magnesia-partially stabilized zirconia
**PEEK** polyetheretherketone
**PSZ** partially stabilized zirconia
**PTFE** polytetrafluoroethylene
**RBSN** reaction bonded silicon nitride
**ROM** range of motion
**S6A** strontium exaluminate
**THR** total hip replacement
**TKR** total knee replacement
**TZP** tetragonal zirconia polycrystal
**UHMWPE** ultra-high molecular weight polyethylene
**Y-TZP** yttria-stabilized tetragonal zirconia polycrystals
**ZPTA** zirconia- and platelets-toughened alumina
**ZTA** zirconia-toughened alumina
**ZTCs** zirconia-toughened ceramics

## 5.1 Introduction

The basic idea to use ceramics in load-bearing application for orthopedics can be attributed to the surgeon Themistocles Gluck in the 1880s. In fact, he designed and manufactured a number of ivory (a natural ceramic material) devices while working in the Tendelenburg Clinic in Berlin (Eynon-Lewis et al., 1992). The most important product was an hinged knee replacement, implanted with cement, a first record too. Ivory was still in clinical use in Burma (now Myanmar) in the 1970s, as reported by Dr. U. San Baw (1970), who implanted at least 100 ivory hip endoprostheses in that country.

Today, ceramics are well-established biomaterials in orthopedics, especially as load-bearing components in joint replacements. Although the best known application of ceramics is in the replacement of the hip joint, today these materials are used in a number of other joints, such as in condyles and tibial plateau for knee replacements, glenoid head for shoulder replacements, finger joints, and disk replacements in the spine.

Among the many hi-tech ceramics (or advanced ceramics, or fine ceramics) available today, only a few are used in load-bearing applications. Among oxides, alumina (alpha-$Al_2O_3$) and zirconia (partially stabilized zirconia, PSZ; tetragonal zirconia polycrystals, TZPs) are the most widely used, while nonoxide ceramics (titanium nitrides, diamond-like carbon) are used as coatings for metallic components. Products for hip and knee joints made of silicon nitride ($Si_3N_4$) are currently under development.

The interest in oxides is justified by their excellent mechanical behavior. The high hardness of oxides is the prerequisite for low wear of the joints as well as for scratch resistance to third bodies. The stiffness of these materials ensures the dimensional stability of the components, a key feature in the design of the head-cup clearance in ceramic-on-ceramic (CoC) bearings. However, the most attractive property is the extreme chemical stability, since they do not undergo oxidative reactions. Due to the covalent or ionic nature of the chemical bonds in their structure, corrosion and ion release are impeded. This is the root of their biological safety, and of the biological safety of their wear debris if locally released. Concerns about the long-term behavior of joint replacement bearings are due to the biological response to wear debris released in the "equivalent joint space," as described by Schmalzried and Callaghan (1999).

The use of ceramics in joint replacements is aimed at minimizing the wear of the joint, a key factor for the long-term survival of the implant. The cellular reactions to the debris released from the joint trigger a cascade of events promoting osteolysis, which is still one of the main reason for reoperation of joint replacements.

Today, joint arthroplasty is performed in a high number of patients worldwide: about 2.1 million total hip replacements (THR) and 1.5 million total knee replacements (TKRs) were performed in 2015 (Organisation for Economic Cooperation and Development FR, 2015), with high clinical success. This increased the expectations of patients—many of them relatively young and active and wishing to improve their lifestyle. The longer survival of today's arthroplasties increases the relevance of primary surgery with respect to revision arthroplasty, which is more difficult to perform, costly, and has poorer outcomes.

Oxide ceramics bearings are especially suited for patients with an active lifestyle and/or long life expectancy, because their debris elicit a lower biological reactions as compared to metallic or polyethylene ones. The combination of small volume of wear with the low biological activity of the debris gives the "functional biological activity of the debris," as defined by Fisher et al. (2006). According to this parameter, the functional biological activity of alumina debris were found to be 20-times lower than cross-linked polyethylene (XLPE) ones and 80-times lower than conventional ultra-high-molecular-weight polyethylene (UHMWPE) debris. In addition, the use of both CoC and ceramic-on-polyethylene (CoP) bearings in place of metal bearings avoids the reactions induced by metallic debris (e.g., metallosis, lymphocytic reactions, or pseudo-tumors) (Daniel et al., 2012).

Evidence of low wear and biological safety supports the diffusion of ceramics in joint replacements. Arthroplasty registers show that in certain European countries (Austria, France, Germany, Italy, and Switzerland) more than 50% of the hip implants are made with ceramic ball heads. The use of ceramic heads in joint replacements is growing also worldwide, especially in United States, China, India, and Russia.

Alumina was the first oxide introduced in clinical use (see Section 5.2.1.1) for the production of ball heads and acetabular inserts for THR, as well as in bipolar heads for hemiprosthetics. In orthopedics, it become the "ceramic" and in scientific literature the use of the term "ceramic"—without any other specification—to indicate alumina is accepted. Nevertheless, this may result in confusion because of the many ceramics used in clinics or under development (e.g., yttria-stabilized tetragonal zirconia polycrystals (Y-TZP), magnesia-partially stabilized zirconia (Mg-PSZ),

$Si_3N_4$, zirconia-toughened alumina (ZTA), alumina-toughened zirconia (ATZ), etc.) besides alumina, to be used as joint replacements.

To date, alumina is being replaced progressively by alumina–zirconia composites because of the better mechanical behavior of these ceramics that allows higher flexibility in device design as well as higher reliability of ceramic components.

The number of companies manufacturing ceramic ball heads for THRs is limited. While some of them are pioneers in this field and have operated in the orthopedics markets for a long time (see Section 5.5), other companies are newcomers attracted by the growing diffusion of ceramics in arthroplasty.

Besides alumina, which is still in clinical use in some markets, some of them are making components made of alumina–zirconia composites.

The use of ceramic components in joints other than the hip is limited (see Section 5.5). Ceramics are taking their first steps by now in shoulder joints, while ceramic knee replacements are still a niche market in orthopedics. Kyocera Medical (Kyoto, Japan)—a pioneer in this field—is making femoral condyles in zirconia (Y-TZP), that have been clinically used in Japan since 2001 and have been tested in the United States by Kinamed (Camarillo, CA). In Europe, only CeramTec (Plochingen, Germany) is manufacturing zirconia- and platelets-toughened alumina (ZPTA) components for the knee implants produced by Lima Corporate now in clinical use (Villanova di San Daniele, Italy) and by Peter Brehm (Weisendorf, Germany).

Figs. 5.1 and 5.2 depict some contemporary load-bearing composite ceramics components.

## 5.2 Development of ceramics for joint replacements

### 5.2.1 Oxide biomaterials

#### 5.2.1.1 Alumina

It is known that the first mention of the use of alumina ($\alpha$-$Al_2O_3$) as a biomaterial was made in 1932 by Max Rock (1933), who issued a patent on alumina for the production of "artificial spare parts ... for humans and animal bodies." This patent had no practical consequence until the use of alumina in dental devices which took place in the 1960s thanks to the work of Dr. Sami Sandhaus inn Lausanne, Switzerland (Sandhaus, 1966). It was only during the 1950s that oxide ceramics were investigated again in load-bearing applications as bone substitutes. This was due to Lyman W. Smith who developed Cerosium, a porous alumina silicate component (65 vol% of porosity) filled with epoxy resin (Smith, 1992), aimed at the replacement of large defects in long bones. During the same era, Eyring and Campbell (1969) from the Ohio State University, developed alumina temporary osteotomy spacers and implanted them in a limited number of patients. A further significant contribution from the United States came from the research by Sam Hulbert and colleagues (Hulbert et al., 1972) from Clemson

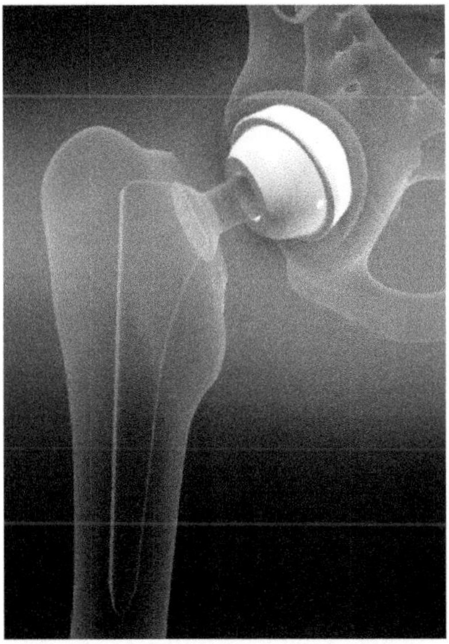

**Figure 5.1** Schematic of a total hip replacement evidencing the ceramic ball head and insert. The metallic stem and the cup shell are shadowed.
Courtesy of CeramTec GmbH, Medical Products Division, Plochingen, Germany.

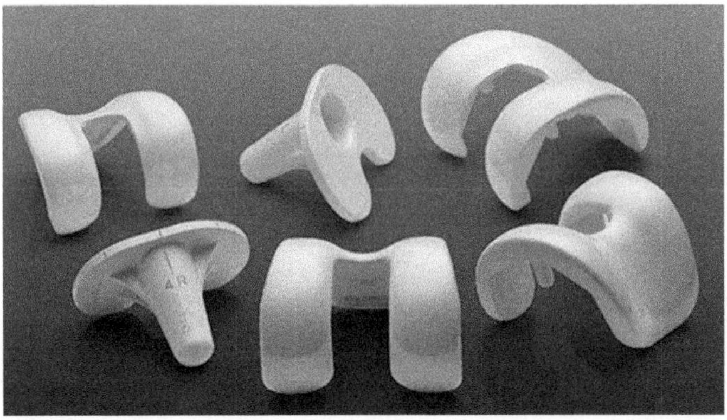

**Figure 5.2** Ceramic femoral components and tibial trays for total knee replacements.
Courtesy of CeramTec GmbH, Medical Products Division, Plochingen, Germany.

University (Clemson, South Carolina). These researchers, in fact, gave a relevant contribution to the understanding of the mechanism of bone ingrowth into porous ceramics and deepened the characteristics of the porosity allowing the implant–bone interlock.

The availability of a high-purity alumina precursor (with only minor impurities of lime)—Degussit AL23—introduced into the market by Degussa (Mannheim,

Germany) in the early 1960s, made feasible the production of pure alpha-alumina devices. Using this precursor, Sandhaus manufactured a dental implant system based on alumina dental fixtures—the CBS dental system (CBS: Crystalline Bone Screw)—which was the first alumina load-bearing implantable medical device (Sandhaus, 1969).

In the United States in 1968, the US Army Medical Research and Development Command, Dental Research Division, funded a wide research program on alumina in medical devices. In this framework, T.A. Driskell developed the Synthodont dental implant system that gained in the following years a significant clinical success (Chess and Babbush, 1980).

Alumina was the most advanced ceramic material in 1960. As an oxide, it fulfills the maximum inertia requirement, which was the key issue in the use of implantable materials at that time. In addition, high-density alumina ceramics are characterized by high hardness, the prerequisite for scratch resistance and extremely low wear. It was during the second half of 1960 that Dr. Pierre Boutin, an orthopedic surgeon practicing in Pau (southern France), started to develop its alumina-on-alumina bearing for hip replacement. It is likely that his attention to alumina was due to the early success of the Sandhaus implants. In addition, he had among his patients a top manager of CGE France, whose factory was manufacturing industrial components of high-purity alumina. Their cooperation originated Boutin's first patent issued in 1970 (Boutin, 1972), and the company Ceraver SA which is still operative in the orthopedics market.

Both the alumina cup and the metallic stem in the Boutin's implants were fixed to the host bone with cement, while the ceramic ball head was fixed by epoxy glue to a cylindrical trunnion at the extremity of the stem. This fixation originated several failures, due to the degradation of the glue. Attempts to replace the glue with a solder were also ineffective.

In Germany, the development of ceramics components for joint replacements was carried out in the framework of a wide research and development programme sponsored by the Federal Government. It involved several Universities and companies like Rosenthal (Lauf, Germany), Friedrichsfeld (Mannheim, Germany) and Feldmuhle (Plochingen, Germany) that in the first half of the 1970s put on the market a number of alumina devices. One of the key concepts in the German devices was to achieve direct-to-bone fixation. In particular, the Feldmuhle and the Friedrichsfeld cups were screwed into the bone, while the Rosenthal cup was stabilized by backside pegs. In addition, some of the stems were designed for cementless fixation.

The most interesting feature of all the German hip-replacement systems was the fixation of the ceramic head to the metallic stem by a Morse-type taper. This technical solution introduced modularity in arthroplasty and it is still used in a number of different devices, besides hip replacements.

Some of the implants with Rosenthal ball heads were fixed to the stem by an original variation of the taper connection designed to minimize the stress transfer to the ceramic head (Zeibig and Luber, 1983). This fixation was aimed at maintaining compressive stresses in the head zone close to the bore rim, and was suitable for the early generation of alumina, in which the variability in tensile properties of the material was an issue.

Rosenthal Technik (Lauf, Germany) developed a number of very innovative devices; an example is provided by the Wagner-type resurfacing devices, made of a cemented alumina femoral cup, coupled with a polyethylene acetabular component. Rosenthal also made alumina ceramic–ceramic resurfacing implants (Piconi, 2011).

A further pioneer company in the development of alumina ceramics for joint arthroplasty was the Keramische Werk Hermsdorf (KWH, Mosdorf, Germany, now Mathys Orthopaedie) in the former German Democratic Republic. Such a company developed biomedical alumina ceramics under the tradename of Bionit (Lang, 1983). Starting from 1978, KWH developed and produced alumina hip heads for joint replacements with CoP bearings. However, the most relevant KWH products were unicondylar alumina tibial replacements. These devices, implanted by Langer in 73 cases from 1972 to 1980 in the Orthopedic Clinic of the University of Jena are the first application of alumina ceramic in knee joints (Langer and Blumentritt, 1987; Langer, 2002).

Japanese researchers were also very active in developing ceramic devices. To improve the mechanical behavior, some of them investigated the feasibility of devices made from alumina single crystal (Kawahara, 1986). This original approach allowed the development of single-crystal alumina modular stems for joint replacements after resection of bone tumors (Yamamuro et al., 1989). In addition, Japanese researchers devoted relevant efforts to the development of ceramic knee replacements (see Section 5.3.5).

In spite of the many advantages of alumina ceramics, clinical results of hip joint replacements with alumina components were unsatisfactory in several cases. In particular, in the United States, the outcomes of implants made by alumina monolithic cups and cementless stems (O'Leary et al., 1988) led to the withdrawal of this system from the market. However, the reasons for this market removal were related more to the design of the implants (large and heavy monolithic devices) than to the ceramic bearing materials. In the absence of standards identifying the minimum requirements for use of alumina ceramic in medical devices, some series used in Europe experienced an unacceptable rate of failures (3%–13%) (Piconi et al., 1999).

The outcomes of early alumina implants were described in the review by Amstutz (1989), showing that the improved and carefully controlled fabrication process was the key to obtaining improved performances. However, the clinical use of these early alumina-on-alumina bearings allowed surgeons and engineers to assess their clinical advantages in terms of wear reduction and absence of particle-induced osteolysis. Notwithstanding the unsatisfactory outcomes due to the component design or to failures in the cementation, in younger patients with good bone quality—in which good primary stability in the cortical bone was achieved—several positive clinical results were reported (Richter et al., 1998; Sedel, 2004; Petzatodis et al., 2010).

Due to this situation, several manufacturers left the market of biomedical alumina, but the ones remaining started a development process aimed at increasing the mechanical properties of the products and their reliability. Namely, the analysis of the outcomes of the early alumina devices allowed learning some lessons, e.g., Piconi and Streicher (2013):

- The failures in the French series were due to (1) the unsatisfactory performances of the acetabular components and (2) the unsatisfactory fixation (glue, solder) of the ceramic head to the metallic stem (glue, solder).
- The failures in German and USA series were due to the bulky design of the acetabular component, and to the "mushroom" design of the femoral component.
- The wear rate of alumina ceramic bearings was very low in comparison with that of metal–polyethylene bearings, which was the standard at that time.
- The application of joint replacements with alumina bearings in younger patients reduced complications related to aseptic loosening of the components.

Since the second half of the 1970s to the present time, it has been possible to observe a continuous development process, aimed at increasing the mechanical properties of alumina for medical devices. Selection of ceramic precursors, optimization of batch preparation and powder consolidation routes allowed the increase in the sintered density and decrease in the alumina grain size. The most significant technological improvement was the introduction in the manufacturing process of hot isostatic pressing (HIP) and of the proof testing (Piconi, 2011). The application of Total Quality System to production allowed alumina ceramics to be produced whose bending strength was almost twice that of early materials (Piconi and Streicher, 2013). The improvement in mechanical properties of alumina—due to processing advances—are illustrated in Table 5.1, while the typical microstructure of a contemporary alumina for medical devices is depicted in Fig. 5.3.

The standards EN ISO 6474 and ASTM F603 state the characteristics of alumina for medical devices (American Society for Testing and Materials, 2016; International Standards Organization, 2010).

### *5.2.1.2 Zirconia*

Although the reliability of alumina heads and inserts increased significantly thanks to the improvements introduced in its technology, the intrinsic brittleness of the material limited the design of components. The discovery of phase transformation toughening in zirconia (zirconium dioxide, $ZrO_2$) offered to engineers the opportunity to overcome the limitations of alumina. Garvie, Hannink and Pascoe in 1975 (Garvie et al., 1975) obtained a material—called PSZ—that at room temperature is formed by cubic grains containing nanometric tetragonal precipitates. This was obtained by a careful processing and by the addition of "stabilizing" oxides to zirconia, such as CaO, MgO, $CeO_2$, and $Y_2O_3$. In particular, the addition of 8 mol% of MgO to $ZrO_2$ allows the development of tetragonal metastable precipitates (depicted in Fig. 5.4) that nucleate during controlled cooling and aging, within the fully cubic microstructure formed at about 1800°C.

The enhancement in toughness in PSZ is due to the ability of the metastable tetragonal precipitates to transform to monoclinic when the constraint

**Table 5.1 Improvements in the characteristics of medical-grade alumina**

| Property | Units | Alumina (1970) | Alumina (1974) | HIP-treated Alumina (1995) |
|---|---|---|---|---|
| $Al_2O_3$ content | vol% | 99.1–99.6 | >99.6 | >99.8 |
| Density | g/cm$^3$ | 3.90–3.95 | 3.94–3.96 | 3.96–3.98 |
| Average grain size | μm | ≤5 | ≤4 | <2 |
| Flexural strength | MPa | >300 | 400 | 550–630 |
| Young's modulus | GPa | 380 | 410 | 400 |
| Hardness | GPa | 18 | 18–19 | 19–20 |

*HIP*, hot isostatic pressing.
From Piconi, C. Alumina. In: Ducheyne, P., Healey, K.E., Hutmacher, D.W., Grainger, D.W., Kirkpatrick, C.J., editors, Comprehensive Biomaterials, vol. 1. New York; Elsevier: 2011. p. 73–94

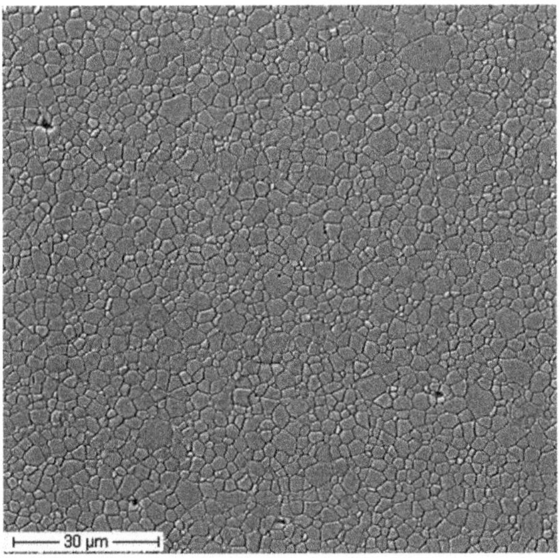


**Figure 5.3** Typical microstructure of a high density, hot isostatic pressed alumina for medical applications.
Courtesy of Dr. Thomas Oberbach, Mathys Medical, Bettlach, Switzerland.

exerted on them by the matrix is relieved, i.e., by a crack advancing in the material. The *t–m* transformation takes places at the expense of the elastic energy leading the advancement of the crack. In addition, the *t–m* transformation implies lattice expansion and shear strains. The energy associated with crack propagation is dissipated both in the *t–m* transformation and in overcoming the compression stresses

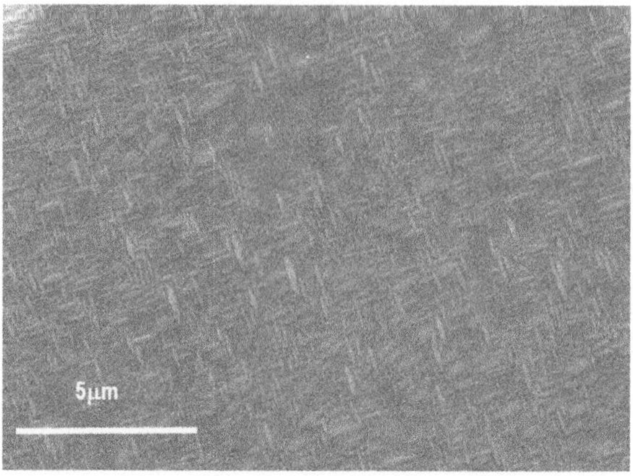


**Figure 5.4** Scanning electron microscope image of magnesia-partially stabilized zirconia (Mg-PSZ) evidencing the lenticular tetragonal precipitates within the cubic matrix. Courtesy of Dr. Goffredo De Portu, ISTEC-CNR, Faenza, Italy.

due to the volume expansion, constrained by the neighboring grains. In this case, the stress field associated with expansion due to the phase transformation acts in opposition to the stress field that promotes the crack propagation, resulting in the enhancement in toughness and strength of the material.

In 1978 Gupta and coworkers (Gupta et al., 1977) developed a zirconia stabilized by yttria, called TZP. Y-TZP containing some 2–3 mol% $Y_2O_3$ and it is almost completely constituted by tetragonal grains, some hundreds of nanometers in size (less than 0.5 μm), the balance being some cubic phase. In Fig. 5.5, a typical Y-TZP microstructure is depicted. The mechanical properties of Y-TZP ceramics depend on the fraction of metastable tetragonal phase retained at room temperature, this latter being dependent on the size of grains, on the yttria content, and on the constraint exerted on them by the matrix due to residual stresses generated on cooling. Table 5.2 illustrate some properties of Mg-PSZ and Y-TZP, in comparison with alumina ones.

However, it was observed that the metastability of the tetragonal phase—which provides the outstanding properties to Y-TZP—is also its main drawback, because the metastable tetragonal phase can transform into monoclinic in the absence of any external stress. This behavior—whose kinetics are enhanced by temperature and by a wet environment—is known as low-temperature degradation (LTD). The progress of LTD causes the decrease in strength of Y-TZP in a relatively short time (Chevalier et al., 1999) and justifies the many studies devoted to investigating this behavior. A first explanation was based on the diffusion of $OH^-$ groups in the zirconia lattice that scavenge the stabilizing yttria from the tetragonal grains (Sato and Shimada, 1985; Yoshimura et al., 1987; Lawson, 1995). More recent models take into account the role of the oxygen vacancies created by the trivalent $Y^{3+}$ cations

**Figure 5.5** Microstructure of yttria-tetragonal zirconia polycrystal (Y-TZP). Courtesy of Dr. Luciano Pilloni, ENEA, Roma, Italy.

**Table 5.2 Comparison of selected properties of yttria-tetragonal zirconia polycrystal and magnesia-partially stabilized zirconia**

| Property | Unit | Alumina | Y-TZP | Mg-PSZ |
|---|---|---|---|---|
| Grain size | μm | <2 | ≤0.5 | 20–40 |
| Density | $g/cm^3$ | 3.96–3.98 | 6.02 | 5.5 |
| Bending strength | MPa | 550–630 | 900–1200 | 400–650 |
| Fracture toughness | $MPa\sqrt{m}$ | 3.5–4 | 8–10 | 8–12 |
| Hardness | GPa | 19–20 | 12–14 | 10–13 |
| Thermal conductivity (298 K) | W/mK | 30 | 3 | 3.1 |

*Mg-PSZ*, magnesia-partially stabilized zirconia; *Y-TZP*, yttria-stabilized tetragonal zirconia polycrystals. Data on alumina are reported as reference.

that enhance the diffusion of water in the lattice (Chevalier et al., 2007; Sergo, 2010; Zhang et al., 2016).

The development of Y-TZP in clinical applications was initiated in France during the second half of 1980s (Christel et al., 1988) and was pursued up to 2000 with applications in hip and knee replacements (Calès and Stefani, 1995; Piconi and Maccauro, 1999). Over this period, many manufacturers worldwide introduced zirconia components into the market, with variable quality and behavior (Piconi et al., 2007; Yoshitomi et al., 2009). Ceramic manufacturers focused on the production on Y-TZP because the technology of PSZ requires the precise control of two process parameters, which are especially difficult to control in the large kilns used in mass production, e.g., the temperature control during cooling at the very low rate and the temperature hold time steps (aging steps) necessary to obtain the nucleation of tetragonal phase. Also the coarse grain size in PSZ was a concern for its use in components subject to wear, like the bearing of joint replacements.

The main zirconia heads manufacturer was Saint Gobain—Advanced Ceramics Desmarquest which sold more than 600,000 Y-TZP ball heads for THR under the trademark Prozyr by the year 2001. In this year, the unexpected high rate of fracture reported by two batches of Prozyr heads led to the worldwide product withdrawal, as requested by the regulatory authorities. Although the problem was limited to only two batches processed by the new tunnel furnace introduced in the production line to increase its throughput (Piconi et al., 2006; Chevalier, 2006), this issue created a lack of confidence in zirconia, which stopped being used in hip joint replacements. It is noted that the first clinical outcomes of THR bearings with zirconia ball heads reported in the literature were not clear, because of the number of different materials used and the behavior of some polyethylene cups coupled to zirconia heads (Piconi et al., 2006). Today, the use of Y-TZP in orthopedics is limited to two TKRs used in Japan, made by Kyocera (Kyoto, Japan) and to ball heads made by Signal Medical Corporation (St Louis, MO, USA). On the other hand, Y-TZP has found a wide field of application in dentistry, especially in dental implants and in the structure of crowns and bridges obtained by computer-aided design/computer-aided manufacture (CAD/CAM) machining of presintered blanks (Piconi et al., 2014).

#### *5.2.1.3 Alumina–zirconia composites*

Claussen (1976) and Becher (1991) clearly showed the increase in strength and toughness achievable in alumina ceramic by the introduction of metastable tetragonal zirconia in the alumina matrix. Nevertheless, little attention was given to these materials with reference to their applications in the medical field. The first mention of alumina–zirconia composites as biomaterials is due to Rieu and Goeuriot (1993), who carried out an early research project led by the Ecole des Mines (St Etienne, France), and aimed to develop new materials for hip-replacement bearings. The results allowed the assessment of the tissue response to these materials and gave some hints about their tribological behavior (Mandrino et al., 1990, 1992).

In the following years, a further research project on alumina–zirconia composites was carried out in the framework of the Eureka initiative (EU294). It was coordinated by Centro Ceramico (Bologna, Italy) and it was focused on the development of a new process for the production of ceramic ball heads using sol-gel synthesis and slip casting techniques (Salomoni et al., 1994; Agathopoulos et al., 1996).

Both these two research projects did not originate marketable products. In the meantime, the disappearance of zirconia from the market at the turn of the century created a technological gap in arthroplasty. The use of ceramics joints was affirmed in arthroplasty and the demand for devices with innovative and challenging design for hip, knee, shoulder, and spine could not be satisfied using alumina.

To satisfy this demand, several ceramists oriented their attention towards zirconia-toughened composite ceramics. The step forward was due to W. Burger and H.G. Ritcher who, in 1997, developed the composite known by the tradename BIOLOXdelta and commercialized by Ceramtec (Plochingen, Germany) (Burger and Richter, 2001). This composite is made by an alumina matrix containing a homogeneous dispersion of fine zirconia grains and of strontium hexaluminate platelets. Due to its excellent behavior, it has allowed the development of several new ceramic devices, and opened the way to a new class of oxide ceramic composites put on the orthopedic market by other manufacturers worldwide (see Section 5.5).

Alumina–zirconia composites used in joint replacements belong to two classes, identified either as ZTA and having alumina as main component, or as ATZ when the main component is zirconia. The ZTA material had the largest application in the last decade, because of highly suitable properties for application in THA bearings, but also due to the concerns about the use of zirconia-rich materials.

The basic concept of a ZTA material is to substantially increase the material fracture toughness and strength with respect to alumina, while maintaining the alumina properties of hardness, stiffness, and thermal conductivity, which are the rationale for its successful clinical use in joint replacements. This is achieved by exploiting the tetragonal to monoclinic phase transformation of zirconia, which is introduced in ZTA as a reinforcing element. The key point for the excellent mechanical properties of ZTA ceramics is the transformability of the tetragonal zirconia. As a consequence, the retention of a significant amount of the zirconia tetragonal phase at body temperature is essential for the desired toughening mechanism. The proper selection of the stabilizing oxide, its concentration, the homogeneous and fine distribution of Y-TZP in the alumina matrix and the control of the microstructure and grain size are key parameters to "tune" the stability of the tetragonal phase. In addition, the compressive residual stresses that develop on cooling due to the mismatch in thermal expansion coefficients between the alumina matrix and the dispersed zirconia phase increase the energy threshold for the $t$–$m$ phase transformation, contributing to the strength of the composite (Piconi and Porporati, 2016).

Besides phase transformation, a well-known method for toughening ceramics is the introduction of short fibers into the matrix. The fiber debonding by an advancing crack constitutes an effective lengthening of the crack path and is an effective mechanism for dissipating the fracture energy (Becher, 1991; Cook and Pharr, 1994).

Cutler et al. (1991) reported the increase in toughness and strength in a ceria-stabilized TZP–alumina composite where strontium hexaluminate ($SrAl_{12}O_{19}$) was nucleated in situ during sintering. As reported by Magnani and Brillante (2005) and by Kern (2014), other oxides have also been found to originate platelet-like grains during sintering of alumina–zirconia composites. This subclass of ZTA ceramics is sometimes called ZPTA, whose microstructure is shown in Fig. 5.6.

The material described in 1997 by Burger (1997, 1998) is based on this feature. It is a ZPTA (known under its tradename BIOLOXdelta) consisting of a fine-grained high-purity alumina matrix (average $Al_2O_3$ grain size about 0.5–0.6 μm), that—as main phase—determines the basic physical properties of the composite, e.g., stiffness, hardness, thermal conductivity, etc. Reinforcing elements to the microstructure determine the fracture toughness and strength. To this aim, the material incorporates about 17 vol% of zirconia in the alumina

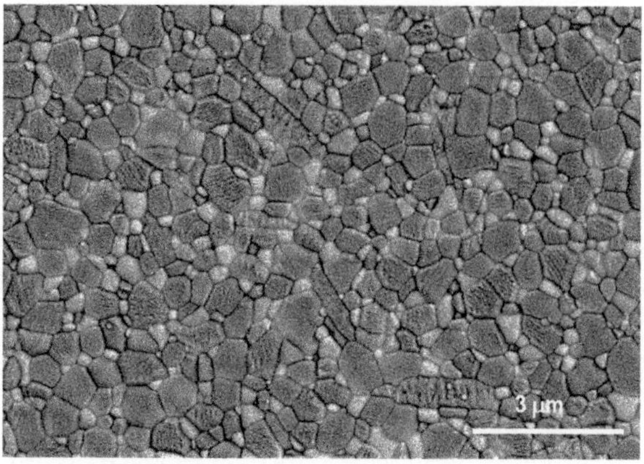


**Figure 5.6** Zirconia- and platelets-toughened alumina. In evidence is the homogeneous distribution of small yttria-stabilized zirconia grains and the elongated, platelet-like grains within the alumina matrix.
Courtesy of Dr. Luciano Pilloni, ENEA, Roma, Italy.

matrix and a further reinforcing element, consisting of elongated strontium hexaluminate (S6A) crystals with a magneto-plumbite structure. The S6A platelet-shaped grains homogenously dispersed in the ceramic composite microstructure provide an additional barrier to crack propagation, changing the path of subcritical cracks that could take place during the ceramic component's lifetime. In this way, two well-known reinforcing effects, transformation toughening and crack deflection, are operating synergistically in this alumina–matrix composite. In addition, yttria ($Y_2O_3$) solubilized in the Y-TZP phase supports its tetragonal stabilization, while chromia ($Cr_2O_3$) completely solubilized in the alumina matrix provides hardness and gives to BIOLOXdelta its characteristic, patented, pink color.

An original approach was followed by Kyocera (Kyoto, Japan) which developed a ZTA component (BioCeram AZ209) in which zirconia is stabilized in the tetragonal state by residual stresses only. This is obtained by the control of the size of zirconia crystals, which should range between the size that hinders the transformation and the size where it spontaneously transforms into monoclinic during cooling, as described by Palmero et al. (2014).

Similarly to ZTA, ATZ is aimed at combining the advantages of the two monolithic materials. So far, the only ATZ for orthopedic applications was presented in 2005 by Begand et al. (2005) and was introduced into the orthopedic marked in 2007 by Mathys Orthopedie (Bettlach, Switzerland) under the tradename Ceramys. The microstructure of this composite material is depicted in Fig. 5.7. As reported by Schneider et al. (2008), a large part of this material (80 vol%) is made by zirconia, but only about 75% of the grains are in the tetragonal state, the balance being cubic and some monoclinic phases. The mechanical behavior of the material is remarkable and in some cases is better than the ZTA alternatives (see Section 5.5).

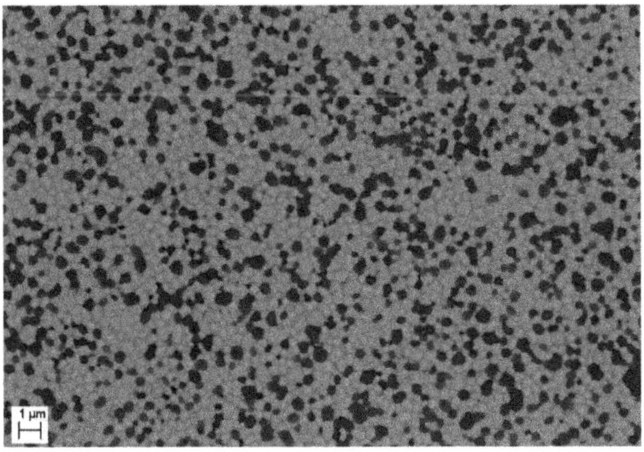

**Figure 5.7** Alumina-toughened zirconia. In evidence is the fine and homogeneous grain size of the zirconia and alumina phases of the material.
Courtesy of Dr. Thomas Oberbach, Mathys Medical, Bettlach, Switzerland.

**Table 5.3 Characteristics of alumina/zirconia ceramic composites**

| Property | Units | HIP alumina | ZTA | ATZ | ZPTA |
|---|---|---|---|---|---|
| Alumina content | vol% | >99.8 | 75 | 20 | 81 |
| Zirconia content | vol% | — | 25 | 80 | 17 |
| Density | $g/cm^3$ | 3.96–3.98 | 4.4 | 5.5 | 4.37 |
| Flexural strength | MPa | 550–630 | >700 | 1050 | >1300 |
| Young's modulus | GPa | 400 | 380 | 300 | 380 |
| Fracture toughness | $MPa\sqrt{m}$ | 4.5 | >5 | 7.5 | 7 |

*ATZ*, alumina-toughened zirconia; *ZPTA*, zirconia- and platelets-toughened alumina; *ZTA*, zirconia-toughened alumina. Data on alumina are reported as reference.

Nevertheless, due to the permanence of concerns regarding zirconia, the diffusion of ATZ in arthroplasty seems limited in favor of ZTA (Table 5.3).

## 5.2.2 Nonoxide bioceramics

Several nonoxide biomaterials are used in joint-replacement bearings. They are applied as coatings on metallic ball heads for improving the hardness of the surface and protecting it from scratches by third bodies. Nitrides (TiN, TiNbN, CrN, ZrN) and diamond-like carbon (DLC) coatings are used in this way (see Section 5.4). Among non-oxides, only silicon nitride ($Si_3N_4$) ceramics have mechanical and tribological properties suitable for use in joint replacements bearings as a bulk material; therefore a number of studies were carried out some years ago to investigate its potential. These early studies allowed the assessment of the biocompatibility of $Si_3N_4$ and its wear behavior, investigated also using hip and knee simulators (Zhou et al., 1997; Streicher et al., 1991; Piconi, 2010; Medri et al., 2016).

Silicon nitride ($Si_3N_4$) was studied for high-temperature engineering applications from 1950. Silicon nitride is difficult to sinter, because of the high degree of covalent bonding that limits the diffusion of silicon and nitrogen both in volume and at grain boundaries. Then, the early works were focused on reaction bonded silicon nitride (RBSN), a class of materials obtained by high-temperature reaction of pure silicon bodies obtained by powders compaction, characterized by high porosity and low bending strength (e.g., 200–400 MPa), then unsuitable for application in joint replacement bearings (Riley, 2000).

Until now, high-performance, fully dense $Si_3N_4$ ceramics have been obtained by liquid-phase sintering (LPS). In this process, some oxides (e.g., $Y_2O_3$ and $Al_2O_3$) are introduced as sintering aids in the powder batch to form a liquid phase that enhances the mass transport during pressure-free sintering at temperatures between 1500°C and 1700°C (Sun et al., 1998). A postsintering treatment, e.g., HIP), allows the development of elongated $Si_3N_4$ grains in a rod-like shape. The resulting material is formed by $Si_3N_4$ grains with length/thickness ratios from 5 to 10, by a crystalline secondary phase, and by an amorphous (glassy) grain boundary phase that forms a thin layer among the grains or at triple joints.

The resulting mechanical properties of LPS-HIP are increased because of the toughening effect due to crack bridging and deflection mechanisms exerted by the elongated grains. Medri et al. (2016) as well as Bal and Ramahan (2012) reported toughness up to 11 $MPa\sqrt{m}$. Some of the main properties of LPS-$Si_3N_4$ are summarized in Table 5.4.

Recently, the development of nanocrystalline DLC-coated $Si_3N_4$ ball heads and inserts was reported by Amaral et al. (2015). DLCs are carbon-based materials, formed by a dispersion of diamond "nodules" in a graphite matrix. Their characteristics are often described by the ratio sp3/sp2, e.g., the concentration of diamond-type bonds versus the graphite bonds, the ratio depending on the film deposition conditions (Yamamuro, 2008). This results in a broad family of DLCs, as recently reported by Nagashima et al. (2016). In DLC coatings, the interfacial residual stresses may reach very high values within the 1–2-μm-thick coating layer, leading to its delamination. To improve the adhesion of the coating, its deposition is made as

**Table 5.4 Liquid-phase sintering silicon carbide: selected properties**

| Property | Unit | Value |
|---|---|---|
| Density | $g/cm^3$ | 3.15–3.26 |
| Bending strength | MPa | 800–1100 |
| Young's modulus | GPa | 300–320 |
| Fracture toughness | $MPa\sqrt{m}$ | 8–11 |
| Vickers hardness | GPa | 13–16 |
| Thermal conductivity | W/mK | 30–40 |

Based on data from Medri, A., Landi, E., Bellosi, A., 2016. Non-oxide ceramics. In: Sonntag, R., Kretzer, J.P., editors, Materials for Total Joint Arthroplasty. London: Imperial College Press. pp. 183–221.

a multigrade multilayer coating, as reported by Almeida et al. (2007) and by Salgureido et al. (2013). The results of tests performed on a hip simulator on a CoC bearing formed by nano-DLC-coated $Si_3N_4$ pairs show promising results.

## 5.3 Requirements of ceramics in joint replacements

The basic requirements of a ceramic biomaterial for the production of bearings for joint replacements are summarized as follows:

1. biological safety of the material, of its debris and of its degradation products, if any;
2. chemical stability in the long term: absence of corrosion/ion release;
3. suitability of the mechanical properties to ensure the component expected behavior;
4. physical stability in the long term: very low wear, absence of swelling, stiffness under load;
5. high surface finish achievable: resistance to third-body scratching;
6. suitability for the geometrical design of the components;
7. workability by common mechanical tooling;
8. contained production costs.

In this subchapter, special emphasis is given to cases related to ball heads for hip replacement bearings, because this is the most common application of load-bearing ceramics in joint replacements.

### *5.3.1 Application of ceramics in hip replacements*

Notwithstanding the high number of THR presently offered by the implants manufacturers on the orthopedic market worldwide, their design is based on several common features. The femoral component is constituted by a stem to be inserted in the femoral canal hosting at its proximal extremity a ball head, the head is articulating into the acetabular component of the implant (the cup, the socket), made by an insert (ceramic or polymeric) fixed into a metallic shell. Both the stem and the cup may be cemented into bone, or cementless positioned. For the extent of this chapter, we are only concerned with ceramic heads; however, we should recall that there is still a widespread use of metallic heads (usually CoCr-alloy) and that all-polyethylene cups are also in clinical use. Consequently, THR bearings are categorized as hard-on-hard or hard-on-soft bearings. The different bearing configurations are summarized in Table 5.5.

The choice of the bearing couple marks the difference among countries: while in the EU, Japan, and Korea there is a prevalence of the use of ceramic heads (e.g., configuration CoP), in the United States and Australia the CoCr-alloy is the material of choice for THR heads. In the acetabular side, cross-linked UHMWPE (XLPE) is the material more used worldwide; however, in France and in Korea CoC is the preferred bearing, as depicted in Fig. 5.8 . It is noted that the market is evolving very quickly, and the use of ceramic heads in arthroplasty is growing, especially coupled with XLPEs.

Table 5.5 **Bearing couples with ceramic components in hip arthroplasty**

| Inserts / Heads | Hard-on-hard | | | | | Hard-on-soft | | | |
|---|---|---|---|---|---|---|---|---|---|
| | **Alumina** | **ZTA** | **ATZ** | **ZPTA** | **$Si_3N_4$ (exp.)** | **UHMWPE** | **XLPE** | **Vit.E-XLPE** | **PEEK (exp.)** |
| Alumina | X | | X | X | | X | X | X | X |
| ZTA | | X | X | | | | X | X | |
| ATZ | | | X | | | | | X | |
| ZPTA | | | | X | | | X | X | X |
| $Si_3N_4$ experimental | | | | | X | | | X | |
| Mg-PSZ | | | | | | X | X | X | |
| Y-TZP | | | | | | X | X | X | |

*ATZ*, alumina-toughened zirconia; *Mg-PSZ*, magnesia-partially stabilized zirconia; *PEEK*, polyetheretherketone; *UHMWPE*, ultra-high-molecular-weight polyethylene; *XLPE*, cross-linked polyethylene; *Y-TZP*, yttria-stabilized tetragonal zirconia polycrystals; *ZPTA*, zirconia- and platelets-toughened alumina; *ZTA*, zirconia-toughened alumina.

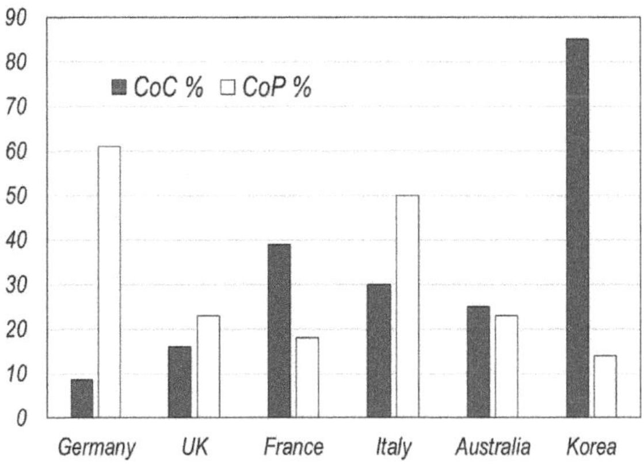


**Figure 5.8** Use of ceramic-on-ceramic (CoC) and ceramic-on-polyethylene (CoP) bearings in total hip replacement in selected countries.

### *5.3.1.1 Design of ceramic bearings*

Ceramic ball heads are manufactured in several diameters depending on the material. The standard series of ball head diameters is 28, 32, 36, 40, 44 mm. For any diameter the depth internal of the conical bore can be selected in four steps, identified by the resulting neck length of the implant, i.e., +5 mm (XL, extra-long neck), +3.5 mm (L, long neck), 0 mm (M, medium neck) and −3.5 mm (S, short neck) (Piconi, 2011). It is noted that with composite ceramics (e.g., BIOLOXdelta, CeramTec GmbH, Plochingen, Germany) it is possible to decrease the diameter down to 22.2 mm (7/8 in) for the Charnley's Low Friction Arthroplasty system and its evolutions but XL necks are not available in these designs. However, not all the manufacturers are offering such a wide array of ball head designs.

Whatever the ball type, the taper connection transfers the loads due to patient activity to the ceramic head generating two main tensile stresses in the ceramic head, e.g., in the head dome, and homoradial (hoop) stresses close to the taper surface (Andrisano et al., 1990; Middleton et al., 1994; Weisse et al., 2003).

As remarked in the introduction of this chapter, the taper connection developed for the head-stem connection in THR by the German researchers in the early 1970s made possible the modularity, which is now widely used in a number of joint replacements. The taper connection allows the insertion of a conical trunnion made on the stem into the bore made inside the ceramic head. Thanks to the modular design, a stem may host metallic or ceramic heads, while a modular acetabular socket can host ceramic or polyethylene inserts. The number of available size gives rise to a family of bearings, providing the selection of the wear couple that suits better the needs and the anatomy of the patients. The taper fitting offers several specific features:

- the connection of the head to the stem is easy and quick to perform, facilitating the handling of the head in the surgical theater;

- the connection is stable in the long term, ball-to-stem movements are eliminated;
- no adhesives or solders are necessary, whose stability may pose problems in the long term.

The taper fitting more common in Europe is the so-called 12/14 taper. This denomination does not correspond to the real geometry of the taper, whose angle, length, upper and lower base diameter may differ widely among the different implant systems, as shown in Fig. 5.9. In addition, implants of different models made by the same manufacturer may have different designs of the taper connection. Kiefer et al. (2014) reported at least eight different taper designs that are called 12/14, although their diameter was in the range from 11.0 mm to 12.7 mm and their angle in the range from 5°20′0″ to 5°40′30″. Calés and Stefani (1998) analyzed 20 different taper designs, observing significant variations between the top of the trunnion with respect to the center of the ball head and of the distance between the top of the trunnion and the bore rim, both parameters relevant for the stress distribution within the ball head. In addition, the variability among the tapers of the different implant systems are enhanced by the machining tolerances and by the surface finish of the taper itself, which are specific to each manufacturer and to each THR system (Munir et al., 2015). In consequence of the many variables that characterize each taper, it is evident that coupling between stem and head is not made at random, but carefully following the instructions given by the implant manufacturer.

It is known that the frequency of fracture of 28-mm heads made of alpha alumina is higher than that of 32-mm heads or bigger, and that the fracture frequency of medium neck (M-neck) heads is lower than the one of L- and S-neck heads. Then, although much of the attention is always devoted to the ceramic, the design of the metallic trunnion also plays a relevant role, because stresses in the ceramic depend on taper characteristics such as, e.g., stiffness, extent of the contact, cone angle, surface roughness, roundness, and straightness. Moreover, the perfect matching of the metal trunnion with the ceramic taper is only an ideal representation of the reality: the unavoidable tolerances in machining the metallic and ceramic surfaces through which the loads are transferred are relevant for the stress distribution in the system (Piconi, 2011; Piconi et al., 2005). To compensate for the deviations due to machining tolerances, implant manufacturers take advantage of the ductility

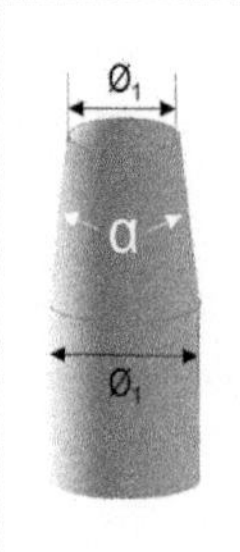


| Type | α | L (mm) | $Ø_1$ (mm) | $Ø_2$ (mm) |
|---|---|---|---|---|
| A | 5°44′ | 16.74 | 12.87 | 13.61 |
| B | 5°40′ | 10.00 | 14.29 | 15.28 |
| C | 5°44′ | 16.13 | 11.66 | 12.46 |
| D | 5°38′ | 17.78 | 12.03 | 14.03 |
| E | 5°38′15′ | 12.19 | 12.03 | 13.74 |
| F | 5°40′ | 10.50 | 11.03 | 12.34 |

**Figure 5.9** Geometrical variation among male tapers for total hip replacement stems.

of metals, i.e., providing grooves in the trunnion surface ("structured" taper). The angle of the bore into the head is slightly wider than the trunnion angle, so that when the head is positioned onto the trunnion and loaded, the tip of the grooves will be deformed progressively. In this way, the contact area is increased and stress concentrations are avoided. Also the head-trunnion friction torque is increased by the plastic deformation of the metal, improving the rotational stability of the coupling (Piconi, 2011). The observation of marks of transferred metal in the bore of retrieved ceramic heads demonstrates the formation of a ceramic–metal diffusion joint at the taper interface (Willmann et al., 2000; Masson, 2009).

In the large majority of hip replacement systems now on the market, the acetabular components (the socket, the cup) also have a modular design, consisting of a metallic shell (the metal back) hosting a ceramic or UHMWPE insert (or inlay) fitted into the shell by a taper connection. To date, the use of inserts made of CoCr alloys has practically been abandoned in hip arthroplasty, due to concerns about the biologic reaction to cobalt debris (Medicine and Healthcare products Regulatory Agency, 2012; Amatullah et al., 2016).

Whatever the design of the implant system, the mechanical interlock between the liner and the metal back has to ensure the stability of the insert, that once seated into the metal back has to resist to pull out, to torsion moments, to lever out moment due to the forces exerted on it during its clinical use. It is noted that the taper must be self-locking, but it must also be possible to remove the components intra-operatively, or at the time of revision surgery, if necessary. For this reason, 1:3 taper (about 18 degrees) was selected for sockets, allowing the ceramic insert removal by, e.g., a stroke on the rim of the metal back (Piconi, 2011). The intraoperative malseating of the insert is the main cause of chipping or fracture of the ceramic inserts. To facilitate the positioning of the insert in the shell, several solutions have been developed, e.g., insert design that include a peg in the apical part, to guide the seating of the component. In addition, the design of ceramic inserts must consider that, when the insert is completely seated into the metal back, the contact will be limited to the tapered part only, because contacts in the dome region will push the insert out of the shell. Opposite considerations may be applied when using UHMWPE inserts in the same metal back. Due to the difference in elastic properties between ceramic and polyethylene, the initial contact of UHMWPE inserts has to take place in the inner part of the taper, and has to be extended to the dome region to achieve the maximum load transmission with minimum deformation, avoiding in such a way a "brake" effect on the ball head.

Not all the manufacturers are offering CoC bearings. The design of CoC bearings has several critical points, the main one being the ball-insert clearance, a design parameter of paramount relevance on the performance of ceramic bearings.

This is determined by the difference in diameter between the ball head and the insert, and by their roundness. Up to the early 1990s, ceramic bearings manufacturers recommended the installation of CoC bearings as "selected pairs" due to the variability in roundness and roughness of the components. Today, thanks to the improvements in the manufacturing process, deviation from roundness are of the order of one micrometer. It is then possible to control the clearance of CoC bearings, whose optimal value is between 10 and 50 μm (Piconi, 2011). The clearance is a key parameter in ensuring the long-lasting performance of the joint: the continuity of the fluid film at the joint interface depends on this parameter, which must be carefully controlled by the prosthesis manufacturer (Piconi and Porporati, 2016).

As the clearance of the joint depends on the machining tolerance on a component's roundness, mixing ceramic balls and inlays from different manufacturers is not permitted, only manufacturer-approved combinations and size must be used.

Artificial joints are to be designed to enable the whole range of physiological movements (flexion, extension, abduction, adduction, and rotation) then THRs are currently designed to allow a range of motion (ROM) at least of 120 degrees. The increase in diameter may allow ROM of 135–140 degrees, and the increase in diameter of THR bearing is a trend clearly observable in hip arthroplasty during recent years. Bearings of 36 or 40 mm are now usual in many THR systems. Large bearings are made both in CoC and CoP bearings, this last exploiting the wear behavior of the new cross-linked polyethylenes and doped by vitamin-E as antioxidant (see Section 5.3.1.3).

Thanks to the higher ROM, the risk of impingement of the cup rim and of the stem neck is decreased, as demonstrated by Willmann et al. (2000). Besides the consequence in terms of component damage and release of wear debris, the increase in bearing diameter increases the "jumping distance" of the joint, e.g., the displacement necessary to permanently dislocate the head from the socket, decreasing the risk of implant dislocations that are among the main complications in THR (Willmann, 1998; Zagra et al., 2004).

This is especially relevant for young and active patients, or for patients demanding high joint mobility due to their resting position (squatting) (Piconi, 2011). Nevertheless, the increase in the diameter of the bearing could provide some drawbacks, because it implies the increase in the overall diameter of the socket. On the contrary, it is important to limit the overall diameter of the implant, both to save the patient's bone stock, and to adapt the implant for smaller anatomies (e.g., female or Asian patients). As a consequence, it is necessary to limit the thickness of the cup, thus limiting the thickness of the shell and of the insert, but without compromising the stiffness of the whole cup. This is a very challenging task in the design of the implant (Amlie et al., 2010).

In light of the above issue, the use of ceramics in larger bearings is very interesting, because of the low friction of CoC surfaces that do not lead to increase in wear or torque for bigger head diameters (Pandorf, 2007). The mechanical behavior of composite ceramics made feasible the design of thinner, stiff inserts in CoC bearings with a high level of reliability, making feasible the introduction in joint arthroplasty of the so-called monoblock cups, devices with ceramic inserts preassembled in the factory (DeltaMotion, DePuy, Leeds, UK).

The unsurpassed mechanical behavior of the ZTA and ATZ composites now available allows further development in the design of cementless all-ceramic cups. Namely, it was demonstrated that it is possible to impart bone bonding behavior to the external surface of ceramic cups, achieving osseointegration of the device, as demonstrated in animal trials (Girard, 2015; Schreiner et al., 2002; Theelke et al., 2009). In these devices, the thickness is the minimum available with the present technology, and if introduced in clinical use, it will allow the maximum part of the patient bone to be kept in the acetabular side. By composite ceramics, it was also possible to rejuvenate the ceramic resurfacing (Schreiner et al., 2012; Randelli et al., 1983), to design and manufacture prototypes of a new ceramic resurfacing device, not in clinical use yet (DeltaSurf, Finsbury Development, Leeds, UK) (Dickinson et al., 2011).

### *5.3.1.2 Hard-on-hard bearings*

The improvement introduced in the in manufacturing process of ceramic components has improved the survival of CoC THRs that in modern implants reach up to 97% at 10 years (Jeffers and Walter, 2012). Taking into account the risk of wear-debris-induced aseptic loosening, the low wear of CoC bearings joined to the high biological safety of ceramic debris makes periprosthetic osteolysis a rare event (Sedel, 2012). Because the patient's bone stock is preserved, the revision surgery of hip replacements with CoC bearings—when occurring—is easier and has better outcomes than those performed in implants with different types of bearings (Sedel, 2012; Hannouche et al., 2011). Thus, CoC bearings are especially suitable for young and active patients, who are the group with the higher expectations after surgery, but also with the higher risk of revision because of their higher activity levels and demands.

The use of alumina ball heads is today limited to niche markets replaced by the better-performing alumina–zirconia composites. The production worldwide of alumina heads of the major manufacturer (Ceramtec, Plochingen, Germany) is about 10% of its total production, whereas the production of alumina inserts has been practically stopped.

This is because the CoC bearings made of composites offer higher reliability in comparison with "pure" alumina, especially when the bearing operates in off-normal conditions. Namely, the suboptimal orientation of the acetabular component (e.g., anteversion or inclination outside, the so-called Lewinnek's safe zone (Lewinnek et al., 1978)) may lead to the concentration of stresses in the rim of the insert. A consequence of edge loading is the so-called stripe wear, the evidence of a narrow zone of high wear in the articulating surface of the ball head due to the concentrated cyclic stresses (Mak et al., 2011). A further off-normal condition that may be experienced by the bearing is due to the microseparation wear. This working condition is due to periprosthetic soft tissue laxity, and consists of the separation of the head from the insert during the gait cycle and its successive relocation. The wear of alumina heads in microseparation is much higher than that of composite ceramics, as demonstrated by Stewart et al. (2003) and by Al-Hajjar et al. (2013), due to the better strength and toughness of the composite ceramic tested.

Although now replaced by ceramic composites in most of the THR systems, the reliability of high-quality alumina in CoC bearing couples is remarkable. Tateiwa et al. (2008) carried out a survey on alumina bearings implanted in the

United States and observed only 24 fractures that took place on more than 35,000 cases followed from 3 to 25 years. A further feared complication of CoC bearings is the intraoperative chipping of the rim of ceramic insert that occurred in 2%–3% of implants.

Absence of osteolysis in implants performed in young and active patients was observed by D'Antonio et al. (2014) in a multicentric perspective clinical study on third-generation CoC bearings with alumina components. The THR 10-year postoperative survival in this cohort was 97%. Similar survival (96.5%) was reported by Imbuldeniya et al. (2013) in a series of 120 arthroplasties in patients younger than 55 years that could go back to sport practice or to heavy work.

The different composite ceramics now on the market—provided that the components of the various manufacturers are not coupled at random —not only provide a reduction in wear of the bearing, but also higher reliability. The most well-known is BIOLOXdelta (Ceramtec, Plochingen, Germany) which is the first of this class of materials, introduced to clinical use in 2004 (Piconi et al., 2005). It can be estimated that by December 2016, about 6.5 million BIOLOXdelta heads and inserts have been released to the market worldwide, and this material can be taken as the reference ceramic in hip arthroplasty.

Massin et al. (2014) reported the data of the French National Agency for Medicines and Health Products Safety (ANSM) on the fracture frequencies of BIOLOXdelta liners (0.025%) and of ball heads (0.0013%), that closely match the 0.001% (1/100.000) for heads and 0.021% for inserts that Sentuerk et al. (2016) reported as a result of the manufacturer's records.

So far, the report of the largest prospective, randomized, multicenter trial carried out on BIOLOXdelta is by Hamilton et al. (2015). They observed similar survival in two groups of CoC THR and in CoP THR, both with BIOLOXdelta heads at an average follow-up of 31.2 months (range: 21–49 months), in good correspondence with the data of other authors (Cai et al., 2012; Aoude et al., 2015).

Since 2007, a new hard-on-hard bearing composed of a ceramic ball head articulating on a CoCr-alloy insert was introduced in hip arthroplasty. The CoMplete Acetabular Hip System (DePuy Intl, Leeds, UK) was approved by the FDA for clinical use in the United States in June 2011. The aim of this device was to avoid the risk of insert chipping and to decrease the overall diameter of the implant by decreasing the thickness of the insert, thus allowing the use of larger-diameter bearings and hence increasing the ROM of the joint. Although first clinical tests were looking promising (Williams et al., 2007; Cigada et al., 2011), poor survival of the implants was evident 5 years postoperatively: patients were showing high levels of metal ions in blood and radiological evidence of loosening (Hill et al., 2015; Zeng Yi et al., 2016). Today, DePuy seems to have abandoned this technology is in favor of large-diameter cups with factory-installed ceramic inserts (DeltaMotion).

### *5.3.1.3 Hard-on-soft bearings with ceramic heads*

The hard-on-soft configuration is a tradition in THR since 1960, when Sir John Charley selected UHMWPE for the acetabular component of low-friction arthroplasty, after that the first attempts made with polytetrafluoroethylene (PTFE) resulted in a series of failures. The UHMWPE debris generated by the wear of the bearing was identified as the origin of the cascade of events leading to aseptic loosening of the implants (Willert and Semlitsch, 1977). The increased number of hip arthroplasties performed in more active patients has enhanced the relevance of the risk of complications related to wear debris. As evidenced in the introductory part of this section, there are several ceramics that can be used for the ball heads, and a number of polymeric materials that can be used for the articular surface of the cup.

Since the first years after the introduction of ceramics in hip arthroplasty, the decrease in wear of CoP bearings in comparison with bearings made with metallic heads has been evident. This is due to the better surface finish achievable in ceramic ball heads as well as to the high scratch resistance of oxide ceramics.

A number of investigations were carried out to improve the tribological behavior of UHMWPE, e.g., by the introduction of second phases (e.g., glass fibers, carbon fibers). Today, the solution that is widespread in arthroplasty consists of improving the mechanical properties of UHMWPE by the increase of the cross-linking of the molecular chains, and a number of different cross-linked polyethylenes were developed (see Table 5.6). The development of this technology was comprehensively illustrated by Brach del Prever et al. (2009) and more recently by Oral and Muratoglu (2016). Alternate approaches consist of the development of inserts made of alternative materials, e.g., polyurethane (PU) and polyetheretherketone (PEEK), which in some cases could be reinforced with carbon fibers (CFR-PEEK).

The number of possible bearing couples makes it difficult to evaluate the behavior of the different materials, due to the high number of variables, as summarized by Kabo et al. (1993): (1) thickness of the insert; (2) bearing diameter; (3) extent of the articular surface; (4) patient activity level; (5) overall design of the cup.

**Table 5.6 Some cross-linked ultra-high-molecular-weight polyethylene (UHMWPE) used in hip arthroplasty**

| Generation | Manufacturer | Tradename |
|---|---|---|
| 1st Generation | Biomet | ArCom |
| | DePuy J&J | Marathon |
| | Smith & Nephew | Reflection |
| | Stryker | Crossfire |
| | Sultzer | Durasul |
| | Zimmer | Longevity |
| 2nd Generation | Stryker | X3 |
| | Biomet | E1 |
| | DJO Surgical | E-plus |
| | DePuy J&J | AOX |
| 3rd Generation | Corin | E-CiMa |
| | Zimmer | Vivacit-E |
| | Mathys | Vitamys |

Moreover, the different modes of implant fixation, different polyethylene materials, and the number of methods for the measure of wear contribute to the complexity of the study. Nevertheless, there is general consensus on the evidence of the reduction of wear by using ceramic ball heads instead of metallic heads in hard-on-soft THR bearings.

The reduction in polyethylene wear was already evident in long-term follow-ups carried out with alumina on standard UHMWPE. Delaunay (2001) reported 13% revision at 20 years in subjects under 40 years of age, while Meftah et al. (2013) at follow-up between 15 and 20 years observed that the mean wear rate in THR with ceramic heads was about half that of THR with metal heads. The introduction of bearings with composite ceramics heads and XLPE inserts further improved the performance. For example, White et al. (2013) observed that in the hip arthroplasties made in the Ranawat Orthopedic Center using BIOLOXdelta-on-highly XLPE bearings, the wear rates were lower than in cases with metal heads running on the same XLPE (0.006 mm/year vs 0.011 mm/year).

Investigation of the wear behavior of CFR-PEEK cups coupled with alumina ball heads gave promising, preliminary results (Wang et al., 1999). Clinical study was performed only in a limited number of patients, using a monolithic CFR-PEEK cup coupled with alumina ball heads (Pace et al., 2008). At the same time, the design of a horseshoe-shaped, flexible acetabular cup (the MITCH-PCR device) (Ahmed et al., 2008) was proposed. Although the results obtained were judged positively by the investigators, both these devices are not in clinical use so far.

### 5.3.2 Applications of ceramic in knee replacements

The issue of wear is becoming more and more relevant in knee replacements, because the number of implants performed each year is growing, and more and more young patients are today candidates for knee-replacement surgery. The use of a ceramic in-knee replacement has several potential advantages: first, an improved lubrication of the articulating surface due to the high wettability of ceramic surface by the synovia liquid and then a lower wear rate of the polyethylene liner on the tibial component. A further reason for the selection of ceramics in knee replacements is linked to the growing incidence of allergic reactions to metal ions, and of the wide metallic surface that patients may develop for the presence of different metallic implants in several anatomical districts of the body. A reduction in polyethylene wear can also be expected for the better scratch resistance of the ceramic surfaces, in comparison with metallic alloys, which will save the status of the polished articulating surfaces (Piconi and Maccauro, 2016).

Although the first use of alumina in the knee is due to Langer, who used unicompartimental tibial plateau replacements (Langer and Blumentritt, 1987; Langer, 2002), the development of ceramic TKR was started in Japan in the 1970s by the late Hironobu Oonishi, a pioneer in the development of ceramic devices. These TKRs (the so-called KOM-1)—made by the company Kyocera

(Kyoto, Japan)—were formed by an alumina femoral component articulating on a polyethylene insert hosted on an alumina tibial plateau, and were cementless implanted in 134 patients (Oonishi, 1990; Oonishi et al., 2006). Kyocera also developed unicompartimental knee replacements that showed high success rates at controls made at an average 42 months after surgery (24–68 months) (Atsui et al., 1997).

Since then, several other TKR designs based on alumina have been developed in Japan, such as the Low Friction Anatomical (LFA-1), the Yokohama Medical Ceramic Knee (YMCK), the Bisurface knee replacement designed by the University of Kyoto all made by the company Kyocera (Kyoto, Japan), and the Kyoto Ceramics-1 (KC-1) (Piconi and Maccauro, 2016).

Other researchers focused their work on the development of TKRs with zirconia femoral components. Payten and Ben Nissan (2000) reported the results achieved in the design and prototyping of a modular knee replacement using Mg-PSZ for its femoral component, made by ICI Advanced Ceramics (Melbourne, Australia).The ceramic condyles were clipped on a metallic baseplate hosting a metallic stump aimed to its cementless fixation in the femur after condyles resection. There are no further mentions of this device in the literature.

Unsatisfactory short-term clinical results were reported by Vavřík et al. (2008) and by Veigl et al., (2011) in a series of 20 TKRs with zirconia femoral condyles implanted in 20 patients in the University Hospital Motol (Praha, Czech Republic), but by now the development of these devices seems to have been abandoned.

A TKR with Y-TZP condyles made by SGCA Desmarquest was used in a clinical trial sponsored by Encore Orthopedics (Austin, Texas) (Blaise et al., 2002). After the abandoning of bioceramics production by SGCA Desmarquest, this project went on with a ceramic component made by Kyocera, which is presently manufacturing for the Japanese market the Bisurface Knee replacement and the LFA THR. The clinical trial of a knee replacement with azirconia femoral component was started in 2004 in the United States by the company Kinamed (Camarillo, CA) (Bal et al., 2005), but the development of this product seems to have now stopped. The contemporary development of femoral components for knee arthroplasty made of alumina matrix composite (CeramTec, Plochingen, Germany (Heimke et al., 2002)) in association with concern for failures, similar to the ones that took place in ball heads for hip replacements, may have contributed to the dismissal of this project.

So far, BIOLOXdelta components are used in two different knee replacements, the Multigen Plus Total Knee Replacement designed by LIMA Corporate (San Daniele del Friuli, Italy) (Dalla Pria et al., 2006) and the BPK-S designed by Peter Brehm (Weisendorf, Germany). The Multigen Plus TKR (depicted in Fig. 5.10) is already available for clinical use, while clinical tests on BPK-S (Fig. 5.11) are still in progress. The early series of the Multigen Plus TKR had a metallic tibial tray, replaced in its current version by a monoblock tibial component made of XLPE. In the BPK-S the BIOLOXdelta tibial tray hosts a semi-constrained XLPE insert, with a stump in its inferior part articulating with the

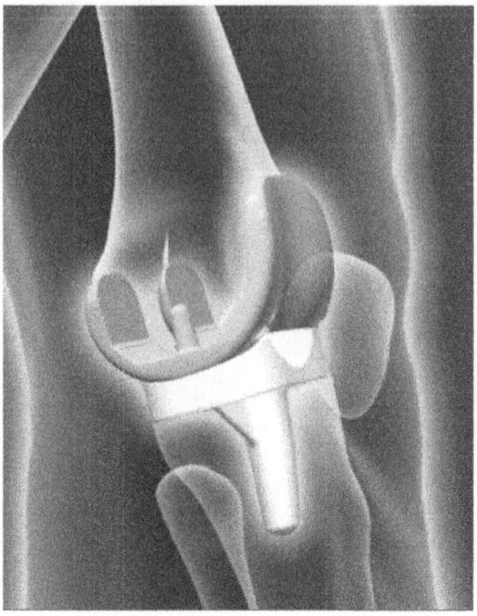

**Figure 5.10** The Multigen total knee replacement with a ceramic femoral component.
Courtesy of CeramTec GmbH, Medical Products Division, Plochingen, Germany.

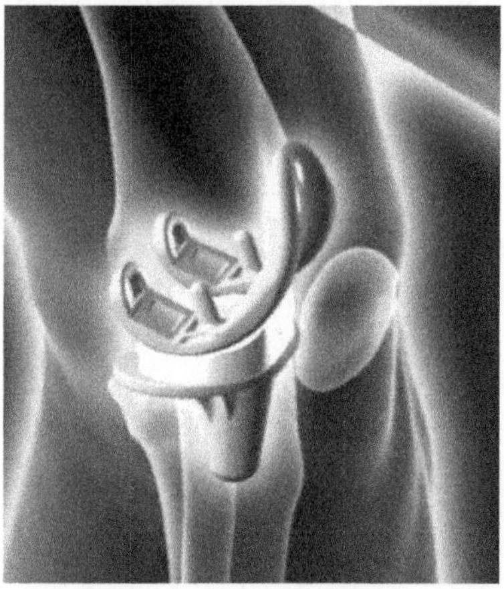

**Figure 5.11** The BPK-S total knee replacement with a ceramic femoral component and tibial tray.
Courtesy of CeramTec GmbH, Medical Products Division, Plochingen, Germany.

tray to control its motion. An international multicenter study is presently in progress on Multigen Plus TKR, involving 107 patients who underwent knee arthroplasty at seven centers in the EU. The report of clinical and radiological outcomes and survival rate of this device after 5-year follow-up shows outcomes comparable to other metallic and ceramic unconstrained TKA systems (Bergschmidt et al., 2015).

### 5.3.3 Application of load-bearing ceramics in other joints

#### 5.3.3.1 Shoulder joints

Besides hip and knee replacements, there is today a growing interest in the use of ceramic components in shoulder replacements, as the glenoid component of the implant. This solution has been attempted in the past. As an examples, Sim et al. (1980) reported the implant of a ceramic humeral component made by Rosenthal (Lauf, Germany) after resection due to bone tumor. Some years later, Huckstep and Sherry (1996) reported in three cases the use of a prosthesis having an alumina head for limb salvage due to bone tumor.

The development achieved in recent years in shoulder replacements stimulated the interest for using ceramic components in total shoulder replacement (TSR) systems. Enomoto (2001) reported the short-term results of 11 cementless artificial humeral head replacements performed between 1993 and 2000, by using alumina-ceramics head Physio-shoulder system (Kyocera, Japan), while a glenoid ball head coupled to a ceramic humeral insert is used in the Unic TSR (Evolutis, Brennon, France). Ceramic glenoids or ceramic humeral heads are also used in the TSRs of the Affinys system (Mathys Orthopedie, Bettlach, Switzerland) (Bell and Coghlan, 2014).

#### 5.3.3.2 Ankle joints

Although the early attempts in ankle arthroplasty were unsatisfactory, advances in surgical techniques and instrumentation as well as in the design of devices more effective from a biomechanical viewpoint is pushing several surgeons into reconsidering this procedure in place of arthrodesis. First attempts for using alumina in an ankle joint replacement were made in Japan in the early 1980s. In the early 1990s Kyocera (Kyoto, Japan) introduced into the Japanese market the TNK total ankle replacement, which is still in clinical use. The tibial and the talar components are made of high-density alumina. The tibial component hosts a UHMWPE insert on the articular surface. The bone-contacting surfaces of the tibial and talar components are coated with alumina beads, forming a porous surface aimed at achieving the cementless fixation of the implant by bone ingrowth. Takakura et al. (2004) reviewed their clinical experience with the two successive generations of alumina devices, remarking on the improved results they achieved using cement to stabilize the implants in situ. Similar results were obtained by Nishikawa et al. (2004).

More recently, Taniguchi et al. (2015) reported the outcomes of a series of alumina patient-specific talar replacements, obtained from computed tomography scans of the contralateral talus, that were implanted in a limited number of patients due to osteonecrosis of the talus.

#### 5.3.3.3 Finger joints

Several prosthetic implants have been designed to treat the proximal interphalangeal and metacarpophalangeal joints affected by posttraumatic conditions or rheumatoid arthritis.

Pyrolytic carbon (or Pyrocarbon—PyC), a synthetic form of carbon with an ordered, layered structure similar to graphite, was used in finger joints. The main use of PyC is in heart valve prostheses thanks to its hemocompatibility. It was proposed as a coating in the joints of orthopedic implants during the second half of the 1990s, as well as in small prosthetic devices for joint replacements in the hand (Cook et al., 1999). Although the first results achieved were promising, most of the literature reports complications, including failure, fracture, and dislocation of the implants (Heers et al., 2013; Squitieri and Chung, 2008; Chan et al., 2013; Pettersson et al., 2015). Wagner et al. consider the use of PyC implants as a risk factor in surgery of the proximal interphalangeal joint (Wagner et al., 2015).

The literature also mentions the use of zirconia in the arthroplasty of finger joints. Zirconia balls (Orthosphere, Wright Medical, Austin TX) were used in the interpositional arthroplasty of the thumb carpometacarpal joint, as reported by Calandruccio and Jobe in the late 1990s (Calandruccio and Jobe, 1997).

### *5.3.3.4 Spine joints*

Ceramics devices are used in spine arthrodesis (the synthesis of two or more adjacent vertebral bodies) and in spine arthroplasty by total disk replacement (TDR). The main advantage of TDR over arthrodesis consists of the preservation of the relative motion of the vertebral bodies. The ceramics used as load-bearing components in arthrodesis are cages (or spacers) made out silicon nitride (Schneider et al., 2008), while apatite-wollastonite glass ceramics (Yamamuro, 2008) are used in intervertebral spacers. In addition, the development of alumina/zirconia composite cages, plates and screws for synthesis in the cervical spine was started by NEVZ Bioceramics (Novosirbisk, Russian Federation), but this activity is now in stand-by.

Recently, Siskey et al. (2016) presented the preliminary results obtained in the development of a PEEK-ceramic cervical TDR making use of a ZTA nucleus articulating between the PEEK endplates, but clinical results of this device are missing so far. A further two TDRs with ceramic components in their bearings device are described in the literature: the Discocerv (Scient'x, Voisin Le Bretonneaux, France) and the Regain (Biomet, Warsaw, IN, USA).

The Discocerv's intended use is to replace discs in the cervical spine (C2−C7). It is formed by two titanium alloy (Ti-6Al-4V) endplates whose external profile fits into the native disc space. In their interior there is the bearing, formed by a convex alumina disc articulating on a concave Y-TZP disc (Ramadan et al., 2007).

The Regain TDR was conceived for implants in the lumbar spine (typically L4−L5 or L5−S1). It was formed by a graphite nucleus coated with PyC. The convex design of the end surfaces was intended for the conformal articulation against the upper and lower vertebrae endplates (Coric and Mummaneni, 2008). This device seems not to have overcome the developmental stage. Similarly, also the development of the Discmaxx C TDR (Maxxspine Ltd, Eltville am Rhein, Germany) with DiamolithDLC-coated bearing surfaces (Wallwork, Manchester, UK) described by Hauert et al. (2013) appears to have stopped. On the other hand, the DLC-coated BagueraC TDR (Spineart, Geneve, Switzerland) is already in clinical use in cervical arthroplasty and the results of clinical studies are promising (see Section 5.4.3).

## 5.4 Ceramic coatings in joint replacements

Several ceramic coatings are used by the orthopedic industry to improve the hardness of metallic components made of Ti-base or in CoCr-alloys. Also, ceramicized bearing surfaces obtained by growing a zirconium dioxide layer on the surface of a zirconium alloy are used to improve the wear of hip and knee prosthetic joints. Nitride coatings are the more widespread, while the development of DLC coatings in joint replacements bearings is still in progress (Suka, 1986).

### *5.4.1 Nitride coatings*

Titanium nitride (TiN) coatings were developed in the 1980s to increase the durability of cutting tools used in mechanics. The golden appearance of TiN coatings soon raised the interest of dental industry that started the use of these materials in the mid-1980s in crowns, in dentures, and in some dental instruments. The ceramic coating forms a barrier against corrosion coupled with the increase in surface hardness, both behaviors making TiN coatings attractive for use in joint replacements. The early studies were focused on coating Ti-alloy ball heads with titanium nitride to improve the poor wear behavior of Ti-alloy-on-UHMWPE bearings (Peterson et al., 1988; McKellop et al., 1990; Piconi et al., 2017). Nevertheless, due to the difference in stiffness between the TiN coating and the Ti-alloy substrate, the delamination of the coating may take place with consequent high wear of the joint.

When Ti-alloy heads were replaced by the stiffer CoCr-alloy the development of ceramicized ball heads was pursued, aimed at approaching the wear behavior of CoP joints. The rationale of the work was to minimize UHMWPE wear, limiting the risk of fractures that, at that time, affected some ceramic products.

During the following years, other types of nitride coatings were developed to improve the wear behavior of hip or knee replacement bearings: titanium nitride (TiN) and titanium niobium nitride (TiNbN) coatings obtained by physical vapor deposition (PVD). To improve the adhesion, coatings are applied by multilayer processes, as reported by Cabañas (2014). This consists of the successive applications of the coating in several layers to grade the transition in elastic properties between the "soft" substrate and the hard surface layer. Moreover, because of the random distribution in each layer of the local defects that are inherent in the PVD process (i.e., microdroplets, pinholes, or other point defects), multilayer coating could be preventive of the corrosion of the substrate and of coating failure.

TiN coatings are applied in hip, knee, ankle and shoulder replacements, but in spite of their extensive use, little exists in the literature concerning their clinical outcomes as evidenced in a comprehensive review by van Hove et al. (2015). Even if most papers report cases of coating failures (Barouk et al., 2004;

Raimondi and Pietrabissa, 2000), the clinical outcomes of nitride coatings in joint replacements bearings is still controversial. The composition of a multilayer zirconium nitride (ZrN) coating applied on a unicompartimental knee implant was reported by Affatato et al. (2011): it was formed by seven layers obtained under nitrogen atmosphere by a PVD process making use of a series of sputtering targets. The resulting coating is formed by a thin Cr bond layer, five layers of CrN−CrCN and a ZrN final layer, with total thickness between 3.5 and 5 μm. This coating, leaving ZrN at its surface, is used clinically in one knee replacement device at least, but there are no reports on its clinical outcomes so far.

### 5.4.2 Zirconium dioxide coatings

Monoclinic zirconium dioxide coatings (Oxinium) are obtained by a proprietary process by Smith & Nephew (Memphis, TN, USA). The coating is an oxide layer of about 5 μm thick, obtained by the oxidation at high temperature (e.g. 600°C/1 hour or 635°C/6 hours) of semifinished components made of Zr-2.5 Nb alloy (e.g., Zircadyne705, ATI, Pittsburgh, PA). Davidson et al. (1992) and Hunter et al. (2005) provided a comprehensive overview of the process. In 2007 the process was improved, as described by Pawar et al. (2011). Briefly, the oxidation in air is followed by a heat treatment in a vacuum, aimed at obtaining a deeper diffusion of oxygen from the $ZrO_2$ surface layer into the substrate. The FDA cleared Oxinium (OxZr) for clinical use 1995 coupled with UHMWPE components. By 2012, about 350,000 TKAs and about 150,000 THAs had been performed using OxZr components.

Laboratory studies demonstrate the improvement in joint replacements wear achievable using OxZr in place of CoCr-alloy components (Good et al., 2003; Ries, 2006; Bourne et al., 2005). Nevertheless, the clinical advantages of OxZr over CoCr ball heads in hip replacements (Kadar et al., 2011; Morison et al., 2014; Jassim et al., 2015; Zaoui et al., 2015) are not yet fully demonstrated. Also in clinical studies on knee replacements, the advantages of OxZr-coated TKRs on the traditional TKRs with CoCr-alloy femoral and tibial trays are under discussion (Petis et al., 2016; Hui et al., 2011; Kim et al., 2010, 2012; Inacio et al., 2013; Minoda et al., 2014). In addition, several reports have provided evidence of cases of damage of the articulating surface of OxZr ball heads due to joint instability or occurring during surgery (Gascoyne et al., 2016; Evangelista et al., 2007; Kop et al., 2007; Mai et al., 2010; McCalden et al., 2011; Tribe et al., 2013; Moussa et al., 2015), due to the scratch sensitivity of this oxide scale (Piconi et al., 2015).

### 5.4.3 Diamond-like carbon coatings

Several comprehensive reviews published in recent years have evidenced the potential application of DLCs in medical devices (Nagashima et al., 2016; Vila, 2014; Love et al., 2013) and the development of nanocrystalline diamond coatings is now in progress (Maru et al., 2015; Choudhury et al., 2015), giving a new momentum to this technology in arthroplasty.

Notwithstanding the number of laboratory tests performed to assess the wear behavior of DLC coatings and to demonstrate its biocompatibility (Piconi et al., 2004), only a few devices were developed with DLC-coated bearing components. In addition, some of them were affected by severe failures once in clinical use.

The knee replacement Diamond Rota Gliding, implanted in about 200 patients in Switzerland, was withdrawn from the market in 2001 due to the delamination of the coating and high wear of the polyethylene insert (Swissmedic, 2001). Alakoski et al. (2008) reported the case of the French company MIL SA that fabricated DLC-coated components for shoulder replacements and ankle joints, but these components were also soon withdrawn from the market. The clinical prospective study carried out by Taeger et al. (2003) compared DLC-coated heads (Adamante) with alumina heads in THR bearings. Both types of heads were coupled with the same UHMWPE cups. The survivorship for aseptic loosening of implants with DLC/UHMWPE bearings at mean 7.5 years postoperatively was significantly lower than that of implants with Alumina/UHMWPE bearings (54% vs 88%). Heads retrieved on revisions for aseptic loosening gave clear evidence of pitting of the DLC coating.

So far, the only device with DLC-coated bearing surfaces in clinical use is the BAGUERAC cervical disk replacement (Spineart AG, Geneve, Switzerland). It is composed of a high-density polyethylene nucleus, articulating against two DLC-coated titanium endplates. According to the manufacturer's press release, this device was implanted in 15,000 cases worldwide by November 2016 (http://www.spineart.com/news/2016/0, 2017).

## 5.5 Commercial ceramics for joint replacements bearings

The market of ceramic components for joint replacement bearings—some of them shown in Fig. 5.12—is characterized by the presence of several ceramic manufacturers that are offering ceramic ball heads. The largest share of the market belongs to CeramTec Gmbh that has sold up to now more than 10 million ceramic components under the brand name BIOLOX. Other major players are Kyocera Medical (Kyoto, Japan), Ceraver (Roissy, France), Mathys (Bettlach, Switzerland). New players are CoorsTech Medical (Golden, CO, USA), and Amedica (Salt Lake City, UT, USA), as shown in Table 5.7. The characteristics of these commercial products are reported in the following. However, due to different characterization techniques which could be used, their properties are not directly comparable.

### *5.5.1 CeramTec*

The products of the CeramTec, Medical Division (Plochingen, Germany) are the mostly used in joint replacements worldwide, marketed under the tradename BIOLOX. The company claims that every minute a BIOLOX ball head is implanted somewhere. Actually, CeramTec products represent about 80% of the worldwide market. This company incorporates the experience of Feldmüle AG and of

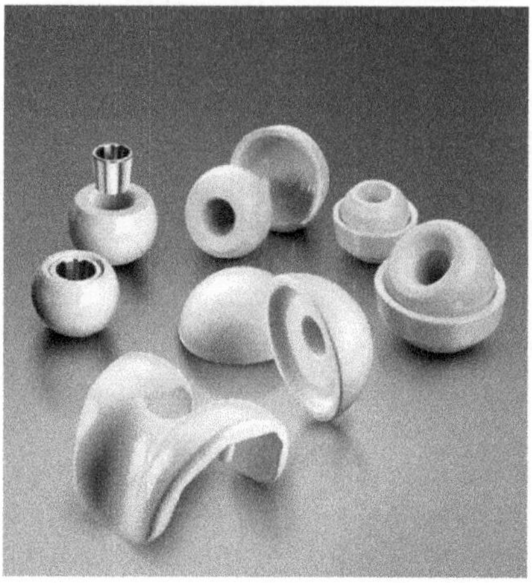

**Figure 5.12** Ceramic components for joint replacements of the hip, the knee, the shoulder. Courtesy of CeramTec GmbH, Medical Products Division, Plochingen, Germany.

Rosenthal Technical Ceramics, both pioneer companies in the field of bioceramics for joint replacement bearings. The product portfolio of CeramTec Medical Division (CT-MD) includes the composite ceramic BIOLOXdelta and the high density, HIPped alumina heads (BIOLOXforte), now used in a limited number of THR systems and in biarticular heads for hemiarthoplasty only (BIOLOXduo). The CT-MD main product is BIOLOXdelta, now in clinical use for more than 10 years. This material, which has been implanted in more than 4 million patients, is considered the gold standard for ceramics in joint replacements. BIOLOXdelta—which is characterized by its pink color, patented in the European market, is presently used for the production of ball heads that are manufactured in nine different diameters from 22 to 44 mm, with four different neck lengths. The production of inserts is more differentiated, because it takes into account not only the inner but also the external diameter of the insert, to comply with the metallic shells of the different cup design now on the market.

In addition to "standard" ball heads, CT-MD also produces ball heads (BIOLOXoption, depicted in Fig. 5.13) expressly designed to be implanted on used THR tapers, e.g., after ball head removal from a stable stem during a revision surgery. The design of these devices (from 28 to 48 mm in diameter) includes a conical sleeve made of Ti6Al4V alloy, that adapts by plasticity the deformations of the stem taper to the ball head deformations. Besides its array of products for hip replacements, CT-MD manufactures ceramic components for knee replacements and humeral heads for shoulder replacements. Table 5.8 is illustrates some of the main properties of BIOLOX ceramics.

## 5.5.2 Mathys

Mathys (Bettlach, Switzerland) is a family-run company that, since 1960, manufactures and sells a wide array of joint replacements for the hip, the knee, the shoulder.

**Table 5.7 Manufacturers of ceramic components for joint replacements, with an indication of the materials released to the market and under development**

| Company | Country | Materials | | | | | | |
|---|---|---|---|---|---|---|---|---|
| | | Alumina | Y-TZP | Mg-PSZ | ZTA | ATZ | ZPTA | Si3N4 |
| CeramTec | Germany | X | | | | | X | |
| Mathys Orthopedie | Switzerland | X | | | X | X | | |
| CoorsTech Medical | USA | X | | | | | X | |
| Kyocera Medical | Japan | X | X | | X | | X | |
| Morgan Technical Ceramics | United Kingdom | X | | | X | | | |
| NEVZ Ceramics | Russia | X | | | | | X | |
| Socièté des Cèramiques Techniques | France | X | | | | | | |
| Ceraver Osteal | France | X | | | | | | |
| Groupe Lépine | France | X | | | | | | |
| IFGL Refractories | India | X | | | | | | |
| Amedica | USA | | | | | | | X |
| Signal Medical Corporation | USA | | | X | | | | |

*ATZ*, alumina-toughened zirconia; *Mg-PSZ*, magnesia-partially stabilized zirconia; *Y-TZP*, yttria-stabilized tetragonal zirconia polycrystals; *ZPTA*, zirconia- and platelets-toughened alumina; *ZTA*, zirconia-toughened alumina.

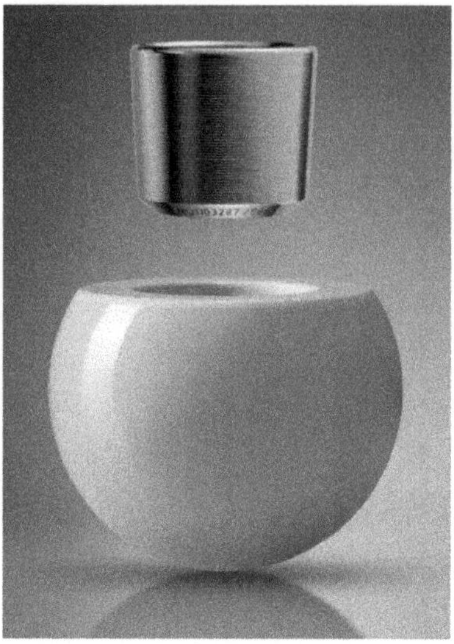

**Figure 5.13** BIOLOXOption head, with Ti-alloy sleeve to adapt damaged stem tapers. Courtesy of CeramTec GmbH, Medical Products Division, Plochingen, Germany.

Table 5.8 **Characteristics of some BIOLOX ceramics**

| Property | Units | BIOLOX forte | BIOLOX delta |
|---|---|---|---|
| $Al_2O_3$ content | vol% | >99.8 | 79 |
| $ZrO_2$ content | vol% | — | 17 |
| Other oxides | vol% | — | 1 |
| Density | $g/cm^3$ | 3.97 | 4.37 |
| Average grain size | μm | 1.75 | 0.56 |
| Young's modulus | GPa | 407 | 358 |
| Vickers hardness | GPa | 20 | 19 |
| Flexural strength | MPa | 631 | 1384 |
| Fracture toughness | $MPa\sqrt{m}$ | 4.5 | 6.5 |

In 2002, Mathys incorporated the activity of the company Keramed (Moesdorf, Germany) and started the development of ceramic components (ball heads, inserts, glenoids) for its own products line and for other implant manufacturers. As reported in the introductory part of this chapter, Keramed (formerly Keramik Werk Hermsdorf—KWK) is among the pioneers in this field since 1972. The alpha-alumina Bionit2, i.e., based on the long experience gained by Keramed in production of alumina heads (since 1978) has been joined in 2007 by the ATZ Ceramys and since 2015 by the ZTA Symarec. Ceramys (see Table 5.9) is presently the composite with the highest toughness on the market. The production of ball heads covers the most significant diameters now in clinical use (29, 32, 36 mm) while the production of inserts for the corresponding diameters is made using Bionit2 and

**Table 5.9 Selected characteristics of ceramics by Mathys. It is noted that the flexural strength is measured with the biaxial (ring) method. These value are not directly comparable with the ones of other manufacturers**

| Property | Units | Bionit 2 | Symarec ZTA | Ceramys ATZ |
|---|---|---|---|---|
| $Al_2O_3$ content | vol% | 100 | 75 | 20 |
| $ZrO_2$ content | vol% | 0 | 25 | 80 |
| Density | $g/cm^3$ | 3.99 | 4.37 | 5.51 |
| Average grain size $Al_2O_3$ | μm | 2.3 | 0.8 | 0.4 |
| Hardness | GPa | 20 (HV1) | 20 (HV1) | 15 (HV20) |
| Flexural strength (Biaxial) | MPa | ≥350 | ≥700 | ≥900 |
| Fracture toughness (SEVNB) | $MPa\sqrt{m}$ | ≥3 | ≥5 | ≥7 |

*ATZ*, alumina-toughened zirconia; *ZTA*, zirconia-toughened alumina.

Ceramys only. It is noted that Mathys is also manufacturing vitamin-E-doped inserts (XPLP Vitamys). Mathys introduced in its shoulder implants the alumina humeral head in the year 2000, and is also manufacturing sleeved ball heads using the ATZ Ceramys, for use in revision surgery or in primary implants thanks to extra-long sleeves.

### 5.5.3 Ceraver

The company Ceraver started to operate in the domain of ceramic bearings for joint replacement around 1970 with the production of alumina ball heads and cups, by following the invention of Dr. Pierre Boutin. After the first series, in 1972 Ceraver developed its own cemented stem (Osteal) made in Ti6Al4V alloy, still in production today. The production of Ceraver alumina heads and inserts is used in his own hip implants.

### 5.5.4 Kyocera

Kyocera (formerly Japan Medical Materials) is a historical manufacturer of fine ceramics for biomedical applications, the first implants of its alumina Bioceram can be traced back to 1976. Some characteristics of Kyocera ceramics used in joint replacement bearings are summarized in Table 5.10. To date, Kyocera is still making alumina heads and sockets, but its most advanced materials for joint replacements are the new ZTA AZ209 and AZUL, this last owing its tradename to its characteristic blue color, due to the presence of cobalt among its additives. Most of the products by Kyocera are for sale only in Japan. They include two TKR systems with zirconia ceramic femoral component (LFA and Bisurface), a total shoulder

Table 5.10 **Selected characteristics of Kyocera ceramics for joint replacement bearings**

| Property | Units | Bionit 2 | Symarec ZTA | Ceramys ATZ |
|---|---|---|---|---|
| $Al_2O_3$ content | vol% | 100 | 75 | 20 |
| $ZrO_2$ content | vol% | 0 | 25 | 80 |
| Density | $g/cm^3$ | 3.99 | 4.37 | 5.51 |
| Average grain size $Al_2O_3$ | μm | 2.3 | 0.8 | 0.4 |
| Hardness | GPa | 20 (HV1) | 20 (HV1) | 15(HV20) |
| Flexural strength (Biaxial) | MPa | ≥350 | ≥700 | ≥900 |
| Fracture toughness (SEVNB) | $MPa\sqrt{m}$ | ≥3 | ≥5 | ≥7 |

*ATZ*, alumina-toughened zirconia; *ZTA*, zirconia-toughened alumina.

replacement with alumina humeral head, and a ceramic humeral capitel for total elbow replacement.

### 5.5.5 CoorsTek medical

CoorsTek is the branch manufacturing medical products of Coors, a century-old family-run business that entered in the production of labware ceramics during the 1930s.

CoorsTek's CeraSurf-p ceramic femoral heads and acetabular liners have been available for clinical use as bearing surfaces for hip implant systems in South America since 2011 and in Europe since 2012. The FDA recognized CeraSurf for use in hip implant systems in February 2016. Also CeraSurf is characterized by the pink color, analogous with BIOLOXdelta. According to the press releases of CoorTek, more than 7000 CeraSurf hip balls and acetabular liners have been sold for distribution across key global markets since 2011. So far, CoorsTek has not released data about the behavior of its ceramic composite, and reports on the outcomes of implants with CeraSurf components are not available in the literature.

### 5.5.6 Amedica

Amedica Corp (Salt Lake City, UT, USA) claims to be the only manufacturer of medical grade silicon nitride that is now in clinical use for interbody fusion device in spine surgery. In addition, Amedica is developing silicon nitride ball heads for hip replacements and femoral and tibial components for knee replacements in cooperation with Kyocera (Kyoto, Japan) and University partners.

### 5.5.7 Groupe Lépine

Groupe Lépine (Genay, France) is an orthopedic implant manufacturer that has introduced in its own hip replacements alumina heads under the tradename CeraLépine. The products are obtained from alumina ALUCER sintered blanks provided by the Société des Céramiques Techniques (SCT, Tarbes, France). Groupe Lépine provides in-house the taper machining, the finish of the surfaces, cleaning, etc.

### 5.5.8 Morgan advanced ceramics

Morgan AC (Windsor, Berkshire, UK) offers HIP Vitox Alumina for implantable medical devices, with long clinical experience. HIP Vitox Alumina femoral heads are available for hip replacements using HIP Vitox Alumina cup inserts for CoC bearings as well as for implants using polyethylene inserts. Morgan has also developed a material called Vitox AMC that can be used to manufacture femoral heads with diameters close to the natural joint and thinner wall section acetabular cups. Table 5.11 illustrates the typical values of these materials.

### 5.5.9 Signal medical corp

Signal Medical Corporation (St Louis, MO, USA) was created in 1996: it manufactures and sells its line of hip and joint replacements as well as orthopedic instrumentation. Signal has been manufacturing since its creation of Mg-PSZ ball heads from 22.2 to 36 mm in diameter under the tradename DuraCer. The main characteristics of this material are illustrated in Table 5.12.

## 5.6 Conclusions

The load-bearing ceramics used in orthopedics today are the result of more than 50 years of continuous development. This development followed the contemporary

Table 5.11 **Selected characteristics of Vitox ceramics**

| Property | Units | Vitox Alumina | Vitox AMC |
|---|---|---|---|
| $Al_2O_3$ content | vol% | 99.9 | — |
| $ZrO_2$ content | vol% | 0 | — |
| Density | $g/cm^3$ | 3.978 | 4.26 |
| Average grain size $Al_2O_3$ | μm | 1.2 | 0.67 |
| Average grain size Y-TZP | μm | — | 0.16 |
| Hardness | GPa | 22 | 17 |
| Flexural strength | MPa | 550 | 700 |
| Fracture toughness (SENB) | $MPa\sqrt{m}$ | 4.0 | 4.5 |

*Y-TZP*, yttria-stabilized tetragonal zirconia polycrystals.

**Table 5.12 Selected properties of DuraCer magnesia-partially stabilized zirconia**

| Property | Units | DuraCer Mg-PSZ |
|---|---|---|
| Density | $g/cm^3$ | 5.83 |
| Average grain size | μm | 0.3 |
| Hardness | GPa | 10.7 |
| Flexural strength | MPa | 620 |
| Fracture toughness (SENB) | $MPa\sqrt{m}$ | 10 |

*Mg-PSZ*, magnesia-partially stabilized zirconia.

development of hip arthroplasty, which is among the surgeries with the better outcomes in the long term. The success of hip arthroplasty entrained the diffusion of ceramic components which, since their introduction in clinical practice, demonstrated their low wear behavior and their effectiveness in the reduction of associated complications in THR. It can be estimated that more than 15 million ceramic components have been implanted worldwide in hip, knee, and other joint replacements. Therefore, the works of Dr. Boutin, and of the many other distinguished scientists in Germany, Japan, Austria, Italy, United States, and United Kingdom who focused their efforts on oxides as load-bearing ceramics for joint arthroplasty, stand as one of the major clinical, scientific, industrial success stories of the last century.

The attention—initially focused on alumina as reference material—shifted soon towards toughened ceramics, especially zirconia (Y-TZP) (Christel et al., 1988) and ZTA composites (Mandrino et al., 1990; Salomoni et al., 1994). A breakthrough characterized the turn of the century, with the introduction of ZPTA (Burger and Richter, 2001). Although alumina is still in clinical use with satisfactory outcomes, ceramic composites are the standard ceramics in arthroplasty today, for their unsurpassed reliability, low wear behavior and high performance, due to the toughening effect of different reinforcing phases (both zirconia and platelets) present in the microstructure (Palmero et al., 2015; Reveron et al., 2017). Therefore, several ceramic manufacturers worldwide now offer components made of ceramic composites. The demand for components for THR is continuously increasing: the demand for hip arthroplasties in OECD Countries increased by 35% from 2000 to 2013, whereas in the same years, the demand knee replacements was almost doubled (Organisation for Economic Cooperation and Development FR, 2015). The increased demand for implants is leading not only to the increase in demand for ceramic components for THRs, but to new ceramic components for other joints like, e.g., the knee, the shoulder, or for small joints.

Although mass production is still concentrated in a few companies worldwide, the increase in demand is opening new markets and several ceramic manufacturers are entering the market of load-bearing ceramics for joint replacements. In some cases, their approach is very innovative like, e.g., the development of silicon nitride components for THR bearings now in progress in the United States, but also approaches based on the use of nanomaterials may give a new momentum to a market that is still on the move. Moreover, further innovative ceramic devices could be expected to enter the orthopedic scene in the coming years, due to the increasing demand of metal-free implantable medical devices.

## References


Affatato, S., Spinelli, M., Lopomo, N., Grupp, T.M., Marcacci, M., Toni, A., 2011. Can the method of fixation influence the wear behavior of ZrN coated unicompartimental mobile knee prostheses? Clin. Biomech. 26, 152–158.

Agathopoulos, S., Nikolopoulos, P., Salomoni, A., Tucci, A., Stamenkovich, I., 1996. Preparation and properties of binary oxide bioceramics. J. Mater. Sci. Mater. Med. 7, 629–636.

Ahmed, M., Latif, A.M.H., Mehats, A., Elcocks, M., Rushton, N., Field, R.E., et al., 2008. Pre-clinical studies to validate the MITCH PCR™ Cup: a flexible and anatomically shaped acetabular component with novel bearing characteristics. J. Mater. Sci. Mater. Med. 19, 1729–1736.

Alakoski, E., Tiainen, V.-M., Soininen, A., Konttinen, Y.T., Konttinen, Y.T., 2008. Load-bearing biomedical applications of diamond-like carbon coatings: current status. Open Orthop. J. 2, 43–50.

Al-Hajjar, M., Fisher, J., Tipper, J.L., Williams, S., Jennings, L.M., 2013. Wear of 36-mm BIOLOX delta ceramic-on-ceramic bearing in total hip replacements under edge loading conditions. Proc. IMechE Part H J. Eng. Med. 227-H, 535–542.

Almeida, F.A., Amaral, M., Oliveira, F.J., Fernandes, A.J.S., Silva, R.F., 2007. Baptista DL. Nano to micrometric HFCVD diamond – adhesion strenght to Si3N4. Vacuum. 81, 1443–1447.

Amaral, M., Maru, M.M., Rodrigues, S.P., Gouvêa, C.P., Trommer, R.M., Oliveira, F.J., et al., 2015. Extremely low wear rates in hip joint bearings coated with nanocrystalline diamond. Tribol. Int. 89, 72–77.

Amatullah, D.F., Sucher, M.G., Bonadurer, G.F., Pereira, G.C., Taunton, M.J., 2016. Metal in total hip arthroplasty: wear particles, biology and diagnosis. Orthopedics 39, 371–379.

American Society for Testing and Materials, 2016. Standard Specification for High-Purity Dense Aluminum Oxide for Medical Application ASTM F603–12.

Amlie, E., Hoevik, O., Reikeras, O., 2010. Dislocation after total hip arthroplasty with 28 and 32.mm femoral head. J. Orthoped. Traumatol. 11, 111–115.

Amstutz, H.C., 1989. Evolution of ceramic total hips. In: Oonishi, H., Aoki, H., Sawai, K. (Eds.), Bioceramics. Ishiyaku Euro America, Tokio, pp. 249–253.

Andrisano, A.O., Dragoni, E., Strozzi, A., 1990. Axysymmetric mechanical analysis of ceramic heads for total hip replacement. Proc. Instn. Mech. Eng. Part H. 204-H, 157–167.

Aoude, A., Antoniou, J., Epure, L.M., Huk, O.L., Zukor, D.J., Tanzer, M., 2015. Midterm outcomes of the recently FDA approved ceramic on ceramic bearing in total hip arthroplasty patients under 65 years of age. J. Arthroplasty. 30, 1388–1392.

Atsui, K., Tateishi, H., Futani, H., Maruo, S., 1997. Ceramic unicompartmental knee arthroplasty for spontaneous osteonecrosis of the knee joint. Bull. Hosp. Jt. Dis. 56, 233–236.

Bal, B.S., Greenberg, D.D., Aleto, T.J., 2005. Primary total knee replacement with a zirconia ceramic femoral component. In: D'Antonio, J.A., Dietrich, M. (Eds.), Bioceramics and Alternative Bearings in Joint Arthroplasty. Steinkoppf, Darmstadt, pp. 83–190.

Bal, B.S., Ramahan, M.N., 2012. Orthopedic applications of silicon nitride ceramics. Acta Biomater. 8, 2889–2898.

Barouk, P., Maynou, C., Hildebrand, H.F., et al., 2004. Frequence élevée des descellement prothétiques après utilisation d'un couple titane implanté-polyéthyléne. Rev. Chir. Ortop. 90, 26–32.

Becher, P.F., 1991. Microstructural design of toughened ceramics. J. Am. Ceram. Soc. 74, 255–269.

Begand, S., Oberbach, T., Glien, W., 2005. ATZ: a new material with a high potential in joint replacement. Key Eng. Mater. 284-286, 983–986.

Bell, S.N., Coghlan, J.A., 2014. Short stem shoulder replacement. Int. J. Shoulder. Surg. 8, 72–75.

Bergschmidt, P., Bader, R., Ganzer, D., Hauzeur, C., Lohmann, C.H., Krüger, A., et al., 2015. Prospective multi-centre study on a composite ceramic femoral component in total knee arthroplasty: five-year clinical and radiological outcomes. The Knee 22, 186–191.

Blaise, L., Webb, J., Calés, B., 2002. Mechanical analysis of a knee prosthesis with a zirconia femoral component. Orthop. Proc. 84-B, 14.

Bourne, R.B., Barrack, R., Rorabeck, C.H., Salehi, A., Good, V., 2005. Arthroplasty options for the young patient, oxinium on cross-linked polyethylene. Clin. Orthop. Rel. Res. 441, 159–167.

Boutin, P., 1972. Arthroplastie totale de la hanche par prostheses en alumine fritté. Rev. Chir. Orthop. 58, 230–246.

Brach del Prever, E.M., Bistolfi, A., Bracco, P., Costa, L., 2009. UHMWPE for arthroplasty: past or future? J. Orthopaed. Traumatol. 10, 1–8.

Burger, W., 1997. Umwadlungs- und plateletverstaerkte Aluminiumoxidmatrixwerkstoffe (teil 1). Keram Z. 49, 1067–1070.

Burger, W., 1998. Umwadlungs- und plateletverstaerkte Aluminiumoxidmatrixwerkstoffe (teil 2). Keram Z. 50, 18–22.

Burger, W., Richter, H.G., 2001. High strength and toughness alumina matrix composites by transformation toughening and "in situ" platelet reinforcement (ZPTA). Key Eng. Mater. 192-195, 545–548.

Cabañas, M.V., 2014. Bioceramic coatings for medical implants. In: Vallet-Regì, M. (Ed.), Bioceramics With Clinical Applications. Wiley, Chichester, pp. 249–289.

Cai, P., Hu, Y., Xie, J., 2012. Large diameter Delta ceramic-on-ceramic vs. common-sized ceramic-on-polyethylene bearings. Orthopedics. 35, e1307–e1313.

Calandruccio, J.H., Jobe, M.T., 1997. Arthroplasty of the thumb carpometacarpal joint. Semin. Arthoplasty. 82, 135–147.

Calés, B., Stefani, Y., 1995. Yttria stabilized zirconia for improved orthopedic prostheses. In: Wise, L., Trantolo, D.J., altobelli, D.E., Yaszemski, M.J., Gresser, J.D., Schwartz, E. R. (Eds.), Encyclopedic Handbook of Biomaterials and Bioengineering. Dekker, New York, pp. 415–452.

Calés, B., Stefani, Y., 1998. Risks and advantages in standardization of bores and cones for heads in modular hip prostheses. J. Biomed. Mater. Res. Appl. Biomater. 43, 62–68.

Chan, K., Ayeni, O., McKnight, L., Ignacy, T.A., Farrokhyar, F., Thoma, A., 2013. Pyrocarbon versus silicone proximal interphalangeal joint arthroplasty: a systematic review. Plast. Reconstr. Surg. 131, 114–124.

Chess, J.T., Babbush, C.A., 1980. Restoration of lost dentition using aluminum oxide endosteal implants. Dent. Clin. North Am. 24, 521–533.
Chevalier, J., Gremillard, L., Deville, S., 2007. Low-temperature degradation of zirconia and implications for biomedical implants. Annu. Rev. Mater. Res. 37, 1–32.
Chevalier, J., 2006. What future for zirconia as a biomaterial? Biomaterials. 27, 535–543.
Chevalier, J., Cales, B., Drouin, J.M., 1999. Low-temperature ageing of Y-TZP ceramics. J. Am. Ceram. Soc. 82, 2150–2154.
Choudhury, D., Urban, F.M., Hartl, M., Krupka, I., 2015. A novel tribological study on DLC-coated micro-dimpled orthopaedics implant interface. J. Mech. Behav. Biomed. Mater. 45, 121–131.
Christel, P., Meunier, A., Dorlot, J.-M., Crolet, J.-M., Witvoet, J., Sedel, L., et al., 1988. Biomechanical compatibility and design of ceramic implants for othopedic surgery. In: Ducheyne, P., Lemons, J.E. (Eds.), Bioceramics: Material Characteristics Versus In Vivo Behavior. The New York Academy of Sciences, New York, pp. 234–256.
Cigada, A., Cotogno, G., Chiesa, R., 2011. The ceramic-on-metal coupling in total hip replacements for young patients: a review study. J. Appl. Biomater. Biomech. 9, 2–10.
Claussen, N., 1976. Fracture toughness of alumina with an unstabilized zirconia dispersed phase. J. Am. Ceram. Soc. 59, 49–51.
Cook, R.F., Pharr, G.M., 1994. Mechanical properties of ceramics. In: Swain, M.V. (Ed.), Structure and Properties of Ceramics (Materials Science and Technology, vol. 11). VCH, Weinheim, pp. 339–407.
Cook, S.D., Beckenbaugh, R.D., Redondo, J., Popich, L.S., Klawitter, J.J., Linsheid, R.L., 1999. Long-term follow-up of pyrolytic carbon metacarpophalangeal implants. J. Bone Joint Surg. Am. 81, 635–648.
Coric, D., Mummaneni, P.V., 2008. Nucleus replacement technologies. J. Neurosurg. Spine. 8, 115–120.
Cutler, A.C., Mayhew, R.J., Prettyman, K.M., Virkar, A.V., 1991. High-toughness Ce-TZP/$Al_2O_3$ ceramics with improved hardness and strength. J. Am. Ceram. Soc. 74, 179–186.
Dalla Pria, P., Giorgini, L., Kuntz, M., Pandorf, T., 2006. Ceramic knee design. In: Benazzo, F., Falez, F., Dietrich, M. (Eds.), Bioceramics and Alternative Bearings in Joint Arthroplasty. Steinkoppf, Darmstadt, pp. 115–123.
Daniel, J., Holland, J., Quigley, L., Sprague, S., Bandhari, M., 2012. Pseudotumours associated with total hip arthroplasty – current concepts review. J. Bone Joint Surg. Am. 94, 86–93.
D'Antonio, J.A., Capello, W.N., Naughton, M., 2014. High survivorship with a titanium-encased alumina ceramic bearing for total hip arthroplasty. Clin. Orthop. Rel. Res. 472, 611–616.
Davidson, J.A., Asgian, C.M., Mishra, A.K., Kovacs, P., 1992. Zirconia (ZrO2)-coated zirconium-2,5Nb alloy for prosthetic knee bearing application. In: Yamamuro, T., Kokubo, T., Nakamura, T. (Eds.), Bioceramics, 5. Kobunshi Kankokai, Kyoto, pp. 389–400.
Delaunay, C., 2001. Couple de frottement des prothèses totales de hanche. Ce qu'un chirurgien orthopédiste devrait savoir. Cahiers SOFCOT. 7, 63–96.
Dickinson, A.S., Browne, M., Wilson, K.C., Jeffers, J.R.T., Taylor, A.C., 2011. Pre-clinical evaluation of ceramic femoral head resurfacing prostheses using computational models and mechanical testing. Proc. IMechE Part H: J. Eng. Med. 225, 866–876.
Enomoto, E., 2001. Cementless artificial humeral head replacement for a comminuted proximal humeral fracture. Katakansetsu 25, 487–490.

Evangelista, G.T., Fulkerson, E., Kummer, F., Di Cesare, P.E., 2007. Surface damage to an Oxinium femoral head prosthesis after dislocation. J. Bone Joint Surg. Br. 89-B, 535–537.

Eynon-Lewis, N.J., Ferry, D., Pearse, M.F., 1992. Themistocles Gluck: an unrecognised genius. BMJ. 305, 1534–1536.

Eyring, E.J., Campbell, W., 1969. Ceramic Prostheses, News in Engineering, Ohio State University Publishing, 1992. pp. 4–7.

Fisher, J., Jin, Z., Tipper, J., Stone, M., Ingham, E., 2006. Tribology of alternative bearings. Clin. Orthop. Rel. Res. 453, 25–34.

Garvie, R.C., Hannink, R.H.J., Pascoe, R.T., 1975. Ceramic steel? Nature 258, 703–704.

Gascoyne, T.C., Teeter, M.G., Guenther, L.E., Burnell, C.D., Bohm, E.R., Naudie, D.R., 2016. *In vivo* wear performance of cobalt-chromium versus oxidized zirconium femoral total knee replacements. J. Arthroplasty. 31, 137–141.

Girard, J., 2015. Femoral head diameter considerations for primary total hip arthroplasty. Orthop. Traumatol. Surg. Res. 101, S25–S29.

Good, V., Ries, M., Barrack, R., Widding, K., Hunter, G., Dan Heuer, D., 2003. Reduced wear with oxidized zirconium femoral heads. J. Bone Joint Surg. Am. 85, 105–110.

Gupta, T.K., Bechtold, J.H., Kuznicki, R.C., Cadoff, L.H., Rossing, B.R., 1977. Stabilization of tetragonal phase in polycrystalline zirconia. J. Mater. Sci. 12, 2421–2426.

Hamilton, W.G., McAuley, J.P., Blumenfeld, T.J., Lesko, J.P., Himden, S., Dennis, D.A., 2015. Midterm results of delta ceramic-on-ceramic total hip arthroplasty. J. Arthroplasty. 30, 110–115.

Hannouche, D., Zaoui, A., Zadegan, F., Sedel, L., Nizard, R., 2011. Thirty years of experience with alumina-on-alumina bearings in total hip arthroplasty. Int. Orthop. 35, 207–213.

Hauert, R., Thorwart, K., Thorwart, G., 2013. An overview on diamondlike carbon coatings in medical applications. Surf. Coat Tech. 233, 119–130.

Heers, G., Springorum, H.R., Baier, C., Götz, J., Grifka, J., Renkawitz, T., 2013. Proximal interphalangeal joint replacement with an unconstrained pyrocarbon prosthesis (Ascension(R)): a long-term follow-up. J. Hand. Surg. Eur. 38, 680–685.

Heimke, G., Leyen, S., Willmann, G., 2002. Knee arthroplasty: recently developed ceramics offer new solutions. Biomaterials 23, 1539–1551.

Hill, J.C., Diamond, O.J., O'Brien, S., Boldt, J.G., Stevenson, M., Beverland, D.E., 2015. Early surveillance of ceramic-on-metal total hip arthroplasty. Bone Joint J. 97-B, 300–305.

http://www.spineart.com/news/2016/0 (last accessed January 13, 2017).

Huckstep, R.L., Sherry, E., 1996. Replacement of the proximal humerus in primary bone tumours. Aust. NZJ Surg. 66, 97–100.

Hui, C., Salmon, L., Maeno, S., Roe, J., Walsh, W., Pinczewski, L., 2011. Five-year comparison of oxidized zirconium and cobalt-chromium femoral components in total knee arthroplasty: a randomized controlled trial. J. Bone Joint Surg. Am. 93-A, 624–630.

Hulbert, S.F., Morrison, J.S., Klavitter, J.J., 1972. Tissue reaction to three ceramics of porous and non-porous structures. J. Biomed. Mater. Res. 1992 (6), 347–374.

Hunter, G., Dickinson, J., Herb, B., Graham, R., 2005. Creation of oxidized zirconium orthopaedic implants. J. ASTM Intl. 2, 216–229.

Imbuldeniya, A., Chana, R., Walter, W., Zicat, B., Walter, W., 2013. Long-term results of third generation alumina -on-alumina ceramic bearings in patients under the age of 55: a ten year minimum follow-up. Bone Joint J. 95-B (SUPP 34), 198.

Inacio, M.C.S., Cafri, G., Paxton, E.W., Kurtz, S.M., Namba, R.S., 2013. Alternative bearings in total knee arthroplasty: risk of early revision compared to traditional bearings. Acta Orthop. 84, 145–152.

International Standards Organization, 2010. Implants for surgery – Ceramic materials – Part 1: Ceramic materials based on high purity alumina. ISO 6474-1.

Jassim, S.S., Patel, S., Wardle, N., Tahmassebi, J., Middleton, R., Shardlow, D., et al., 2015. Five-year comparison of wear using oxidised zirconium and cobalt–chrome femoral heads in total hip arthroplasty. Bone Joint J. 97-B, 883–889.

Jeffers, J.R.T., Walter, W.L., 2012. Ceramic-on-ceramic bearings in hip arthroplasty. J. Bone Joint Surg. Br. 94-B, 735–745.

Kabo, J.M., Gebhard, J.S., Loren, G., Amstutz, H.C., 1993. *In vivo* wear of polyethylene acetabular components. J. Bone Joint Surg. Br. 75, 254–258.

Kadar, T., Hallan, G., Aamodt, A., Indrekvam, K., Badawy, M., Skredderstuen, A., et al., 2011. Wear and migration of highly cross-linked and conventional cemented polyethylene cups with cobalt chrome or Oxinium femoral heads: a randomized radiostereometric study of 150 patients. J. Orthop. Res. 29, 1222–1229.

Kawahara, H., 1986. Materials for hard tissue replacement. In: Lin, O.C.C., Chao, E.Y.S. (Eds.), Perspectives on Biomaterials. Elsevier, Amsterdam, pp. 167–206.

Kern, F., 2014. A comparison of microstructure and mechanical properties of 12Ce-TZP reinforced with alumina and in situ formed strontium- or lanthanum hexaaluminate precipitates. J. Eur. Ceram. Soc. 34, 413–423.

Kiefer, H., Usbeck, S., Scheuber, L.F., Atzrodt, V., 2014. Clinical Management of Hip Arthroplasty. Springer Medizin, Heidelberg, 22 p.

Kim, Y.-H., Kim, J.-S., Huh, W., Lee, K.-H., 2010. Weight of polyethylene wear particles is similar in TKAs with oxidized zirconium and cobalt-chrome prostheses. Clin. Orthop. Rel. Res. 468, 1296–1304.

Kim, Y.H., Park, J.W., Kim, J.S., 2012. Comparison of the Genesis II total knee replacement with oxidised zirconium and cobalt-chromium femoral components in the same patients. J. Bone Joint Surg. Br. 94-B, 1221–1227.

Kop, A.M., Whitewood, C., Johnston, D.J.L., 2007. Damage of oxinium femoral heads subsequent to hip arthroplasty dislocation - three retrieval cases. J. Arthoplasty. 22, 775–779.

Lang, H., 1983. Tibialplateauprothesen aus Aluminiumoxid – Indikation und Egebnisse. Hermsdorfer Technische Mitteilungen. 23, 1974–1975.

Langer, G., 2002. Ceramic tibial plateau of the 70s. In: Garino, J.P., Willmann, G. (Eds.), Bioceramics in Joint Arthroplasty. Thieme, Stuttgart, pp. 128–130.

Langer, G., Blumentritt, S., 1987. Our ceramic endoprostheses programme – investigations and results. In: Vincenzini, P. (Ed.), Ceramics in Clinical Applications. Elsevier, Amsterdam, pp. 313–319.

Lawson, S., 1995. Environmental degradation of zirconia ceramics. J. Eur. Ceram. Soc. 15, 485–502.

Lewinnek, G.E., Lewis, J.L., Tarr, R., Compere, C.L., Zimmermann, J.R., 1978. Dislocations after total hip-replacement arthroplasties. J. Bone Joint Surg. Am. 60-A, 217–220.

Love, C.A., Cook, R.B., Harvey, T.J., Dearnley, P.A., Wood, R.J.K., 2013. Diamond like coatings for potential applications in biological implants: a review. Tribol. Int. 63, 141–150.

Magnani, G., Brillante, A., 2005. Effect of the composition and sintering process on mechanical properties and residual stresses in zirconia–alumina composites. J. Eur. Ceram. Soc. 25, 3383–3392.

Mai, K.T., Verioti, C., D'Lima, D., Colwell Jr, C.W., Ezzet Jr., K.A., 2010. Surface roughness of femoral head prostheses after dislocation. Am. J. Orthop. 39, 495–500.

Mak, M., Jin, Z., Fisher, J., Stewart, T.D., 2011. Influence of acetabular cup rim design on the contact stress during edge loading in ceramic-on-ceramic hip prostheses. J. Arthrop. 26, 131–136.

Mandrino, A., Eloy, R., Moyen, B., Lerat, J.-L., Treheux, D., 1992. Base alumina ceramics with dispersoids: mechanical behaviour and tissue response after in-vivo implantation. J. Mater. Sci. Mater. Med. 3, 457–463.

Mandrino, A., Moyen, B., Ben Abdallah, A., Treheux, D., Orange, D., 1990. Aluminas with dispersoids. Tribological properties and in-vivo aging. Biomaterials. 11, 88–91.

Maru, M.M., Amaral, M., Rodrigues, S.P., Santos, R., Gouvea, C.P., Archanjo, B.S., et al., 2015. The high performance of nanocrystalline CVD diamond coated hip joints in wear simulator test. J. Mech. Behav. Biomed. Mater. 49, 175–185.

Massin, P., Lopes, R., Masson, B., Mainard, D., the French Hip & Knee Society (SFHG), 2014. Does Biolox®delta ceramic reduce the rate of component fractures in total hip replacement?. Orthop. Traumatol. Surg. Res. 100, S317–S321.

Masson, B., 2009. Emergence of alumina composite in hip arthroplasty. Intl. Orthop. 33, 359–363.

McCalden, R.W., Charron, K.D., Davidson, R.D., Teeter, M.G., Holdsworth, D.W., 2011. Damage of an Oxinium femoral head and polyethylene liner following routine total hip replacement. J. Bone Joint Surg. Br. 93-B, 409–413.

McKellop, H., Sarmiento, A., Schwinn, C.P., Ebramzadeh, E., 1990. *In vivo* wear of titanium-alloy hip prostheses. J. Bone Joint Surg. Am. 72-A, 512–517.

Medicine and Healthcare products Regulatory Agency. Medical Device Alert. MDA/2012/036 (June 25, 2012).

Medri, A., Landi, E., Bellosi, A., 2016. Non-oxide ceramics. In: Sonntag, R., Kretzer, J.P. (Eds.), Materials for Total Joint Arthroplasty. Imperial College Press, London, pp. 183–221.

Meftah, M., Klingenstein, G.G., Yun, R.J., Ranawat, A.S., Ranawat, C.S., 2013. Long-term performance of ceramic and metal femoral heads on conventional polyethylene in young and active patients: a matched-pair analysis. J. Bone Joint Surg. Am. 95, 1193–1197.

Middleton, J., Pande, G.N., Richter, H.G., Willmann, G., 1994. Investigation into the mechanical reliability of ceramic femoral heads for hip joints. J. Mater. Sci. Mater. Med. 5, 503–506.

Minoda, Y., Hata, K., Iwaki, H., Ikebuchi, M., Hashimoto, Y., Inori, F., et al., 2014. No difference in in vivo polyethylene wear particles between oxidized zirconium and cobalt-chromium femoral component in total knee arthroplasty. Knee Surg. Sports Traumatol. Arthrosc. 22, 680–686.

Morison, Z.A., Patil, S., Khan, H.A., Bogoch, E.R., Schemitsch, E.H., Waddell, J.P., 2014. A randomized controlled trial comparing oxinium and cobalt-chrome on standard and cross-linked polyethylene. J. Arthop. 29, 164–168.

Moussa, M.E., Esposito, C.I., Elpers, M.E., Wright, T.M., Padgett, D.E., 2015. Hip dislocation increases roughness of oxidized zirconium femoral heads in total hip arthroplasty: an analysis of 59 retrievals. J. Arthrop. 30, 713–717.

Munir, S., Walter, W.L., Walsh, W.R., 2015. Variations in trunnion surface topography between different commercially available hip replacement stems. J. Orthop. Res. 33, 98–105.

Nagashima, S., Moon, M.W., Lee, K.-R., 2016. Diamond-like carbon coatings for joint arthroplasty. In: Sonntag, R., Kretzer, J.P. (Eds.), Materials for Total Joint Arthroplasty. Imperial College Press, London, pp. 395–412.
Nishikawa, M., Tomita, T., Fujii, M., Watanabe, T., Hashimoto, J., Sugamoto, K., et al., 2004. Total ankle replacement in rheumatoid arthritis. Intl. Orthop. 28, 123–126.
O'Leary, J.F., Mallory, T.H., Kraus, T.J., Lombardi Jr, A.V., Lye, C.L., 1988. Mittelmeier ceramic total hip arthroplasty. A retrospective study. J. Arthrop. 3, 87–96.
Oonishi, H., 1990. Knee and ankle joint replacements, vol. 1. In: Heimke, G. (Ed.), Osseo-Integrated Implants. CRC Press, Boca Raton, pp. 171–186.
Oonishi, H., Oonishi, H., Kim, S.C., Kyomoto, M., Iwamoto, M., Masuda, S., et al., 2006. Ceramic knee arthroplasty: advanced clinical experiences of 26 years. Semin. Arthop. 17, 134–140.
Oral, E., Muratoglu, O.K., 2016. Crosslinked polyethylene. In: Sonntag, R., Kretzer, J.P. (Eds.), Materials for Total Joint Arthroplasty. Imperial College Press, London, pp. 133–182.
Organisation for Economic Cooperation and Development (FR). Health at a Glance 2015: OECD indicators. 2015. 220 p. ISBN 978-92-64-23257-0.
Pace, N., Marinelli, M., Spurio, S., 2008. Technical and histologic analysis of a retrieved carbon fiber–reinforced Poly-Ether-Ether-Ketone composite alumina-bearing liner 28 months after implantation. J. Arthrop. 23, 151–155.
Palmero, P., Montanaro, L., Reveron, H., Chevalier, J., 2014. Surface coating of oxide powders: a new synthesis method to process biomedical grade nano-composites. Materials. 7, 5012–5037.
Palmero, P., Fornabaio, M., Montanaro, L., Reveron, H., Esnouf, C., Chevalier, J., 2015. Towards long lasting zirconia-based composites for dental implants. Part I: innovative synthesis, microstructural characterization and in vitro stability. Biomaterials. 50, 38–46.
Pandorf, T., 2007. Wear of Large ceramic bearings. In: Chang, J.D., Billau, K. (Eds.), Bioceramics and Alternative Bearings in Joint Arthroplasty. Steinkopff, Darmstadt, pp. 91–98.
Pawar, V., Weaver, C., Jani, S., 2011. Physical characterization of a new composition of oxidized zirconium-2,5 wt% niobium produced used a two-step process for biomedical applications. Appl. Surf. Sci. 257, 6118–6124.
Payten, W.M., Ben Nissan, B., 2000. Development of a modular ceramic knee prosthesis. In: Wise, D., Trantolo, D.J., Lewandrowski, K.-U., Gresser, J.D., Cattaneo, M.V., Yaszemski, M.J. (Eds.), Biomaterials Engineering and Devices: Human Applications, vol. 2. Humana Press, Totowa, NJ, pp. 309–336.
Peterson, C.D., Hillberry, B.M., Heck, D.A., 1988. Component wear of total knee prostheses using Ti-6Al-4V, titanium nitride coated Ti-6Al-4V, and cobalt chromium molybdenum femoral components. J. Biomed. Mater. Res. 22, 887–903.
Petis, S.M., Vasarhelyi, E.M., Lanting, B.A., Howard, J.L., Naudie, D.D.R., Somerville, L.E., et al., 2016. Mid-term survivorship and clinical outcomes of cobalt-chrome and oxidized zirconium on highly crosslinked polyethylene. Can. J. Surg. 59, 48–53.
Pettersson, K., Amilon, A., Rizzo, M., 2015. Pyrolytic carbon hemiarthroplasty in the management of proximal interphalangeal joint arthritis. J. Hand Surg. Am. 40, 462–468.
Petzatodis, G.E., Papadoupoulos, P.P., Papavasiliou, K.A., Hatzokos, I.G., Agathangelidis, F. G., Christodoulou, A.G., 2010. Primary cementless total hip arthroplasty with an alumina ceramic-on-ceramic bearing: results after a minimum of twenty years of follow-up. J. Bone Joint Surg. Am. 92-A, 639–644.

Piconi, C., De Santis, V., Maccauro, G., 2017. Clinical outcomes of ceramicized ball heads in total hip replacement bearings: a literature review. J. Appl. Biomater. Funct. Mater. [Internet] Jan [cited 2017 feb 16]; 15(1):e1-e9. Available from: http://www.jab-fm.com/article/eb5c25ba-d78d-44c0-9032-706500f37e2b.

Piconi, C., Kosmac, T., Condò, S.G., 2014. Alumina- and zirconia-based ceramics for load bearing applications. In: Shen, J.Z., Kosmac, T. (Eds.), Advanced Ceramics for Dentistry. Butterworth-Heinemann, Waltham, MA, pp. 220–225.

Piconi, C., Maccauro, G., Angeloni, M., Rossi, B., Learmonth, I.D., 2007. Zirconia heads in perspective: a survey of zirconia outcomes in total hip replacement. Hip. Intl. 17, 119–130.

Piconi, C., Maccauro, G., Muratori, F., 2005. Alumina matrix composites in arthroplasty. Key Eng. Mater. 284-6, 979–982.

Piconi, C., Maccauro, G., Muratori, F., 2004. Ceramic coating in Metal-PE joints: where are we now? In: Lazennec, J.-Y., Dietrich (Eds.), Bioceramics in Joint Arthroplasty. Steinkopff, Darmstadt, pp. 105–109.

Piconi, C., Maccauro, G., Pilloni, L., Burger, W., Muratori, F., Richter, H.G., 2006. On the Fracture of a Zirconia Ball Head. J. Mater. Sci. Mater. Med. 17, 289–300.

Piconi, C., 2011. Alumina. In: Ducheyne, P., Healey, K.E., Hutmacher, D.W., Grainger, D. W., Kirkpatrick, C.J. (Eds.), Comprehensive Biomaterials, vol. 1. Elsevier, Amsterdam, pp. 73–94.

Piconi, C., 2010. Non oxide ceramics: status quo and future options. In: Cobb, J. (Ed.), Modern Trends in THA Bearings. Springer, Berlin, pp. 37–44.

Piconi, C., Maccauro, G., 1999. Zirconia as a ceramic biomaterial. Biomaterials. 20, 1–25.

Piconi, C., Porporati, A., 2016. Bioinert ceramics: zirconia and alumina. In: Antoniac, I. (Ed.), Handbook of Bioceramics and Biocomposites, vol. 1. Springer, Berlin, pp. 59–90.

Piconi, C., Maccauro, G., 2016. Perspective and trends on bioceramics in joint replacements. In: Antoniac, I. (Ed.), Handbook of Bioceramics and Biocomposites, vol. 2. Springer, Berlin, pp. 821–858.

Piconi, C., Streicher, R., 2013. Forty years of ceramic-on-ceramic THR bearings. Semin. Arthropl. 24, 188–192.

Piconi, C., Porporati, A.A., Streicher, R.M., 2015. Ceramics in THR bearings: behavior in off-normal conditions. Key Eng. Mater. 631, 1–7.

Piconi, C., Labanti, M., Magnani, G., Caporale, M., Maccauro, G., Magliocchetti, G., 1999. Analysis of a failed alumina THR ball head. Biomaterials. 20, 1637–1646.

Piconi, C., Maccauro, G., Logroscino, G., 2005. Safety issues in the use of ceramic heads and cups. Key Eng. Mater. 284-286, 975–978.

Raimondi, M.T., Pietrabissa, R., 2000. The in-vivo wear performance of prosthetic femoral heads with titanium nitride coating. Biomaterials. 21, 907–913.

Ramadan, A.S., Mitulescu, A., Schmitt, P., 2007. Total cervical disc replacement with the Discocerv® (Cervidisc Evolution) cervical prosthesis: early results of a second generation. Eur. J. Orthop. Surg. Traumatol. 17, 513–520.

Randelli, G., Lonati, F., D'Imporzano, M., Cucciniello, C., 1983. Wagner's bioceramic superficial prosthesis in the hip surgery. In: Vincenzini, P. (Ed.), Ceramics in Surgery. Elsevier, Amsterdam, pp. 341–350.

Reveron, H., Fornabaio, M., Palmero, P., Furderer, T., Adolfsson, E., Lughi, V., et al., 2017. Towards long lasting zirconia-based composites for dental implants: transformation induced plasticity and its consequence on ceramic reliability. Acta Biomater. 48, 424–432.

Richter, H.G., Willmann, G., Weick, K., 1998. Improving the reliability of the ceramic-on-ceramic wear couple in THR. In: Jacobs, J.J., Craig, T.L. (Eds.), Alternative Bearing Surfaces in Total Joint Replacements - ASTM STP 1346. American Society for Testing and Materials, West Conshohoken, pp. 173−185.

Ries, M., 2006. Oxidized zirconium in total joint arthroplasty. Semin. Arthropl. 17, 161−164.

Rieu, J., Goeuriot, P., 1993. Ceramic composites for biomedical applications. Clin. Mater. 12, 211−217.

Riley, F.L., 2000. Silicon nitride and related materials. J. Am. Ceram. Soc. 83, 245−265.

Rock, M. Künstliche Ersatzteile für das Innere und Aussere des menschliche und tierische Körpers, German Patent DRP 583.589:1933.

Salgureido, E., Abreu, C.S., Amaral, M., Oliveira, F.J., Gomes, J.R., Silva, R.F., 2013. Self-mated tribological systems based on multilayer nano/microcrystalline CVD diamond coatings. Wear 303, 225−234.

Salomoni, A., Tucci, A., Esposito, L., Stamenkovich, I., 1994. Forming and sintering of multiphase bioceramics. J. Mater. Sci. Mater. Med. 5, 651−653.

San Baw, U., 1970. Ivory prosthesis for ununited fractures of the neck of femur. J. Bone Joint Surg. Br. 52B, 177−178.

Sandhaus, S. Materiau pour implants, prothèses et outils. 11 Mars 1966. Brevet Inv. N. 1.471.090, P.V.53.006.

Sandhaus, S. Noveaux aspects de l'implantologie: l'implant CBS. Lausanne, 1969.

Sato, T., Shimada, M., 1985. Control of the tetragonal-to-monoclinic phase transformation of yttria partially stabilized zirconia in hot water. J. Mater. Sci. 20, 3899−3992.

Schmalzried, T.P., Callaghan, J.J., 1999. Current concepts review: wear in total hip and knee replacements. J. Bone Joint Surg. Am. 81-A, 115−136.

Schreiner, U., Schroeder-Boersch, H., Schwarz, M., Scheller, G., 2002. Verbesserung der knöchernen Integration bioinerter Keramiken durch Modifikation der Oberfläche - Ergebnisse eines Tierversuchs. Biomed. Technik. 47, 164−168.

Schneider, J., Begand, S., Kriegel, R., Kaps, C., Glien, W., Oberbach, T., 2008. Low-temperature aging behavior of alumina-toughened zirconia. J. Am. Ceram. Soc. 91, 3613−3618.

Schreiner, U., Schulze, A., Scheller, G., Apruzzese, C., Schwarz, M.L., 2012. Osteointegration zementfreier Hüftpfannen aus Keramik. Z Othop. Unf. 150, 32−39.

Sedel, L., 2004. Thirty year experience with all ceramic bearings. In: Lazennec, J.-Y., Dietrich, M. (Eds.), Bioceramics in Joint Arthroplasty. Steinkopff, Darmstadt, pp. 17−20.

Sedel, L., 2012. Evolution of alumina-on-alumina implants: a review. Clin. Orthop. Rel. Res. 379, 48−54.

Sentuerk, U., von Roth, P., Perka, C., 2016. Ceramic on ceramic arthroplasty of the hip. Bone Joint J. 98-B (2 Suppl. A), 14−17.

Sergo, L.V., 2010. Low temperature degradation -aging- of zirconia: a critical review of the relevant aspects in dentistry. Dent. Mater. (26), 807−820.

Sim, F.H., Chao, E.Y., Pritchard, D.J., Salzer, M., 1980. Replacement of the proximal humerus with a ceramic prosthesis: a preliminary report. Clin. Orthop. Rel. Res. 146, 161−174.

Siskey, R., Ciccarelli, L., Lui, M.K.C., Kurtz, S.M., 2016. Are PEEK-on-ceramic bearings an option for total disc arthroplasty? an in vitro tribology study. Clin. Orthop. Rel. Res. 474, 2428−2440.

Smith, L.W., 1992. Ceramic-plastic material as a bone substitute. Clin. Orthop. Rel. Res. 282, 4–9.

Squitieri, L., Chung, K.C., 2008. A systematic review of outcomes and complications of vascularized toe joint transfer, silicone arthroplasty, and PyroCarbon arthroplasty for posttraumatic joint reconstruction of the finger. Plast. Reconstr. Surg. 121, 1697–1707.

Stewart, T.P., Tipper, J.L., Insley, G., Streicher, R.M., Ingham, E., Fisher, J., 2003. Long-term wear of ceramic–matrix composite material for hip prostheses under severe swing phase microsimulation. J. Biomed. Mater. Res. App. Biomater. 66B, 567–573.

Streicher, R.M., Semlitsch, M., Schön, R., 1991. Ceramic surfaces as wear partners for polyethylene. In: Bonfield, W., Hastings, G.W., Tanner, L. (Eds.), Bioceramics 4. Butterworth–Heinemann, Oxford, pp. 9–16.

Suka, T., 1986. Experimental study on biomaterials coated with titanium-nitride ceramic for orthopaedics. Nihon Seikeigeka Gakkai Zasshi. 60, 637–647.

Sun, E.Y., Becher, P.F., Plucknett, K.P., Hsueh, C.-H., Alexander, K.B., Waters, S.B., et al., 1998. Microstructural design of silicon nitride with improved fracture toughness: II effects of yttria and alumina additives. J. Am. Ceram. Soc. 81, 2831–2840.

Swissmedic. Retrait de Protése de genou Diamond Rota Gliding. Bull Office Federal Santé Publique 35 (27. 8. 2001).

Taeger, G., Podleska, L.E., Schmidt, B., Ziegler, M., Nast-Kolb, D., 2003. Comparison of diamond-like-carbon and alumina-oxide articulating with polyethylene in total hip arthroplasty. Materialwiss Werkst. 34, 1094–1100.

Takakura, Y., Tanaka, Y., Kumai, T., Sugimoto, K., Ohgushi, H., 2004. Ankle arthro plasty using three generations of metal and ceramic prostheses. Clin. Orthop. Rel. Res. 424, 130–136.

Taniguchi, A., Takakura, Y., Tanaka, Y., Kurokawa, H., Tomiwa, K., Matsuda, T., et al., 2015. An alumina ceramic total talar prosthesis for osteonecrosis of the talus. J. Bone Joint Surg. Am. 97, 1348–1353.

Tateiwa, T., Clarke, I.C., Williams, P.A., Garino, J., Manaka, M., Shishido, T., et al., 2008. Ceramic total hip arthroplasty in the United States: safety and risk issues revisited. Am. J. Orthop. 37, E26–E31.

Theelke, B., Kuntz, M., Eichhorn, S., Boxleitner, T., Pandorf, T., Burgkart, R., 2009. Development of osseointegrative ceramic coatings based on ZPTA– mechanical characterization and influence on the substrate. In: Kim, S. (Ed.), Bioceramics 22. Korean Society for Biomaterials, Seoul, pp. 145–149.

Tribe, H., Malek, S., Stammers, J., Ranawat, V., Skinner, J.A., 2013. Advanced wear of an oxinium femoral head implant following polyethylene liner dislocation. Ann. R Coll. Surg. Engl. 95, e133–e135.

van Hove, R.P., Sierevelt, I.N., van Royen, B.J., Nolte, P.A., 2015. Titanium-nitride coating of orthopaedic implants: a review of the literature.. BioMed. Res. Intl. Article ID 485975, 9 pages. http://dx.doi.org/10.1155/2015/485975.

Vavřík, P., Landor, I., Denk, F., 2008. Clinical evaluation of the ceramic femoral component used for reconstruction of total knee replacement. Acta. Chir. Orthop. Traumatol. Cech. 75, 436–442.

Veigl, D., Vavřík, P., Pokorný, D., Slouf, M., Pavlova, E., Landor, I., 2011. Comparison of in vivo characteristics of polyethylene wear particles produced by a metal and a ceramic femoral component in total knee replacement. Acta Chir. Orthop. Traumatol. Cech. 78, 49–55.

Vila, M., 2014. Carbon-based materials in biomedicine. In: Vallet-Regi, M. (Ed.), Bio-Ceramics With Clinical Applications. Wiley, Chichester, pp. 175–192.

Wagner, E.R., Van Demark, R., Kor, D.J., Moran, S.L., Rizzo, M., 2015. intraoperative periprosthetic fractures in proximal interphalangeal joint arthroplasty. J. Hand Surg. Am. 40, 2149–2154.

Wang, A., Lin, R., Stark, C., Dumbleton, J.H., 1999. Suitability and limitations of carbon fiber reinforced PEEK composites as bearing surfaces for total joint replacements. Wear 225–229, 724–727.

Weisse, B., Zahner, M., Weber, W., Rieger, W., 2003. Improvement of the reliability of ceramic hip joint implants. J. Biomech. 36, 1633–1639.

White, P.B., Ranawat, A.S., Ranawat, C.S., 2013. Ceramic-on-polyethylene: the experience of the Ranawat Orthopaedic Center. Sem. Arthrop. 24, 206–210.

Willert, H.G., Semlitsch, M., 1977. Reactions of the articular capsule to wear products of artificial joint prostheses. J. Biomed. Mater. Res. 11, 157–164.

Williams, S., Schepers, A., Isaac, G., Hardaker, C., Ingham, E., van den Jagt, D., et al., 2007. Ceramic-on-metal hip arthroplasties. Clin. Orthop. Rel. Res. 465, 23–32.

Willmann, G., 1998. Ceramic cups for hip endoprostheses. Part 5: considerations on cup design. Biomed. Technik. 43, 342–349.

Willmann, G., Brodbeck, A., Richter, H.G., 2000. Untersuchung von explantierten BIOLOX Kopfen: analyse der metallische Abdrücke in der konischen Bohrung. In: Willmann, G., Zweimüller, K. (Eds.), Bioceramics in Hip Joint Replacements. Thieme, Stuttgart, pp. 81–87.

Yamamuro, T., Kotoura, Y., Nakamura, T., Kakutani, Y., Kitsugi, T., 1989. Rationales for orthopedic applications of bioceramics. In: Oonishi, H., Aoki, H., Sawai, K. (Eds.), Bioceramics. Ishiyaku Euro America, Tokio, pp. 19–24.

Yamamuro, T., 2008. Clinical application of bioactive glass-ceramics. In: Kokubo, T. (Ed.), Bioceramics and Their Clinical Applications. Woodhead, Cambridge, pp. 583–605.

Yoshimura, M., Noma, T., Kawabata, K., Somiya, S., 1987. Role of $H_2O$ on the degradation process of Y-TZP. J. Mater. Sci. Lett. 6, 465–467.

Yoshitomi, H., Shikata, S., Ito, H., Nakayama, T., Nakamura, T., 2009. Manufacturers affect clinical results of THA with zirconia heads: a systematic review. Clin. Orthop. Relat. Res. 467, 2349–2355.

Zagra, L., Giacometti-Ceroni, R., Corbella, M., 2004. THA ceramic-ceramic coupling: the evaluation of the dislocation rate with bigger heads. In: Lazennec, J.-Y., Dietrich (Eds.), Bioceramics in Joint Arthroplasty. Steinkopff, Darmstadt, pp. 163–168.

Zaoui, A., El Hage, S., Langlois, J., Scemama, C., Courpied, J.P., Hamadouche, M., 2015. Do oxidized zirconium femoral heads reduce polyethylene wear in cemented THAs? A blinded randomized clinical trial. Clin. Orthop. Rel. Res. 473, 3822–3828.

Zeng Yi, Z., Bo, Z., Bin, S., Jing, Y., Zongke, Z., Fuxing, P., 2016. Clinical results and metal ion levels after ceramic-on-metal total hip arthroplasty: a mean 50-month prospective single-center study. J. Arthrop. 31, 38–441.

Zeibig, A., Luber, H., 1983. Bioceramic hip joint components. In: Vicenzini, P. (Ed.), Ceramics in Surgery. Elsevier, Amsterdam, pp. 267–275.

Zhang, F., Batuk, M., Hadermann, J., Manfredi, G., Mariën, A., Vanmeensel, K., et al., 2016. Effect of cation dopant radius on the hydrothermal stability of tetragonal zirconia: grain boundary segregation and oxygen vacancy annihilation. Acta Mater. 106, 48–58.

Zhou, Y.S., Ohashi, M., Tomita, N., Ikeuchi, K., Takashima, K., 1997. Study on the possibility of silicon nitride-silicon nitride as a material for hip prostheses. Mater. Sci. Eng. C 5, 1295–1299.

# Ceramics for dentistry: Commercial devices and their clinical analysis

# 6

*Loredana Cerroni*
University of Rome "Tor Vergata", Rome, Italy

**Chapter Outline**

**Abbreviations 181**
**6.1 Introduction 182**
**6.2 Dental applications of load-bearing ceramics 182**
6.2.1 Blanks for the CAD/CAM technology system 182
6.2.2 Dental implants 186
6.2.3 Other applications 200
**6.3 Commercial load-bearing ceramics: a comparative analysis 217**
6.3.1 Toughened ceramics 217
6.3.2 Glass ceramics 227
6.3.3 Load-bearing polymer–ceramic composites 231
**6.4 Conclusions 232**
**References 232**
**Further reading 248**

## Abbreviations

| | |
|---|---|
| **ATZ** | alumina toughened zirconia |
| **CAD/CAM** | computer assisted design/computer assisted manufacture |
| **Ca-PSZ** | calcia-partially stabilized zirconia |
| **CEREC** | chairside economical restoration of esthetic ceramics, or ceramic reconstruction |
| **CICERO** | computer integrated ceramic reconstruction |
| **CTE** | coefficient of thermal expansion |
| **FDP/FDPs** | fixed dental prosthesis/prostheses |
| **FRC** | fibre reinforced composite |
| **HIP** | hot isostatic pressing |
| **ITI** | international team for oral implantology |
| **LTD** | low temperature degradation |
| **PICN** | polymer infiltrated ceramic network |
| **Y-PSZ** | yttria-partially stabilized zirconia |
| **Y-TZP** | yttria-stabilized tetragonal zirconia polycrystals |
| **SEM** | scanning electron microscopy |
| **TZP** | tetragonal zirconia polycrystals |
| **VHN** | Vickers hardness number |
| **ZTA** | zirconia toughened alumina |

**Advances in Ceramic Biomaterials.**
**DOI: http://dx.doi.org/10.1016/B978-0-08-100881-2.00006-3**

# 6.1 Introduction

In recent years, the demand for esthetic restorations in dentistry has increased and the research has focused the interest on high-strength ceramics. Crowns and fixed dental prostheses (FDPs) can be constructed from a variety of dental materials and laboratory processes, but metal-free prostheses are more frequently requested both for esthetics and for biosafety.

Ceramics are considered the best class of materials able to mimic the natural appearance of teeth; in spite of this, until some years ago ceramics were used only for veneers, due to their inherent brittleness. Major advances in ceramic dental materials started in the 1960s with the development of porcelains, which could be fired on dental casting alloys, giving rise to the metal–ceramic restorations. This system, however, showed limitations due to the corrosion of metal, the possible release of metal ions, the discoloration, and chipping phenomena.

Therefore, the interest was increasingly focused on materials charcaterized by both esthetic properties and mechanical performance.

Different approaches and materials were investigated: for instance, some materials appeared to be more suitable for teeth of the anterior group, where esthetics is more important compared to strength. In this case, the evolution started from pressed and cast ceramics, to porous ceramics infiltrated with glasses, followed by pressing of the filled glass. Glass ceramics can be used in restorative dentistry as inlays, onlays, veneers, and crowns for their excellent esthetic properties. In the posterior area, the mechanical strength is more important than esthetics. Therefore, the research has focused on computer assisted design/computer assisted manufacture (CAD/CAM) technology to achieve high-strength and nonshrinking ceramics. In addition, glassy-free materials such as polycrystalline ceramics are used, as they satisfy load-bearing requirements.

This chapter presents an overview of commercial polycrystalline and glassy ceramics, focusing on composition, laboratory production, and literature review. In the first part, the state-of-the-art in load-bearing ceramics will be described with respect to different clinical applications. In the following part, the technical characteristics of the main load-bearing ceramics are systematically analysed and compared, even if the use of different characterization techniques makes difficult a clear and direct comparison between their properties.

# 6.2 Dental applications of load-bearing ceramics

## 6.2.1 *Blanks for the CAD/CAM technology system*

The fabrication of FDPs in dental practice is one of the most common procedures for replacing missing teeth. The clinical survival rates of FDPs are 72%–87% after 10 years, 69%–74% after 15 years, and 53% after 30 years (Miyazaki et al., 2013). Long-term survival (>8 years) of all-ceramic crowns ranged from 84% to 100% (Canadian Agency for Drugs and Technologies in Health, 2015). Transmission of light by the substructure directly influences the final appearance of veneer porcelain, as the metal substructure blocks the light. High-strength ceramics are opaque and can substitute metallic frameworks; because of color, finish line can be at the gingival margin or 0.5 mm subgingival, without compromising esthetics. All-ceramic systems have reduced thermal conductivity, resulting in less thermal sensitivity and pulpal irritation (more biocompatible) (Pilathadka and Vahalová, 2007). Similar to the metal–ceramic technique, the construction of all-ceramic-based restorations uses a high-strength ceramic material for the framework to provide sufficient resistance against cyclic loading.

Conventional porcelains that best mimic the optical properties of enamel and dentine are predominantly glass materials with a flexural strength of about 100 MPa, indicating that they are not suitable for load-bearing restorations. Reinforced glassy materials were successfully used to make full-contour crowns for the anterior region, in which the fillers are usually crystalline phases, but can also be particles of a higher-temperature-melting glass. Polycrystalline ceramics with improved translucency have been used for full-contour crowns in the molar region. In the polycrystalline ceramics, the atoms are densely packed into regular arrays and are much stronger than glassy ceramics, so they are more resistant to fracture (Kelly and Benetti, 2011).

#### *6.2.1.1 CAD/CAM systems*

CAD/CAM technology is particularly used in prosthodontic and restorative dentistry and includes various methods and techniques for scanning, designing and fabrication of indirect restorations. Mormann et al. developed the CEREC system (Sirona Dental), and succeeded in producing a ceramic inlay restoration using computer-assisted technology (Mormann et al., 1989). The inlay cavity is digitized directly in the mouth using a compact intraoral camera; design and fabrication of the ceramic inlays are performed using a compact machine set at the chairside in the dental surgery. This application was limited to inlays and occlusal morphology and contour was initially not available. The original idea of in-office restoration fabrication is still currently practised. The evolution of the system can produce not only inlays and onlays, but also crowns and the cores/frameworks of bridges in both clinical and laboratory settings (Miyazaki and Hotta, 2011).

The first generation of application of the dental CAD/CAM system was introduced by Duret and colleagues (Duret and Preston, 1991). The intraoral abutment can be scanned by an intraoral digitizer to obtain an optical impression, the digitized data are reconstructed as a three-dimensional (3D) graphic and the better morphology of the crown can be "virtually designed" on the monitor. The final crown is fabricated by milling a block using a numerically controlled machine (Miyazaki and Hotta, 2011).

The second generation of the application of dental CAD/CAM systems uses the conventional stone model to begin the CAD/CAM process for the fabrication of crowns, especially for dental laboratory use. In more detail, a teeth stone model is made from an impression and the stone model is then scanned and converted to digital data. These types of CAD/CAM systems are able to fabricate many varieties of restorations, including metallic and ceamic restorations, at a lower cost while maintaining good quality (Miyazaki and Hotta, 2011).

The CAD/CAM systems can be classified into:

1. Chairside system: the dentist digitally scans the prepared tooth and creates restorations in office.
2. Laboratory system: laboratories scan tooth-prepared models made from physical impressions, designing the single coping or framework using a particular company's construction software, and using CAD/CAM to produce restorations or electronically sending the information to the company's milling center;
3. Centralized production: the dentist obtains a digital impression and then the data is sent via the internet to the laboratory (Baroudi and Ibraheem, 2015).

If the ceramic framework is fabricated using a CAD/CAM system in the machining center, final restorations are often completed by veneering porcelain using traditional layering of porcelain, a pressing technique, and the CAD-on veneering technique (Alghazzawi, 2016).

Three different approaches were developed in the last years to provide structural nonshrinking ceramics:

1. Filled glass (leucite or lithium or disilicate) (IPS Empress CAD, e.maxCAD).
2. Lightly sintered ceramics to form necks between touching particles and then infiltrating the porous structures with glass (VITA In-Ceram spinell/alumina/zirconia, manufacturing process for inLab).
3. Milling/machining of blocks of polycrystalline ceramics. The subtractive technique, which is the most commonly used, involves cutting the coping or framework from a solid block to achieve the desired geometry (CEREC, Cercon, 3 M Espe Lava, Ivoclar e.max zirCAD).

Dense polycrystalline ceramics such as alumina ($Al_2O_3$), zirconia ($ZrO_2$) and in particular yttria-stabilized tetragonal zirconia ($Al_2O_3$-$ZrO_2$) polycrystals (Y-TZP) and alumina–zirconia composites are available for CAD/CAM technology. Polycrystalline ceramics tend to be relatively opaque compared to glass ceramics and so they are used as substructure materials upon which glass ceramics are veneered to obtain the desired esthetics. CAD/CAM processing allows the use of partially stabilized zirconia for thinner core layers and the use of all-ceramic FDPs in posterior locations (Griggs, 2007). Y-TZP has a high fracture toughness (5–10 $MPa\sqrt{m}$) and a flexural strength of 900–1400 MPa (Miyazaki et al., 2013; Guazzato et al., 2004). Zirconia is provided to dental laboratories in various-sized blocks and can be milled into single-unit copings or multiple-unit fixed-bridge frameworks. Polycrystalline ceramics are formed from powders that can be packed to around 70% of their theoretical density, and during firing the shrinkage is about 30% by volume. In these systems, each block is bar coded with the density for the shrinkage calculation and the milling machines can automatically change milling tools to obtain accuracy of fit (Kelly and Benetti, 2011; Guazzato et al., 2004). Zirconia presents superior mechanical properties as compared with alumina.

Y-TZP frameworks for FDP can be produced in two ways:

1. Framework with final dimensions can be milled directly from fully sintered ceramic blanks (CEREC-Sirona, DC-Zirkon, Digident).
   a. Advantages: higher fit
   b. Disadvantages: wear of tools, chipping of the material

2. Frameworks with enlarged dimensions can be milled from partially sintered blanks (green) followed by a postsintering at high temperature (1350–1550°C) (Cercon, 3 M Espe Lava, Ivoclar e.max zirCAD, Denzir). Correction for 20%–30% firing shrinkage is calculated during the CAD phase. The soft machining process is the most common manufacturing system for 3Y-TZP. Addition of metal oxides to zirconia powder or immersing cores in metal salt solutions might yield colored cores. This coloration does not affect mechanical properties of zirconia cores (Khamverdi and Moshiri, 2012).
   a. Advantages: better machinability
   b. Disadvantages: shrinkage during subsequent high-temperature firing

CAD/CAM technology can be applied to zirconia–alumina composites as well. The materials of this class are called zirconia-toughened alumina (ZTA) when alumina is the main component, and alumina-toughened zirconia (ATZ), when zirconia is the main component. ZTA has not yet found much application in dentistry, it is much more opaque with respect to zirconia and probably not appreciated from an esthetic point of view (Fabbri et al., 2014). There is an exception however: a porous TZP infiltrated with glass and known as InCeramZirconia system (described in Section 6.3.2.2).

The properties of alumina–zirconia composites are the combination of the characteristics of alumina (high hardness, high stiffness) with the properties of zirconia (high-strength, toughness, improvement of slow crack growth resistance (DeAza et al., 2002)). In ZTA, the positive effect of adding zirconia into an alumina matrix (ZTA) is well known: enhancement of flexural strength, fracture toughness, and fatigue resistance are clearly shown. In ATZ, the addition of alumina increases the hydrothermal stability of the tetragonal phase of the zirconia structure, because alumina acts as a barrier for the propagation of phase transformation into the bulk (Affatato et al., 2006). This is due to the elastic modulus of alumina, higher than that of Y-TZP, which allows maintenance of the zirconia particles in the metastable tetragonal state, thus acting as a "mechanical stabilizer" (Fabbri et al., 2014; Affatato et al., 2006; Zhao et al., 2012; Kohorst et al., 2012). Both ZTA and ATZ materials showed much better aging resistance than monolithic Y-TZP.

### 6.2.1.2 Marginal fit

From a clinical point of view, zirconia restoration fit represents a focal point for marginal precision. Marginal gap is the main cause for plaque accumulation or marginal leakage, which can lead to periodontal disease, bone loss, or secondary dental caries (Song et al., 2013). The accuracy of the CAD/CAM technology and the control of the sintering shrinkage are the most important variables for marginal precision. When using CAD/CAM technology, the fit can be set for each abutment tooth in the software, which customizes the marginal gap for each clinical situation. The accuracy and ability of CAD/CAM technologies to implement the predetermined 3D fit of zirconia copings depends on the accuracy and precision of the scanning device, milling material, and milling unit. In the case of presintered ceramic (e.g., zirconia), the homogeneity of the material is especially important as it controls shrinkage during the final sintering process (Song et al., 2013; Moldovan et al., 2011). The grinding process and the preparation design may affect the internal adaptation, while the diameter of the preparation is determined by the smallest diameter of the bur used for machining the internal surface. In structures smaller than the narrowest bur diameter, more internal substance may be removed than necessary (Torabi Ardekani et al., 2012).

The absolute marginal fit of zirconia FDPs have been reported to be between 9 and 206.3 μm and most of the available systems provide clinically acceptable marginal adaptation (Boening et al., 2000). Gaps of up to 150 μm are commonly considered as being clinically tolerable (Li et al., 2014).

### 6.2.2 Dental implants

Titanium is the most commonly used dental implant material, due to its excellent biocompatibility. Although the crown that abuts the titanium implant may be esthetically optimal, the grayish color of the titanium implant could be detected through the thin peri-implant mucosa, thus impairing the esthetic result (Caglar et al., 2010). With highly sensitive immunologic tests, sensitization to titanium can be observed in some cases (Sicilia et al., 2008). The rising popularity of metal-free reconstructions motivates clinicians to offer implants of alternative materials. Ceramic implants can feature esthetic benefits in both supra- and subcrestal areas (Borgonovo et al., 2013), in particular in the presence of a thin biotype or gingival recession. Bioinert and not resorbable metal oxides such as alumina or zirconia can be used as dental implants. Zirconia is radiopaque and clearly visible on radiographs, its color is similar to that of natural teeth, rendering it extremely useful in esthetically critical areas of the oral cavity (Caglar et al., 2010).

The first use of alumina as a dental implant material dates back to 1965, when Sandhaus (Sandhaus, 1969) patented a dental implant screw composed of high-density alumina Degussit AL23 (Fig. 6.1).

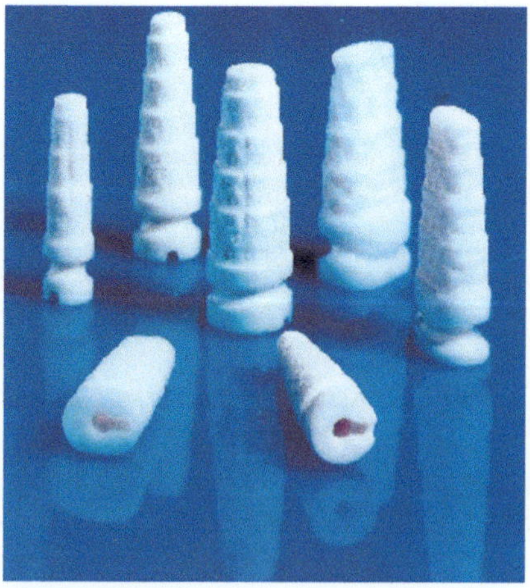

**Figure 6.1** Sandhaus dental implant, 1969.
From Piconi, C., Rimondini, L., Cerroni, L., Donati, C., Mutone, V. La zirconia in odontoiatria. Milano: Elsevier, 2008.

The Tubingen (Frialit) implants, made from polycrystalline α-alumina, were introduced in 1974. However, these implants do not withstand tensile forces and are susceptible to brittle fractures, the connector area is especially prone to failure. For this reason, zirconia was introducd in the dental field as an alternative to titanium (Reinhardt and Beikler, 2014). No clinical follow-up studies on alumina implants have been published since 2000.

Concerning zirconia impants, the behavior in terms of biomechanical properties, biocompatibility and in vitro behavior was thoroughly investigated, as reported in the following.

### 6.2.2.1 Biomechanical properties of zirconia implants

Ceramic implant failure can be due to physical, chemical, and mechanical properties. Failure analysis of fractured dental zirconia implants revelead that many fractured implants were located on the anterior side of the maxilla and mandibula (mechanical overloading). Manufacturing imperfections or flaws created during ceramic implant fabrication and subsequent surface treatment may compromise their strength. Material flaws usually assume the form of pores or microcracks of a submillimeter scale (Osman et al., 2013; Zhang et al., 2013; Gahlert et al., 2012).

Yttria partially stabilized zirconia (Y-PSZ) implants showed stress distribution similar to that of commercially pure Ti implants in the anterior maxilla (Kohal et al., 2002). Three different thread-form configurations in zirconia implants were evaluated in the study by Caglar et al. (2010), Z-implants (V-shape threads), Ziterion (Buttress-shaped threads), and White-Sky (square and V-shape threads combined) (Bredent Medical). The 3D finite element analysis showed that Von Mises, compressive, and tensile stress in the cortical bone in the White-Sky implants were lower with respect to the other implants under oblique and horizontal loading conditions, since there is no thread in the neck region. The highest stress occurred on the cortical bone of the Z-system design.

### 6.2.2.2 Biocompatibiliy of zirconia implants

The biocomapatibility of zirconia implants was thoroughly investigated, and the main results in terms of lymphocytes, fibroblasts, chondrocytes, osteoblasts, and macrophage responses are summarized in the following.

*Lymphocytes*: the presence of zirconia (Calcia-Partially Stabilize Zirconia, Ca-PSZ) particles (30−106 μm) showed a dose-dependent inhibitory effect; even if at high concentrations the cytotoxic effect did not exceed 50% and was below the oxide titanium ($TiO_2$) (Bukat et al., 1990). Alumina and zirconia powders showed similar effects on mitogenesis (Piattelli et al., 1992; Schierano et al., 2010).

*Fibroblasts*: the zirconia powders were much more toxic in the dense form. This effect was related to different surface reactivity and the release of the yttrium ion (Li et al., 1993). Dion et al. (1994) have shown the lack of toxic effects both on 3T3 fibroblasts and on HUVEC endothelial cells cultured with the medium previously incubated with Y-ZTP. The analysis by scanning electron microscopy (SEM) showed the adhesion and spreading of 3T3 fibroblasts on the material.

*Chondrocytes*: the cells in direct contact with the zirconia produce collagen and noncollagen protein similar to that detected for cells grown on titanium surfaces, but a reduced activity of alkaline phosphatase was detected (Hambleton et al., 1994).

*Osteoblasts*: zirconia and alumina showed absence of cytotoxicity, cells exhibited good adhesion and colonization, presenting the characteristic morphological aspect. The osteoblasts were able to process the extracellular matrix before the mineral deposition (collagen type I/V, osteonectin, osteocalcin, fibronectin, sialoproteins) (Josset et al., 1999; Cerroni, 2008b).

*Macrophage*: the ceramic powders (both alumina and zirconia) have no toxic effects, however, they induce apoptosis as a function of the concentration of the particles (80–150 particles/cell). Macrophages exposed to the particles of zirconia undergo to a change of cell permeability, with a slight damage of all cells, unlike alumina which causes more severe damage. The alumina and zirconia particles increase the concentration of intracellular sodium in cultured macrophages, while decreasing the concentration of potassium (Catelas et al., 1999; Nkamgueu et al., 2000).

The phagocytic activity (Tullio et al., 2010) of macrophages is inhibited (27%) because the cells initially have swallowed too many particles of zirconia. The reduction of the phagocytic activity also corresponds to the reduced biomaterials intracellular generation of hydrogen peroxide, determined by an alteration of the NADPH oxidase system.

The zirconia powder and dense purified zirconia did not elicit mutagenicity and/or carcinogenicity (Nicoli Aldini et al., 2004; Ruby and McNally, 1995; Reznikoff et al., 1973; Covacci et al., 1999). The study of Josset et al. (Josset et al., 1999) demonstrated the absence of mutagenicity and carcinogenicity of alumina and zirconia on osteoblast cells cultured in vitro for up to 30 days. Recently, research has focused the attention on a ceria-stabilized zirconia/alumina nanocomposites (NANOZR), which shows higher strength and fracture toughness when compared to 3Y-TZP (Yamashita et al., 2009). Cell attachment of mouse-osteoblast-like-cells on NANOZR was comparable to that of Ti; surface roughness significantly influenced the attachment of cells with a better initial response and expression of integrins. Setzer et al. (2009) used human fetal osteoblasts to study adhesion on different materials (Zi-Unit and Metoxit). The behavior of zirconia materials was similar to that of titanium with respect to histology, gene expression, and morphology; cells were modulated by surface roughness during the early stage of proliferation (Assal, 2013). A summary of main research on zirconia biocompatibility is reported in Table 6.1.

### *6.2.2.3 In vivo behavior of the main zirconia implant systems*

The main data on different implant systems will be reported below, whereas in Table 6.2 the more consistent clinical trials on zirconia implants are collected. Many of these studies report the use of one-piece zirconia implants.

#### Incermed SA, Losanna

In 1984, Sandhaus developed the zirconia implant SIGMA 1, with internal hexagonal abutment connection. The osseointegration of implants SIGMA has been studied

**Table 6.1 Summary of main in vitro experiments on different cell types in the presence of zirconia**

| Cells | References | Sample | Test | Results |
|---|---|---|---|---|
| Fibroblasts 3T3, primary, gingival | Bukat et al. (1990); Li et al. (1993); Dion et al. (1994); Uo et al. (2003); Raffaelli et al. (2008) | Dish, powder, eluate | Direct contact, 3-(4,5-dimethylthiazol-2-yl)-2,5-diphenyltetrazolium bromide (MTT), SEM, DNA | Good adhesion and proliferation. Cytotoxicity of powder > cytotoxicity wear particles |
| Lymphocytes | Bukat et al. (1990); Piattelli et al. (1992); Nkamgueu et al. (2000); Demir et al. (2013) | Powder 30−175 μm<br>Nanoparticles | Mitogenesis<br>X-Ray microanalysis, cytometry, modified alkaline comet assay | Inhibition $ZrO_2$ <$TiO_2$, reduced viability (8%), reduced phagocytic activity, no genotoxicity |
| Endothelial cells HUVEC | Dion et al. (1994) | Powder | Direct contact, MTT, SEM | No cytotoxicity |
| Chondrocytes | Hambleton et al. (1994) | Ultra-thin film | DNA-RNA, extracellular matrix (ECM) proteins synthesis | Good collagen production, alkaline phosphatase inhibition |
| Macrophages J774 | Catelas et al. (1999); Nkamgueu et al. (2000); Obando-Pereda et al. (2014) | Powder 80−150 μm | Apoptosis, fluorescent microscopy, X-ray microanalysis, flow cytometry, expression of Toll-like receptors | Apoptosis as a function of particles concentration, reduction of phagocytic activity caused by $ZrO_2$ particles. $ZrO_2$ ceramic particles are less bioactive than Ti particles |
| Heparinized blood | Fischer et al. (2007) | Dish | Emocompatibility | < partial thromboplastin time (PTT),> partial thromboplastin time (TAT), reduced protein adsorption respect to Ti |

*(Continued)*

**Table 6.1 (Continued)**

| Cells | References | Sample | Test | Results |
|---|---|---|---|---|
| Osteoblasts: human primary, MG63, HOB, CAL72, SAOS2, MC3T3-E1 | Josset et al. (1999); Lohmann et al. (2002); Oum'hamed et al. (2004); Carinci et al. (2004); Hao et al. (2005); Bachle et al. (2007); Depprich et al. (2008a); Hempel et al. (2010); Watanabe et al. (2012); Ito et al. (2013); Bergemann et al. (2015) | Dish, powder | MTT, SEM, immunohistochemistry, metalloproteases, DNA microarray, RT PCR | Good adhesion and colonization, ECM production. Inhibition $ZrO_2 < TiO_2$. MMP9 expression. Increase of GSPT1, IL8, HDS11B1, PLOD2, reduction of MAP4, CYLN2, CDH11, GPC1. Surface treatment with laser 2.25 kW/cm (Canadian Agency for Drugs and Technologies in Health, 2015) increases cell adhesion. $ZrO_2$ treated with $Al_2O_3$ and etched with HVl-$H_2SO_4$ = Ti. Topographical differences of $ZrO_2$ have minor effects on osteoblast biology. Blast/Etch, $O_2$-Plasma, or UV treatment could create and maintain superhydrophilic surfaces and enhance initial attachment of osteoblast-like cells. Micro- and nano-topographies on TZP by surface treatment offers a promising method of enhancing the proliferation and differentiation. Sandblasting, acid etching and additionally heat treatment increase osteocalcin production |

*ECM*, extra cell matrix; *MTT*, Mossman's tetrazole test; *PTT*, Partial Thromboplastin Time; *RT PCR*, reverse transcriptase-polymerase chain reaction; *SEM*, scanning electron microscopy; *TAT*, thrombin-antithrombin III complex.

**Table 6.2** Clinical studies on zirconia implants

| | No. of implants | Prosthetic reconstruction | Follow-up years | Clinical parameters | Bone loss | Survival % | AMBL | Results |
|---|---|---|---|---|---|---|---|---|
| Blaschke and Volz (2006) | 66Vollzirkon1,2, Z-Look3 (Z.system) | After 4–6 months SC | 2 | ND | ND | 99 | ND | |
| Oliva et al. (2007) | 100 Ceraroot (Oral Iceberg) | After 4–11 months All ceramic (LAVA) SC | 1 | BOP | ND | 98 | ND | |
| Oliva et al. (2010) | 831 CeraRoot (Oral Iceberg) | After 4–11 months All ceramic (LAVA) SC | 3 | BOP | ND | 95 | ND | High success rate for implants with roughened surfaces, especially by acid-etching |
| Cannizzaro et al. (2010) | 40 Z-Look3 (Z-System) | After 4–6 months ceramic SC | 1 | | | 87.5 | 0.7–0.9 | Immediately loaded implants placed in postextractive sites had high failure rates |
| Borgonovo et al. (2012) | 29 White-Sky (Bredent) | After 6 months all-ceramic $ZrO_2$ SC or bridges (LAVA) | 4 | BOP, PD, PI | ≥2 mm (6.9%) | 100 | 1.21 | The reduction of marginal bone is mainly due to the one-piece morphology |
| Kohal et al. (2012) | 65 ZiUnite (Nobel Biocare) | After 6–14 weeks SC | 1 | PD, CAL | ≥2 mm (34%); ≥3 mm (14%) | 95.4 | 1.31 | The frequency of increased radiographic bone loss (>2 mm) after 1 year was considerably higher as compared to conventional two-piece Ti implants |
| Kohal et al. (2013) | 28 ZiUnite (Nobel Biocare) | After 6–14 weeks three-unit FDPs | 1 | PD, CAL, mPI mBI | ≥2 mm (40%); ≥3 mm (28%) ≥4 mm (12%) | 98.2 | 1.95 | $ZrO_2$ implant seems to perform inferior to Ti implant after 1 year when applied for FDPs and cannot be recommended for clinical routine due to the increased frequency of bone loss more than 2 mm |
| Gahlert et al. (2007) | 170 Z-Look3 (Z-System) | After 3 months 87 SC, 25 with FDP and 7 with RHD. | 3 | PI, PD, BOP | | 82.4 | | The survival rate was lower for the anterior versus posterior area, for maxilla versus mandible |
| Payer et al. (2013) | 20 White-Sky (Bredent) | After 4–6 months all ceramic crowns (e. max CAD-Blocks, Ivoclar-Vivadent | 2 | BOP, PD, PI, Periotest, PES | | 95 | 1.29 | The main focus of the present pilot was to evaluate the applicability of an immediate adhesive and microgap- less CAD/CAM restoration of Y-TZP implants without using removable protection devices |

*(Continued)*

**Table 6.2 (Continued)**

| | No. of implants | Prosthetic reconstruction | Follow-up years | Clinical parameters | Bone loss | Survival % | AMBL | Results |
|---|---|---|---|---|---|---|---|---|
| Osman et al. (2014) | 56 Ti (Southern Implants)<br>73 $ZrO_2$ (Southern Implants) | After 3–4 months acrylic overdentures | 1 | | | 82.1<br>71.2 | 0.18<br>0.42 | Increased marginal bone loss and higher fracture rate were observed for $ZrO_2$ implants compared with Ti implants, their use should only be limited to cases with proven allergy to Ti or those requesting a metal-free prosthodontic rehabilitation |
| Cionca et al. (2015) | 76 ZERAMEX_T Implants system (Dentalpoint) | After 6 months $ZrO_2$ abutments and Ceramic SC | 2 | PD, mBI, mPI | | 86% | | |
| Payer et al. (2015) | 16 Ziterion vario z,<br>15 Ziterion vario t | After 4–6 months Straight or angulated prefabricated standard ceramic abutments (Ziterion $ZrO_2$ Abutment) and all-ceramic lithium disilicate SC (e.maxCADBlocks) | 2 | BI, PI, Periotest, PES | | 93.3<br>100 | 1.48<br>1.43 | A rubber dam application at crestal levels is a prerequisite for a proper adhesive fixation of the $ZrO_2$ abutment to the $ZrO_2$ implant |
| Spies et al. (2015) | 53 Ziraldent FR1 | | 3 | PD, CAL, mBI > | $\geq$2 mm (8.1%) | 94.2% | 0.79 mm | |
| Roehling et al. (2016) | 161 Z-Look3 (Z-System | After 3 months 112 SC, 31 FDP, 4 RHD | 7 | GI, mPI, mBI | | 77.3 | 0.97 | Fractures were associated with decreasing implant diameter (3.25 mm) and with bruxism. During the loading period were observed in 11 implants with single tooth reconstructions, seven implants with FDP reconstructions. All implant fractures occurred at the sandblasted part (threads) of the coronal part of the implant body |

*AMBL*, average marginal bone loss; *BI*, bleeding index; *BOP*, bleeding on probing; *GI*, Gingival Index; *mBI*, modified bleeding index; *mPI*, modified plaque index; *PD*, probing depth; *PES*, pink esthetic score; *PI*, plaque index; *RHD*, removable hybrid denture; *SC*, single crown.

after 10 months from insertion in the mandible of dogs in comparison with implants in alumina Cerasand and experimental titanium Grade 1. The implants were placed after 6 months from the filling of surgical defects with coralline derived calcium carbonate (BIOCORAL, Inoteb, Saint Gonnery, France). The bone–implant contact was higher than that of titanium implants (Piconi, 2008).

For manufacturing Y-TZP BIO-HIP (Hot Isostatic Pressing) Sigma implants, the crystalline products are processed into powder by grinding and compressed by an isostatic process at high temperature, up to approximately 2000°C. The pure powder of zirconium is processed through pressure in high-temperature molds. This results in homogenous implants of exact dimensions. The chemical composition is >99.9% $ZrO_2$ + $HfO_2$+ $Y_2O_3$, of which 5.2% is $Y_2O_3$ and 0.1% are other oxides (Assal, 2013).

## Goei implants (Goei Industry, Akitsu-Hiroshima, Japan)

Akagawa et al. have placed 12 one-stage loaded and unloaded Y-TZP implants in beagles (dogs). After 3 months, the bone–implant contact was 69.8% for the loaded group (Akagawa et al., 1993). The same implants were observed under different load conditions after 2 years of function in monkeys. The prosthesis was divided into single implant, connection of two implants, and connection of one natural tooth and one implant. The authors reported the exposure of thread and evident marginal bone resorption in the initially loaded Y-TZP implants. There was no significant difference in groups with different loads. Marginal bone resorption was relatively high (1.7 ~ 2.1 mm) and the average bone–implant interface was 54% ~ 82% without significant difference between the different groups (Akagawa et al., 1998).

## Z-systems AG, Konstanz, Germany

Between 1998 and 2000, the first licensed and certified ceramic implant-system (Z-system) made of zirconium oxide was developed. Volz in 2003 reported the case of eight one-piece zirconia (Vollzirkon 1) implants on which within 6 months were cemented all-ceramic crowns (Piconi, 2008). Between 2001 and 2002 30 Vollzirkon 1 implants were inserted equipped with an apical cut for inserting the screw and characterized by a shoulder of support for small amplitude crown. The next evolution (Vollzirkon 2), used in over 80 cases, was equipped with a thread and a shoulder of greater amplitude. In the version produced from 2003 (Zlock3), the design of the neck and shoulder was optimized, and introduced a hexagonal connection at abutment level. Clinical results at 2 and 5 years after the inclusion of 66 fixtures of the above types inserted in 34 patients were reported by Blaschke and Volz (2006). After 4–6 months, 98% of implants had reached a good osteointegration; at the end of follow-up there was a good density in the newly formed cortical bone of 97.5% of the implants, with the absence of inflammation in the peri-implant soft tissue (Piconi, 2008).

Mellinghoff reported a survival rate of 93% at 12 months in a series of 189 Z-Look3 implants inserted between 2003 and 2005 in 71 patients, 53 of whom

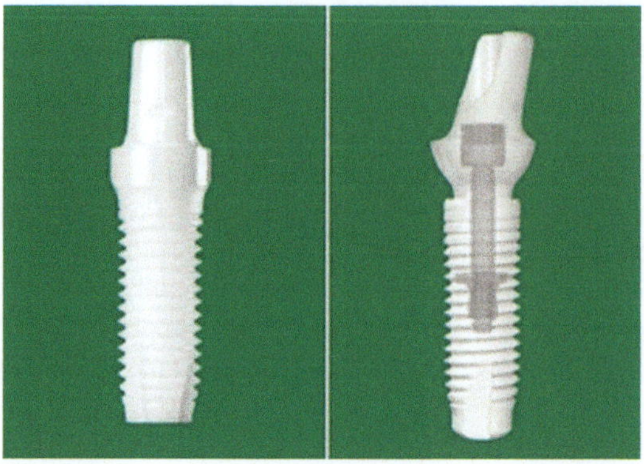

**Figure 6.2** Z5m Zirkolith implant-Z5s Zirkolith implant. http://zsystems.com.

received a fixed prosthesis (Mellinghoff, 2006). Immediately loaded zirconia implants placed in postextractive sites had high failure rates (12.5%) (Cannizzaro et al., 2010).

In the study of Gahlert et al. (2012) a fracture rate of nearly 10% (13 fractured implants out of a total of 170 implants) within a follow-up period of mean $36.8 \pm 5.3$ months (20 up to a maximum of 56 months) triggered a systematic analysis of the failed implants. Twelve of the 13 fractured implants had a diameter of 3.25 mm, the smallest size available within this implant system (ZLook3, Z-Systems AG). Only one failed implant had a diameter of 4 mm. After 7 years (Roehling et al., 2016) the overall longitudinal survival rate was 77.3%. The observed fracture rate of almost 10% seems to be in contrast to the publication by Mellinghoff (2006). Z-Look3 with a roughened surface were compared to Osseotite (Biomet 3i); the results of the hystologic study after 2 and 4 weeks after implant placement demonstrated a similar rate of bone apposition on surface-modified zirconia and titanim implants after 2 weeks, but after 1 month the bone apposition was higher in titanium (69%–91%) than in zirconia (62%–80%) (Hoffmann et al., 2008). Z-Look3 is the most analyzed implant in clinical trials present in international literature, with a survival rate of 77.3% after 7 years of follow-up. A new generation of Z-system implants was introduced to the market (Fig. 6.2); all Z5 implants are made from TZP-A Bio-HIP zirconium oxide; the SLM surface, which has been developed and patented by Z-Systems, achieves a surface enlargement through increased macro- and microroughness.

## BIO-HIP Metoxit AG, Thayngen, Switzerland

The main steps of the manufacturing process for dental HIP Y-TZP-A implants are: (1) material compaction, (2) sintering, (3) hot isostatic pressed (HIP), (4) reoxidizing, followed by (5) machining (grinding), (6) measurement proof testing, and (7) quality control. The chemical composition is >95.0% $ZrO_2$, 4.0% is $Y_2O_3$ and

0.25% is $Al_2O_3$. Adding 0.25% of $Al_2O_3$ diminishes the rate of conversion from tetragonal to monoclinic by a factor 10. Kohal et al. (2010) showed, by an in vitro study, that ATZ implants have an increased mechanical stability compared with TZP implants. By modifications of the implant geometry, especially at the highly loaded neck and abandonment of sandblasting at this region, an improvement in the implant strength is possible due to the reduction of detrimental stress concentrations at notches. ATZ ceramics seem to be advantageous compared with Y-TZP regarding the susceptibility to the tetragonal/monoclinic transformation and aging-induced fatigue (Spies et al., 2015a).

A prospective cohort investigation evaluated a one-piece implant made of ATZ (Ziraldent FR1). The surface was modified using the Zircapore surface technology (Metoxit AG). This coating was generated by an initial sandblasting procedure in terms of a "priming" followed by the application of a ceramic slurry that produces a porous surface after a final sintering process (Sennerby et al., 2005). A total of 27 patients received one ATZ implant each in a one-stage implant surgery with immediate temporization. The cumulative survival rate of the presented ceramic implant was slightly below (88.9%) the reported survival rates of titanium implants when immediately restored. The early failure can possibly be accounted for by the treatment with immediately temporized one-piece-implants. The average marginal bone loss after 1 year was 0.77 mm (Spies et al., 2016). The restoration type seemed to have a significant effect on bone resorption after 3 years follow-up (single crown: 0.47 mm; 3-unit FDPs: 1.07 mm; $P < 0.001$) with an average bone loss of 0.79 mm (Spies et al., 2015b).

## Bredent (Senden Germany)

White-Sky implants are fabricated in Brezircon, a zirconium dioxide tetragonal polycrystal ceramic, hot isostatically pressed (Fig. 6.3). It is a one-piece implant, with a design characterized by a conical body with double threads and a rounded apex. The endosseous implant surface is treated with a sandblasting process that determines microscopical surface characteristics of medium rugosity (Ra = 0.9−1). Borgonovo et al. (2012) evaluated survival and success rates of 29 zirconia implants

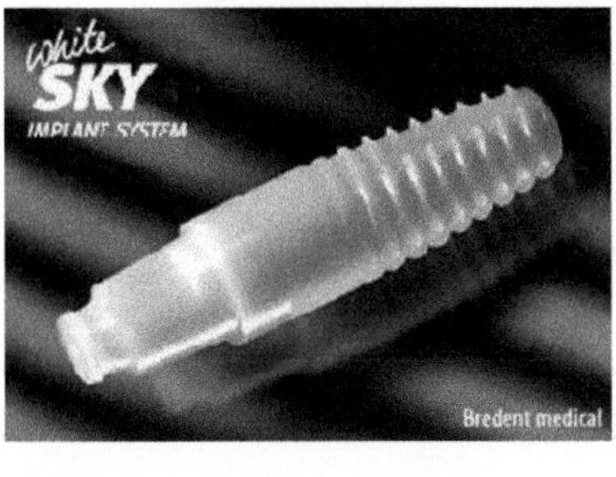


**Figure 6.3** White-Sky. Bredent. http://www.bredent.com.

that received immediate temporary restorations: the mean marginal bone loss at 4 years from the implants insertion was 1.63 mm, a bone losing between 1 and 2.6 mm has been reported in successfully osseointegrated dental implants. The survival rate was 100%. One-piece zirconia dental implants are characterized by high biocompatibility, low plaque adhesion, and absence of microgap that can be related to the clinical success of these implants even in the esthetic areas (Borgonovo et al., 2015).

### CeraRoot-Oral Iceberg Barcelona, Spain

Oliva et al. (2007) reported the first clinical evaluation of 100 zirconia implants with two different surface roughnesses in humans after 1 year of follow-up. Two implants placed with sinus elevation failed after 15 days. The overall success rate was reported as 98%. Pirker and Kocher (2009) placed an immediate zirconia implant to the maxillary first premolar region and evaluated the clinical outcome. At 2-year follow-up, a stable implant and an unchanged peri-implant marginal bone level were observed. No bleeding was detected on probing. The most recent work on CeraRoot Implants was about 5 years' survival of 831 fixtures (Oliva et al., 2010). The zirconium implant has an acid-etched surface, providing and optimal macro-, micro-, and nano-roughness. This new ICE Surface helps achieve optimal conditions for the integration between implant and bone. It is a rough surface specially designed for achieving faster and stronger osseointegration compared to machined zirconia implants (Fig. 6.4).

### Ziterion

Cylindrical screw type subgingival, platform switched two-piece zirconia implants (Zit-vario $4.0 \times 11.5$ mm) were inserted into the maxillary incisor region. They were left for 6 months to osseointegrate. Panoramic and periapical radiographs were obtained and examined for bone–implant osseointegration. During the follow-up period the patients were satisfied with their prostheses and no complications were observed (Bankoğlu Güngör et al., 2014). An overall survival and success rate of 93.3% for 16 zirconia/Ziterion vario Z two piece implant after 24 months and a bone loss of $1.48 \pm 1.05$ mm was observed (Payer et al., 2015).

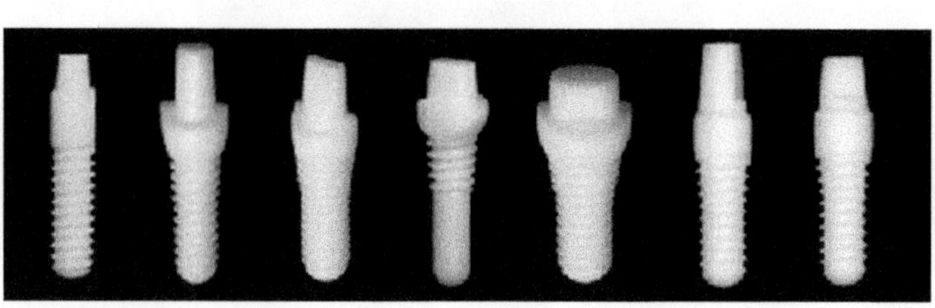

**Figure 6.4** CeraRoot Implants. http://www.ceraroot.com.

## ReImplant; Hagen Germany

The osseointegration of sandblasted zirconia implants compared with sandblasted and acid-etched titanium implants was evaluated in primates, the average bone implant interface after 9 months was 72.9% ± 14% for titanium and 67.4% ± 17% for zirconia. There was no significant difference in the average height of the outer surface of soft tissue around the implant (titanium: 5.2 ± 1.0 mm; zirconia: 4.5 ± 0.6 mm (Kohal et al., 2004).

## Konus dental

Twenty-four screw-type zirconia implants (3.5 × 9 mm) with roughened surfaces (Ra 0.598) produced by acid etching were compared to 24 implants of commmercially pure titanium with acid-etched surfaces (Konus Dental Implant; Bingen, Germany). Twenty minipigs were used for implant surgery. After 12 weeks, successful osseointegration of the zirconia as well as the titanium implants was visualized at the ultrastructural level. No interposition of interfacial layer or foreign-body reaction was detected, no significant difference in strength and stiffness was observed (Depprich et al., 2008b).

## Axis Biodental

Available either in two-piece or in one-piece, the Axis two-piece implant has an internal thread (Fig. 6.5). This ensures a reversible assembly between abutment and implant since no glue is needed. The surface of the Axis implant's body has been specially structured to obtain a relatively high roughness (1.6 μm) (Figs. 6.6 and 6.7), while the implant's collar surface has been specially developed to achieve low roughness (0.5 μm) (http://www.axis-biodental.ch).

## ZiUnite; Nobel Biocare

This is the only system that seems to add a porous surface on zirconia; however, there is little or no information about the chemical structure of the implant. Seventy-two threaded zirconia ceramic implants were manufactured by isostatically cold -ressing zirconia powder (TZ-3YSB-E, Tosoh Corporation, Tokyo, Japan) into rods. These rods were presintered and then turned into threaded implants. To achieve a porous surface, the implants were coated with a slurry containing zirconia powder and a pore former (Ra 0.489) on the surface of the not-yet sintered implant. During sintering to full density, the pore-former burns off and leaves a porous surface (Assal, 2013).

In the study by Sennerby et al. (2005) two slurries, each with a different pore former, were used to create two different surface structures. After the coating was applied, the implants were sintered to full density during which the pore former burned off and left a porous surface. As a control, 24 noncoated zirconia implants and 24 modified oxidized implants (TiUnite) were used. The study showed a strong bone tissue response to surface-modified zirconia implants after 6 weeks of healing. The nonmodified zirconia implants showed statistically lower removal torque values than all other implants tested. All of the modified zirconia implants

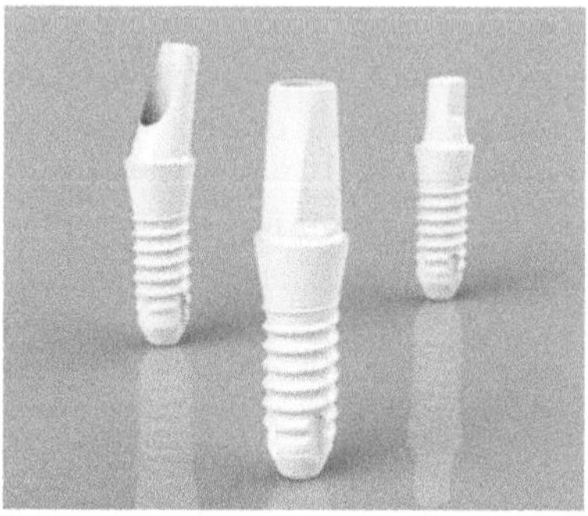

**Figure 6.5** Axis Implants. http://www.axis-biodental.ch.

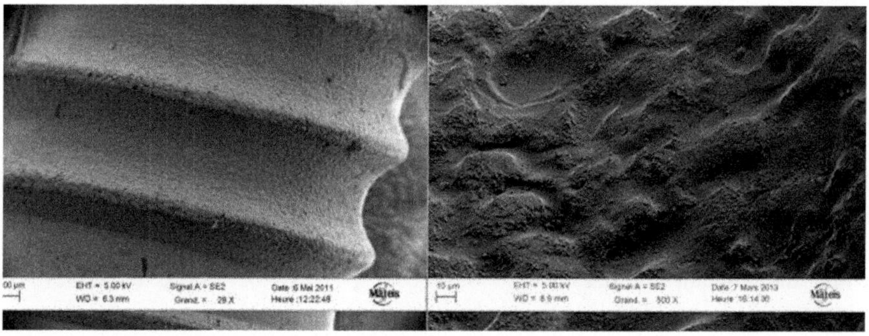

**Figure 6.6** Axis Rough from Sanon et al. (2015).

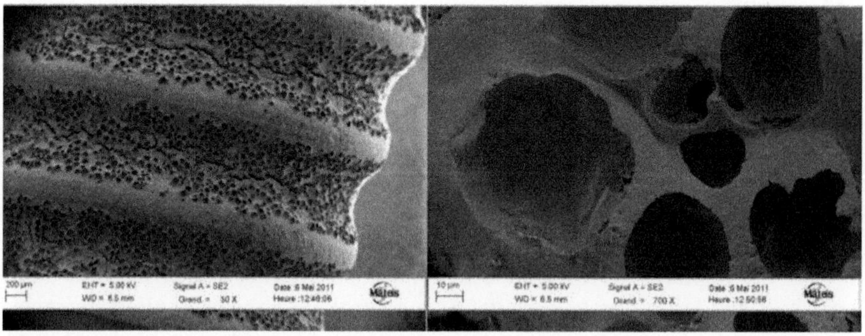

**Figure 6.7** Prototype Axis Alveolar. (Ra = 11 ± 2 μm), from Sanon et al. (2015).

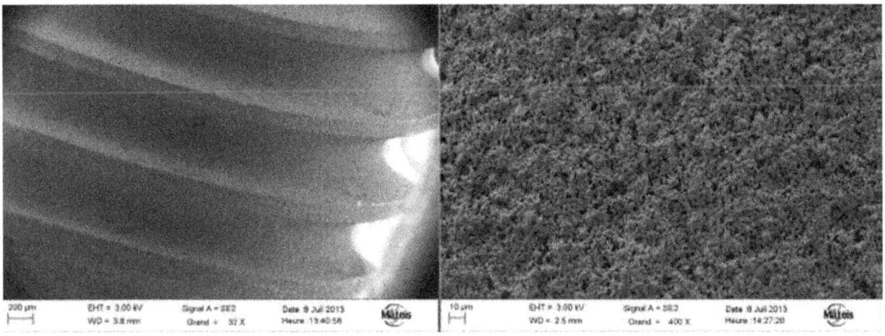

**Figure 6.8** Prototype ZiUnite from Sanon et al. (2015).

and the oxidized titanium implants showed similar resistance to torque forces. After removal torque testing, the SEM examination of the implant surfaces showed bone interface fracture rather than bone separation from the implant surface. However, Rocchietta et al. (2009) concluded that chemical addition to zirconia implants does not seem to be beneficial while Abhoushelib showed that nanoporous selected infiltration-etched zirconia could improve osteontegration in rabbits (Aboushelib et al., 2013). This implant (Fig. 6.8) is not available on the market.

## Straumann

The removal torque values for zirconia implants with either a machined (smooth) or a sandblasted (rough) surface, manufactured with exactly the same cylindrical shape with the same standard international team for implantology (ITI) thread configuration as the sandblasted and acid-etched (SLA) titanium implants (Gahlert et al., 2007). The zirconia implants were manufactured by Metoxit AG (Thayngen, Switzerland) under the control of Straumann AG (Basel, Switzerland).

The zirconia implants were processed as follows: (1) isostatic dry pressing, (2) sintering, (3) HIP, (4) shaping, and (5) polishing by a diamond tool. Half of the zirconia implants were sandblasted ($Al_2O_3$, Ø 250 μm) under 5 bars of pressure to generate a rough surface. The results of the study showed that rough zirconia implants had significantly higher removal torque values than smooth zirconia implants, although standard SLA titanium implants had significantly higher removal torque values than rough zirconia implants. The Straumann PURE Ceramic Implant features the (Zirconia Sandblasted and Acid-Etched ZLA®) surface, which is based on the SLA® surface (Fig. 6.9).

## ZERAMEX T Implants system (Dentalpoint AG, Zurich, Switzerland)

The all-ceramic implant system is intended to replace missing teeth in partially edentulous patients. The product consists of an implantable device and an

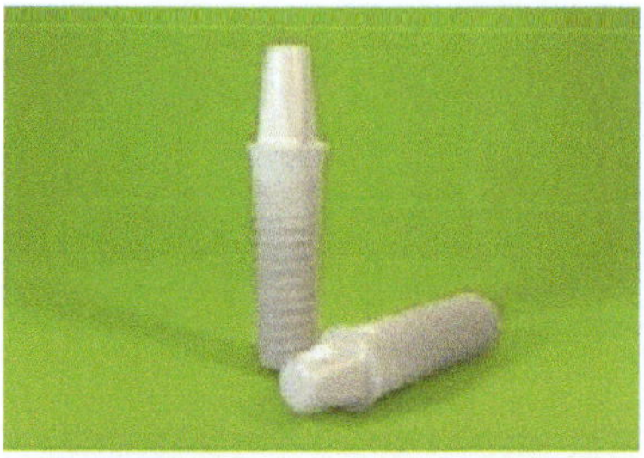

**Figure 6.9** Straumann® PURE Ceramic Implant. http://www.straumann.co.uk.

abutment, both made from highly dense zirconium dioxide ($ZrO_2$-ATZ-Bio-HIP, Metoxit AG, Thayngen, Switzerland). Thirty-two partially edentulous patients were treated with 49 two-piece zirconia implants. All patients were reevaluated 1 year after loading. The cumulative survival rate was 87% of implants. In the present study, the 1-year clinical exam evidenced healthy conditions of the peri-implant tissues throughout the entire cohort. No sites showed suppuration, redness, swelling, or marked bleeding upon probing (Cionca et al., 2015).

#### 6.2.2.4 Conclusions

The data in the literature can confirm the biocompatibility of the zirconia in the dense form, but we must be pay attention to the possible release of particles resulting from the degradation of the devices: they may cause inflammatory and immunological reactions.

Since each dental implant company has its own process, zirconia implants may behave differently, even if the starting powder is the same. Roughening the turned zirconia implants seems to enhance osteoconduction and bone apposition by increasing available surface area for fibrin attachment.

Surface topography has a beneficial effect on the interfacial shear strength but surface modification has a large influence on strength and sensitivity to aging. A protocol is needed to validate zirconia implant functionality and safety prior to its clinical use as proposed by Sanon et al. (2015).

### 6.2.3 Other applications

#### 6.2.3.1 Endodontic post

Endodontically treated teeth with a considerable coronal destruction, are more prone to fracture and need of a post-and-core system providing a substructure able to increase retention of the restoration to the tooth surface (Pfeiffer et al., 2006; Dikbas and Tanalp, 2013). Posts are recommended to strengthen weakened endodontically treated teeth against intraoral forces by distributing torquing forces along the roots (Dilmener et al., 2006); for this reason, research has focused on post materials and design, resin–post interface, and ferrule effect (Qing et al., 2007; Mannocci et al., 2008). Prefabricated posts of the same color as the teeth are preferred for the restoration of anterior teeth, which undergo to endodontic therapy (Rosentritt et al., 2000; Cerroni, 2008a), to avoid alterations in the transmission and reflection of light (Paul and Werder, 2004). Despite the high number of in vitro studies carried out regarding fiber-reinforced composite (FRC) posts, it is difficult to directly extrapolate the results to clinical conditions; the survival rate of glass fibers was found to be 71.9% over a period of 5 years (Schmitter et al., 2011). The ceramic posts are very stiff and strong, with no plastic behavior (Asmussen et al., 1999). In particular, there is today widespread use of zirconia ceramic post systems. The avalaible techniques for zirconia post and core reconstruction are: direct composite build-ups, adhesively luted ceramic core, ceramic core heat-pressing, and one-piece ceramic post-and-core restorations. Mechancial properties (in terms of fracture strength, retentive strength and bond strength to core) as well as clinical studies of zirconia endodonic posts are described in the following.

## Fracture strength of zirconia endodonic posts

The use of a rigid material as zirconia can lead to a concentration of stress at the apical portion of the endodonic post. The fracture strength of teeth with zirconia posts and composite cores ranged between 300 and 700 N. However, when ceramic cores were used, these values ranged between 800 and 1500 N (Ozkurt et al., 2010). Zirconia posts exhibited higher fracture strength when used with bonded prefabricated ceramic cores (1495 N) than with heat-pressed custom-made ceramic cores (463 N), as a result of change in the inner structure of the zirconia material during the heating process (Strub et al., 2001).

The evaluation of the 0%–2% yield strength of Cerapost ISO 50,90,110 was tested by Pfeiffer et al. (2006). The mean 0%–2% yield strength was $58 \pm 4$ N, $117 \pm 4$ N, and $166 \pm 23$ N for zirconia posts and $141 \pm 12$ N for titanium posts (control group). The stiffness and resistance to fracture of zirconia posts are similar to prefabricated titanium posts and can be recommended as an alternative to cast metal posts and cores.

Many authors believe that the fracture strength of a zirconia post is higher than that of a fibre reinforced composite (FRC) post, even if zirconia posts are more predisposed to cause root and crown fracture. According to other authors, the fracture resistance of a zirconia post when subjected to static load applied to 2 mm below the incisal margin of the palatal surfaces was similar to that of FRC. The type of core (direct or indirect technique) did not change the results (Cerroni, 2008a). Dilmener et al. (2006) compared the fracture resistance to compressive loading of two esthetic post-and-core system: Cosmopost and IPS Empress Cosmo Ingot (Ivoclar) (ZCER) exhibited the higher resistance to fracture (710 N) against

Cosmopost and Charisma ZCOM (450 N). The control group (metal post-and-core) exibited only root fracture, ZCOM displayed post and core fracture and ZCER more root and post fracture.

In 2007, a new post composed of glass fibers (43%), zirconia (17%) and resin (40%) (Fibio) ($E = 15$ GPa) was analyzed. The glass–zircon post showed failure loads significantly lower than those of the control group (NiCr) with a mean failure load of paired differences between the groups of −261 N. All the failures were in the form of root fractures (Qing et al., 2007). Table 6.3 summarizes the in vitro tests on the mechanical behavior of different types of zirconia post.

## Retentive strength of zirconia endodonic posts

FRC posts with a reduced diameter, for a given load and modulus of elasticity (40 GPa), have a higher tendency to deform than those of the upper diameter (Cerroni, 2008a). This problem could be resolved with a post of higher rigidity and lower deformability such as, e.g., metal and zirconia ($E = 200–220$ GPa) (Musikant et al., 2001).

Zirconia posts can be built up using composites as well as heat-pressed ceramic cores (Schulz et al., 2006; Rosentritt et al., 2000; Koutayas and Kern, 1999). A more stable and rigid core material may decrease the apical stress and prevent the intrusion of the post subjected to load, but stability is only partially achieved with a strong link between post and core (Cerroni, 2008a; Yaman and Thorsteinsson, 1992). Some authors have suggested that the system ceramic post/composite core should be avoided to insufficient bonding strength to dentin (Al-harbi and Nathanson, 2003).

The retention of the ceramic posts turns out to be rather difficult; the force required to detach the CosmoPost from the roots was lower than that required for FRC posts (89 N) (Hedlund et al., 2003). The integrity of cement used for endodontic post luting can be modified by the difference in modulus of elasticity between post and cement, which is due to the different distribution of stress on the adhesive system when a mechanical load is applied.

Cosmopost luted with the resin cement (Variolink II) presented statistically higher tensile bond strength (228.1 N) than those retained with glass-ionomer Fuji I (121.8 N). The post failed adhesively at the cement/post interface, because the lack of a long-term durable chemical bond between resin cements and zirconia ceramics. The higher values of resin luting cement can be attributed to its better tensile and shear strength (Marchan et al., 2005). Similar results were obtained with Cerapost-Ketac Cem (243 N) and Cerapost-Panavia F (304 N) (Gernhardt et al., 2005).

The bond between resin cement and zirconia is affected by the concentration of stress, because zirconia (as the metal) has an elastic modulus greater than that of dentin (Bottino et al., 2007; Galhano et al., 2008).

## Table 6.3 In vitro evaluation of the mechanical behaviour of $ZrO_2$ posts

| References | Samples | Materials | Test conditions | Results |
|---|---|---|---|---|
| Mannocci et al. (1999) | 40 single-rooted premolars: quartz fiber, carbon-quartz fiber, $ZrO_2$ posts | Composite crown build up-Ceramic crown (Empress) | Cyclic loading test, 45 degrees- 2 million cycles, wet environment | One crown fracture and five root fractures + post fractures |
| Rosentritt et al. (2000) | 40 incisors<br>Cosmopost, Ti, cast gold alloy, FRC | Core composite<br>Cement: Variolink | Thermal cycling and mechanical loading | 338 N, higher than other groups |
| Maccari et al. (2003) | 30 single-rooted teeth<br>Aestheti-Post, FibreKor Post, CosmoPost | All-Bond 2, C&B, Bisco, Tetric Ceram for crown build up | Compressive load, 45 degree at the lingual middle third of the crown, crosshead speed 0.5 mm/min | Fracture strength of CosmoPost was significantly lower than that of the other posts (36.5 kgf) and presented 30% of root fracture |
| Oblak et al. (2004) | 120 $ZrO_2$ posts (60-diam 1.3 and 60 diam 1.5 mm). Three groups (Control, sandblasted, grounded with diamond bur) | Clearfil-Panavia21 | Fracture load, 45 degree with loading tip on the coronal retentive ring, crosshead speed 1 mm/min | Sandblasting increases fracture resistance (993.6 vs 622.7 N). $ZrO_2$ post with 1.5 mm of diameter showed higher resistance |
| Toksavul et al. (2005) | 30 incisors | Cosmopost-Tetric Ceram<br>Cosmopost-Cosmo Ingot<br>FRC Postec-Tetric Ceram<br>Variolink2 cement | Static load applied to 2 mm below the incisal edge on the palatinal surface | There were no statistically significant differences (475–498 N) |
| Dilmener et al. (2006) | 40 incisors | Cast metal post-an-core (Ni-Cr)<br>Parapost-Charisma<br>Cosmopost-Charisma<br>Cosmopost-IPS Empress | Thermal cycling 5–55°C—crosshead speed 1 mm/min, 45 degrees | Cosmopost-IPS Empress and Cast metal post-and-core (Ni-Cr) exhibited similar fracture resistance (710 vs 739 N) |
| Xible et al. (2006b) | 30 canines<br>Cosmopost -IPS Empress Cosmopost<br>FibreKor- Build It FR Resin Composite<br>AZthecAnchor- Build It FR Resin Composite | Crown: IPS Empress 2 | Mechanical load of 250 N for 500,000 cycles at a frequency of 1.7 Hz and then to static load until failure-crosshead speed 0.5 mm/min, 45 degrees | Fracture strength: 886.5 N<br>Equivalent fracture strength values and mode of failure |

(Continued)

**Table 6.3 (Continued)**

| References | Samples | Materials | Test conditions | Results |
|---|---|---|---|---|
| Pfeiffer et al. (2006) | Cerapost ISO50/90/110 | | Two-point bending test. Crosshead speed 2.5 mm/min, 45 degrees | 58/117/166 N |
| | Glass FRC-ISO50/90/110 | | | 27/52/73 N |
| | Ti ISO50-90-110 | | | 54/117/141 N |
| Bottino et al. (2007) | 40 single-rooted human teeth | All Bond 2 + resin cement Duo-link CoJet-Sand + ESPE-Sil | Fatigue testing. 2,000,000 cycles; load: 50 N; angle: 45 degrees; frequency: 8 Hz<br>Push-out at a crosshead speed of 1 mm/min | The bond strength of the $ZrO_2$ post was significantly affected by fatigue |
| | D.T. Light-Post | | | 6.9 ± 1.9 MPa |
| | Cosmopost | | | 3.3 ± 2.3 MPa |
| Qing et al. (2007) | 30 incisors and canines | Cement: Panavia F | Compressive load, crosshead speed 0.5 mm/min, 135 degrees to the long axis of the root | (Ni-Cr)1308 N |
| | Fibio (43%glass fiber,17% $ZrO_2$, 40% resin) | | | Fibio 1045 |
| | Cast metal post-and-core (Ni-Cr) | | | All specimens displayed root fracture |
| Bittner et al. (2010) | Maxillary central incisors and canines | The posts and cores were cemented | Shear strength test, crosshead speed 0.5 mm/min, 135 degrees | |
| | 17 cast gold post and core (Au) | With dual-polymerized composite resin cement (Multilink) | | 443 ± 150 N |
| | 17 one-piece milled $ZrO_2$ post and core (Zr) | | | 443 ± 123 N |
| | 17 prefabricated $ZrO_2$ post with heat-pressed ceramic core (Zr/Cer) | | | 413 ± 143 N |
| | 17 Ti post and composite resin core (Ti) | | | 556 ± 154 N |
| | 17 combined fiber/$ZrO_2$ post with composite resin core (Fiber/Zr) | | | 606 ± 202 N<br>Prefabricated posts (Ti and fiber posts) showed higher load-bearing values than custom posts |
| Mortazavi et al. (2012) | Structurally compromised endodontically treated teeth | Bonding resin: Clearfill SE Bond, hybrid composite (Clearfill AP-X) | 1500 thermal cycles intermittently between 5 and 55°C for 30 s with 12-s intervals crosshead speed 0.5 mm/min, 45 degrees | The fiber post treated teeth showed more desirable fracture patterns compared to those restored with $ZrO_2$ posts |
| | Double taper light posts (DT.Light-Post) | | | 732.44 N |
| | Double taper Light posts and Ribbond fibers | | | 603.44 N |
| | Cosmopost, Ivoclar | | | 573.67 N |

| | | | | |
|---|---|---|---|---|
| Rotunno and Rotunno (2012) | Maxillary central incisors | Cement: Panavia 21, Kuraray | Combined compression and bending | Carbon fiber posts were seen to fracture above the cement-root interface, in $ZrO_2$ post the fracture was located below the cement–root interface |
| | 5 Carbon fiber Tech.2000 | | | 18–26 daN |
| | 5 $ZrO_2$ post-Komet | | | 15–25 daN |
| Ozcan and Sahin (2013) | Maxillary central incisors | Cement: RelyX ARC. $ZrO_2$ post were abraded with $Al_2O_3$ particles | 6000 cycles (5–55°C, 20 s dwell time). A compressive load was applied to the posts at 45 degrees to the long axis of the tooth, at a crosshead speed of 1 mm/min, 4 mm from the incisal edge | Cervical teeth fractures |
| | Cerec 3D milled $ZrO_2$ blanks to one-piece postcore restorations | | | 577 N |
| | Feldspathic cores (prefabricated CAD/CAM) adhesively luted to CosmoPost $ZrO_2$ posts | | | 586 N |
| | and IPS Empress cores directly pressed to CosmoPost $ZrO_2$ posts | | | 585 N |
| Kaya and Ergun (2013) | Maxillary central incisors | All of the $ZrO_2$ posts received an airborne-particle abrasion with 30-mm silicatized $Al_2O_3$ particles (CoJet_Sand; 3 M Espe, Seefeld, Germany) at 280 kPa pressure from a distance of 10 mm for 20 s. self-adhesive luting agent (Clearfil SA Cement; metal crowns | A compressive load was applied on the lingual surface (2 mm below the incisal edge) at a 45 degrees angle and crosshead speed of 0.5 mm/min | Longer $ZrO_2$ posts with $ZrO_2$- or resin-based cores can be recommended as an alternative to FRC posts with resin-based cores<br>10 mm length / 15 mm length |
| | One-piece milled $ZrO_2$ post and core | | | 108 N / 191 N |
| | $ZrO_2$ post with resin core | | | 167 N / 157 N |
| | $ZrO_2$ post with resin composite core | | | 197 N / 157 N |
| | FRC post with resin core | | | 75 N / 98 N |
| | FRC post with resin composite core | | | 101 N / 91 N |

(*Continued*)

**Table 6.3 (Continued)**

| References | Samples | Materials | Test conditions | Results |
|---|---|---|---|---|
| Soundar et al. (2014) | Maxillary central incisor teeth | Cement: Multilink K, post diameter: 1.7 mm | Increasing oblique compressive load was applied, 2 mm below the tip. crosshead speed of 1.00 mm/min, 40 degrees | |
| | 12 Cast metal post (NiCr) | | | 294.33 ± 1.02 N |
| | 12 Pressable ceramic E-max- Lithium disilicate ($LS_2$) glass–ceramic | | | 375.00 ± 1.57 N |
| | 12 Cosmo Postlithium disilicate glass ceramic core | | | 638.67 ± 0.81 N |
| | 12 Milled $ZrO_2$ - Ceramill Zi-presintered | | | 415.00 ± 0.89 N |
| Kurthukoti et al. (2015) | Maxillary central incisors | | Compressive load, 135 degree to the long axis of the teeth, crosshead speed 0.5 mm/min | Teeth restored with the dentin post system and the FRC post system demonstrated more favorable, teeth restored with the $ZrO_2$ post system demonstrated more catastrophic fractures making them difficult for retreatment |
| | Cosmo Post | | | 522 ± 110 N |
| | FRC posts (Postec Plus) | | | 661 ± 161 N |
| | Dentin posts | | | 721 ± 127 N |

*FRC*, fiber reinforced composite.

## Bond strength of zirconia post to core

The chemical bonding of bisphenol A glycidyl methacrylate (bis-GMA)-based composite to zirconia is difficult to achieve, therefore the bond must rely on macroretention only (Kern and Wegner, 1998). Many authors believe that adhesion of composite might benefit from a retentive coronal portion of endodontic post (Kosmac et al., 2000). A zirconia endodontic post system with a retentive coronal portion was introduced by Oblak et al. (2004) (Fig. 6.10); three retentive rings were designed, running perpendicular to the long axis, with the apical ring being the widest.

Before cementation, the zirconia post and core often must be reshaped to achieve accurate fit between the material and the prepared root canal. Chairside grinding with diamond burs may affect the mechanical properties of the post and lead to a significant drop in load to fracture of zirconia posts, whereas airborne-particle abrasion increases the fracture load.

Locally developed temperatures when diamond burs are used could exceeded the tetragonal-monoclinic transformation temperature below which zirconia is thermodynamically stable (Kosmac et al., 1999, 2000).

Many pretreatments of zirconia were tested and most of these were on zirconia posts. Edelhoff and Sorensen (Edelhoff and Sorensen, 2002) have evaluated in vitro the retention of selected core materials to zirconia posts dependent on different surface treatments and bonding procedures. CeraPost and CosmoPost were employed for the study and the cores were fabricated of either heat-pressed, zirconia-containing glass ceramic (IPS Empress Cosmo (EMC), Ivoclar Vivadent), highly filled hybrid composite (Tetric Ceram (TEC), Ivoclar Vivadent) or an experimental, high-strength glass ceramic (OHSU-RWTH (EX), Ivoclar Vivadent). Prior to core

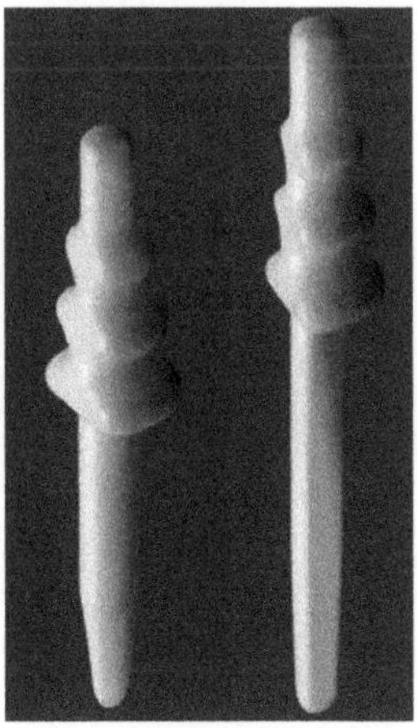

**Figure 6.10** Experimental posts with diameters of 1.5 mm (left) and 1.3 mm (right), showing retentive post heads with apical, middle, and coronal ring structures (Oblak et al., 2004). From Piconi C, Rimondini L, Cerroni L. La zirconia in odontoiatria. Milano: Elsevier Masson; 2008. p. 164.

application, the post surfaces were preconditioned by alumina abrasion or tribochemical silicoating and silanation. The push-out test did not determine significant differences between the separation loads. For both post systems tested with the combinations alumina abrasion/zirconia-containing glass ceramic and tribochemical silicoating and silanation/highly filled hybrid composite, a reliable retention was achieved. Teeth restored with the system Cosmopost-IPS-Empress Cosmo exhibited higher level of microleakage compared to metal and glass fiber post (Snowpost). This can probably be attributed to the higher elastic modulus of zirconia with respect to the luting cement (Variolink) and the creation of high-stress zones (Usumez et al., 2004).

Xible et al. (2006a) conducted a study on the effect of tribochemical tratment (Rocatec) on bond strength between Cosmopost and composite core Tetric Ceram (Fig. 6.11).

The use of a tribochemical silica coating process and silanization on zirconia-based ceramic posts increased both the bond strength to composite resin as well as the fracture strength of posts. These results have been partially confirmed by Bitter et al. (2006), who showed that Cosmopost treated with Rocatec system resulted in a higher bond strength than with Cojet system. Bond strengths to post were significantly affected by the type of luting agent, Panavia produced better results if the Rocatec system is used while PermafloDC (Ultradent) is better improved by Cojet treatment (Sahafi et al., 2003) (Fig. 6.12).

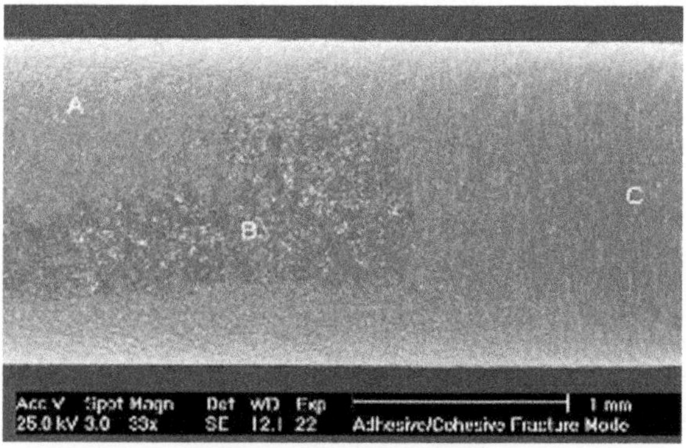


**Figure 6.11** Photomicrograph of tribochemical-treated zirconia dowel confirming cohesive/adhesive fracture mode observed (original magnification 333). Composite resin can be observed on only small percentage of visible area. (A) Nontreated ceramic surface area; (B) tribochemically treated ceramic surface area; (C) composite resin adhered to tribochemically treated ceramic surface area (Xible et al., 2006a).
From Xible, A.A., de Jesus Tavarez, R.R., de Araujo Cdos, R., Bonachela, W.C., Effect of silica coating and silanization on flexural and composite-resin bond strengths of zirconia posts: an in vitro study. J. Prosthet. Dent. 2006a; 95: 224-229; Piconi C, Rimondini L, Cerroni L. La zirconia in odontoiatria. Milano: Elsevier Masson; 2008. p. 166.

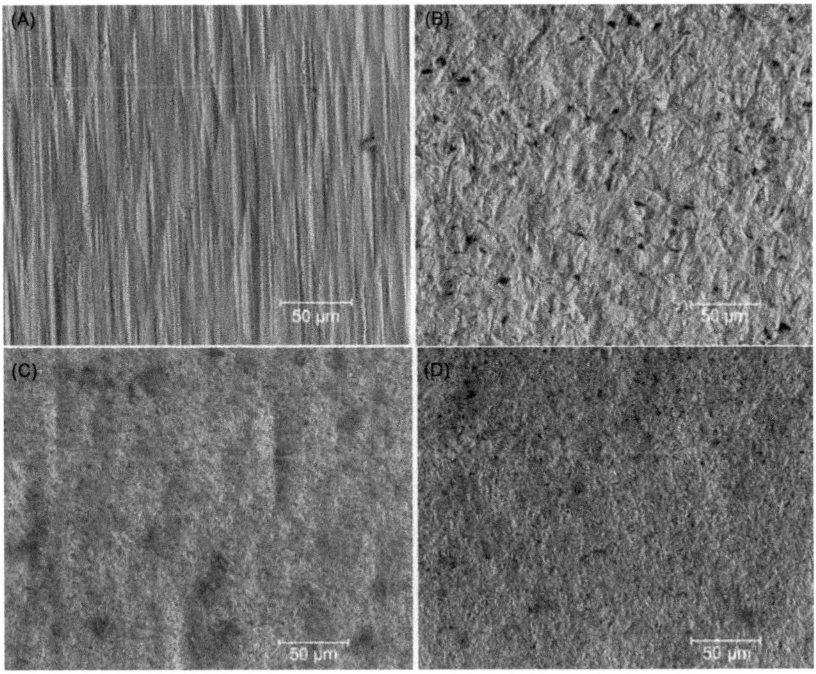


**Figure 6.12** Representative surface of (A) untreated zirconium-oxide post revealing smooth grooves; (B) airborne-particle–abraded surface indicating micromechanical retentive areas after treatment with aluminum-oxide particles (110 mm diameter); (C) CoJet-treated surface revealing smaller microretentive areas compared to airborne-particle–abraded surface; (D) after pretreatment with Rocatec System. Surface appears smoother compared to airborne particle brasion alone. Original magnification ×300.
From Bitter, K., Priehn, K., Martus, P., Kielbassa, A.M., In vitro evaluation of push-out bond strengths of various luting agents to tooth-colored posts. J. Prosthet. Dent. 2006 Apr;95(4): 302-310. Piconi C, Rimondini L, Cerroni L. La zirconia in odontoiatria. Milano: Elsevier Masson; 2008. p. 168.0

## Clinical studies of zirconia endodonic posts

In a retrospective study, 79 zirconia posts (52 patients) with direct composite cores and 34 zirconia posts (19 patients) with indirect glass ceramic cores (IPS-EMPRESS Cosmo), were evaluated after 4 years (Paul and Werder, 2004). No failures were observed for the tooth reconstructed with direct composite cores, while three failures were observed in the second group for loss of retention of post from glass ceramic cores. The clinical study confirmed in vitro studies that consider the composite core more resistant than the glass ceramic core. In the prospective study of Nothdurft and Pospiech (2006), 25 zirconia posts with heat-pressed ceramic cores (Empress) cemented with GI Ketac Cem or resin modified GI (ProTecCem) were observed for a variable time of 8–44 months. The authors reported no failures in terms of loss of retention, fracture, or dislodgement, confirming the results obtained by Koutayas and Kern (1999) in an obervational study of 6–16 months.

Ozkurt et al. (2010) reported a case in which a fractured fiber post was replaced with a custom-made zirconia post in order to improve adaptation and retention. The zirconia postcore was fabricated by means of manual milling system (MAD/MAM) system (Zyrkonzahn).

As a conclusion, zirconia endodonic posts have revealed good mechanical properties in static experiments but mechanical cycling appears to damage the bond strength to cores, probably due to stress concentrations. Zirconia posts can cause root fractures, due to the high modulus of elasticity. It is very difficult to remove zirconia posts from the root canal and it is a problem when a tooth must be retreated.

### *6.2.3.2 Ceramic implant abutments*

The abutment material over the implant could be visible, by transparency, when soft tissue discoloration happens in the cervical third of the implant portion of the restorations (Gomes and Montero, 2011). Intrasulcural abutment design is critical to reduce the risk of metallic blue shimmer through thin soft tissue. Ceramic transgingival components have been introduced by many manufacturers to provide abutments more esthetic than those fabricated from titanium (Ti). Ceramic abutments allow for optimal adaptation between the margins of the restoration and the soft tissue (Manicone et al., 2007).

The first ceramic abutments were the CerAdaptTM (Nobel Biocare, Goteborg, Sweden) made of alumina and designed to fit the extern hexagon of Brånemark implant type. Andersson et al. (1999) inserted 105 implants in 32 patients: after 2 years, the cumulative survival rate was of 97.1% for the implants and 97.2% for the restorations over the implants (94.7% for ceramic and 100% for titanium abutments). A higher loss of marginal bone around the titanium abutments than around the ceramic ones (0.4 mm vs 0.2 mm) was observed. The same results were shown after 5 years (Andersson et al., 2003).

However, since these products are generally made of very stiff material such as alumina, they are often affected by unpleasant technologic problems because of their low resistance to bending forces (Sadowsky, 2006). Procera abutments based on CAD/CAM technology has provided new opportunities for single-tooth esthetic restorations in zirconia. The Procera abutments in zirconia showed a precision and a rotational freedom between the implant and the abutment similar to that of Procera abutments in titanium (Yildirim et al., 2003).

In a comparative study, zirconia abutments showed fracture loads more than twice those recorded for alumina abutments (Gomes and Montero, 2011; Yildirim et al., 2003). One paper presented the clinical success of 36 experimental zirconia abutments on single-tooth implants. No abutment fractures were observed during clinical loading, resulting in a cumulative survival rate of 100% after 49 months. Healthy peri-implant mucosa and stable marginal bone levels were documented at zirconia abutments (Andersson et al., 2003; Canullo, 2007). Under the mastication simulator and static loads, the strength of the zirconia abutments was comparable to those of titanium (281 N vs 305 N) (Butz et al., 2005).

Conversely, Att et al. (2006) found a similar strength between zirconia and alumina abutments subjected to artificial aging.

The success rate of 37 zirconia–alumina composite abutments (ZirAce, Acucera Inc., Reno, NV) was evaluated (nine single-tooth implants and 28 FDPs implants). No abutment fractures, cracks, screw loosening, peri-implant infection, or adverse soft tissue reactions were reported after 12 months (Bae et al., 2008). The clinical success of zirconia abutments are confirmed by many authors but few randomized clinical trials have been performed (Canullo, 2007; Glauser et al., 2004; Kollar et al., 2008; Zembic et al., 2013; Román-Rodríguez et al., 2010). A recent prospective clinical trial showed a success rate of 100% for titanium abutments and 88% for zirconia abutments at a 3-year recall. The hypothesis is that the fracture of the internal connection was due to imprecision of milling or micromotion, with a possible deformation of the implant shape (Ferrari et al., 2015).

## Implant/abutment fitting

Zirconia abutments are available prefabricated or custom-made; prefabricated zirconia abutments are a practical solution, but CAD/CAM technology can optimize the manufacturing of individualized zirconia abutments. The gap between implant and the implant-supported prosthesis has been described as a relevant factor in stress transference and a biological answer for peri-implant tissues. The adjustment between the external hexagon of implant and the internal hexagon of the abutment will have to allow less than 5 degrees of rotational movement to maintain a stable screw union (Gomes and Montero, 2011).

The misalignment determines extra loads to the different prosthetic components, to the implant, and to the bone, causing loosening of the prosthesis retention, abutment fractures, bone microfractures, loss of crestal bone, and implant failure. Titanium and zirconia Procera abutments did not have significant differences in rotational freedom (<3 degrees), and their values were significantly smaller with respect to alumina abutments (Vigolo et al., 2006). Totally ceramic abutments had a superior rotational misalignment when compared with the ceramic abutments with a metallic ring (Garine et al., 2007). Zirconia is about 10-times harder than titanium and may damage the titanium interface of implants during function (Stimmelmayr et al., 2013).

Zirconia abutments can be the cause of wearing down and abrasion of the connection metallic part, thus, as a result of positioning/removal of the zirconia abutments during their individualization, a smoothing of the corners of the external hexagon could occur (Gomes and Montero, 2011; Andersson et al., 2003; Stimmelmayr et al., 2013). Zirconia abutments connected to titanium cores determined a higher fracture resistance when compared to one-piece zirconia abutments (Vigolo et al., 2006). However Peixoto et al., in a 3D model, showed that zirconia abutments do not concentrate higher stress values with respect to titanium abutments; the peak stresses are concentrated in the first threads of the prosthetic screw and are independent of the materials used in the abutments (Peixoto et al., 2016).

## Zirconia abutments strength

The cervical part of the abutment is the area with a concentrated stress (torque) generated by the screwing (Att et al., 2006).

Adatia et al. (2009) measured in vitro the effect of different preparations of zirconia abutments on their resistance to fracture, submitted to clinically similar conditions. Original zirconia abutments (without preparation) fractured in the cervical region, at the abutment/analog interface; the design of the interface implant/pillar seems to have a main role in the fracture mode (Gomes and Montero, 2011). The zirconia abutments registered values of strength at least 15% higher than the anterior bite force, and it was checked that the abutments preparation did not adversely affect their resistance to the fracture (Adatia et al., 2009).

The flexion strength of the zirconia abutments when used in a cantilever structure is greater than or similar to the titanium abutments (Sundh and Sjögren, 2008).

The zirconia abutments under static load exhibited maximum fracture values of 672 N, and after 80,000 cycles values of 269 N, supporting loads that exceed the established maximum values of force at incisal level (Gehrke et al., 2006).

Wall thickness does not affect the resistance to fracture of zirconia abutments (Att et al., 2012) but circumferential preparation might negatively affect the fracture strength within the implant/abutment internal connection (Koutayas et al., 2012). A summary of in vitro studies on fracture resistance of zirconia abutments is reported in Table 6.4.

## Bacterial adherence and response of the tissues

Dental implants require a biological sealing to inhibit the epithelial recession and the bacterial invasion of the subepithelial conjunctive tissue and of implant interfaces. The need to promote the formation of an adhered gingival tissue to create a biological barrier to the bacterium migration and toxins to the biological space has been emphasized (Rimondini et al., 2002; Banche et al., 2010).

Scarano et al. (2004) registered a degree of bacterial coating of 12.1% in the zirconia, compared to 19.3% in the titanium. Rimondini et al. (2002) confirmed these results with an in vivo and in vitro study in which Y-TZP accumulated fewer bacteria than titanium, in terms of total number of bacteria. The different free surface energy of titanium and zirconia abutments had no influence on *Aggregatibacter actinomycetemcomitans, Porphyromonas gingivalis*, and total bacteria adhesion (de Oliveira et al., 2012; Nascimento et al., 2014).

As a conclusion, zirconia abutments could be suitable for clinical application because of low bacterial colonization potential.

The majority of the studies consider that the ceramic abutments failure is more frequent in the cervical region, very close to the interface implant/abutment Zirconia abutments milled by means of CAD/CAM systems can be modified by the clinician to obtain a better marginal adaptation.

The fracture strength of the implant abutment increased with the implant diameter. Zirconia abutments are able to support single-tooth implant restoration in the anterior and premolar regions.

Table 6.4 **In vitro performance of Y-TZP abutment**

| Author | Samples | Mean fracture load (*N*) | Implant | Restoration | AFV | Conditions | Conclusions |
|---|---|---|---|---|---|---|---|
| Yildirim et al. (2003) | 10 $ZrO_2$-Wohlwend Innovative Switzerland<br>10 $Al_2O_3$- CerAdapt | 737.6 ± 245.0<br>280.1 ± 103.1 | Branemark | Glass ceramic crowns (IPS Empress) | 30 | Static load: 5 N | $ZrO_2$ abutments were more than twice as resistant to fracture as the $Al_2O_3$ abutments. Inhomogeneous fracture pattern |
| Butz et al. (2005) | 16 Zireal (Biomet 3i Palm Beach Garden, Florida, US) with Ti insert<br>16 $Al_2O_3$<br>16 Ti | 294 ± 53<br>239 ± 83<br>324 ± 85 | Osseotite | Dentitan crown (Krupp, Essen, Germany) | 30 | Thermocycling 1.2 million loading cycles | Ti-reinforced ZrO(2) abutments showed a similar to Ti abutments |
| Att et al. (2006) | Esthetic $ZrO_2$ (Nobel Biocare)<br>Esthetic $Al_2O_3$<br>Esthetic Ti | 443.6<br>422.5<br>1454 | Replace select | $Al_2O_3$ crowns (Procera) | 45 | Thermocycling 1.2 million loading cycles | $ZrO_2$ abutments have the potential to withstand occlusal forces applied in the anterior region. Failure at the implant interface |
| Gehrke et al. (2006) | 7 Cercon (Dentsply) (straight) | 672 (static load)<br>403 ($10^4$ cycles)<br>269 ($8 \times 10^5$ to $5 \times 106$ cicles) | XiVE | Spherical caps | 30 | Loads 100–450 N<br>5 million loading cycles at 15 Hz | Fracture strength exceeded the established values for maximum incisal bite forces reported in the literature |
| Canullo et al. (2007) | 20 Zircozahn (custom-made)<br>Ti insert | 436 | None | None | 30 | Static load | Bi-component $ZrO_2$ abutments have mechanical properties similar to esthetic abutments |
| Aramouni et al. (2008) | 20 ZiReal<br>20 UCLA-Ti | 792.2 ± 122.5<br>793.6 ± 162.3 | 3i | IPS Empress 2 full ceramic crowns | 45 | Static load | The mean load-to-failure values was above the reported normal maximal incisal load range |
| Kerstein and Radke (2008) | 29 Atlantis AAZ<br>29 Procera AllZirkon | 831<br>740 | Nobel Biocare | None | 40 | Incremental loads | Both types of $ZrO_2$ abutments demonstrated failure loads that exceed maximum human bite force |

(*Continued*)

Table 6.4 **(Continued)**

| Author | Samples | Mean fracture load (*N*) | Implant | Restoration | AFV | Conditions | Conclusions |
|---|---|---|---|---|---|---|---|
| Adatia et al. (2009) | 10 Y-TZP (Astra Tech) | 429–576 ± 140 | Implant analog | None | 60 | Fracture load, crosshead speed 0.1 mm/min | The preparation of $ZrO_2$ abutments (0.5- to 1-mm reduction) did not significantly impair the fracture resistance of simulated implant assemblies |
| Kim et al. (2009) | 10 Procera AllZirkon<br>10 CAD/CAM-designed $ZrO_2$ -based ceramic | 480.01 ± 174.46<br>902 ± 102 | Implant analog | Lithium disilicate pressable ceramic (IPS e.max Press). | 30 | Fracture load, crosshead speed 0.1 mm/min | Procera abutments are stronger than $ZrO_2$ abutments |
| Mitsias et al. (2010) | 18 Astra Tech Y-TZP<br>18 Ti | 690 ± 430<br>1475 ± 625 | | Metal crowns | 30 | Monotonic stress 400 N (5 × 105 cicles) | Strength and reliability were significantly higher for the Ti abutments compared to the $ZrO_2$ |
| Nothdurft et al. (2010) | 8 ZirDesign (Astra Tech) straight<br>8 angled | 233.68 ± 30.68<br>324.62 ± 108.07 | ZirDesign (Astra Tech) | FDPs (chromium-cobalt alloy) | NA | Static load. 105 cycles between 5°C and 55°C | Compensation for angulated implant positions with an angulated $ZrO_2$ abutment is possible without reducing the load-bearing capacity of implant/tooth-supported anterior FDPs |
| Nothdurft et al. (2011) | (FRIADENT CERCON abutments, DENTSPLY Friadent (implant–implant supported)<br>(implant–tooth supported) | 472.75 ± 24.71<br>736.25 ± 82.23 | XiVe® S plus screw implants (DENTSPLY Friadent) | FDP (all-ceramic) | NA | Thermomechanical load, 5,000 thermal cycles between 5° and 55°C and chewing simulations (1,200,000 cycles − 50 N) | Implant–tooth-supported FDP restorations did exhibit an increased fracture load compared to implant–implant-supported FDP restorations |

| | | | | | | | |
|---|---|---|---|---|---|---|---|
| Canullo et al. (2013) | 10 (custom-made) Sweden & Martina, Padua, Italy<br>0.3 mm thikness at the connection area<br>STRAIGHT | 237.4 | Ti screw-Ti connection-PEEK ring-All Stone Cement | None | 30 | Fatigue test, 15 Hz for 5 million cycles in dry conditions at 20 ± 5°C. | A straight bi-component abutment did not present different maximum load than an angled abutment under fatigue<br>The failure of straight abutment happened at cervical region |
| | 10 ANGLED 25 degrees | 240 | | | | Dynamic | |
| Stimmelmayr et al. (2013) | 8 BeCe CAD Zircon XH-diameter 3.75 mm<br>8 BeCe CAD Zircon XH-Ti core—diameter 3.75 mm | 526 ± 32<br>1241 ± 269 | Bego-Semados S | None | 30 | 1000 thermal cycles 5–55°C 250 N for 100,000 cycles at a frequency of 1.2 Hz. Loading speed 10 mm/s, lifting speed 60 mm/s | The fracture strength of $ZrO_2$ abutments connected to Ti cores was significantly higher than the fracture strength of one-piece $ZrO_2$ abutments |
| Kim et al. (2013) | 20 Aadva CAD/CAM $ZrO_2$ Abutment<br>20NobelProcera Abutment $ZrO_2$-Ti insert fiction-fitted<br>20 Lava $ZrO_2$ abutment Ti insert bonded | 503.9 (46.3)<br>484.6 (56.6)<br>729.2 (35.9) | Dummy NobelReplace Tapered Groovy | $ZrO_2$ copings (Lava $ZrO_2$) | 30 | Thermomechanical loading, 20,000 cycles between 5°C and 55°C. Static load crosshead speed of 1 mm/min (ISO-Norm 14801). | Lava abutment was significantly higher than that of the Aadva or NobelProcera abutment |
| Mühlemann et al. (2014) | 12 Straumann Bone level, one-piece internal connection<br>12 Astra Tech AB OsseoSpeed one-piece internal connection<br>12 Nobel Biocare Replace Select), two-piece external connection<br>12 Branemark MkIII external connection<br>12 Straumann StandardPlus two-piece internal connection | 464.9 ± 106.6<br>216.4 ± 90.0<br>581.8 ± 172.8<br>556.7 ± 128.4<br>605.4 ± 54.7 | Respective implant | Glass–ceramic crowns | 30 | Thermocycling (ISO-Norm 14801). Fracture load was analyzed by calculating the bending moments | The type of connection had a minor effect on the bending moments of restored $ZrO_2$ abutments |

*(Continued)*

**Table 6.4 (Continued)**

| Author | Samples | Mean fracture load (*N*) | Implant | Restoration | AFV | Conditions | Conclusions |
|---|---|---|---|---|---|---|---|
| Jiménez-Melendo et al. (2014) | 8 Zireal Post, External connection<br>8 Internal connection | 378 ± 53<br>326 ± 32 | Osseotite, Biomet 3i | Fluroapatite ceramic [IPS e-max Ceram] | 30 | Cycling load between 150 and 400 N at a frequency of 1 Hz with an upper cycle limit of $4 \times 10^5$ and cross-speed of 1 mm/min | There are no significant differences in mechanical behavior under static and dynamic loading conditions neither between internal and external geometries, nor between bare (as-received) and one-layer ceramized abutments |
| Gehrke et al. (2015) | 7 prefabricated $ZrO_2$ (Xive CERCON)<br>7 One-piece CAD/CAM $ZrO_2$ (Compartis) | 251.8 ± 23.2<br>232.1 ± 29.8 | Conexao Implant | | 30 | Thermocycling, followed by fracture resistance test. The maximum load was applied to the tapered occlusal area, crosshead speed of 0.5 mm/min | Superior resistance was achieved for two-piece hybrid CAD/CAM $ZrO_2$ abutments. These abutments might be clinically beneficial in high-load areas, such as premolar and molar regions |
| | 7 two-piece CAD/CAM $ZrO_2$ (Compartis) | 291.4 ± 27.8 | Xive S, Dentsply | | | | |

Maximum incisal forces reported in the literature: 90–370 N. Maximal occlusal forces in the area of the first-molar: 180 and 850 N. *AFV*, angle force to vertical; *FDPs*, fixed dental prostheses.

## 6.3 Commercial load-bearing ceramics: a comparative analysis

### 6.3.1 Toughened ceramics

#### 6.3.1.1 Fully sintered polycrystalline alumina ceramics

Procera AllCeram (Nobel Biocare) is the first fully dense polycrystalline ceramic introduced in 1993 in dental marketing (Andersson and Odén, 1993). This core material contains 99.9% high-purity polycrystalline $Al_2O_3$. It has a flexural strength between 464 and 650 MPa (Zeng et al., 1996; Esquivel-Upshaw et al., 2001) and a fracture toughness of 4.2–6 MPa$\sqrt{m}$ (Wagner and Chu, 1996; Lazar et al., 2008). Limited long-term data of its use for single crowns on natural and implant-supported abutments are available; it is recommended for the fabrication of anterior and posterior crowns, but its use for three-unit FDPs is still questionable (Sorrentino et al., 2012b; Raigrodski, 2005).

The accuracy of fit achieved by the Procera AllCeram system is within the range of clinical acceptance (Boening et al., 2000). The core can be produced in different colors (translucent and white) and thicknesses (0.6–0.4 mm), with different optical properties. This variation can be helpful to mask any discolored teeth without compromising the strength of the ceramic material (Pilathadka and Vahalová, 2007).

#### 6.3.1.2 Fully sintered polycrystalline zirconia ceramics

All-ceramic restorations were used at first in anterior regions because of their excellent esthetic properties and biocompatibility. In recent years, they have been introduced for the treatment of posterior regions. The zirconia material used today by most manufacturers is Y-TZP. Although 3Y-TZP has the same chemical composition, there are differences in strength and translucency, based on the powder type and the production conditions. Y-TZP has allowed the fabrication of frameworks of crowns or FDPs because of its great flexural strength (900–1400 MPa) and high fracture toughness (5–10 MPa$\sqrt{m}$) (Miyazaki et al., 2013; Nakamura et al., 2012). They are suitable for monolithic crowns and bridges in anterior and posterior regions. Bridges have to be limited to six units with a maximum of two pontics.

It is known that Y-TZP is subject to degradation in a humid atmosphere, even in low ambient temperatures (Nakamura et al., 2012).

Some of the zirconia materials on the market have a strength of 900 MPa, whereas others exhibit strength values over 1200 MPa. Many zirconia materials present differences in machinability (e.g., wet milling and dry milling) and in sintering. The available zirconia powders can have different distributions of the various grain sizes, and different additives.

The powder is first pressed, which can be accomplished by different procedures (HIP or axial pressing) (http://glidewelldental.com). In HIP, the isostatic pressing is

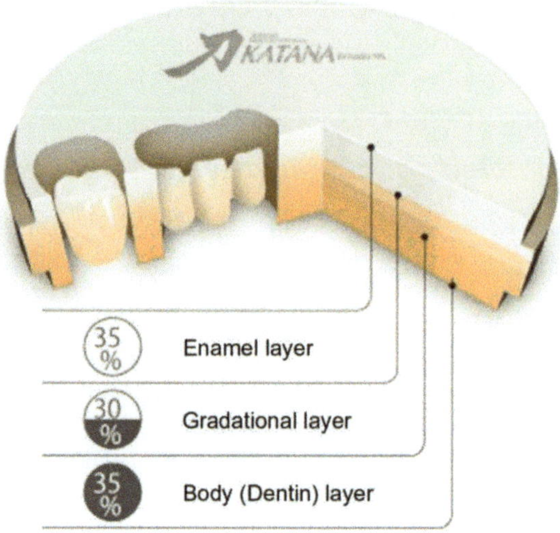


**Figure 6.13** Multi Layered, KATANA Zirconia (ML). Specialized for FCZ (Full Contour Zirconia). Kuraray.

combined with high-temperature sintering, producing a block that is easier to mill. This reduces the stress on the machine's drills and spindle.

The pressed zirconia powder is then presintered in a furnace with an optimized temperature profile to generate a blank with suitable strength and millability. After sintering, the device can be veneered. Some zirconia materials can be colored in the presintered state by immersing copings and frameworks in a dyeing liquid (http://www.zirkonzahn.com), while others are disposable in a multilayered form (Fig. 6.13).

Y-TZP can be manufactured as green stage (diamonds with cooling liquid), presintered stage (dry carbide burs), and completely sintered stage (diamonds with cooling liquid), The main features of commercially available Y-TZP are depicted in Table 6.5.

In the case of presintered pieces, the dental laboratory mills the blank and then sinters the coping or framework to achieve full density. In the case of fully sintered blanks, during milling, there is the danger of having irregular surfaces and creating structural defects on the ceramic, which could also negatively impact the permanent strength of the ceramics. Compared with green processing, the hard processing of dense sintered zirconia with diamond burs is more time and labor intensive and also involves increased wear on the milling instruments.

In addition, the main causes of structural failures in ceramics (and, particularly, in polycrystalline zirconia) are described below.

The most common causes of all-ceramic structural failures are fractures initiated in the connector area of FDPs, either at the core—veneer interface or at the gingival embrasure, and *chipping* of the porcelain veneer (Della Bona et al., 2015). Zirconia has little translucency and elevated hardness, so porcelain must be veneered by layering or press techniques. The difference in thermal expansion

## Table 6.5 Commercially available $ZrO_2$

| $ZrO_2$ | Manufacturer | $ZrO_2$ (%) | $Al_2O_3$(%) | $Y_2O_3$ (%) | Flexural strength (MPa) | T °C sintering | CTE x$10^{-6}$ /K | Toughness (MPa$\sqrt{m}$) | Veneering |
|---|---|---|---|---|---|---|---|---|---|
| **Partially sintered** | | | | | | | | | |
| $ZrO_2$ Bettini DB + (white) DB + LUX (traslucent) | Bettini srl Monte Marenzo (LC) Italy | 94.6 | 0.15–0.25 | 4.4–5.4 | 1400 | 1450 | 10.5 | ≥5 | |
| NexxZr S | Sagemax Bioceramics, Inc. WA, USA | 94–96 | | 4–6 | 1100–1300 | 1520 | 10 | | |
| Lava Plus | 3 M | 79–97 | | 3–15 | 1100 | 1500 | 10.5 + 0.2 | 5.9 | |
| Ceramill zolid | (Amann Girrbach (Koblach, AU) | 88–90 | | 9.15–9.55 | 700 ± 150 | | 10.1 ± 0.5 | | Multilayered |
| Cercon base | Degudent, Frankfurt, Germany | 95 | | 5 | | 1450 | 10.5 | 6–8 | |
| Cercon ht | Dentsply | 94–95 | <1 | 5 | 1200 | 1500 | 10.5 | 9 | |
| Copran | Whitepeaks Dental Solutions GmbH & Co. Essen, Germany | 93,99 – 94,89 | 0.15 – 0.35 | 4.95 – 5.35 | 1250 – 1400 | 1500 | | | |
| KATANA ZIRCONIA MULTI-LAYERED DISC | Kuraray Noritake | 97 | | 3 | 1200 | 1400 | 10.5 | | Multilayered |
| Incoris TZI | Sirona | 94–95.5 | <0.5 | 4.5–6 | >900 | 1500 | 10 | ≥5 | |
| In Ceram YZ Cube | VITA | 94–95 | <3 | 5 | 1200 | 1530 | 10.5 | 5.9 | |
| Procera AllZirkon | Nobel Biocare | 94–95 | | 4.5–5.5 | 1120 | 1550 | 10.4 | 6–9 | |
| IPS emax ZirCAD | Ivoclar | 87–95 | <1 | 4–6 | 900 ± 50 | 1500 | 10.8 | 5.5 | Coloring |
| Everest ZS-blanks | Kavo | 93–94 | <0.5 | | 1155 | | | | |
| DC-Shrink | Bien-Air | 95.5 | | | 1000 | | 10 | | |
| Z-CAD | METOXIT-Dental | 93–94.5 | <0.5 | 4.5–6 | 1200 | 1450–1500 | 10.5 | 8 | |

(*Continued*)

Table 6.5 (Continued)

| $ZrO_2$ | Manufacturer | $ZrO_2$ (%) | $Al_2O_3$(%) | $Y_2O_3$ (%) | Flexural strength (MPa) | T °C sintering | CTE x$10^{-6}$ /K | Toughness (MPa$\sqrt{m}$) | Veneering |
|---|---|---|---|---|---|---|---|---|---|
| Zenostar | Wieland Dental + Technik GmbH & Co. KG Pforzheim Germania | >99 | <1 | 4.5–6 | 1200 | 1600 | 10.5 | >5 | |
| Zerion | (Straumann Etkon) | 94–96 | 0.5 | 4.5–6 | >800 | | 10.5 | | |
| $ZrO_2$ Prettau | ZirkonZahn (Steger) | 94–96 | <1 | 4–6 | 1000–1200 | 1600 | 10 | | Colored |
| Zirtooth | Hass | 95–99 | 0.05 | <5 | 1005 | 1500 | 10.3 | | Multilayered |
| ZYTTRIA WT | Concept Busseto (PR) Italy | 94–95% | 0.25 | 5.15 ± 0.2 | >1200 | 1450 | 10.5 | 9 | |
| **Fully sintered** | | | | | | | | | |
| DC-Zirkon—DC-Zirkon Col | Bien Air | 95 | | 5 | 1200 | | 10 | | |
| ZH-Blanks (Everest) | KAVO | | | | 1200 | | 10 | 8 | |

HfO < 5%.

coefficient (CTE) between the zirconia core and veneering porcelain is about 5–10 ppm. The difference in the CTE between the ceramic core and the esthetic porcelain produces a compressive stress in the veneering porcelain and a tensile stress in the core (Baldassarri et al., 2012). The greater the difference in CTE, the stronger the bond between the core material and the veneering ceramic. This difference could probably impair the fracture strength of zirconia crowns (Kwon et al., 2013). The clinical survival of all-ceramic crowns depends on: (1) the surface quality of the veneering (strength, fracture toughness, surface roughness), (2) the veneering-core bond, and (3) the strength of the underlying core structure (Rosentritt et al., 2009).

The rate of fracture for porcelain-veneered zirconia restorations has been evaluated as 6%–15% after 3–5 years compared to metal–ceramic restorations (4% after 10 years) (Tan et al., 2012; Agustín-Panadero et al., 2014). Elevated functional impact forces on implants might further exacerbate veneer fractures determined by fixture rigidity and impaired proprioception (Guess et al., 2011). Chipping or fracturing of the veneering porcelain is observed at a relatively high rate in posterior zirconia-based ceramic restorations; Table 6.6 shows the clinical survival and complications of tooth-supported three- to five-piece zirconia frameworks.

The frameworks made of LavaFrame/Lava Ceram showed a survival rate of 96%–100% after 2–3 years and 90%–92% after 4–6 years while that made of Cercon/Cercon CeramS showed a survival rate of 91%–100% after 2 years and 83%–96% after 4–6 years. The fracturing of the veneering porcelain (minor and major) makes up 10%–25% of complications in three- to five-piece zirconia frameworks after 2 years and increases to 23%–29% after 5–6 years of permanence.

The possible explanations for veneer fractures may be:

1. *Occlusal function*

   The zirconia cores and ceramic veneers appear to bond by means of mechanical engagement and the formation of compressive strength resulting from thermal contraction during cooling after sintering, without any type of chemical bond (Guess et al., 2011). The most frequent reasons for failures within the veneering ceramic are the cohesive fractures (71.7%–88.8%) (Agustín-Panadero et al., 2012; Saito et al., 2010). Fractographic analysis of clinically failed veneered zirconia restorations revealed cracks originating from the occlusal surface and propagating to the core–veneer interface, leaving an intact core (Aboushelib et al., 2009). These veneer failures were associated with roughness in the veneering ceramic depending on occlusal function (the occlusal zone adjacent to the point of contact with the antagonist) or occlusal adjustment (Guess et al., 2011; Sailer et al., 2009; Hobkirk and Wiskott, 2009). Adjustments should be performed only with fine-grain diamonds under water irrigation followed by a thorough polishing sequence (Guess et al., 2011).

2. *Unsupported porcelain*

   The lack of a uniform support of the veneering ceramic has been discussed as a possible reason for chipping fractures. With CAD/CAM technologies, excessive veneer layer thickness (>2.5 mm) was created because of the uniform layer thickness of the copings for crowns and bar-shaped connectors for FDPs. Improved customized zirconia coping design derived from the conventional porcelain fused to metal technique has been

**Table 6.6** **Clinical survival and complications of tooth supported 3–5 piece $ZrO_2$ frameworks. Mean time of clinical studies > 24 months. Sample size > 20**

| | % Chipping ≥24 months | % Chipping ≥36 months | % Chipping ≥48 months | % Chipping ≥60 months | System | Survival rate% (satisfactory) | FDPs 3–5 piece | Other complications |
|---|---|---|---|---|---|---|---|---|
| Vult von Steyern et al. (2005) | 15 | | | | DC-Zirkon/VitaD | 100 | 20 | 0 |
| Raigrodski et al. (2006) | 25 | | | | LavaFrame/Lava Ceram | 100 | 20 | 1 ET |
| Sailer et al. (2007) | | | 15.2 | | Cercon/prototype veneering ceramic | 73.9 | 33 | 1CP-7C |
| Tinschert et al. (2008) | | 6.1 | | | DC-Zircon/VitaD | 100 | 58 | 2AF-3ET |
| Edelhoff et al. (2008) | | 9.1 | | | Digizon/Zr-Keramik | 90.5 | 22 | 1 AF-1 ET |
| Molin and Karlsson (2008) | 0 | | | | Denzir/IPS Empress | 100 | 19 | 1 AF |
| Sailer et al. (2009) | | 25 | | | Cercon/Cercon CeramS | 100 | 36 | 1ET |
| Schmitt et al. (2009) | 10 | | | | LavaFrame/Lava Ceram | 96.3 | 30 | 1ET |

| | | | | | | | | |
|---|---|---|---|---|---|---|---|---|
| Wolfart et al. (2009) | | | 12.5 | | Cercon/Cercon CeramExpress | 96 | 24 | 1C-2ET-2AF |
| Beuer et al. (2009) | | 0 | | | Cercon/Cercon CeramExpress | 90.5 | 21 | 1CP-1AF |
| Tsumita et al. (2010) | | 7.4 | | | Cercon/ Creation ZI | 100 | 21 | 0 |
| Roediger et al. (2010) | | | 13.1 | | Cercon/Cercon CeramS | 94 | 99 | 1ET-3C-6AF-1PL |
| Tartaglia et al. (2011) | | 0 | | | Zirite/CZR | 98.2 | 81 | 3 CP |
| Peláez et al. (2012) | | 10 | | | LavaFrame | 95 | 20 | 1PL |
| Schmitt et al. (2012) | | | | 23 | LavaFrame/Lava Ceram | 92 | 30 | 2ET, 1AF |
| Raigrodski et al. (2012) | | | | 25 | LavaFrame/Lava Ceram | 90 | 20 | 1RF-1PL |
| Sorrentino et al. (2012a) | | | | 6.3 | (Procera All Zircon, | 100 | 48 | 0 |
| Crisp et al. (2012) | | 5.8 | | | LavaFrame/Lava Ceram | 100 | 34 | 3ET |
| Burke et al. (2013) | | 26.5 | | | LavaFrame/Lava Ceram | 97 | 33 | 3ET |

*(Continued)*

**Table 6.6 (Continued)**

| | % Chipping ≥24 months | % Chipping ≥36 months | % Chipping ≥48 months | % Chipping ≥60 months | System | Survival rate% (satisfactory) | FDPs 3–5 piece | Other complications |
|---|---|---|---|---|---|---|---|---|
| Rinke et al. (2013) | | | | 28.8 | Cercon/ Cercon CeramS | 83.4 | 80 | 12CP-1RF-2PL-3C-4CP-4ET |
| Naenni et al. (2015) | | 40 | | | CEREC/ IPS e.max ZirPress | 100 | 20 | 0 |
| | | 20 | | | CEREC/ IPS e.max Ceram | | 20 | |
| Ioannidis and Bindl (2016) | | | | 27 | In-Ceram 2000YZ-Cubes/Vitadur Alpha | 85 | 59 | 2RF-5ET-3PL |

*AF*, decementation; *C*, caries; *CP*, complete fracture; *ET*, endodontic complication; *PL*, periodontal loss or periapical lesion; *RF*, root fracture; *VF*, veneer fracture.

recommended to provide adequate support for the veneering ceramic (Andreiuolo et al., 2013; Lorenzoni et al., 2010).

Preliminary in vitro studies showed that cohesive fractures within the veneering ceramic could not be avoided with the improvement of support, but the size of the fractures was significantly decreased (Rosentritt et al., 2009; Lorenzoni et al., 2010) and failure initiation was shifted toward higher loads (Andreiuolo et al., 2013; Lorenzoni et al., 2010; Bonfante et al., 2010).

3. *Thermal expansion/contraction and residual stress*

   The CTE is frequently discussed as a contributing factor for veneer failure. Residual stresses in bilayer crowns and FDPs are associated with the possibility of thermal gradients being developed in these structures during cooling. For zirconia veneer all-ceramic systems, the low thermal conductivity of the zirconia results in the highest temperature difference and, therefore, very high residual stresses. Thick layers of veneering ceramics on zirconia cores are highly susceptible to generating high tensile subsurface residual stresses, resulting in unstable cracking or chipping (Rosentritt et al., 2009). Cooling too rapidly causes a residual stress within the porcelain, with a thermal gradients of up to 160°C; many dental materials companies recommend slow cooling (Kelly and Benetti, 2011).

   The restorations must be slowly cooled above the glass transition temperature of the porcelain, this could prevent the development of high tensile subsurface residual stresses in the porcelain. Most manufacturers recommend a reduced cooling rate after final firing or glazing; an additional 6 minutes has been shown to be effective (Agustín-Panadero et al., 2014). Slow cooling and slow heating regimens should be used when firing porcelain to zirconia. Cooling regimens were found to be more influential than heating rates. Failure was localized to the porcelain adjacent to the porcelain–zirconia interface, not to the interface itself, indicating that the residual stresses of thermal origin within the porcelain dominated. The preparation of zirconia with 50-μm aluminum oxide at a pressure of 0.34 MPa was sufficient to prevent interfacial failure (Agustín-Panadero et al., 2014).

4. *Weaker porcelain*

   The veneering ceramic material (flexural strength, approx 90–120 MPa) is weak when compared with the high strength of core material and seems to be prone to failure at low loads during masticatory function (Guess et al., 2011).

   The veneer chippings/fractures could be reduced by higher-strength veneering ceramic. The development of glass ceramic ingots for pressing veneering ceramics onto zirconia frameworks did not result in an increased resistance of the veneering ceramic. The same chip-failure patterns were observed and spherical porosities were noted within the veneer layer and also at the interface (Bonfante et al., 2010; Tsalouchou et al., 2007; Guess et al., 2009b).

5. *Auto-catalytic transformation*

   Zirconia-based devices are susceptible to low-temperature degradation (LTD): an autocatalytic transformation of the crystals from tetragonal to monocline starts at surface grain boundaries and the transformation of crystal continues through the entire body, leading to microcrack formation and strength reduction (Kelly and Denry, 2008).

Recent alternatives could be:

- CAD/CAM porcelain veneering;
- full-contoured zirconia without porcelain veneering (Fig. 6.13).

## Zirconia cementation

Resin cementation of zirconia restorations showed a shear bond strength between 5.1 and 15.7 MPa depending on the luting agent. The internal surface treatment seems to be unnecessary to obtain good adhesion (Manicone et al., 2007) but other authors suggest that surface roughness has a key role on zirconia-cement bonding (Aboushelib, 2011). After zirconia coping fabrication using a CAD/CAM system and before veneering, the surface treatments are typically performed. The main surface treatement are briefly described in the following:

1. *Sandblasting*. Since mechanical adhesion alone is not enough to obtain an optimal resin bond strength to zirconia, several authors suggest particle abrasion as a mandatory treatment. Improved michromechanical retention and fracture strength was obtained by sandblasting zirconia posts (Oblak et al., 2004; Sahafi et al., 2003); air abrasion with 50−110 μm aluminum oxide particles is effective in roughening and cleaning the zirconia surface and increasing the bond strength (Wolfart et al., 2007; Yun et al., 2010). Because of its relatively high hardness (400 VHN), sandblasting produced minimal roughness with a detrimental effect on bond strength (Kern and Wegner, 1998). Mechanical stress is known to induce phase transformation from tetragonal to monoclinic $ZrO_2$, subsequently resulting in compressive stress. Therefore, heat treatment is recommended after sandblasting in dental practice (Kosmač, 2004). Such treatments, however, are not recommended overall, most likely because a sandblasting too deeply can lead to the formation of craters and defects, which act as stress concentrators decreasing the flexural strength and resistance to fracture under stress. It has been reported that particle abrasion creates structural defects that are conducive to radial cracking during function, then reduced particle size and pressure are recommended (Guess et al., 2010b).
2. *Tribochemical treatment*. In order to establish a strong chemical bond between resin cements and hard ceramics, Ozcan et al. (2008) recommended a cover with silica by means of air abrasion devices. Zirconia has no specific groups to bond to the silanization agent, therefore the zirconia has to be pretreated. This method is usually applied in dental laboratories using $Al_2O_3$ particles of 110 μm particle size coated with silica. The blasting pressure results in silica-coated alumina particles being embedded on the ceramic surface, rendering the silica surface modified to be chemically more reactive to the resin through silane coupling agents. Silane coupling agents lower the surface tension of a substrate, wet it, and make its surface energy higher, and hence accessible for effective bonding.
3. *Rocatec treatment*. This consists of sandblasting with aluminum oxide (Rocatec Pre-110 mm, 3 M ESPE) to clean the surface and tribochemical treatment with silicates (Rocatec-soft 30 mm, 3 M ESPE), or Rocatec Plus (coated with aluminum oxide dioxide silicon) and subsequent treatment with silane. The treatment is able to increase the bonding strength between the zirconia and composite material. This effect can be explained in two ways: the microscopic irregularities increase the micromechanical retention and a special coating generated by the application of silane creates a silicon adhesive layer. Some studies have shown that a tribochemical treatment can increase the bonding strength to the composite, but others are conflicting (Piascik et al., 2009, 2011; Wegner and Kern, 2000; Inokoshi et al., 2013; Chai et al., 2011; Oguri et al., 2012; Della Bona et al., 2007; Sriamporn et al., 2014; Vult von Steyern et al., 2005; Raigrodski et al., 2006, 2010, 2012; Sailer et al., 2007; Tinschert et al., 2008; Edelhoff et al., 2008; Molin and Karlsson, 2008; Schmitt et al., 2009, 2012; Wolfart et al., 2009; Beuer et al., 2009; Tsumita et al., 2010; Tartaglia et al., 2011; Peláez et al., 2012).

4. *Cojet treatment.* Cojet treatment and sandblasting are the two most effective treatments and comparable results in increasing the degree of adhesion were shown. The Cojet treatment improves the adhesion of the zirconia at BisGMA-based composite cement; while the bonding of Panavia F improves only when treated with sandblasting and subsequent application of silane (Aboushelib, 2011; Wegner and Kern, 2000; Inokoshi et al., 2013). Chai et al. (2011) reported that In-Ceram Zirconia treated with CoJet had significantly higher shear bond strengths than untreated In-Ceram Zirconia or treated with Rocatec. Surface treatment did not affect the shear bond strength of Zirconia significantly. The bonding strength is modified by the type of cement used and this can be explained by differences in the surface energy of the components (Bitter et al., 2006).
5. *Silica coating process.* This surface modification process can be appropriate for joining dental porcelain to zirconia-based ceramics increasing shear bond strength, e.g., P-NANOZR (Panasonic Health Care, Osaka) and the porcelain Cerabien ZR (Noritake Dental Supply Co, Nagoya) (Oguri et al., 2012).
6. *Hydrofluoric acid etching.* Etching with hydrofluoric acid and subsequent silanization can increase the mechanical strength of the bond of the glass ceramic materials to the composite resin. The acid etching partially removes the vitreous matrix and creates mechanically retentive areas where the silane molecules are positioned and link the inorganic molecules of the crystalline phase of the ceramics to resin molecules present in the composite material. However, this technique does not increase the bonding strength between resin cement and high-strength ceramics such as alumina and zirconia (Aboushelib, 2011; Della Bona et al., 2007). Zirconia is a silica-free ceramic, and is resistant to conventional etching techniques. Immersing zirconia under moderate conditions (9.5% hydrofluoric acid at 80°C for 1 minute or at 25°C for 1 hour) can create surface roughness by corroding the zirconia grains. After etching with hydrofluoric acid under any of the above conditions, all the materials used exhibited a monoclinic zirconia peak in the X-ray diffraction analysis. This indicates hydrofluoric acid etching can induce the LTD (Sriamporn et al., 2014).

## 6.3.2 Glass ceramics

### 6.3.2.1 Reinforced glass ceramics

#### Leucite reinforced glass ceramics ($SiO_2$-$Al_2O_3$-$K_2O$)

These core materials use crystalline filler to reinforce glass ceramic structures. Leucite glass ceramics consist of 35%–45% volume fraction of 1- to 5-μm crystals densely distributed in the glassy matrix and arranged like strings of beads along the glass grain boundaries. The finer particle size helps resist machining damage. Tetragonal leucite ($KAlSi_2O_6$) nucleates and grows in the glass system by a surface crystallization mechanism initiated at the surface of the glass construct and propagating inward toward the bulk (Saint-Jean, 2014). The strength increase is attributed to a good dispersion of the fine leucite crystals as well as the tangential compressive stresses that develop around the crystals on cooling because of the difference in the CTE between leucite crystals and the glassy matrix (Denry et al., 1996). These stresses contribute to crack deflection and improved mechanical performance (Guess et al., 2011). Copings may be fabricated using either a heat-pressing procedure or via CAD/CAM technology. The restorations are highly translucent and are recommended for moderately translucent teeth (Heffernan et al., 2002). They are not recommended when the underlying abutment is a discolored tooth or a metallic substructure. The strength of these restorations depends on a successful bond to the tooth structure and, therefore, must be adhesively cemented. Their indication is restricted only for veneers or crowns at the front region giving survival rates of up to 95% after 11 years of clinical service (Fradeani and Redemagni, 2002). Adhesively luted IPS Empress crowns showed a low fracture rate for incisors and premolars and a somewhat higher rate for molars and canines (Heintze and Rousson, 2010).

Multicolored blocks were recently developed to reproduce color transitions and shading as well as different levels of translucency to reproduce natural teeth.

*1986-IPS-Empress (Ivoclar)*-heat pressed: veneers, onlay, inlay, crowns. These were used for anterior restorations of teeth of low value, requiring high translucency.

The reported flexural strength of this core material ranges between 105 and 120 MPa, and the fracture toughness from 1.5 to 1.7 ($MPa\sqrt{m}$) (Seghi and Sorensen, 1995; Seghi et al., 1995). Survival of inlays and onlays was 91% at 7 years and the survival of crowns ranged from 92% to 99% at 3 years. Use of IPS-empress crown is not recommended in the posterior region of the mouth (El-Mowafy and Brochu, 2002).

*1998-IPS ProCAD*-milled: used with CEREC inLab system (Sirona). The marginal gap, internal fit and fracture load was comparable with Empress in an in vitro study (Keshvad et al., 2011). A mid-term evaluation of a clinical split-mouth investigation of all ceramic partial coverage on molars reported a survival rate of 97% after 3 years (Denissen et al., 2002; Guess et al., 2009a, 2010a).

*2006-IPS-Empress CAD:* developed for chair-side single-unit restorations and has a flexural strength of 160 MPa, the milled restorations can be stained and glazed in the next step (Li et al., 2014).

## Lithium disilicate glass ceramics ($SiO_2$-$Li_2O$-$K_2O$)

Lithium disilicate consist of a large volume fraction of up to 70% fine rod-like ($5 \times 0.8$ μm) entangled $Li_2Si_2O_5$ crystals and a minor amount of lithium orthophosphate crystals that are randomly oriented and uniformly dispersed in the glassy matrix. Crystal alignement after heat pressing of the lithium disilicate glass ceramic leads to multiple crack deflections. The framework can be fabricated either with the lost-wax and heat-pressure technique, or can be milled out of prefabricated blanks. Its flexural strength ranges from 350 to 450 MPa, this is higher than that of leucite-reinforced dental ceramics and its fracture toughness is between 2.8 and 3.5 $MPa\sqrt{m}$) (Höland et al., 2006). These restorations should be etched and adhesively luted to enhance their strength and longevity.

*1998-IPS Empress2-IPS e.max (Ivoclar)*: an ingot is plasticized at 920°C and pressed into an investment mold under vacuum and pressure. It is used for crowns, and anterior FDPs. This material, thanks to its high fracture toughness, permits the extension of the range of indications of glass ceramics from inlay and crowns to three-unit bridges (Affatato et al., 2006). A survival rate of 86.7% was reported for posterior Empress II FDPs after 4 years and a survival rate of 100% for single crowns and 70% for FDPs extending up to the second premolar after 5 years of function was reported (Esquivel-Upshaw et al., 2008; Marquardt and Strub, 2006).

After 10 years, high survival rate (95.5%) was observed on 261 anterior and posterior crowns (Valenti and Valenti, 2009).

*2006-IPS e.max CAD (Ivoclar-Vivadent)*: chair-side monolithic restorative material. Recommended for inlays, onlays, veneers, anterior and superior crowns, and implant-supported crowns. The lithium disilicate blanks are exposed to a two-stage crystallization process, in the first stage 40% of lithium metasilicate crystals (1.5 μm) are produced. The resulting glass ceramic has a flexural strength such that milling and intraoral adjustment are simplified. The material, which is supplied in a typically blue shade, has been especially designed for the milling process in the CAD/CAM technique. After the milling process, the material is subjected to thermal treatment, which results in a lithium disilicate glass ceramic that demonstrates a characteristic tooth color. The resulting dental restorations can be polished and completed with glazing and characterization materials. Laboratory studies have shown that fully anatomical crowns may be resistant to fatigue in cyclic loading and their fracture load is higher than the PROCAD and EmpressCAD (Guess et al., 2011; Asai et al., 2010). Clinical trials on single crowns showed a survival rate of between 97.4% and 100% after 2 years (Reich et al., 2010; Fasbinder et al., 2010). Lithium disilicate suffers from fatigue failure during clinical service; microcracks usually initiate in load-bearing and/or stress-concentration areas, eventually fusing under dynamic loads and creating major flaws that could weaken the lithium disilicate structure; when the ultimate mechanical strength is overcome, catastrophic failures occur (Zhao et al., 2014; Zarone et al., 2016).

### 6.3.2.2 Glass-infiltrated ceramics

The glass-infiltrated ceramics consist of a porous presintered ceramic core that is infiltrated with a low-viscosity lanthanum aluminosilicate glass fired at 1100°C for 4–6 hours to eliminate porosity and increase strength. In-Ceram is primarily crystalline in nature.

*In-Ceram Alumina-Slip-cast or milled*: introduced in 1989, this is a high-alumina-content, glass-infiltrated ceramic core material containing 75% polycrystalline alumina and 25% infiltration glass. Four-point flexural strength values of bend bars of In-Ceram infused alumina core were reported to be between 236 and 429 MPa (Giordano et al., 1995; Tinschert et al., 2000). Mean biaxial flexure strengths of In-Ceram Alumina was 600 MPa, mean fracture toughness measured according to indentation strength was 3.2 $MPa\sqrt{m}$, whereas the mean fracture toughnesses measured according to indentation fracture was 2.7 $MPa\sqrt{m}$ (Guazzato et al., 2002). It is recommended for anterior and posterior crowns, and is the first all-ceramic system available for three-unit anterior FDPs. In-Ceram Alumina crowns had a significantly higher fracture strength than In-Ceram Spinell crowns in both conventional and copy-milling methods

(Hwang and Yang, 2001). Because of its core, the ceramic is semiopaque and does not allow full transmission of light and therefore provides limited esthetic results (Heffernan et al., 2002). In-Ceram Alumina can be milled in combination with *CEREC.*

*Synthoceram*: a high-strength glass impregnated aluminum oxide ceramic core fabricated through CICERO technology (Computer Integrated Ceramic Reconstruction) in four steps: laser scanning, ceramic sintering, computer-integrated milling, the core is then veneered with leucite freeglass ceramic.

*1993 Vita-CAD/CAM InCeram*-Alumina -Single anterior and posterior crowns: the blocks are manufactured by dry pressing the ceramic powder into a mold and compacted until the open pore microstructured is reached (Apholt et al., 2001); the material is then sintered and infiltrated by La-glass.

A survival rate of 92% was reported after 5 years for premolar and molar crowns fabricated with a CEREC2 sytem (Bindl and Mörmann, 2002).

*In-Ceram Spinell*: this material was designed to improve the light reflection and light transmission. It consists of 78% $MgAl_2O_4$ core infiltrated with 22% glass. The fabrication procedures are the same as those for In-Ceram Alumina. The flexural strength is lower than that of In Ceram Alumina (280–377 MPa) (Hwang and Yang, 2001; Magne and Belser, 1997; Chong et al., 2002), but its translucency is twice that of In Ceram Alumina. In-Ceram Spinell can be recommended for anterior crowns, especially if highly esthetic results are required (Fradeani et al., 2002; Wassermann et al., 2006).

*1994-CEREC inLab*-inlay, crown-anterior restorations, vital teeth: this been reported to yield survival rates of 92%–100% after 5 years (Bindl and Mörmann, 2002; Fradeani et al., 2002; Bindl and Mörmann, 2004).

*In-Ceram Zirconia*: this consists of In-Ceram Alumina (67 wt%) alumina with the addition of 33 wt% of ceria-stabilized zirconia (Saint-Jean, 2014). Its flexural strength ranges from 421 to 800 MPa and its fracture toughness from 5 to 8 $MPa\sqrt{m}$) (Hwang and Yang, 2001; Apholt et al., 2001; Chong et al., 2002; Guazzato et al., 2004; Bottino et al., 2009). The fabrication may be carried out either with the slip-casting technique or with CAD/CAM technology. The high opacity of its core (Heffernan et al., 2002; Fradeani and Redemagni, 2002; Heintze and Rousson, 2010; Seghi and Sorensen, 1995; Seghi et al., 1995; El-Mowafy and Brochu, 2002; Keshvad et al., 2011; Denissen et al., 2002; Guess et al., 2009a, 2010a; Li et al., 2014; Höland et al., 2006; Esquivel-Upshaw et al., 2008; Marquardt and Strub, 2006; Valenti and Valenti, 2009; Asai et al., 2010; Reich et al., 2010; Fasbinder et al., 2010; Zhao et al., 2014; Zarone et al., 2016; Giordano et al., 1995; Tinschert et al., 2000; Guazzato et al., 2002, 2004; Hwang and Yang, 2001; Apholt et al., 2001; Bindl and Mörmann, 2002; Magne and Belser, 1997; Chong et al., 2002; Fradeani et al., 2002; Wassermann et al., 2006; Bindl and Mörmann, 2004; Bottino et al., 2009; Chen et al., 2008) restricts its application to the fabrication of posterior FDPs, with an outcome comparable to metal–ceramic FDPs (Suárez et al., 2004; Eschbach et al., 2009; Kern et al., 2012). It offers the possibility of masking discolored teeth, ideal for more opaque and high-value teeth. In vitro studies showed that posterior FDPs made of CAD/CAM InCeramZirconia produce a better fit than the slip-cast In Ceram Zirconia and the accuracy is similar to ceramo-metal conventional FDPs (Bindl and Mörmann, 2007).

### 6.3.3 Load-bearing polymer–ceramic composites

The major drawback of ceramics used for dental restorations is their clinical failure rate in posterior sites (Alshehri, 2011), all-ceramic crowns are often replaced because of bulk fracture. Resin-based composites have a Young's modulus which is similar to that of the dentin; associating them with the long-lasting esthetics of ceramics would result in a better restorative material. New CAD/CAM restorative materials have been introduced which do not require heat treatment to achieve acceptable strength.

The main polymer ceramic composites for dental restorations, and some key charcateristics are reported below. In general, such materials present a lower flexural strength than the glass ceramics.

*Paradigm MZ100 (3 M ESPE, St Paul, MN, USA)*: this is based on the resin composite Z100 (3 M ESPE), which is filled with 85 wt% zirconia and silica particles ranging from 0.01 to 3.5 m.

*Lava Ultimate CAD/CAM Restorative*: This is a nano-filled resin composite (80 wt%) based on Filtek Supreme Ultra (3 M ESPE) (Lawson et al., 2016). The resin nano-ceramic material, Lava Ultimate Restorative is designed for precision, speed, and single-appointment efficiency. Because the resin nano-ceramic material is less brittle than glass ceramic, it resists chipping and cracking when milled. CEREC dentists and other chairside CAD/CAM dentists can achieve better edge quality and smooth margins for a brilliant finish. There is no post firing, so the restoration is finished faster: simply polish to a high-quality luster. The material showed lower tensile stress when compared to the ceramic model (Chen et al., 2014). Its use is indicated for crowns, onlays/inlays, and veneers. Both Paradigm MZ100 and Lava Ultimate have higher flexural strength and fracture toughness than resin composites polymerized by a dental curing light (Lawson et al., 2016).

*Cerasmart (GC America, Alsip, IL, USA):* this is a filled nano-composite (71 wt%); it is a material similar to Lava Ultimate.

*PICN-Vita Enamic, Vita Zahnfabrik*: this newly developed polymer-infiltrated-ceramic-network material showed mechanical properties between porcelains and resin-based composites, reflecting its microstructural components (Della Bona et al., 2014). In this material, ceramic particles are partially sintered and then infiltrated with a low-viscosity polymer by capillary action (Lawson et al., 2016). Compositional analyses revealed a major leucite-based phase of feldspar origin and a minor crystalline phase of zirconia, which could function as a strengthening component interconnected with a polymer-based network. The improvements of the novel PICN CAD/CAM materials are reduced brittleness, rigidity and hardness, coupled with improved flexibility, fracture toughness, and better machinability with respect to ceramics (Coldea et al., 2013). Its use is indicated for crowns, onlays/inlays, and veneers.

## 6.4 Conclusions

Dental devices such as veneers, and crown and bridge restorations are fabricated using various materials to restore the morphology and function of the stomatognathic apparatus. In addition, the esthetic properties and appearance of the dental devices have key importance. For this reason there is today a growing demand for all-ceramic restorations that can couple bioinertness, mechanical strength, and esthetics. The evolution of ceramic materials has proceeded in parallel with the evolution of digital dentistry and milling systems. The application of CAD/CAM technology is promising for the delivery of high-esthetics and biocompatibile ceramic devices in all fields of dentistry.

Glass ceramics can be used in restorative dentistry as inlays, onlays, veneers, crowns, and bridges; their excellent esthetic properties and good mechanical strength are bringing about the gradual decline of metallic restorations. In particular, lithium disilicate glass is indicated for single anterior and posterior crowns; application for anterior four-unit FDP is possible, but further clinical and scientific validation are needed.

Zirconia-based restorations exhibit excellent esthetics and optimal mechanical properties; in fact, zirconia-based posterior three-unit FDPs demonstrate good performance in terms of clinical fracture resistance.

Future research is needed to ameliorate the problem of cementation and veneer chipping. The research is active to ameliorate the ceramics present in the market and the possible suitability of $ZrO_2$-$Al_2O_3$ composites in the biomedical field, especially in dentistry applications such as implantology.

## References

Aboushelib, M.N., Feilzer, A.J., Kleverlaan, C.J., 2009. Bridging the gap between clinical failure and laboratory fracture strength tests using a fractographic approach. Dent. Mater. 25 (3), 383–391.

Aboushelib, M.N., Salem, N.A., Taleb, A.L., El Moniem, N.M., 2013. Influence of surface nano-roughness on osseointegration of zirconia implants in rabbit femur heads using selective infiltration etching technique. J. Oral Implantol. 39 (5), 583–590.

Aboushelib, M.N., 2011. Evaluation of zirconia/resin bond strength and interface quality using a new technique. J. Adhes. Dent. 13 (3), 255–260.

Adatia, N.D., Bayne, S.C., Cooper, L.F., Thompson, J.Y., 2009. Fracture resistance of yttria-stabilized zirconia dental implant abutments. J. Prosthodont. 18, 17–22.

Affatato, S., Torrecillas, R., Taddei, P., Rocchi, M., Fagnano, C., Ciapetti, G., et al., 2006. Advanced nanocomposite materials for orthopaedic applications. I. A long-term in vitro wear study of zirconia-toughened alumina. J. Biomed. Mater. Res. B Appl. Biomater. 78 (1), 76–82.

Agustín-Panadero, R., Fons-Font, A., Roman-Rodriguez, J.L., Granell-Ruiz, M., del Rio-Highsmith, J., Sola-Ruiz, M.F., 2012. Zirconia versus metal: a preliminary comparative analysis of ceramic veneer behavior. Int. J. Prosthodont. 25, 294–300.

Agustín-Panadero, R., Román-Rodríguez, J.L., Ferreiroa, A., Solá-Ruíz, M.F., Fons-Font, A., 2014. Zirconia in fixed prosthesis. A literature review. J. Clin. Exp. Dent. 6 (1), e66–e73.
Akagawa, Y., Ichikawa, Y., Nikai, H., Tsuru, H., 1993. Interface histology of unloaded and early loaded partially stabilized zirconia endosseous implant in initial bone healing. J. Prosthodont. Dent. 69, 599–604.
Akagawa, Y., Hosohawa, R., Sato, Y., Kamayama, K., 1998. Comparison between freestanding and tooth-connected partially stabilized zirconia implants after two years function in monkeys: a clinical and hystologic study. J. Prosthodont. Dent. 80, 551–558.
Alghazzawi, T.F., 2016. Advancements in CAD/CAM technology: options for practical implementation. J. Prosthodont. Res. 60 (2), 72–84.
Al-harbi, F., Nathanson, D., 2003. In vitro assessment of retention of four esthetic dowels to resin core foundation and teeth. J. Prosthet. Dent. 90 (6), 547–555.
Alshehri, S.A., 2011. An investigation into the role of core porcelain thickness and lamination in determining the flexural strength of In-Ceram dental materials. J. Prosthodont. 20 (4), 261–266.
Andersson, B., Schärer, P., Simion, M., Bergström, C., 1999. Ceramic implant abutments used for short-span fixed partial dentures: a prospective 2-year multicenter study. Int. J. Prosthodont. 12, 318–324.
Andersson, B., Glauser, R., Maglione, M., Taylor, A., 2003. Ceramic implant abutments for short-span FPDs: a prospective 5-year multicenter study. Int. J. Prosthodont. 16, 640–646.
Andersson, M., Odén, A., 1993. A new all-ceramic crown. A dense-sintered, high-purity alumina coping with porcelain. Acta Odontol. Scand. 51 (1), 59–64.
Andreiuolo, R.F., Sabrosa, C.E., Dias, K.R., 2013. Dual-scan technique for the customization of zirconia computer-aided design/computer-aided manufacturing frameworks. Eur. J. Dent. 7 (Suppl. 1), S115–S118. Available from: http://dx.doi.org/10.4103/1305-7456.119088.
Apholt, W., Bindl, A., Lüthy, H., Mörmann, W.H., 2001. Flexural strength of Cerec 2 machined and jointed InCeram-Alumina and InCeram-Zirconia bars. Dent. Mater. 17 (3), 260–267.
Aramouni, P., Zebouni, E., Tashkandi, E., Dib, S., Salameh, Z., Almas, K., 2008. Fracture resistance and failure location of zirconium and metallic implant abutments. J. Contemp. Dent. Pract. 9, 41–48.
Asai, T., Kazama, R., Fukushima, M., Okiji, T., 2010. Effect of overglazed and polished surface finishes on the compressive fracture strength of machinable ceramic materials. Dent. Mater. J. 29, 661–667.
Asmussen, E., Peutzfeldt, A., Heitmann, T., 1999. Stiffness, elastic limit, and strength of newer types of endodontic posts. J. Dent. 27, 275–278.
Assal, P.A., 2013. The osseointegration of zirconia dental implants. Schweiz Monatsschr Zahnmed. 123 (7-8), 644–654.
Att, W., Kurun, S., Gerds, T., Strub, J.R., 2006. Fracture resistance of single tooth implant-supported all-ceramic restorations: an in vitro study. J. Prosthet. Dent. 95, 111–116.
Att, W., Yajima, N.D., Wolkewitz, M., Witkowski, S., Strub, J.R., 2012. Influence of preparation and wall thickness on the resistance to fracture of zirconia implant abutments. Clin. Implant. Dent. Relat. Res. 14 (Suppl. 1), e196–e203.
Bachle, M., Butz, F., Hubner, U., Bakalinis, E., Kohal, R.J., 2007. BCAL 72 osteoblast-like cells cultured on zirconia ceramics with different surface topographies. Clin. Oral Impl. Res. 18, 53–59.

Bae, K.H., Han, J.S., Seol, Y.J., et al., 2008. The biologic stability of alumina–zirconia implant abutments after 1 year of clinical service: a digital subtraction radiographic evaluation. Int. J. Periodont. Restorat. Dent. 28, 137–143.

Baldassarri, M., Stappert, C.F., Wolff, M.S., Thompson, V.P., Zhang, Y., 2012. Residual stresses in porcelain-veneered zirconia prostheses. Dent. Mater. 28 (8), 873–879.

Banche, G., Tullio, V., Allizond, V., Mandras, N., Roana, J., Scalas, D., et al., 2010. Synergistic effect of erythromycin on polymorphonuclear cell antibacterial activity against erythromycin-resistant phenotypes of *Streptococcus pyogenes*. Int. J. Antimicrob. Agents. 36, 319–323.

Bankoğlu Güngör, M., Aydın, C., Yılmaz, H., Gül, E.B., 2014. An overview of zirconia dental implants: basic properties and clinical application of three cases. J. Oral. Implantol. 40 (4), 485–494.

Baroudi, K., Ibraheem, S.N., 2015. Assessment of chair-side computer-aided design and computer-aided manufacturing restorations: a review of the literature. J. Int. Oral. Health. 7 (4), 96–104.

Bergemann, C., Duske, K., Nebe, J.B., Schöne, A., Bulnheim, U., Seitz, H., et al., 2015. Microstructured zirconia surfaces modulate osteogenic marker genes in human primary osteoblasts. J. Mater. Sci. Mater. Med. 26 (1), 5350.

Beuer, F., Edelhoff, D., Gernet, W., Sorensen, J.A., 2009. Three-year clinical prospective evaluation of zirconia-based posterior fixed dental prostheses (FDPs). Clin. Oral Investig. 13 (4), 445–451.

Bindl, A., Mörmann, W.H., 2002. An up to 5-year clinical evaluation of posterior in-ceram CAD/CAM core crowns. Int. J. Prosthodont. 15 (5), 451–456.

Bindl, A., Mörmann, W.H., 2004. Survival rate of mono-ceramic and ceramic-core CAD/CAM-generated anterior crowns over 2–5 years. Eur. J. Oral Sci. 112 (2), 197–204.

Bindl, A., Mörmann, W.H., 2007. Fit of all-ceramic posterior fixed partial denture frameworks in vitro. Int. J. Periodont. Restorat. Dent. 27 (6), 567–575.

Bitter, K., Priehn, K., Martus, P., Kielbassa, A.M., 2006. In vitro evaluation of push-out bond strengths of various luting agents to tooth-colored posts. J. Prosthet. Dent. 95 (4), 302–310.

Bittner, N., Hill, T., Randi, A., 2010. Evaluation of a one-piece milled zirconia post and core with different post-and-core systems: an in vitro study. J. Prosthet. Dent. 103 (6), 369–379.

Blaschke, C., Volz, U., 2006. Soft and hard tissue response to zirconium dioxide dental implants—a clinical study in man. Neuro Endocrinol. Lett. 27 (Suppl. 1), 69–72.

Boening, K.W., Wolf, B.H., Schmidt, A.E., Kästner, K., Walter, M.H., 2000. Clinical fit of Procera AllCeram crowns. J. Prosthet. Dent. 84 (4), 419–424.

Bonfante, E.A., Rafferty, B., Zavanelli, R.A., Silva, N.R., Rekow, E.D., Thompson, V.P., et al., 2010. Thermal/mechanical simulation and laboratory fatigue testing of an alternative yttria tetragonal zirconia polycrystal core-veneer all-ceramic layered crown design. Eur. J. Oral Sci. 118, 202–209.

Borgonovo, A.E., Censi, R., Vavassori, V., Arnaboldi, O., Maiorana, C., Re, D., 2015. Zirconia Implants in Esthetic Areas: 4-Year Follow-Up Evaluation Study. Int. J. Dent. 2015, 415029, doi:10.1155/2015/415029. Epub 2015 Jun 1.

Borgonovo, A.E., Fabbri, A., Vavassori, V., Censi, R., Maiorana, C., 2012. Multiple teeth replacement with endosseous one-piece yttrium-stabilized zirconia dental implants. Med. Oral Patol. Oral Cir. Bucal. 17 (6), e981–e987.

Borgonovo, A.E., Corrocher, G., Dolci, M., Censi, R., Vavassori, V., Maiorana, C., 2013. Clinical evaluation of zirconium dental implants placed in esthetic areas: a case series study. Eur. J. Esthet. Dent. 8 (4), 532–545, Winter.

Bottino, M.A., Baldissara, P., Valandro, L.F., Galhano, G.A., Scotti, R., 2007. Effects of mechanical cycling on the bonding of zirconia and fiber posts to human root dentin. J. Adhes. Dent. 9 (3), 327–331.

Bottino, M.A., Salazar-Marocho, S.M., Leite, F.P., Vásquez, V.C., Valandro, L.F., 2009. Flexural strength of glass-infiltrated zirconia/alumina-based ceramics and feldspathic veneering porcelains. J. Prosthodont. 18 (5), 417–420.

Bukat, A., Fassina, P., Greco, F., Piattelli, S., Piconi, C., Zaghini, N., 1990. GSP-made Ca-PSZ for biomedical applications. In: Hulbert, J.E., Hulbert, S.F. (Eds.), Bioceramics 3. Rose-Hulman Institute of Technology Publ., Terre Haute (Indiana, USA), pp. 355–366.

Burke, F.J., Crisp, R.J., Cowan, A.J., Lamb, J., Thompson, O., Tulloch, N., 2013. Five-year clinical evaluation of zirconia-based bridges in patients in UK general dental practices. J. Dent. 41 (11), 992–999.

Butz, F., Heydecke, G., Okutan, M., Strub, J.R., 2005. Survival rate, fracture strength and failure mode of ceramic implant abutments after chewing simulation. J. Oral Rehabil. 32, 838–843.

Caglar, A., Bal, B.T., Aydin, C., Yilmaz, H., Ozkan, S., 2010. Evaluation of stresses occurring on three different zirconia dental implants: three-dimensional finite element analysis. Int. J. Oral Maxillofac Implants. 25 (1), 95–103.

Cannizzaro, G., Torchio, C., Felice, P., Leone, M., Esposito, M., 2010. Immediate occlusal versus non-occlusal loading of single zirconia implants. A multicentre pragmatic randomised clinical trial. Eur. J. Oral Implantol. 3 (2), 111–120.

Canullo, L., 2007. Clinical outcome study of customized zirconia abutments for single-implant restorations. Int. J. Prosthodont. 20, 489–493.

Canullo, L., Morgia, P., Marinotti, F., 2007. Preliminary laboratory evaluation of bicomponent customized zirconia abutments. Int. J. Prosthodont. 20 (5), 486–488.

Canullo, L., Coelho, P.G., Bonfante, E.A., 2013. Mechanical testing of thin-walled zirconia abutments. J. Appl. Oral Sci. 21 (1), 20–24.

Carinci, F., Pezzetti, F., Volinia, S., Francioso, F., Arcelli, D., Farina, E., et al., 2004. Zirconium oxide: analysis of MG63 osteoblast-like cell response by means of a microarray technology. Biomaterials. 25, 215–228.

Catelas, I., Petit, A., Zukor, D.J., Marchand, R., Yahia, L., Huk, O.L., 1999. Induction of macrophage apoptosis by ceramic and polyethylene particles in vitro. Biomaterials. 20, 625–630.

Cerroni, L., 2008a. Altre applicazioni. In: Piconi, C., Rimondini, L., Cerroni, L. (Eds.), La zirconia in odontoiatria. Elsevier Masson, Milano, pp. 158–179.

Cerroni, L., 2008b. Biocompatibilità. In: Piconi, C., Rimondini, L., Cerroni, L. (Eds.), La zirconia in odontoiatria. Elsevier, Milano, pp. 46–61.

Chai, J., Chu, F.C., Chow, T.W., 2011. Effect of surface treatment on shear bond strength of zirconia to human dentin. J. Prosthodont. 20 (3), 173–179.

Chen, C., Trindade, F.Z., de Jager, N., Kleverlaan, C.J., Feilzer, A.J., 2014. The fracture resistance of a CAD/CAM Resin Nano Ceramic (RNC) and a CAD ceramic at different thicknesses. Dent. Mater. 30 (9), 954–962.

Chen, Y.M., Smales, R.J., Yip, K.H., Sung, W.J., 2008. Translucency and biaxial flexural strength of four ceramic core materials. Dent. Mater. 24 (11), 1506–1511.

Chong, K.H., Chai, J., Takahashi, Y., Wozniak, W., 2002. Flexural strength of In-Ceram alumina and In-Ceram zirconia core materials. Int. J. Prosthodont. 15 (2), 183–188.

Cionca, N., Müller, N., Mombelli, A., 2015. Two-piece zirconia implants supporting all-ceramic crowns: a prospective clinical study. Clin. Oral Implants Res. 26 (4), 413–418.

Coldea, A., Swain, M.V., Thiel, N., 2013. In-vitro strength degradation of dental ceramics and novel PICN material by sharp indentation. J. Mech. Behav. Biomed. Mater. 26, 34–42.

Covacci, V., Bruzzese, N., Maccauro, G., Andreassi, C., Ricci, G.A., Piconi, C., et al., 1999. In vitro evaluation of the mutagenic end carcinogenic power of high purità zirconia ceramic. Biomaterials. 20, 371–376.

Crisp, R.J., Cowan, A.J., Lamb, J., Thompson, O., Tulloch, N., Burke, F.J., 2012. A clinical evaluation of all-ceramic bridges placed in patients attending UK general dental practices: three-year results. Dent. Mater. 28 (3), 229–236.

de Oliveira, G.R., Pozzer, L., Cavalieri-Pereira, L., de Moraes, P.H., Olate, S., de Albergaría, et al., 2012. Bacterial adhesion and colonization differences between zirconia and titanium implant abutments: an in vivo human study. J. Periodontal. Implant Sci. 42 (6), 217–223.

DeAza, A.H., Chevalier, J., Fantozzi, G., Schehl, M., Torrecillas, R., 2002. Crack growth resistance of alumina, zirconia and zirconia toughened alumina ceramics for joint prostheses. Biomaterials. 23, 937–945.

Della Bona, A., Donassollo, T.A., Demarco, F.F., Barrett, A.A., Mecholsky Jr., J.J., 2007. Characterization and surface treatment effects on topography of a glass-infiltrated alumina/zirconia-reinforced ceramic. Dent. Mater. 23 (6), 769–775.

Della Bona, A., Corazza, P.H., Zhang, Y., 2014. Characterization of a polymer-infiltrated ceramic-network material. Dent. Mater. 30 (5), 564–569.

Della Bona, A., Pecho, O.E., Alessandretti, R., 2015. Zirconia as a dental biomaterial. Materials. 8, 4978–4991.

Demir, E., Burgucu, D., Turna, F., Aksakal, S., Kaya, B., 2013. Determination of TiO2, ZrO2, and Al2O3 nanoparticles on genotoxic responses in human peripheral blood lymphocytes and cultured embyronic kidney cells. J. Toxicol. Environ. Health A. 76 (16), 990–1002.

Denissen, H.W., El-Zohairy, A.A., van Waas, M.A., Feilzer, A.J., 2002. Porcelain-veneered computer-generated partial crowns. Quintessence Int. 33, 723–730.

Denry, I.L., Mackert Jr, J.R., Holloway, J.A., Rosenstiel, S.F., 1996. Effect of cubic leucite stabilization on the flexural strength of feldspathic dental porcelain. J. Dent. Res. 75 (12), 1928–1935.

Depprich, R., Ommerborn, M., Zipprich, H., Naujoks, C., Handschel, J., Wiesmann, H.P., et al., 2008a. Behavior of osteoblastic cells cultured on titanium and structured zirconia surfaces. Head Face Med. 4, 29, Dec 8.

Depprich, R., Zipprich, H., Ommerborn, M., Naujoks, C., Wiesmann, H.P., Kiattavorncharoen, S., et al., 2008b. Osseointegration of zirconia implants compared with titanium: an in vivo study. Head Face Med. 4, 30, Dec 11.

Dikbas, I., Tanalp, J., 2013. An overview of clinical studies on fiber post systems. Sci. World J.Oct 23;2013:171380. doi: 10.1155/2013/171380. eCollection 2013.

Dilmener, F.T., Sipahi, C., Dalkiz, M., 2006. Resistance of three new esthetic post-and-core systems to compressive loading. J. Prosthet. Dent. 95 (2), 130–136.

Dion, I., Bordenave, L., Lefebvre, F., Bareille, R., Baquey, C., Monties, J.R., et al., 1994. Physico-chemistry and cytotoxicity of ceramics. J. Mater. Sci. Mater. Med. 5, 18–24.

Duret, F., Preston, J.D., 1991. CAD/CAM imaging in dentistry. Curr. Opin. Dent. 1, 150–154.

Edelhoff, D., Sorensen, J.A., 2002. Retention of selected core materials to zirconia posts. Oper. Dent. 27 (5), 455–461.

Edelhoff, D., Florian, B., Florian, W., Johnen, C., 2008. HIP zirconia fixed partial dentures—clinical results after 3 years of clinical service. Quintessence Int. 39 (6), 459–471.

El-Mowafy, O., Brochu, J.F., 2002. Longevity and clinical performance of IPS-Empress ceramic restorations—a literature review. J. Can. Dent. Assoc. 68 (4), 233–237.

Eschbach, S., Wolfart, S., Bohlsen, F., Kern, M., 2009. Clinical evaluation of all-ceramic posterior three-unit FDPs made of In-Ceram Zirconia. Int. J. Prosthodont. 22 (5), 490–492.

Esquivel-Upshaw, J.F., Chai, J., Sansano, S., Shonberg, D., 2001. Resistance to staining, flexural strength, and chemical solubility of core porcelains for all-ceramic crowns. Int. J. Prosthodont. 14 (3), 284–288.

Esquivel-Upshaw, J.F., Young, H., Jones, J., Yang, M., Anusavice, K.J., 2008. Four-year clinical performance of a lithia disilicate-based core ceramic for posterior fixed partial dentures. Int. J. Prosthodont. 21 (2), 155–160.

Fabbri, P., Piconi, C., Burresi, E., Magnani, G., Mazzanti, F., Mingazzini, C., 2014. Lifetime estimation of a zirconia–alumina composite for biomedical applications. Dent. Mater. 30 (2), 138–142.

Fasbinder, D.J., Dennison, J.B., Heys, D., Neiva, G., 2010. A clinical evaluation of chairside lithium disilicate CAD/CAM crowns: a two-year report. J. Am. Dent. Assoc. 141 (Suppl. 2), 10S–14SS.

Ferrari, M., Vichi, A., Zarone, F., 2015. Zirconia abutments and restorations: from laboratory to clinical investigations. Dent. Mater. 31 (3), e63–e76.

Fischer, H., Luk, M., Oedekoven, B., Telle, R., Mottaghy, K., 2007. Hemocompatibility of high strength oxide ceramic materials. An in vitro study. J. Biomed. Mater. Res. 81A, 982–986.

Fradeani, M., Aquilano, A., Corrado, M., 2002. Clinical experience with In-Ceram Spinell crowns: 5-year follow-up. Int. J. Periodont. Restorat. Dent. 22 (6), 525–533.

Fradeani, M., Redemagni, M., 2002. An 11-year clinical evaluation of leucite-reinforced glass-ceramic crowns: a retrospective study. Quintessence Int. 33 (7), 503–510.

Gahlert, M., Gudehus, T., Eichhorn, S., Steinhauser, E., Kniha, H., Erhardt, W., 2007. Biomechanical and histomorphometric comparison between zirconia implants with varying surface textures and a titanium implant in the maxilla of miniature pigs. Clin. Oral Implants Res. 18 (5), 662–668.

Gahlert, M., Burtscher, D., Grunert, I., Kniha, H., Steinhauser, E., 2012. Failure analysis of fractured dental zirconia implants. Clin. Oral Implants Res. 23 (3), 287–293.

Galhano, G.A., Melo, R.M., Pavanelli, C.A., Baldissara, P., Scotti, R., Valandro, L.F., et al., 2008. Adhesive cementation of zirconia posts to root dentin: evaluation of the mechanical cycling effect. Braz Oral Res. 22 (3), 264–269.

Garine, W.N., Funkenbusch, P.D., Ercoli, C., Wodenscheck, J., Murphy, W.C., 2007. Measurement of the rotational misfit and implant-abutment gap of all-ceramic abutments. Int. J. Oral Maxillofac Implants. 22, 928–938.

Gehrke, P., Dhom, G., Brunner, J., WolfD, Degidi, M., Piattelli, A., 2006. Zirconium implant abutments: fracture strength and influence of cyclic loading on retaining-screw loosening. Quintessence Int. 37, 19–26.

Gehrke, P., Johannson, D., Fischer, C., Stawarczyk, B., Beuer, F., 2015. In vitro fatigue and fracture resistance of one- and two-piece CAD/CAM zirconia implant abutments. Int. J. Oral Maxillofac Implants. 30 (3), 546–554.

Gernhardt, C.R., Bekes, K., Schaller, H.G., 2005. Short-term retentive values of zirconium oxide posts cemented with glass ionomer and resin cement: an in vitro study and a case report. Quintessence Int. 36 (8), 593–601.

Giordano, R.A., Pelletier, L., Campbell, S., Pober, R., 1995. Flexural strength of an infused ceramic, glass ceramic, and feldspathic porcelain. J. Prosthet. Dent. 73 (5), 411–418.

Glauser, R., Sailer, I., Wohlwend, A., et al., 2004. Experimental zirconia abutments for implant-supported single-tooth restorations in esthetically demanding regions: 4-year results of a prospective clinical study. Int. J. Prosthodont. 17, 285–290.

Gomes, A.L., Montero, J., 2011. Zirconia implant abutments: a review. Med. Oral Patol. Oral Cir. Bucal. 16 (1), e50–e55.

Griggs, J.A., 2007. Recent advances in materials for all-ceramic restorations. Dent. Clin. North Am. 51 (3), 713–727.

Guazzato, M., Albakry, M., Ringer, S.P., Swain, M.V., 2004. Strength, fracture toughness and microstructure of a selection of all-ceramic materials. Part II. Zirconia-based dental ceramics. Dent. Mater. 20 (5), 449–456.

Guazzato, M., Albakry, M., Swain, M.V., Ironside, J., 2002. Mechanical properties of In-Ceram Alumina and In-Ceram Zirconia. Int. J. Prosthodont. 15 (4), 339–346.

Guazzato, M., Albakry, M., Ringer, S.P., Swain, M.V., 2004. Strength, fracture toughness and microstructure of a selection of all-ceramic materials. Part II. Zirconia-based dental ceramics. Dent. Mater. 20 (5), 449–456.

Guess, P.C., Strub, J.R., Steinhart, N., Wolkewitz, M., Stappert, C.F., 2009a. All-ceramic partial coverage restorations – midterm results of a 5-year prospective clinical splitmouth study. J. Dent. 37, 627–637.

Guess, P.C., Zhang, Y., Thompson, V.P., 2009b. Effect of veneering techniques on damage and reliability of Y-TZP trilayers. Eur. J. Esthet. Dent. 4 (3), 262–276.

Guess, P.C., Zavanelli, R.A., Silva, N.R., Bonfante, E.A., Coelho, P.G., Thompson, V.P., 2010a. Monolithic CAD/CAM lithium disilicate versus veneered Y-TZP crowns: comparison of failure modes and reliability after fatigue. Int. J. Prosthodont. 23, 434–442.

Guess, P.C., Zhang, Y., Kim, J.W., Rekow, E.D., Thompson, V.P., 2010b. Damage and reliability of Y-TZP after cementation surface treatment. J. Dent. Res. 89 (6), 592-6. 21.

Guess, P.C., Schultheis, S., Bonfante, E.A., Coelho, P.G., Ferencz, J.L., Silva, N.R., 2011. All-ceramic systems: laboratory and clinical performance. Dent. Clin. North Am. 55 (2), 333–352.

Hambleton, J., Schwartz, Z., Khare, A., Windeler, S.W., Luna, M., Brooks, B.P., et al., 1994. Culture surface coated with various implant materials affect chondrocyte growth and metabolism. J. Orthop. Res. 12, 542–552.

Hao, L., Lawrence, J., Chian, K.S., 2005. Osteoblast cell adhesion on a laser modified zirconia based bioceramic. J. Mater. Sci. Mater. Med. 16, 719–726.

Hedlund, S.O., Johansson, N.G., Sjögren, G., 2003. Retention of prefabricated and individually cast root canal posts in vitro. Br. Dent. J. 195 (3), 155–158.

Heffernan, M.J., Aquilino, S.A., Diaz-Arnold, A.M., Haselton, D.R., Stanford, C.M., Vargas, M.A., 2002. Relative translucency of six all-ceramic systems. Part I: core materials. J. Prosthet. Dent. 88 (1), 4–9.

Heintze, S.D., Rousson, V., 2010. Fracture rates of IPS Empress all-ceramic crowns—a systematic review. Int. J. Prosthodont. 23 (2), 129–133.

Hempel, U., Hefti, T., Kalbacova, M., Wolf-Brandstetter, C., Dieter, P., Schlottig, F., 2010. Response of osteoblast-like SAOS-2 cells to zirconia ceramics with different surface topographies. Clin. Oral Implants Res. 21 (2), 174–181.

Hobkirk, J.A., Wiskott, H.W., 2009. Ceramics in implant dentistry (Working Group 1). Clin. Oral Implants Res. 20 (Suppl. 4), 55–57.

Hoffmann, O., Angelov, N., Gallez, F., Jung, R.E., Weber, F.E., 2008. The zirconia implant-bone interface: a preliminary histologic evaluation in rabbits. Int. J. Oral Maxillofac Implants. 23 (4), 691–695.

Höland, W., Rheinberger, V., Apel, E., van 't Hoen, C., Höland, M., Dommann, A., et al., 2006. Clinical applications of glass-ceramics in dentistry. J. Mater. Sci. Mater. Med. 17 (11), 1037–1042.

Hwang, J.W., Yang, J.H., 2001. Fracture strength of copy-milled and conventional In-Ceram crowns. J. Oral Rehabil. 28 (7), 678–683.

Inokoshi, M., Kameyama, A., De Munck, J., Minakuchi, S., Van Meerbeek, B., 2013. Durable bonding to mechanically and/or chemically pre-treated dental zirconia. J. Dent. 41 (2), 170–179.

Ioannidis, A., Bindl, A., 2016. Clinical prospective evaluation of zirconia-based three-unit posterior fixed dental prostheses: up-to ten-year results. J. Dent. 47, 80–85.

Ito, H., Sasaki, H., Saito, K., Honma, S., Yajima, Y., Yoshinari, M., 2013. Response of osteoblast-like cells to zirconia with different surface topography. Dent. Mater. J. 32 (1), 122–129.

Jiménez-Melendo, M., Llena-Blasco, O., Bruguera, A., Llena-Blasco, J., Yáñez-Vico, R.M., García-Calderón, M., et al., 2014. Mechanical behavior of single-layer ceramized zirconia abutments for dental implant prosthetic rehabilitation. J. Clin. Exp. Dent. 6 (5), e485–e490.

Josset, Y., Oum'Hamed, Z., Zarrinpour, A., Lorenzato, M., Adnet, J.J., Maquin, D., 1999. In vitro reactions of human osteoblasts in culture with zirconia and alumina ceramics. J. Biomed. Mater. Res. 47, 481–493.

Kaya, B.M., Ergun, G., 2013. The effect of post length and core material on root fracture with respect to different post materials. Acta Odontol. Scand. 71 (5), 1063–1070.

Kelly, J.R., Denry, I., 2008. Stabilized zirconia as a structural ceramic: an overview. Dent. Mater. 24 (3), 289–298.

Kelly, J.R., Benetti, P., 2011. Ceramic materials in dentistry: historical evolution and current practice. Aust. Dent. J. 56 (Suppl. 1), 84–96.

Kern, M., Wegner, S.M., 1998. Bonding to zirconia ceramic: adhesion methods and their durability. Dent. Mater. 14, 64–71.

Kern, T., Tinschert, J., Schley, J.S., Wolfart, S., 2012. Five-year clinical evaluation of all-ceramic posterior FDPs made of In-Ceram Zirconia. Int. J. Prosthodont. 25 (6), 622–624.

Kerstein, R.B., Radke, J., 2008. A comparison of fabrication precision and mechanical reliability of 2 zirconia implant abutments. Int. J. Oral Maxillofac Implants. 23 (6), 1029–1036.

Keshvad, A., Hooshmand, T., Asefzadeh, F., Khalilinejad, F., Alihemmati, M., Van Noort, R., 2011. Marginal gap, internal fit, and fracture load of leucite-reinforced ceramic inlays fabricated by CEREC inLab and hot-pressed techniques. J. Prosthodont. 20, 535–540.

Khamverdi, Z., Moshiri, Z., 2012. Zirconia: an up-to-date literature review. DJH. 4 (1), 1–15.

Kim, J.S., Raigrodski, A.J., Flinn, B.D., Rubenstein, J.E., Chung, K.H., Mancl, L.A., 2013. In vitro assessment of three types of zirconia implant abutments under static load. J. Prosthet. Dent. 109 (4), 255–263.

Kim, S., Kim, H.I., Brewer, J.D., Monaco Jr., E.A., 2009. Comparison of fracture resistance of pressable metal ceramic custom implant abutments with CAD/CAM commercially fabricated zirconia implant abutments. J. Prosthet. Dent. 101 (4), 226–230.

Kohal, R.J., Papavasiliou, G., Kamposiora, P., Tripodakis, A., Strub, J.R., 2002. Three-dimensional computerized stress analysis of commercially pure titanium and yttrium-partially stabilized zirconia implants. Int. J. Prosthodont. 15 (2), 189–194.

Kohal, R.J., Weng, D., Bächle, M., Strub, J.R., 2004. Loaded custom-made zirconia and titanium implants show similar osseointegration: an animal experiment. J. Periodontol. 75 (9), 1262–1268.

Kohal, R.J., Wolkewitz, M., Mueller, C., 2010. Alumina-reinforced zirconia implants: survival rate and fracture strength in a masticatory simulation trial. Clin. Oral Implants Res. 21 (12), 1345–1352.

Kohal, R.J., Knauf, M., Larsson, B., Sahlin, H., Butz, F., 2012. One-piece zirconia oral implants: one-year results from a prospective cohort study. 1. Single tooth replacement. J. Clin. Periodontol. 39 (6), 590–597.

Kohal, R.J., Patzelt, S.B., Butz, F., Sahlin, H., 2013. One-piece zirconia oral implants: one-year results from a prospective case series. 2. Three-unit fixed dental prosthesis (FDP) reconstruction. J. Clin. Periodontol. 40 (5), 553–562.

Kohorst, P., Borchers, L., Strempel, J., Stiesch, M., Hassel, T., Bach, F.W., et al., 2012. Low-temperature degradation of different zirconia ceramics for dental applications. Acta Biomater. 8 (3), 1213–1220.

Kollar, A., Huber, S., Mericske, E., Mericske-Stern, R., 2008. Zirconia for teeth and implants: a case series. Int J Periodont. Restorat. Dent. 28, 479–487.

Kosmac, T., Oblak, C., Jevnikar, P., Funduk, N., Marion, L., 1999. The effect of surface grinding and sandblasting on flexural strength and reliability of Y-TZP zirconia ceramic. Dent. Mater. 15 (6), 426–433.

Kosmac, T., Oblak, C., Jevnikar, P., Funduk, N., Marion, L., 2000. Strength and reliabiliy of surface treated Y-TZP dental ceramics. J. Biomed. Mater. Res. 53, 304–313.

Kosmač, T., 2004. The effect of dental grinding and sandblasting on the biaxial flexural strength and Weibull modulus of tetragonal zirconia. Key Eng. Mater. 254-256, 683–686.

Koutayas, S.O., Kern, M., 1999. All-ceramic posts and cores: the state of the art. Quintessence Int. 30 (6), 383–392.

Koutayas, S.O., Mitsias, M., Wolfart, S., Kern, M., 2012. Influence of preparation mode and depth on the fracture strength of zirconia ceramic abutments restored with lithium disilicate crowns. Int. J. Oral Maxillofac Implants. 27 (4), 839–848.

Kurthukoti, A.J., Paul, J., Gandhi, K., Rao, D.B., 2015. Fracture resistance of endodontically treated permanent anterior teeth restored with three different esthetic post systems: an in vitro study. J. Indian Soc. Pedod. Prev. Dent. 33 (4), 296–301.

Kwon, T.K., Pak, H.S., Yang, J.H., Han, J.S., Lee, J.B., Kim, S.H., et al., 2013. Comparative fracture strength analysis of Lava and Digident CAD/CAM zirconia ceramic crowns. J. Adv. Prosthodont. 5 (2), 92–97.

Lawson, N.C., Bansal, R., Burgess, J.O., 2016. Wear, strength, modulus and hardness of CAD/CAM restorative materials. Dent. Mater.pii: S0109-5641(16)30371-2.

Lazar, D.R., Bottino, M.C., Ozcan, M., Valandro, L.F., Amaral, R., Ussui, V., et al., 2008. Y-TZP ceramic processing from coprecipitated powders: a comparative study with three commercial dental ceramics. Dent. Mater. 24 (12), 1676–1685.

Li, J., Liu, Y., Hermansson, L., Soremark, R., 1993. Evaluation of biocompatibility of various ceramic powders with human fibroblasts in vitro. Clin. Mat. 12 (197), 201.

Li, R.W., Chow, T.W., Matinlinna, J.P., 2014. Ceramic dental biomaterials and CAD/CAM technology: state of the art. J. Prosthodont. Res. 58 (4), 208–216.

Lohmann, C.H., Dean, D.D., Köster, G., Casasola, D., Buchhorn, G.H., Fink, U., et al., 2002. Ceramic and PMMA particles differentially affect osteoblast phenotype. Biomaterials. 23 (8), 1855–1863.

Lorenzoni, F.C., Martins, L.M., Silva, N.R., Coelho, P.G., Guess, P.C., Bonfante, E.A., et al., 2010. Fatigue life and failure modes of crowns systems with a modified framework design. J. Dent. 38 (8), 626–634, http://dx.doi.org/10.1016/j.jdent.2010.04.011. Epub 2010 May 5.

Maccari, P.C., Conceição, E.N., Nunes, M.F., 2003. Fracture resistance of endodontically treated teeth restored with three different prefabricated esthetic posts. J. Esthet. Restor. Dent. 15 (1), 25–30.

Magne, P., Belser, U., 1997. Esthetic improvements and in vitro testing of In-Ceram Alumina and Spinell ceramic. Int. J. Prosthodont. 10 (5), 459–466.

Manicone, P.F., Rossi Iommetti, P., Raffaelli, L., 2007. An overview of zirconia ceramics: basic properties and clinical applications. J. Dent. 35 (11), 819–826.

Mannocci, F., Ferrari, M., Watson, T.F., 1999. Intermittent loading of teeth restored using quartz fiber, carbon-quartz fiber, and zirconium dioxide ceramic root canal posts. J. Adhes. Dent. 1 (2), 153–158.

Mannocci, F., Machmouridou, E., Watson, T.F., Sauro, S., Sherriff, M., Pilecki, P., et al., 2008. Microtensile bond strength of resin-post interfaces created with interpenetrating polymer network posts or cross-linked posts. Med. Oral Patol. Oral Cir. Bucal. 1;13 (11), E745-52.

Marchan, S., Coldero, L., Whiting, R., Barclay, S., 2005. In vitro evaluation of the retention of zirconia-based ceramic posts luted with glass ionomer and resin cements. Braz. Dent. J. 16 (3), 213–217.

Marquardt, P., Strub, J.R., 2006. Survival rates of IPS empress 2 all-ceramic crowns and fixed partial dentures: results of a 5-year prospective clinical study. Quintessence Int. 37 (4), 253–259.

Mellinghoff, J., 2006. Erste klinische ergebnisse zur dentale schraubenimplantate aus zirkonoxid. Z Ahnartl. Implantol. 22, 288–293.

Mitsias, M.E., Silva, N.R., Pines, M., Stappert, C., Thompson, V.P., 2010. Reliability and fatigue damage modes of zirconia and titanium abutments. Int. J. Prosthodont. 23 (1), 56–59.

Miyazaki, T., Hotta, Y., 2011. CAD/CAM systems available for the fabrication of crown and bridge restorations. Aust. Dent. J. 56 (Suppl. 1), 97–106.

Miyazaki, T., Nakamura, T., Matsumura, H., Ban, S., Kobayashi, T., 2013. Current status of zirconia restoration. J. Prosthodont. Res. 57 (4), 236–261.

Moldovan, O., Luthardt, R.G., Corcodel, N., Rudolph, H., 2011. Three-dimensional fit of CAD/CAM-made zirconia copings. Dent. Mater. 27 (12), 1273–1278.

Molin, M.K., Karlsson, S.L., 2008. Five-year clinical prospective evaluation of zirconia-based Denzir 3-unit FPDs. Int. J. Prosthodont. 21 (3), 223–227.

Mormann, W.H., Brandestini, M., Lutz, F., Barbakow, F., 1989. Chairside computer-aided direct ceramic inlays. Quintessence Int. 20, 329–339.

Mortazavi, V., Fathi, M., Katiraei, N., Shahnaseri, S., Badrian, H., Khalighinejad, N., 2012. Fracture resistance of structurally compromised and normal endodontically treated teeth restored with different post systems: an in vitro study. Dent. Res. J. (Isfahan). 9 (2), 185–191.

Mühlemann, S., Truninger, T.C., Stawarczyk, B., Hämmerle, C.H., Sailer, I., 2014. Bending moments of zirconia and titanium implant abutments supporting all-ceramic crowns after aging. Clin. Oral Implants Res. 25 (1), 74–81.

Musikant, B.L., Cohen, B.I., Deutsch, A.S., 2001. The relationship of post design to the long-term success of endodontically restored teeth. Compendium. 22, 974–988.

Naenni, N., Bindl, A., Sax, C., Hämmerle, C., Sailer, I., 2015. A randomized controlled clinical trial of 3-unit posterior zirconia-ceramic fixed dental prostheses (FDP) with layered or pressed veneering ceramics: 3-year results. J. Dent. 43 (11), 1365–1370.

Nakamura, T., Usami, H., Ohnishi, H., Nishida, H., Tang, X., Wakabayashi, K., et al., 2012. The relationship between milling a new silica-doped zirconia and its resistance to low-temperature degradation (LTD): a pilot study. Dent. Mater. J. 31 (1), 106–112.

Nascimento, C.D., Pita, M.S., Fernandes, F.H., Pedrazzi, V., de Albuquerque Junior, R.F., Ribeiro, R.F., 2014. Bacterial adhesion on the titanium and zirconia abutment surfaces. Clin. Oral Implants Res. 25 (3), 337–343.

Nicoli Aldini, N., Fini, M., Giavaresi, G., Martini, L., Dubini, B., Ponzi-Bossi, M.G., et al., 2004. Osteointegration of bioactive glass-coated and uncoated zirconia in osteopenic bone: an in vivo experimental study. J. Biomed. Mater. Res. 68, 264–272.

Nkamgueu, E.M., Adnet, J.J., Bernard, J., Zierold, K., Kilian, L., Jallot, E., et al., 2000. In vitro effects of zirconia and alumina particles on human blood monocyte-derived macrophages: X-ray microanlysis and flow cytometric studies. J. Biomed. Mater. Res. 52, 587–594.

Nothdurft, F.P., Doppler, K.E., Erdelt, K.J., Knauber, A.W., Pospiech, P.R., 2010. Influence of artificial aging on the load-bearing capability of straight or angulated zirconia abutments in implant/tooth-supported fixed partial dentures. Int. J. Oral Maxillofac Implants. 25 (5), 991–998.

Nothdurft, F.P., Pospiech, P.R., 2006. Clinical evaluation of pulpless teeth restored with conventionally cemented zirconia posts: a pilot study. J. Prosthet. Dent. 95 (4), 311–314.

Nothdurft, F.P., Merker, S., Pospiech, P.R., 2011. Fracture behaviour of implant-implant- and implant-tooth-supported all-ceramic fixed dental prostheses utilising zirconium dioxide implant abutments. Clin. Oral Investig. 15 (1), 89–97.

Obando-Pereda, G.A., Fischer, L., Stach-Machado, D.R., 2014. Titanium and zirconia particle-induced pro-inflammatory gene expression in cultured macrophages and osteolysis, inflammatory hyperalgesia and edema in vivo. Life Sci. 97 (2), 96–106.

Oblak, C., Jevnikar, P., Kosmac, T., Funduk, N., Marion, L., 2004. Fracture resistance and reliability of new zirconia posts. J. Prosthet. Dent. 91 (4), 342–348.

Oguri, T., Tamaki, Y., Hotta, Y., Miyazaki, T., 2012. Effects of a convenient silica-coating treatment on shear bond strengths of porcelain veneers on zirconia-based ceramics. Dent. Mater. J. 31 (5), 788–796.

Oliva, J., Oliva, X., Oliva, J.D., 2007. One-year follow-up of first consecutive 100 zirconia dental implants in humans: a comparison of 2 different rough surfaces. Int. J. Oral Maxillofac Implants. 22 (3), 430–435.

Oliva, J., Oliva, X., Oliva, J.D., 2010. Five-year success rate of 831 consecutively placed Zirconia dental implants in humans: a comparison of three different rough surfaces. Int. J. Oral Maxillofac Implants. 25 (2), 336–344.

Osman, R.B., Ma, S., Duncan, W., de Silva, R.K., Siddiqi, A., Swain, M.V., 2013. Fractured Zirconia implants and related implant designs: scanning electron microscopy analysis. Clin. Oral Implants Res. 24, 592–597.

Osman, R.B., Swain, M.V., Atieh, M., Ma, S., Duncan, W., 2014. Ceramic implants (Y-TZP): are they a viable alternative to titanium implants for the support of overdentures? A randomized clinical trial. Clin. Oral Implants Res. 25 (12), 1366–1377.

Oum'hamed, Z., Garnotel, R., Josset, Y., Trenteseaux, C., Laurent-Maquin, D., 2004. Matrix metalloproteinases MMP-2,-9 and tissue inhibitors TIMP-1.-2 expression and secretion by primary human osteoblast cell in response to titanium, zirconia, and alumina ceramics. J. Biomed. Mater. Res. 68A, 114–122.

Ozcan, M., Nijhuis, H., Valandro, L.F., 2008. Effect of various surface conditioning methods on the adhesion of dual-cure resin cement with MDP functional monomer to zirconia after thermal aging. Dent. Mater. J. 27 (1), 99–104.
Ozcan, N., Sahin, E., 2013. In vitro evaluation of the fracture strength of all-ceramic core materials on zirconium posts. Eur. J. Dent. 7 (4), 455–460.
Ozkurt, Z., Işeri, U., Kazazoğlu, E., 2010. Zirconia ceramic post systems: a literature review and a case report. Dent. Mater. J. 29 (3), 233–245.
Paul, S.J., Werder, P., 2004. Clinical success of zirconium oxide posts with resin composite or glass-ceramic cores in endodontically treated teeth: a 4-year retrospective study. Int. J. Prosthodont. 17 (5), 524–528.
Payer, M., Arnetzl, V., Kirmeier, R., Koller, M., Arnetzl, G., Jakse, N., 2013. Immediate provisional restoration of single-piece zirconia implants: a prospective case series - results after 24 months of clinical function. Clin. Oral Implants Res. 24 (5), 569–575.
Payer, M., Heschl, A., Koller, M., Arnetzl, G., Lorenzoni, M., Jakse, N., 2015. All-ceramic restoration of zirconia two-piece implants--a randomized controlled clinical trial. Clin. Oral Implants Res. 26 (4), 371–376.
Peixoto, H.E., Bordin, D., Del Bel Cury, A.A., da Silva, W.J., Faot, F., 2016. The role of prosthetic abutment material on the stress distribution in a maxillary single implant-supported fixed prosthesis. Mater. Sci. Eng. C Mater. Biol. Appl. 65, 90–96.
Peláez, J., Cogolludo, P.G., Serrano, B., Lozano, J.F., Suárez, M.J., 2012. A prospective evaluation of zirconia posterior fixed dental prostheses: three-year clinical results. J. Prosthet. Dent. 107 (6), 373–379.
Pfeiffer, P., Schulz, A., Nergiz, I., Schmage, P., 2006. Yield strength of zirconia and glass fibre-reinforced posts. J. Oral Rehab. 33, 70–74.
Piascik, J.R., Swift, E.J., Thompson, J.Y., Grego, S., Stoner, B.R., 2009. Surface modification for enhanced silanation of zirconia ceramics. Dent. Mater. 25 (9), 1116–1121.
Piascik, J.R., Wolter, S.D., Stoner, B.R., 2011. Development of a novel surface modification for improved bonding to zirconia. Dent. Mater. 27 (5), E99–E105.
Piattelli, S., Maccauro, G., Specchia, N., Maggiano, N., Piconi, C., Greco, F. Effects of ceramic precursors on human lynphocyte mitogenesis. In 4$^{th}$ World Biomaterials Congress Transactions. Berlin, Germania, 24–28 April 1992:343.
Piconi, C., 2008. La zirconia negli impianti dentali. In: Piconi, C., Rimondini, L., Cerroni, L. (Eds.), La zirconia in odontoiatria. Elsevier, Milano, pp. 136–156.
Pilathadka, S., Vahalová, D., 2007. Contemporary all-ceramic systems, part-2. Acta Medica (Hradec Kralove). 50 (2), 105–107.
Pirker, W., Kocher, A., 2009. Immediate, non-submerged, root-analogue zirconia implants placed into single-rooted extraction sockets: 2-year follow-up of a clinical study. Int. J. Oral Maxillofac Surg. 38 (11), 1127–1132.
Porcelain-Fused-to-Metal Crowns versus All-ceramic Crowns: A Review of the Clinical and Cost-Effectiveness [Internet]. Ottawa (ON): Canadian Agency for Drugs and Technologies in Health; 2015 May 29.
Qing, H., Zhu, Z., Chao, Y., Zhang, W., 2007. In vitro evaluation of the fracture resistance of anterior endodontically treated teeth restored with glass fiber and zircon posts. J. Prosthet. Dent. 97 (2), 93–98.
Raffaelli, L., Rossi Iommetti, P., Piccioni, E., Toesca, A., Serini, S., Resci, F., et al., 2008. Growth, viability, adhesion potential, and fibronectin expression in fibroblasts cultured on zirconia or feldspatic ceramics in vitro. J. Biomed. Mater. Res. A. 86 (4), 959–968.
Raigrodski, A.J., 2005. All-ceramic full-coverage restorations: concepts and guidelines for material selection. Pract. Proced. Aesthet. Dent. 17 (4), 249–256, quiz 258. Review.

Raigrodski, A.J., Chiche, G.J., Potiket, N., Hochstedler, J.L., Mohamed, S.E., Billiot, S., et al., 2006. The efficacy of posterior three-unit zirconium-oxide-based ceramic fixed partial dental prostheses: a prospective clinical pilot study. J. Prosthet. Dent. 96 (4), 237–244.

Raigrodski, A.J., Yu, A., Chiche, G.J., Hochstedler, J.L., Mancl, L.A., Mohamed, S.E., 2012. Clinical efficacy of veneered zirconium dioxide-based posterior partial fixed dental prostheses: five-year results. J. Prosthet. Dent. 108 (4), 214–222.

Reich, S., Fischer, S., Sobotta, B., Klapper, H.U., Gozdowski, S., 2010. A preliminary study on the short-term efficacy of chairside computer-aided design/computer-assisted manufacturing-generated posterior lithium disilicate crowns. Int. J. Prosthodont. 23 (3), 214–216.

Reinhardt, B., Beikler, T. Dental Implants. In Advanced Ceramics for Dentistry. Shen JZ and Kosmač Eds. 2014:51–73.

Reznikoff, C.A., Bertram, J.S., Bronkow, D.W., Heidelberger, C., 1973. Quantitative and qualitative studies of chemical transformation of cloned C3H mouse embryo cells sensitive to postconfluence inhibition of cell division. Cancer Res. 33, 3239–3249.

Rimondini, L., Cerroni, L., Carrassi, A., Torricelli, P., 2002. Bacterial colonization of zirconia ceramic surfaces: an in vitro and in vivo study. Int. J. Oral Maxillofac Implants. 17, 793–798.

Rinke, S., Gersdorff, N., Lange, K., Roediger, M., 2013. Prospective evaluation of zirconia posterior fixed partial dentures: 7-year clinical results. Int. J. Prosthodont. 26 (2), 164–171.

Rocchietta, I., Fontana, F., Addis, A., Schupbach, P., Simion, M., 2009. Surface-modified zirconia implants: tissue response in rabbits. Clin. Oral Implants Res. 20 (8), 844–850.

Roediger, M., Gersdorff, N., Huels, A., Rinke, S., 2010. Prospective evaluation of zirconia posterior fixed partial dentures: four-year clinical results. Int. J. Prosthodont. 23 (2), 141–148.

Roehling, S., Woelfler, H., Hicklin, S., Kniha, H., Gahlert, M., 2016. A retrospective clinical study with regard to survival and success rates of zirconia implants up to and after 7 years of loading. Clin. Implant Dent. Relat. Res. 18 (3), 545–558.

Román-Rodríguez, J.L., Roig-Vanaclocha, A., Fons-Font, A., Granell-Ruiz, M., Solá-Ruiz, M.F., Bruguera-Alvarez, A., 2010. Full maxillary rehabilitation with an all-ceramic system. Med. Oral Patol. Oral Cir. Bucal. 15, e523–e525.

Rosentritt, M., Fürer, C., Behr, M., Lang, R., Handel, G., 2000. Comparison of in vitro fracture strength of metallic and tooth-coloured posts and cores. J. Oral Rehabil. 27 (7), 595–601.

Rosentritt, M., Behr, M., Thaller, C., Rudolph, H., Feilzer, A., 2009. Fracture performance of computer-aided manufactured zirconia and alloy crowns. Quintessence Int. 40 (8), 655–662.

Rotunno, F., Rotunno, E., 2012. In vitro comparison of the mechanical strength of carbon fiber and zirconia ceramic posts and cores. Int. J. Periodont. Restorat. Dent. 32 (2), e75–e81.

Ruby, S.G., McNally, A.C., 1995. Quality control of imprint and tissue section DNA ploidy analysis in image anlysis systems utilizing cell culture-based control materials. Am. J. Clin. Pathol. 104, 167–171.

Sadowsky, S.J., 2006. An overview of treatment considerations for esthetic restorations: a review of the literature. J. Prosthet. Dent. 96, 433–442.

Sahafi, A., Peutzfeldt, A., Asmussen, E., Gotfredsen, K., 2003. Bond strength of resin cement to dentin and to surface-treated posts of titanium alloy, glass fiber, and zirconia. J. Adhes. Dent. 5 (2), 153–162, Summer.

Sailer, I., Fehér, A., Filser, F., Gauckler, L.J., Lüthy, H., Hämmerle, C.H., 2007. Five-year clinical results of zirconia frameworks for posterior fixed partial dentures. Int. J. Prosthodont. 20 (4), 383–388.

Sailer, I., Gottnerb, J., Kanelb, S., et al., 2009. Randomized controlled clinical trial of zirconia ceramic and metal-ceramic posterior fixed dental prostheses: a 3-year follow-up. Int. J. Prosthodont. 22 (6), 553–560.

Saint-Jean, S.J. Dental Glasses and Glassceramics. In Advanced Ceramics for Dentistry. Shen JZ and Kosmač Eds. 2014. 255–275.

Saito, A., Komine, F., Blatz, M., Matsumura, H., 2010. A comparison of bond strength of layered veneering porcelains to zirconia and metal. J. Prosthet. Dent. 104, 247–257.

Sandhaus, S., 1969. Noveaux aspects de l'implantologie. Julien Prelat, Paris.

Sanon, C., Chevalier, J., Douillard, T., Cattani-Lorente, M., Scherrer, S.S., Gremillard, L., 2015. A new testing protocol for zirconia dental implants. Dent. Mater. 31 (1), 15–25.

Scarano, A., Piattelli, M., Caputi, S., Favero, G.A., Piattelli, A., 2004. Bacterial adhesion on commercially pure titanium and zirconium oxide disks: an in vivo human study. J. Periodontol. 75, 292–296.

Schierano, G., Pejrone, G., Roana, J., Scalas, D., Allizond, V., Martinasso, G., et al., 2010. A split-mouth study on microbiological profile in clinical healthy teeth and implants related to key inflammatory mediators. Int. J. Immunopathol. Pharmacol. 23 (1), 279–288.

Schmitt, J., Holst, S., Wichmann, M., Reich, S., Gollner, M., Hamel, J., 2009. Zirconia posterior fixed partial dentures: a prospective clinical 3-year follow-up. Int. J. Prosthodont. 22 (6), 597–603.

Schmitt, J., Goellner, M., Lohbauer, U., Wichmann, M., Reich, S., 2012. Zirconia posterior fixed partial dentures: 5-year clinical results of a prospective clinical trial. Int. J. Prosthodont. 25 (6), 585–589.

Schmitter, M., Hamadi, K., Rammelsberg, P., 2011. Survival of two post systems—five-year results of a randomized clinical trial. Quintessence Int. 42, 843–850.

Seghi, R.R., Denry, I.L., Rosenstiel, S.F., 1995. Relative fracture toughness and hardness of new dental ceramics. J. Prosthet. Dent. 74 (2), 145–150.

Seghi, R.R., Sorensen, J.A., 1995. Relative flexural strength of six new ceramic materials. Int. J. Prosthodont. 8 (3), 239–246.

Sennerby, L., Dasmah, A., Larsson, B., Iverhed, M., 2005. Bone tissue responses to surface-modified zirconia implants: a histomorphometric and removal torque study in the rabbit. Clin. Implant Dent. Relat. Res. 7 (Suppl. 1), S13–S20.

Setzer, B., Bächle, M., Metzger, M.C., Kohal, R.J., 2009. The gene-expression and phenotypic response of hFOB 1.19 osteoblasts to surface-modified titanium and zirconia. Biomaterials. 30 (6), 979–990.

Sicilia, A., Cuesta, S., Coma, G., Arregui, I., Guisasola, C., Ruiz, E., et al., 2008. Titanium allergy in dental implant patients: a clinical study on 1500 consecutive patients. Clin. Oral Implants Res. 19 (8), 823–835.

Song, T.J., Kwon, T.K., Yang, J.H., Han, J.S., Lee, J.B., Kim, S.H., et al., 2013. Marginal fit of anterior 3-unit fixed partial zirconia restorations using different CAD/CAM systems. J. Adv. Prosthodont. 5 (3), 219–225.

Sorrentino, R., De Simone, G., Tetè, S., Russo, S., Zarone, F., 2012a. Five-year prospective clinical study of posterior three-unit zirconia-based fixed dental prostheses. Clin. Oral Investig. 16 (3), 977–985, Jun.

Sorrentino, R., Galasso, L., Tetè, S., De Simone, G., Zarone, F., 2012b. Clinical evaluation of 209 all-ceramic single crowns cemented on natural and implant-supported abutments with different luting agents: a 6-year retrospective study. Clin. Implant Dent. Relat. Res. 14 (2), 184–197, Apr.

Soundar, S.I., Suneetha, T.J., Angelo, M.C., Kovoor, L.C., 2014. Analysis of fracture resistance of endodontically treated teeth restored with different post and core system of variable diameters: an in vitro study. J. Indian Prosthodont. Soc. 14 (2), 144–150.

Spies, B.C., Sauter, C., Wolkewitz, M., Kohal, R.J., 2015a. Alumina reinforced zirconia implants: effects of cyclic loading and abutment modification on fracture resistance. Dent. Mater. 31 (3), 262–272, Mar.

Spies, B.C., Sperlich, M., Fleiner, J., Stampf, S., Kohal, R.J., 2015b. Clinical and patient-reported outcomes of a zirconia oral implant: three-year results of a prospective cohort investigation. J. Dent. Res. 94 (10), 1385–1391, Oct.

Spies, B.C., Sperlich, M., Fleiner, J., Stampf, S., Kohal, R.J., 2016. Alumina reinforced zirconia implants: 1-year results from a prospective cohort investigation. Clin. Oral Implants Res. 27 (4), 481–490.

Sriamporn, T., Thamrongananskul, N., Busabok, C., Poolthong, S., Uo, M., Tagami, J., 2014. Dental zirconia can be etched by hydrofluoric acid. Dent. Mater. J. 33 (1), 79–85.

Stimmelmayr, M., Sagerer, S., Erdelt, K., Beuer, F., 2013. In vitro fatigue and fracture strength testing of one-piece zirconia implant abutments and zirconia implant abutments connected to titanium cores. Int. J. Oral Maxillofac Implants. 28 (2), 488–493.

Strub, J.R., Pontius, O., Koutayas, S., 2001. Survival rate and fracture strength of incisors restored with different post and core systems after exposure in the artificial mouth. J. Oral Rehabil. 28 (2), 120–124.

Suárez, M.J., Lozano, J.F., Paz Salido, M., Martínez, F., 2004. Three-year clinical evaluation of In-Ceram Zirconia posterior FPDs. Int. J. Prosthodont. 17 (1), 35–38.

Sundh, A., Sjögren, G., 2008. A study of the bending resistance of implant supported reinforced alumina and machined zirconia abutments and copies. Dent. Mater. 24, 611–617.

Tan, J.P., Sederstrom, D., Polansky, J.R., McLaren, E.A., White, S.N., 2012. The use of slow heating and slow cooling regimens to strengthen porcelain fused to zirconia. J. Prosthet. Dent. 107 (3), 163–169.

Tartaglia, G.M., Sidoti, E., Sforza, C., 2011. A 3-year follow-up study of all-ceramic single and multiple crowns performed in a private practice: a prospective case series. Clinics (Sao Paulo). 66 (12), 2063–2070.

Tinschert, J., Zwez, D., Marx, R., Anusavice, K.J., 2000. Structural reliability of alumina-, feldspar-, leucite-, mica- and zirconia-based ceramics. J. Dent. 28 (7), 529–535.

Tinschert, J., Schulze, K.A., Natt, G., Latzke, P., Heussen, N., Spiekermann, H., 2008. Clinical behavior of zirconia-based fixed partial dentures made of DC-Zirkon: 3-year results. Int. J. Prosthodont. 21 (3), 217–222.

Toksavul, S., Toman, M., Uyulgan, B., Schmage, P., Nergiz, I., 2005. Effect of luting agents and reconstruction techniques on the fracture resistance of pre-fabricated post systems. J. Oral Rehabil. 32 (6), 433–440.

Torabi Ardekani, K., Ahangari, A.H., Farahi, L., 2012. Marginal and internal fit of CAD/CAM and slip-cast made zirconia copings. J. Dent. Res. Dent. Clin. Dent. Prospects. Spring;6(2):42-8. Epub 2012 Jun 6.

Tsalouchou, E., Cattell, M.J., Knowles, J.C., et al., 2007. Fatigue and fracture properties of yttria partially stabilized zirconia crown systems. Dent. Mater. 24 (3), 308–318.

Tsumita, M., Kokubo, Y., Ohkubo, C., Sakurai, S., Fukushima, S., 2010. Clinical evaluation of posterior all-ceramic FPDs (Cercon): a prospective clinical pilot study. J. Prosthodont. Res. 54 (2), 102–105.

Tullio, V., Mandras, N., Scalas, D., Allizond, V., Banche, G., Roana, J., et al., 2010. Synergy of caspofungin with human polymorphonuclear granulocytes for killing *Candida albicans*. Antimicrob. Agents Chemother. 54 (9), 3964–3966.

Uo, M., Sjogren, G., Sundh, A., Watari, F., Bergman, M., Lerner, U., 2003. Cytotoxicity and bonding property of dental ceramics. Dent. Mater. 19, 487–492.

Usumez, A., Cobankara, F.K., Ozturk, N., Eskitascioglu, G., Belli, S., 2004. Microleakage of endodontically treated teeth with different dowel systems. J. Prosthet. Dent. 92 (2), 163–169.

Valenti, M., Valenti, A., 2009. Retrospective survival analysis of 261 lithium disilicate crowns in a private general practice. Quintessence Int. 40 (7), 573–579.

Vigolo, P., Fonzi, F., Majzoub, Z., Cordioli, G., 2006. An in vitro evaluation of titanium, zirconia, and alumina procera abutments with hexagonal connection. Int. J. Oral Maxillofac Implants. 21, 575–580.

Vult von Steyern, P., Carlson, P., Nilner, K., 2005. All-ceramic fixed partial dentures designed according to the DC-Zirkon technique. A 2-year clinical study. J. Oral Rehabil. 32 (3), 180–187.

Wagner, W.C., Chu, T.M., 1996. Biaxial flexural strength and indentation fracture toughness of three new dental core ceramics. J. Prosthet. Dent. 76 (2), 140–144.

Wassermann, A., Kaiser, M., Strub, J.R., 2006. Clinical long-term results of VITA In-Ceram Classic crowns and fixed partial dentures: a systematic literature review. Int. J. Prosthodont. 19 (4), 355–363.

Watanabe, H., Saito, K., Kokubun, K., Sasaki, H., Yoshinari, M., 2012. Change in surface properties of zirconia and initial attachment of osteoblastlike cells with hydrophilic treatment. Dent. Mater. J. 31 (5), 806–814.

Wegner, S.M., Kern, M., 2000. Long-term resin bond strength to zirconia ceramic. J. Adhes. Dent. 2 (2), 139–147.

Wolfart, M., Lehmann, F., Wolfart, S., Kern, M., 2007. Durability of the resin bond strength to zirconia ceramic after using different surface conditioning methods. Dent. Mater. 23 (1), 45–50.

Wolfart, S., Harder, S., Eschbach, S., Lehmann, F., Kern, M., 2009. Four-year clinical results of fixed dental prostheses with zirconia substructures (Cercon): end abutments vs. cantilever design. Eur. J. Oral Sci. 117 (6), 741–749.

Xible, A.A., de Jesus Tavarez, R.R., de Araujo Cdos, R., Bonachela, W.C., 2006a. Effect of silica coating and silanization on flexural and composite-resin bond strengths of zirconia posts: an in vitro study. J. Prosthet. Dent. 95, 224–229.

Xible, A.A., de Jesus Tavarez, R.R., de Araujo Cdos, R., Conti, P.C., Bonachella, W.C., 2006b. Effect of cyclic loading on fracture strength of endodontically treated teeth restored with conventional and esthetic posts. J. Appl. Oral Sci. 14 (4), 297–303, Aug.

Yaman, P., Thorsteinsson, T.S., 1992. Effect of core materials on stress distribution of posts. J. Prosthet. Dent. 68, 416–420.

Yamashita, D., Machigashira, M., Miyamoto, M., Takeuchi, H., Noguchi, K., Izumi, Y., et al., 2009. Effect of surface roughness on initial responses of osteoblast-like cells on two types of zirconia. Dent. Mater. J. 28 (4), 461–470.

Yildirim, M., Fischer, H., Marx, R., Edelhoff, D., 2003. In vivo fracture resistance of implant-supported all-ceramic restorations. J. Prosthet. Dent. 90, 325–331.

Yun, J.Y., Ha, S.R., Lee, J.B., Kim, S.H., 2010. Effect of sandblasting and various metal primers on the shear bond strength of resin cement to Y-TZP ceramic. Dent. Mater. 26 (7), 650–658.

Zarone, F., Ferrari, M., Mangano, F.G., Leone, R., Sorrentino, R., 2016. Digitally oriented materials: focus on lithium disilicate ceramics. Int. J. Dent. 2016, 9840594.

Zembic, A., Bösch, A., Jung, R.E., Hämmerle, C.H., Sailer, I., 2013. Five-year results of a randomized controlled clinical trial comparing zirconia and titanium abutmentssupporting single-implant crowns in canine and posterior regions. Clin. Oral Implants Res. 24 (4), 384–390.

Zeng, K., Odén, A., Rowcliffe, D., 1996. Flexure tests on dental ceramics. Int. J. Prosthodont. 9, 434–439.

Zhang, Y., Sailer, I., Lawn, B.R., 2013. Fatigue of dental ceramics. J. Dent. 41, 1135–1147.

Zhao, K., Wei, Y.R., Pan, Y., Zhang, X.P., Swain, M.V., Guess, P.C., 2014. Influence of veneer and cyclic loading on failure behavior of lithium disilicate glass-ceramic molar crowns. Dent. Mater. 30, 164–171.

Zhao, Y.Q., Li, J., Zhang, J.C., Liao, Y.M., Lu, J.J., Li, W., 2012. Shear bond strengths between alumina-toughened zirconia cores and veneering ceramics and their susceptibility to aging. Asian Pac. J. Trop. Med. 5 (5), 402–405.

## Further reading

Ozkurt, Z., Duygu, G., Canpolat, C., Kazazoğlu, E., 2008. Reconstruction of edentulous maxillary and mandibular arches with implant-supported fixed restorations using a digital treatment planning technique: a clinical report. J. Oral. Implantol. 34 (3), 161–168.

# Ceramics for bone replacement: Commercial products and clinical use

7

*Francesco Baino*
Politecnico di Torino, Torino, Italy

**Chapter Outline**

**7.1 Introduction 249**
**7.2 Bone substitutes of human and animal origin 250**
**7.3 Bone substitutes of nonanimal biological origin: Ceramics from corals 252**
**7.4 Calcium orthophosphates of synthetic origin 254**
**7.5 Bioactive glasses and glass ceramics 256**
**7.6 Composites 262**
**7.7 Moldable and injectable ceramic-based cements 264**
**7.8 Conclusions and outlook 269**
**References 271**

## 7.1 Introduction

Bioceramics are a large class of specially designed crystalline, semicrystalline, or amorphous materials used for the repair and reconstruction of diseased or damaged parts of the body (Hench, 1991). The use of ceramics in medical applications has a long and honorable history that dates back to the 10th century AD when calcium sulfate was found to be useful to repair broken bones of cadavers and mummies (Dorozhkin, 2013a). Calcium sulfate (also known as "plaster of Paris") was firstly implanted as a bone void filler in living humans suffering from tuberculous osteomyelitis in 1892 (Dreesmann, 1892). More recently, it was reintroduced as a bone substitute in the form of high-purity pellets by Peltier in 1959 (Peltier, 1961).

It is instructive to point out that bone is currently the second most common tissue requiring repair after blood (Shegarfi and Reikeras, 2009). Today, bone reconstruction can be performed using transplant tissues or man-made implants. Over the years, tens of ceramic compositions have been experimented with as bone grafting materials, ranging from inert ceramics (e.g., alumina and zirconia) to hydroxyapatite (HA) and bioactive glasses (Chevalier and Gremillar, 2009). Current forms of application for bone repair mainly include monolithic devices (used, for instance, in the reconstruction of small bones in the middle ear), porous granules and rigid scaffolds for filling bone voids, and moldable pastes (e.g., injectable cements for spine surgery).

**Advances in Ceramic Biomaterials.**
**DOI: http://dx.doi.org/10.1016/B978-0-08-100881-2.00007-5**

The ability to create a stable bond with the host tissue is of primary importance in the selection of ceramics for bone substitution: in this regard, bioactive and bioresorbable ceramics represent a valuable solution (Tan et al., 2013; Baino et al., 2015). Furthermore, bioresorbable ceramics possess the added value of degrading gradually over time while being replaced by natural bone and, therefore, disappear once they have performed their function of acting as templates for new tissue (Carrodeguas and De Aza, 2011).

The following sections focus on the main types of ceramic products that are currently available on the market for clinical use; a short perspective for improvement and future research, which will be comprehensively discussed in the third part of the book, is also provided at the end of this chapter.

## 7.2 Bone substitutes of human and animal origin

From a materials scientist's viewpoint, bone is a biocomposite material made of a calcium phosphate mineral matrix (mainly HA) and an organic fraction (mainly type I collagen) (Boskey, 2007) that are finely organized according to a complex three-dimensional (3D) hierarchical structure (Reznikov et al., 2014). Hence, bone transplant materials from human to human (autografts or allografts) or from animal to human (xenografts) can be considered particular types of ceramic-based natural composites (Schlickewei and Schlickewei, 2007).

At present, autologous bone transplantation is the "gold standard" strategy for repairing osseous defects (Pryor et al., 2009). Autologous bone is obtained from the same patient receiving the graft and is usually harvested from nonload-bearing regions of the skeleton such as iliac crest, ribs, chin, and even parts of the skull (Schlickewei and Schlickewei, 2007). Despite excellent biocompatibility and tissue-regenerative properties (high osteoinductivity, no risk of immune responses or infections), autologous bone is associated with some drawbacks, including the slow rate of new bone formation at the harvesting site, the risk of pain or postoperative complications (hemorrhage, local cosmetic deformity, infections), and the limited availability (especially in pediatric and elderly populations) (Kline and Wolfe, 1995; Pape et al., 2010; Baumhauer et al., 2014).

Bone harvested from either living donors (e.g., patients undergoing total hip replacement surgery) or cadavers represents a suitable alternative to autologous bone, being derived from humans as well. Allograft bone is stored in bone tissue banks hosted at medical universities and hospitals and can be considered a very particular type of "commercial" product available to surgeons. Sustainability of bone banks has been repeatedly advocated and castigated due to concerns related to cost and effectiveness of donor bone compared to other available solutions (e.g., man-made bioceramics) (Benninger et al., 2014; Calvo et al., 2011); furthermore, ethical concerns may arise in some patients (Lomas et al., 2013). Bone allografts are osteoconductive but weakly osteoinductive (growth factors may be inactivated depending on the processing) and require sterilization ($\gamma$- or $\beta$-irradiation), which has detrimental effects on the mechanical properties of the graft and can deactivate the proteins normally found in healthy bone. Concerns on the risk of HIV transmission also exist, although only two cases of infection have been reported since the discovery of this immune disease in the 1980s (Khan et al., 2005). Current protocols for allograft procurement and processing are designed to strongly limit the possible transmission of pathogenic agents from donor to patient (Manyalich et al., 2009).

Another alternative to autologous tissue is represented by bone xenografts harvested from animals (Fig. 7.1). Before being used in humans, xenografts have to be freeze-dried or demineralized and deproteinized (Campana et al., 2014; Ramani et al., 1975; Siqueira and Kranzler, 1982; Malca et al., 1996; Lofgren et al., 2000). Commercially available products include Bio-Oss (Geistlich Biomaterials, Zurich, Switzerland), Symbios Osteograf (Cera-Med Co., Denver, CO, USA), and Endobon (Merck Co., Darmstadt, Germany), which are all derived from bovine HA and sold in the form of granules of different sizes. Advantages of xenografts encompass easy availability, osteoconductivity, and low cost (Laurencin and El-Amin, 2008). Xenografts have also been shown to be useful for bone augmentation during total hip arthroplasty in selected cases (Charalambides et al., 2005). However, ethical issues may occur for some patients and concerns have arisen about the risk of disease transmission from animal to patient (e.g., bovine spongiform encephalopathy).

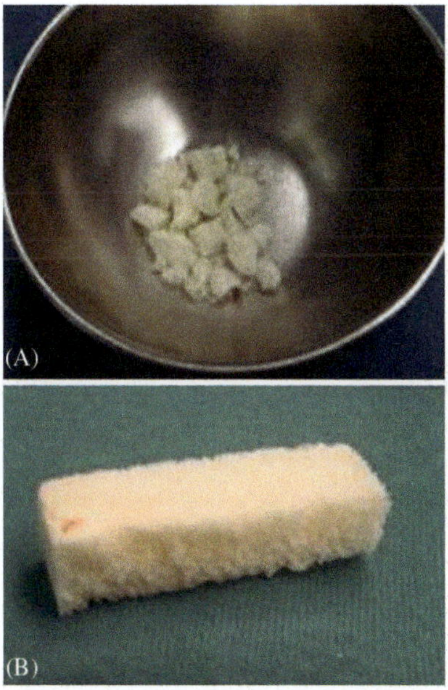


**Figure 7.1** Bovine bone substitute (xenograft) in the form of (A) chips and (B) porous blocks.
*Source*: Adapted from Campana, V., Milano, G., Pagano, E., Barba, M., Cicione, C., Salonna, G., et al., 2014. Bone substitutes in orthopaedic surgery: from basic science to clinical practice. J. Mater. Sci. Mater. Med. 25, 2445–2461, Copyright © The Authors.

Furthermore, bone xenografts are often associated with an unpredictable resorption rate, usually higher than that of autologous bone, which leads to problems of mechanical support in the defect site (Schlickewei and Schlickewei, 2007). Current EU directives discourage the use of xenografts and recommend other options, such as synthetic biomaterials.

## 7.3 Bone substitutes of nonanimal biological origin: Ceramics from corals

Coralline bioceramics are manufactured from particular types of marine corals which possess an exquisite trabecular structure similar to that of cancellous bone. Specifically, corals used for bone substitutions belong to the genera *Porites* (total porosity below 60 vol%, pore size range within 140–160 μm with all the pores interconnected) and *Goniopora* (total porosity above 70 vol%, pore size ranging from 200 to 1000 μm) (Damien and Revell, 2004). An overview of commercial products is reported in Table 7.1.

Coralline calcium carbonate ($CaCO_3$), which is marketed under the commercial name of Biocoral (Biocoral Inc., France) in the form of porous granules and 3D blocks, showed good results as a bone substitute for the repair of infrabony defects in periodontal surgery and alveolar bone augmentation in the jaw (Yukna and Yukna, 1998; Piattelli et al., 1997). A large study was also reported by Nam et al. (2006) who reviewed the postoperative outcomes associated with the use of Biocoral porous blocks for the repair of orbital bone fractures in human patients. Specifically, the results found in 191 patients receiving Biocoral were compared to those assessed for patients (214 cases) implanted with porous polyethylene (Medpor). Postoperative enophthalmos (i.e., recession of the ocular globe within the orbit) was statistically more frequent in Biocoral-treated patients than in those receiving a Medpor implant but no other significant differences in postoperative outcomes were observed between the two groups.

Coral skeletons as such, however, have a different composition compared to that of the mineral matrix of bone ($CaCO_3$ vs HA, a calcium orthophosphate). Coralline HA can be obtained by a multistep hydrothermal conversion of $CaCO_3$ according to a process pioneered in the 1970s (Roy and Linnehan, 1974; White et al., 1975). Commercial products include Interpore and Pro-Osteon lines (Interpore International, Inc., Irvine, Canada); these biomaterials are osteoconductive as new bone formation was found in the pore surfaces which are in direct contact with bone, but no bone ingrowth was observed into the pores that are far from the interface with viable bone (Damien and Revell, 2004). Interpore-200 and Interpore-500 are available as granules or blocks with mean pore size of 200 and 500 μm, respectively, and are especially recommended to treat periodontal defects. Interpore-500 is resorbable and is available in the form of granules with a diameter in the range of 0.4–1.0 mm for general applications in oral surgery and in the range of 0.4–6.0 mm for alveolar bone repair. In the latter case, rapid vascularization of the

Table 7.1 **Commercially available coral-based bioceramics**

| Product name | Coral source (genus) | Product type | Porosity (vol%) | Pore size (μm) | Producer |
|---|---|---|---|---|---|
| Biocoral | Aeropora or Porites | Calcium carbonate (>98%) porous granules, blocks and plates | 20 or 50 | 150 −500 | Biocoral Inc. (France) |
| Interpore-200 | Porites | Hydroxyapatite porous granules and blocks | 60 | 200 | Interpore International Inc. (Canada) |
| Interpore-500 | Goniopora | Hydroxyapatite porous granules and blocks | >70 | 500 | Interpore International Inc. (Canada) |
| Pro-Osteon 200 | Porites | Hydroxyapatite porous blocks for spine surgery | 60 | 200 | Interpore International Inc. (Canada) |
| Pro-Osteon 500 | Goniopora | Hydroxyapatite porous blocks for spine surgery | >70 | 500 | Interpore International Inc. (Canada) |

implant material was observed along with the transformation of newly formed fibrovascular tissue into bone (Kenney et al., 1985; Ayers et al., 1998). Interpore-500 has shown advantages over nonporous HA particles in terms of increased bone bonding and graft fixation (Kenney et al., 1985). Interpore-200 was also successfully experimented with to treat craniofacial bone defects (Reedy et al., 1999).

Using Pro-Osteon porous blocks is indicated in the management of vertebral fractures. Furthermore, coralline HA is a suitable bone graft material in oncological surgery as demonstrated by the promising postoperative outcome of 71 patients receiving Pro-Osteon 500 to replace bone tumors over a 2.4-year follow-up (Irwin et al., 2001). Coral-derived HA blocks were also successfully used as bone graft at the calcaneocuboid joint to achieve distraction in a calcaneal fracture (Elsinger and Leal, 1996).

The use of coralline HA is associated with two peculiar problems: first, there are some environmental concerns due to the harvesting of natural corals and possible damage to marine ecosystems, and secondly coralline implants are usually more expensive than other options available for the same application (e.g., Medpor for orbital floor repair). Problems of mechanical integrity due to the high porosity of coralline structures were also pointed out in some studies, especially when there is the need for implant contouring to match the defect size during surgery (Elmazar et al., 2003) or load-bearing properties after surgery are required (Baino, 2011). Hence, synthetic porous calcium phosphates have gained increasing popularity over coralline bioceramics due to lower cost and higher versatility.

## 7.4 Calcium orthophosphates of synthetic origin

Calcium orthophosphates are probably the most widely used class of bioceramics for bone tissue repair and regeneration. This is due to their favorable properties that include similarity to the mineral phase of bone (biological apatite) in terms of composition and crystal structure, as well as osteoconductivity, i.e., the ability to provide a biocompatible interface along which bone migrates and bonds to the implant without the formation of scar tissue (LeGeros, 2002).

Synthetic HA has a stoichiometric Ca/P molar ratio of 1.67 and, from a crystallographic viewpoint, is the calcium phosphate phase most similar to natural bone apatite. Because of its excellent biocompatibility and osteoconductivity, HA is successfully employed as a bone filler in the form of granules or moldable paste; its use as a 3D porous scaffold is limited due to its low mechanical properties and extremely slow resorption rate (Barrere et al., 2006). It is partly for the latter limitation that other calcium phosphates, such as $\alpha$- and $\beta$-tricalcium phosphate (TCP), have emerged with different degrees of solubility depending mainly on the crystallographic structure and on the Ca/P ratio (the rate of dissolution increases with decreasing Ca/P ratio: $\alpha$-TCP $>$ $\beta$-TCP $>$ HA) (Cao and Hench, 1996; Legeros et al., 2003).

As already mentioned in the case of coralline HA (Elmazar et al., 2003; Baino, 2011), a common drawback to all calcium phosphate bioceramics produced in a porous form is their low mechanical properties (brittleness, low fatigue strength) that largely limit their clinical use to nonload-bearing parts of the skeleton. We have to consider that calcium phosphate scaffolds are often consolidated by a sintering process that, however, does not occur under a viscous flow regime, and thus may not lead to full densification of scaffold struts.

The use of calcium orthophosphates in clinics has been comprehensively described and discussed by Dorozhkin in a series of review papers (Dorozhkin, 2007, 2010a,b, 2012), and a picture for the future was recently provided by Habraken et al. (2016). Dorozhkin also reported the existence of about 150 registered commercial trademarks (current and past) of calcium orthophosphate-based biomaterials (Dorozhkin, 2013b). However, despite the large number of marketed products worldwide as well as the abundance of scientific literature about calcium phosphates for medical applications, there is a relative paucity of reports dealing clearly with commercial devices. The tradename of the implant as well as the manufacturer may be not mentioned in the scientific articles or are difficult to find out, and often the only data about the clinical performance of the materials are the technical information at the producer's websites. A selection of available studies is discussed below.

Kasten et al. (2008) implanted β-TCP porous blocks (Cerasorb, Curasan, Germay) in an animal model (adult mouse) and studied the influence of different porosities (25, 65, and 75 vol%) on osteogenesis (Fig. 7.2). Cerasorb is produced by a solid-state reaction from calcium carbonate and calcium hydrogen phosphate. It was suggested that the distribution and size of the pores, as well as the surface structure, might play an important role in osteogenic differentiation in vivo, but the exact mechanisms were not determined; however, calcification was found to be greater in the scaffolds with higher porosity (65 and 75 vol% vs 25 vol%). In another study, Cerasorb granules (particle size within the range 0.5–2 mm) were implanted in 152 human patients from 1997 to 2002 to reconstruct osseous defects in the jaw (Horch et al., 2006). Results were generally favorable (only 2% of total failures were reported) but Cerasorb resorption rate and bone regeneration often depended on individual patient's factors, such as defect size, implant site, and individual osteogenetic bone potential. Furthermore, combination of Cerasorb granules with autologous bone was necessary if the osseous defect exceeded 2 cm in diameter.

β-TCP porous blocks (OSferion, Olympus, Tokyo Japan; total porosity of 75 vol%, macropores from 100 to 500 μm, micropore size of less than 5 μm) were found to possess superior osteoconductivity in comparison to HA (Bonfil, Mitsubishi Materials, Chichibu, Japan; total porosity of 70 vol%, macropores within 90–200 μm without micropores) in human patients (Ogose et al., 2006). However, the extent to which the superior bone regenerative potential is due to either different materials used or different pore characteristics still needs clarification.

In a preclinical study in rabbit femur condyles, Hing et al. (2007) compared the osteogenic potential of Vitoss (pure β-TCP with a total porosity of 80 vol%;

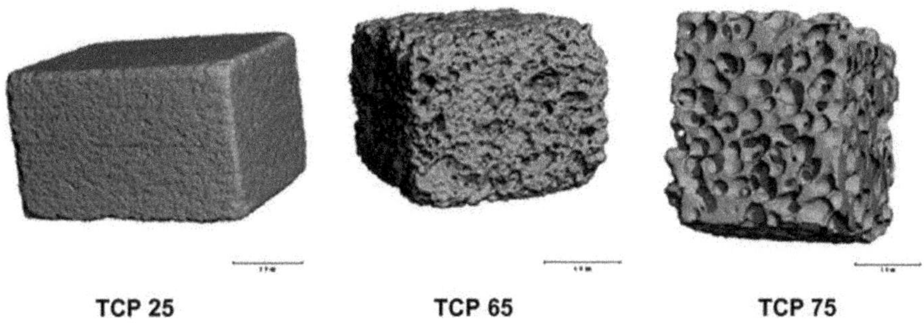


**Figure 7.2** Three-dimensional microtomographic reconstructions of Cerasorb block with different porosities (25, 65, or 75 vol%).
*Source:* Adapted from Kasten, P., Beyen, I., Niemeyer, P., Luginbuhl, R., Bohner, M., Richter, W., 2008. Porosity and pore size of b-tricalcium phosphate scaffold can influence protein production and osteogenic differentiation of human mesenchymal stem cells: an in vitro and in vivo study. Acta Biomater. 4, 1904–1915, Copyright © Elsevier.

Orthovita Inc., Malvern, PA, USA) and Actifuse (Si-substituted HA having a Si content of 0.8 wt% and a total porosity of 70 vol%; ApaTech Ltd., London, UK) pellets. Actifuse appeared to provide a more stable osteoconductive scaffold, which supported faster bone apposition and angiogenesis throughout the defect site, with the development of a functionally adaptive trabecular structure through resorption and remodeling of both scaffold and new bone. There was rapid formation of mineralized tissue after 1 week within the center of the defect and complete infiltration with mature bone by the sixth postoperative week.

Some companies started commercializing calcium phosphate products fabricated by additive manufacturing, such as 3D scaffolds with an oriented architecture to promote bone ingrowth in a specific direction. An example is OsteoFlux (Vivos-Dental AG, Switzerland), a 3D-printed porous block of layered strands of β-TCP and HA, which was shown to stimulate greater bone regeneration compared to a reference substitute (Bio-Oss) in a sheep calvarial model (Carrel et al., 2016). Another approach involves the fabrication of custom-made implants that are very helpful for achieving accurate anatomical correction of osseous defects and good functional results (Oka et al., 2010).

Macroporous biphasic calcium phosphate ceramics (HA/β-TCP in a 60:40 wt% ratio; Triosite, Zimmer Co., Rungis, France) (Fig. 7.3) were found to be suitable to act as a delivery vehicle for osteogenic cells derived from human mesenchymal stem cells (Toquet et al., 1999). This approach may be particularly useful for large osseous defects created by trauma or tumor removal or for elderly patients for whom the number and renewal capability of osteoprogenitor cells are lower.

## 7.5 Bioactive glasses and glass ceramics

Bioactive glasses are not only osteoconductive, like calcium orthophosphates, but also osteoinductive, i.e., they are able to stimulate living cells to produce new healthy bone, thus accelerating tissue healing kinetics (Jones, 2013). A selection of today's commercially available bioactive glass compositions and products is reported in Table 7.2. The first bioactive glass (45S5 Bioglass), invented by Hench and coworkers at the University of Florida in 1969, has been used in over a million patients worldwide to repair bone defects in various sites of the skeleton (Hench, 2006). From a historical viewpoint, the first 45S5 Bioglass device cleared for marketing in the USA aimed to treat conductive hearing loss by replacing the small bones of the middle ear (Merwin, 1986). This implant, called "Bioglass Ossicular Reconstruction Prosthesis" and commercialized under the tradename MEP, was approved by the Food and Drug Administration (FDA) for clinical use in 1985. It was a melt-derived nonporous structure similar to a truncated cone that allowed sound conduction from the tympanic membrane to the cochlea. This was possible due to the ability of 45S5 Bioglass to bond tightly both to calcified tissues (bone) and to soft collagenous tissues (eardrum) (Hench and Greenspan, 2013). While short-term and mid-term results showed superior performance of 45S5 Bioglass

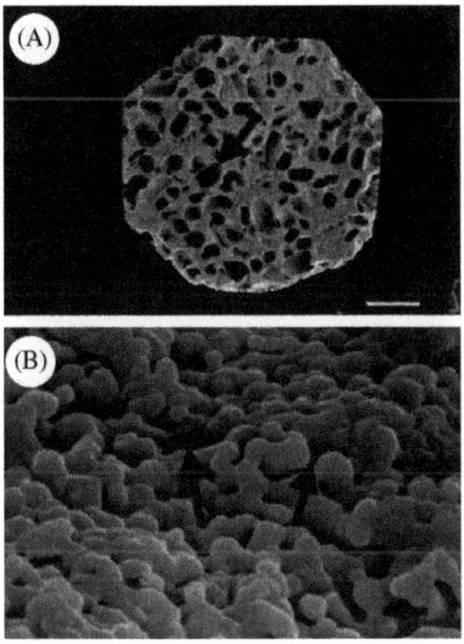


**Figure 7.3** Scanning electron micrograph observation of a commercial Triosite pellet (biphasic calcium phosphate). (A) Cross-sectional micrograph (diameter 5 mm, thickness 2 mm) showing large macropores (*black* arrow) and (B) detail of the surface exhibiting a diffused microporosity. Scale bar = 1 mm in both pictures.
*Source:* Adapted from Toquet, J., Rohanizadeh, R., Guicheux, J., Couillaud, S., Passuti, N., Daculsi, G., et al., 1999. Osteogenic potential in vitro of human bone marrow cells cultured on macroporous biphasic calcium phosphate ceramic. J. Biomed. Mater. Res. 44, 98–108, Copyright © Wiley Periodicals.

compared to almost-inert implants (e.g., alumina prosthetic ossicles) (Wilson et al., 1995), long-term clinical reviews reported that MEP tended to be progressively reabsorbed within the middle ear and break down into small fragments after more than 10 years from operation (Bahmad and Merchant, 2007). This was the reason why MEP implants were taken off the American market; however, these devices are still distributed in some European countries with a slightly modified design (Douek-MED; 45S5 Bioglass cones of three different size are available).

Another option to reconstruct the small bones of the middle ear was Ceravital, which identifies a set of silicate glass–ceramic formulations. The use of Ceravital in otology was debated as, despite the good clinical performance in terms of auditory rehabilitation, the implant tended to slowly resorb over time (Reck et al., 1988) and, therefore, at present the production of such a device has been stopped.

45S5 Bioglass was also experimented with in otology to anchor cochlear implants to the temporal bone of deaf patients who underwent irreversible damage to the cochlea. This device, commercialized under the tradename of Bioglass-EPI (extracochlear percutaneous implant) since the 1980s, comprised a 45S5 Bioglass sleeve that bonded to the temporal bone and protruded through the skin (forming a strong bond with collagenous soft tissues, too), thus acting as a percutaneous and stable seal that protected the interior electronics (Walliker et al., 1987).

**Table 7.2 Overview of commercial bioactive glasses approved for clinical use**

| Glass name | Composition | Commercial products | Producer |
|---|---|---|---|
| 45S5 Bioglass | $45SiO_2-24.5CaO-24.5Na_2O-6P_2O_5$ (wt%) | NovaBone Putty and NovaBone Dental Putty: moldable glass-based paste that can be also injected into the bone/dental defect site by a syringe<br>NovaBone particulate (90–710 μm) for orthopedics<br>NovaBone Morsels (porous granulate)<br>PerioGlas particulate (90–710 μm) for repairing jaw bone defects<br>NovaBone porous blocks<br>Biogran particulate (300–360 μm)<br>NovaMin particulate (18 μm) | Novabone (USA); Mo-Sci Corp. (USA); Biomet 3i (USA) |
| TheraGlass | $70SiO_2-30CaO$ (mol%) | Sol-gel powders | MedCell (UK) |
| S53P4 (BoneAlive) | $53SiO_2-20CaO-23Na_2O-4P_2O_5$ (wt%) | Particulate, monolithic pieces of adjustable size and dimensions that can be processed according to a custom-made approach | Abmin Technologies Ltd/Vivoxid (Finland); Mo-Sci Corp. (USA) |
| 13–93 | $53SiO_2-6Na_2O-12K_2O-5MgO-20CaO-4P_2O_5$ (wt%) | Cast monolithic pieces, quenched frit, rods, fibers, disks, spheres, and microsized powders | Mo-Sci Corp. (USA) |
| S55F5 | $52SiO_2-11.7CaO-19.6Na_2O-5.8P_2O_5-10.9CaF_2$ (wt%) | Cast monolithic pieces, quenched frit, rods, fibers, disks, spheres, and microsized powders | Mo-Sci Corp. (USA) |
| SP-17Sr-17Ca (StronBone) | $44.5SiO_2-4Na_2O-4K_2O-7.5MgO-17.8CaO-4.5P_2O_5-17.8SrO$ (mol%) | Powders and porous granules | RepRegen (UK) |

Bioglass-EPI underwent a fate similar to that of MEP, being taken off the market in the late 1990s due to some concerns about glass resorption over time, and the 45S5 Bioglass sleeve was replaced by a simple titanium pedestal in next models (Downing et al., 1997).

The third commercial device made of 45S5 Bioglass was the Endosseous Ridge Maintenance Implant (ERMI), placed on the market in 1988 and still currently used in periodontal surgery. This device is a cone of 45S5 Bioglass to be inserted into fresh tooth extraction sites for repairing tooth roots and providing a stable ridge for dentures. ERMI proved to be extremely stable over a 5-year follow-up study involving the placement of 242 implants in 29 patients (Stanley et al., 1997).

None of the products described above is in widespread clinical use, as surgeons often claim to cut or shape the implant to match the patient's anatomy better, which is impossible with rigid glass cones of fixed size; this is a common problem already pointed out for calcium orthophosphates scaffolds. Monolithic bioactive glass is more suited to implants that are custom-made for the patient's needs. In this regard, an interesting example was provided by a set of studies dealing with the treatment of orbital bone fractures. Thompson (2011) reported the clinical trials on 30 patients suffering from severe orbital floor damage for which conventional treatment with bone autograft was ineffective. Implantation of melt-derived 45S5 Bioglass plates led to cosmetic and functional rehabilitation of all patients who regained full movement of their eyes at a 5-year follow-up. A similar approach was described in a series of clinical studies carried out in Finland from the late 1980s to the early 2000s by implanting melt-derived S53P4 (commercially known as BoneAlive) plates for the repair of orbital floor fractures (Suominen and Kinnunen, 1996; Kinnunen et al., 2000; Aitasalo et al., 2001; Peltola et al., 2008). Results showed that S53P4 glass was able to stimulate the growth of new orbital bone (Fig. 7.4), was slowly biodegradable (thus no problems of mechanical support occurred) and, if the glass implant size and shape were properly selected, excellent functional and esthetic results comparable to the use of bone/cartilage autografts could be achieved. Furthermore, this approach was associated with reduced morbidity as no donor site operation was needed. These examples show that bioactive glasses can be successfully used for repairing tissues in context, even far from "classical" bone substitution like mere filling of bone defects (Baino, 2015).

Usually, orthopedic and maxillofacial surgeons prefer to use bioactive glass particles rather than monolithic implants as the former can be pressed easily into a bone defect. The first commercial 45S5 Bioglass particulate was approved by FDA in 1993 and marketed under the tradename of PerioGlas (NovaBone Products LLC, Alachua, FL, USA) in more than 35 countries worldwide to repair jaw bone defects resulting from periodontal disease (Hench et al., 2004). Specifically, PerioGlas (particle size within 90–710 μm) is used either to regenerate bone around the root of a healthy tooth to save the tooth, or to repair osseous defects in the jaw so that the quality and quantity of bone becomes sufficient for anchoring titanium implants (Zamet et al., 1997).

A 45S5 Bioglass particulate for repairing osseous defects of maxillofacial or orthopedic nonload-bearing sites was cleared in 1999 under the tradename of

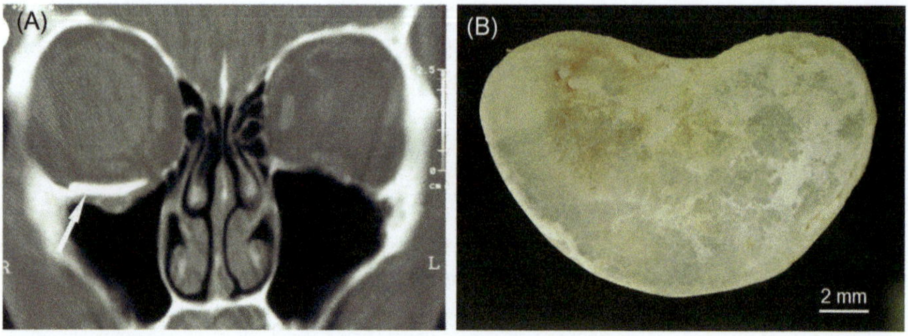


**Figure 7.4** Use of bioactive glass plates (S53P4 composition, BoneAlive) for the repair of orbital floor defect. (A) Tomographic scan taken 2 years after orbital floor reconstruction with a 25 × 2 mm glass implant (arrow). (B) Photograph of a glass plate harvested from the orbit due to revision surgery after 2 years from primary operation (slight resorption of the original margins of the plate was observed).
*Source*: Adapted from Peltola, M., Kinnunen, I., Aitasalo, K., 2008. Reconstruction of orbital wall defects with bioactive glass plates. J. Oral Maxillofac. Surg. 66, 639–646, Copyright © Elsevier.

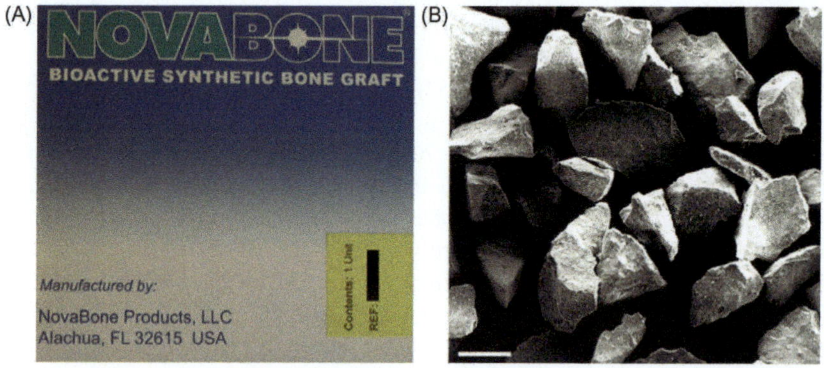


**Figure 7.5** NovaBone: (A) packaging and (B) scanning electron micrograph image of the glass particles (scale bar = 200 μm).
*Source*: Adapted from Jones, J.R., 2013. Review of bioactive glass: from Hench to hybrids. Acta Biomater. 9, 4457–4486, Copyright © Elsevier.

NovaBone (NovaBone Products LLC) (Fig. 7.5) (Hench et al., 2004). Prior to being surgically implanted, NovaBone is often mixed with blood from the defect or a physiological solution so that it assumes a putty-like consistency to be pushed easily into the defect.

NovaBone, which exhibits a particle size distribution analogous to PerioGlas, was compared to iliac crest bone autograft (40 vs 48 patients, respectively) in posterior spinal fusions surgery for the treatment of idiopathic scoliosis

(Ilharreborde et al., 2008). The glass particulate was mixed with the patient's blood and secured in place by compressing the neighboring vertebrae with metal screws and wires. Compared to the autograft, NovaBone was associated with fewer infections (2% vs 5%) and mechanical failures (2% vs 7.5%) over a 4-year follow-up.

Another 45S5 Bioglass-based product is Biogran (Biomet 3i, Palm Beach Gardens, FL, USA), which is used in jaw bone defect repair and is characterized by a narrower particle size distribution (300–360 μm) compared to PerioGlas (Tadjoedin et al., 2002).

Apart from 45S5 Bioglass, other FDA-approved or CE-marked bioactive glasses are available on the market as different products from particulate to porous blocks (Table 7.2). From a general viewpoint, commercial bioactive glasses exhibit a silicate composition containing modifier oxides in specific amounts for enhancing the bioactivity or imparting special characteristics to the material (e.g., SrO is introduced in StronBone to reduce bone resorption (Hill and Stevens, 2009; Fujikura et al., 2012)). The most commonly used are 13–93 and S53P4 (BoneAlive), for which a higher number of studies has been reported in the literature. Clinical trials with both these glasses in a particulate form (diameter within 0.5–1 mm) showed improved bone repair, in terms of quality and quantity of regenerated bone in the frontal sinus, compared to synthetic HA (Peltola et al., 2006). It was also observed that BoneAlive stimulates a faster bone regeneration compared to 13–93, probably due to the magnesium content of the latter glass which decreases bioactivity. BoneAlive granules (1–4 mm) were effective for the repair of quite large bone defects (up to 30 $cm^3$) following benign bone tumor removal in hands, tibia, and humerus (Lindfors et al., 2010). Another application of both 45S5 Bioglass and BonAlive particulate was the obliteration of surgically created cavities in the mastoid bone, a procedure that follows the treatment of chronic suppurative otitis and cholesteatoma (Stoor et al., 2010; Silvola, 2012).

45S5 Bioglass is also commercially available in the form of porous glass ceramic sintered blocks. This product is less bioactive than the parent glass as crystallization is associated with a decrease in bioactivity (Chen et al., 2006). On the other hand, 45S5 Bioglass cannot be sintered without crystallizing as its sintering windows is very small; however, the bioactivity is not totally suppressed (Baino et al., 2013). Other glasses, such as 13–93, have been designed not to crystallize upon sintering and can be produced in a totally amorphous macroporous form (Fu et al., 2008).

In order to complete the overview of 45S5 Bioglass-based products available on the market, a brief mention should be dedicated to oral care; this topic is treated in more detail in another chapter of the present book. Since 2004, a very fine 45S5 Bioglass particulate (mean size 18 μm) called NovaMin (NovaMin Technology, FL, USA; now owned by GlaxoSmithKline, UK) was added to a toothpaste for treating tooth hypersensitivity, which affects about one-third of world population (Gillam et al., 2002; Tai et al., 2006; Pradeep and Sharma, 2010). NovaMin aimed to occlude dentinal tubules and remineralize the surface of teeth, thereby eliminating the cause of dentinal hypersensitivity (Vahid Golpayegani et al., 2012). This particulate was also used for bleaching treatments of teeth. Dentists usually employ ceramic particles (traditionally sodium bicarbonate) as abrasives carried by a high-pressure air flow to remove stains on the tooth; however, this operation can be difficult on patients suffering from dental hypersensitivity. Air polishing with NovaMin (Sylc, OSspray Ltd, UK) was clinically compared to the traditional procedure (Prophy-Jet, Dentsply, UK) and patients reported that the former treatment resulted in a significant reduction (44%) in tooth sensitivity according to their subjective scoring (Banerjee et al., 2010). Teeth treated with glass particulate were also whiter than those treated with sodium bicarbonate.

The full potential of bioactive glasses in medicine still has to be fully exploited, and the relevant market is expected to grow in the coming years. Hench et al. (2010) reported that the 1 millionth dose of NovaBone product and the 1 millionth tube of NovaMin-containing toothpaste were sold in 2009 (40th anniversary of 45S5 Bioglass discovery). A forecast on the impact of bioactive glasses in healthcare over the coming years was provided by Jones et al. (2016). Moreover, although glasses and glass ceramics have traditionally been used for bone repair, some new applications in contact with soft tissues have recently attracted the interest of biomaterials scientists and further expanded the versatility of these bioactive materials; an overview of this emerging field of research has been reported elsewhere (Baino et al., 2016).

## 7.6 Composites

Taking inspiration from Nature and observing that bone is a natural composite, biomaterials scientists hypothesized that an implant manufactured from a polymer enriched with a calcium phosphate phase was likely to behave better than other bone substitutes made as single-material devices.

In the 1980s, Bonfield and associates (Tanner et al., 1994) developed a bioactive composite constituted by a high-density polyethylene matrix in which HA particles were uniformly dispersed at a concentration of 40 vol%. The combination of stiff, osteoconductive but brittle HA with low-modulus, tough, and bioinert polyethylene (PE) produced a highly attractive biomaterial for bone substitution (Tanner, 2010). Following FDA approval in 1994, this composite became commercially available under the tradename of HAPEX (Smith and Nephew, Richards, USA), and since then has been widely used for the reconstruction of orbital bone as well as small bones in the middle ear. In both applications, HAPEX offers the advantage of in situ shaping, so a surgeon can easily cut or mold it to optimize fitting with the patient's anatomy (Rea and Bonfield, 2004).

The major production stages of HAPEX include blending, compounding, and centrifugal milling; then, a bulk material or device is created by compression and injection molding of the composite powder (Wang, 2003). Modern processing of HAPEX also includes a hot rolling step that facilitates uniform dispersion and blending of the ceramic phase in the matrix (Pandey et al., 2006). Fabrication of HA/PE composites by selective laser sintering has also been studied (Fig. 7.6) (Zhang et al., 2008).

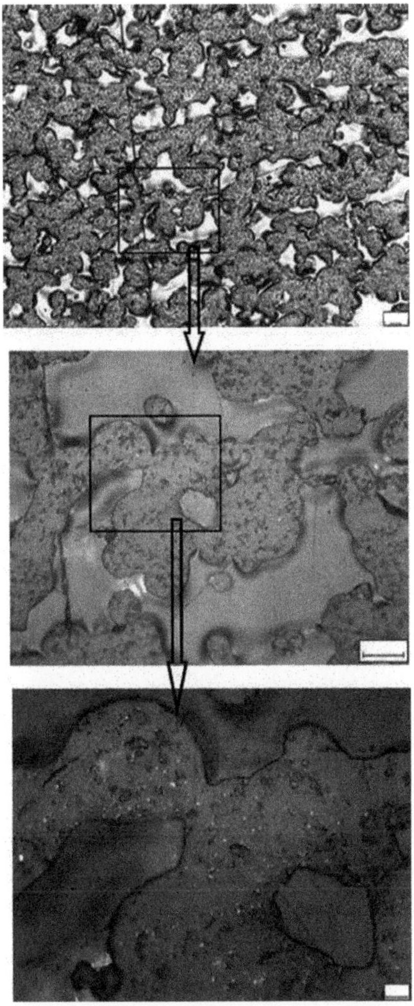

**Figure 7.6** Optical cross-sections of sintered hydroxyapatite/PE composite showing the porous structure with interconnected pores after selective laser sintering (the particles are well fused to each other and form strong boundaries between them). Scale bars (from top to bottom): 50, 50, and 10 μm.
*Source*: Adapted from Zhang, Y., Hao, L., Savalani, M.M., Harris, R.A., Tanner, K.E., 2008. Characterization and dynamic mechanical analysis of selective laser sintered hydroxyapatite-filled polymeric composites. J. Biomed. Mater. Res. A 86, 606–616, Copyright © Wiley Periodicals.

A mechanical interlock between the two phases of HAPEX is obtained by the shrinkage of PE onto the HA particles during cooling (Rea and Bonfield, 2004; Sousa et al., 2003). Smaller ceramic particles generate stiffer composites due to the increase of interfaces between PE and HA; furthermore, rigidity of HAPEX is proportional to the ceramic volume fraction (Wang et al., 1994). The Young's modulus of HAPEX is within 1–8 GPa, which is quite close to that of cortical bone.

On the other hand, HAPEX suffers from a few limitations. The material is non-biodegradable, the surface area of osteoconductive HA available for contact with bone may be quite low, and the presence of bioinert PE decreases the ability to bond to bone (Dorozhkin, 2009). Furthermore, only a mechanical bond exists between the two phases and the low porosity limits the ingrowth of osteoblasts when the implant is placed into the body (Suchanek and Yoshimura, 1998).

Other composite materials have been developed over the years in the effort to mimic more closely the composition of natural bone. Among collagen/calcium phosphate composites, perhaps the most popular is Bio-Oss Collagen (90 wt% Bio-Oss + 10 wt% porcine collagen; Geistlich Biomaterials, Zurich, Switzerland) which exhibits an excellent biocompatibility but tends to resorb very quickly, with consequent loss of the mechanical properties and migration of the inorganic particles into the surrounding environment (Araújo et al., 2010). Another example is Collagraft, which is made of mixed calcium phosphates (HA/β-TCP in a 65:35 wt% ratio) and purified bovine collagen (Zimmer, Warsaw, IN, USA) and is available in the form of paste or soft strips for low-weight-bearing applications (Cornell et al., 1991). Healos (Orquest, Canada) is sold as mineralized (HA-coated) collagen fibers and is indicated for spinal fusions (Kunakornsawat et al., 2013). In general, the performance of these composites depends on the source of collagen from which it was processed (Murugan and Ramakrishna, 2005).

Other polymers (e.g., pectin/chitosan hydrogels) have been recently proposed as matrices for the development of moldable ceramic-reinforced composites (Iviglia et al., 2016a) or as bioactive coatings on calcium phosphate porous scaffolds (Iviglia et al., 2016b).

The combination of HA with $TiO_2$ was also suggested as an interesting strategy to improve the toughness of ceramic-based materials for clinical applications (Martinez et al., 2015).

## 7.7 Moldable and injectable ceramic-based cements

Biocompatible cements for orthopedic surgery include acrylic cements, which are mainly used in the fixation of joint prostheses to bone (Lewis, 2009), and ceramic cements that are employed to fill osseous defects. The latter class grossly encompasses calcium sulfate and calcium phosphate cements.

Calcium sulfate has a long history of use in medicine as a bone graft substitute in various skeletal sites, as reviewed by Thomas et al. (2005). This material offers some important advantages, including wide availability, inexpensiveness, and the ability to stimulate osteoblast activity due to the creation of a Ca-rich environment upon dissolution in the biological environment. Despite these benefits, calcium sulfate has never attracted the same degree of research interest as other biomaterials, probably due to its low working time and fast resorption rate which limit its versatility.

Surgical-grade calcium sulfate cements are currently marketed with the powder constituent being calcium sulfate hemihydrate (Thomas and Puleo, 2009). When mixed with an aqueous medium, the powder is converted to calcium sulfate dihydrate, producing a paste or putty with a solid or partially solid structure (Thomas and Puleo, 2009). Once injected in situ, calcium sulfate cement inhibits fibrous tissue ingrowth, creates a slightly acidic environment that encourages osteogenesis and angiogenesis and, while the material dissolves, bone forms and occupies the voids left by the cement reabsorbed (Kelly and Wilkins, 2004). Depending on the defect volume and location, calcium sulfate cements totally dissolve in vivo within 2 months from implantation (Tay et al., 1999).

Commercial products include BonePlast and MIIG X3 (Table 7.3): both are sold as a calcium sulfate hemihydrate powder which, after being mixed with water, forms a paste that sets in about 5 minutes. The compressive and tensile strength of MIIG X3, determined after hardening at room temperature for 24 hours, are $96.4 \pm 5.9$ MPa and $16.0 \pm 0.2$ MPa, respectively (Carroll et al., 2004).

The second class of ceramic cements encompasses calcium phosphate cements that were first experimented on for clinical use in the 1980s and FDA-approved one decade later (Campana et al., 2014; Lewis, 2006). These cements are marketed as a white calcium phosphate powder that forms a workable paste after being mixed with an aqueous saline solution. This putty can be easily shaped during surgery to fit the dimensions and contour of the bone defect prior to set within 10–20 min. Upon setting, the reactants are reprecipitated until the entire material is converted to finely porous HA. After being implanted in vivo, calcium phosphate cements are gradually resorbed over time and replaced with new bone. Hardened bioceramic cements are brittle and have to be used cautiously in load-bearing applications due to their low tensile, compressive, and bending strength; however, their ability to be precisely sculpted and shaped has made them extremely useful in craniomaxillofacial surgery, in which precise fitting of the bone cavity is required to obtain a good esthetic outcome (Pryor et al., 2009). Furthermore, calcium phosphate putties are injectable through a syringe, which makes them ideal materials for spine surgery as well as for minimally invasive and tissue-sparing procedures in order to reduce morbidity and costs (Lewis, 2006).

An overview of the most commonly used calcium phosphate-based cements is reported in Table 7.3. Norian Bone Cement line (Synthes, PA, USA) was originally approved by FDA for use in distal radius fractures; at present, it has found broad application in craniofacial surgery (Norian CRS) (Pryor et al., 2009) and spine surgery for vertebroplasty and kyphoplasty (Norian SRS) (Lewis, 2006). Norian cement powder is typically mixed with a sodium phosphate solution to form dahllite, a carbonated apatite similar to the mineralogical component of bone and enamel (Constantz et al., 1995). Norian has a mixing time of 2 minutes, a working time of 5 minutes and a setting time of 10–15 minutes. An exothermic reaction associated with a temperature increment up to 42°C occurs upon setting; maximum

**Table 7.3 Overview of commercially available ceramic-based or ceramic-containing cements for bone repair**

| Product name | Composition | Producer |
|---|---|---|
| BonePlast | $CaSO_4 \cdot 0.5\ H_2O$ powder | Interpore Cross International Inc. (Irvine, Canada) |
| MIIG X3 | $CaSO_4 \cdot 0.5\ H_2O$ powder | Wright Medical Technology Inc. (Arlington, TN, USA) |
| Norian | α-TCP, $CaCO_3$, MCPM | Synthes Inc. (West Chester, PA, USA) |
| Bone Source | TTCP, DCP | Stryker (MI, USA) |
| Mimix | α-TCP, TTCP (a vial of dilute citric acid is provided along with the ceramic powder) | Biomet Microfixation (Jacksonville, FL, USA) |
| Biobon | Amorphous calcium phosphate + DCPD | ETEX (Cambridge, MA, USA) |
| Biopex | 75% α-TCP + 18% TTCP + 5% DCPD + 2% hydroxyapatite | Mutsubishi Materials Co. (Saitama, Japan) |
| ChronOS Inject | 42 wt% β-TCP + 21 wt% MCPM + 3 wt% β-TCP granules + 5 wt% magnesium hydrogen phosphate + <1 wt% sodium hydrogen pyrophosphate and $MgSO_4$ | Synthes Inc. (West Chester, PA, USA) |
| Calcibon | α-TCP + $CaHPO_4$ + $CaCO_3$ + hydroxyapatite | Biomet (Dordrecht, The Netherlands) |
| Eurobone | TCP | F-H Orthopedics (Heimsbrum, France) |
| SintLife | Mg-substituted hydroxyapatite | Finceramica (Faenza, Italy) |
| Palacos | Acrylic cement + 15 wt% $ZrO_2$ + 10 ml of dye | Haereus Medical GmbH (Germany) |
| Cortoss | bis-GMA/bis-EMA/TEGDMA monomer matrix (59 vol%) reinforced with glass ceramic particles | Orthovita Inc. (Malvern, PA, USA) |

*bis-EMA*, 2,2-bis [4-(2-methacryloxyethoxy)] phenyl propane; *bis-GMA*, 2,2-bis [4-(2-hydroxymehacryloxypropyl) phenyl] propane; *DCPD*, dicalcium phosphate dihydrate; *MCPM*, monocalcium phosphate monohydrate; *TCP*, tricalcium phosphate; *TEGDMA*, triethylene glycol dimethacrylate; *TTCP*, tetracalcium phosphate.

strength is not achieved until 24 hours from operation (compressive strength ~50 MPa, tensile strength ~2 MPa, bending strength ~0.5 MPa) (Lewis, 2006). Norian is slowly absorbable over time and is not recommended for use in the presence of active infection. Its use to repair tibial bone fractures has also been experimented on successfully (Fig. 7.7) (Campana et al., 2014).

Bone Source (Stryker, MI, USA) is a self-setting calcium phosphate cement originally approved by FDA for use in filling burr holes and for facial skeleton

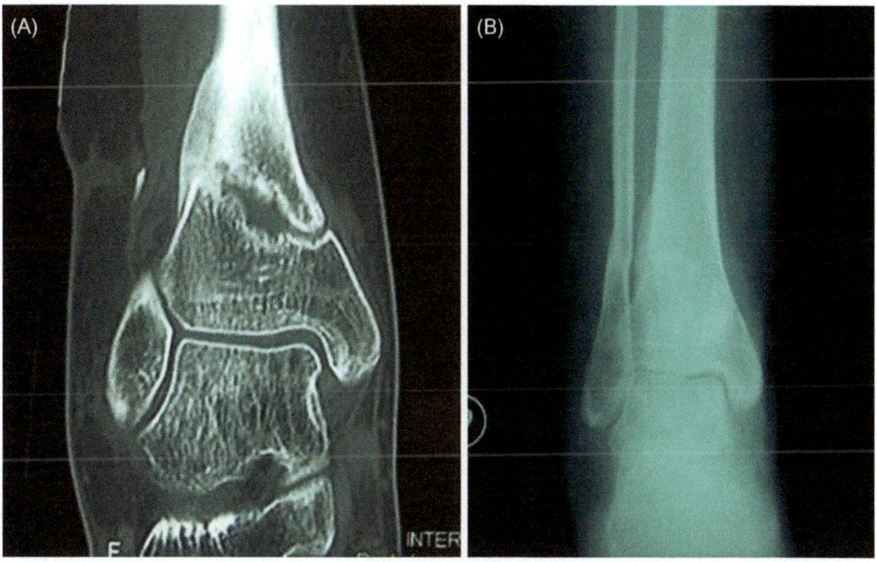


**Figure 7.7** Use of calcium phosphate cement to treat bone fractures. (A) Bone loss in a distal tibial open fracture with delayed union (tomographic scan), and (B) postoperative follow-up (radiographic imaging) showing bone consolidation and osteointegration of the cement at 1 year from surgery.
*Source*: Adapted from Campana, V., Milano, G., Pagano, E., Barba, M., Cicione, C., Salonna, G., et al., 2014. Bone substitutes in orthopaedic surgery: from basic science to clinical practice. J. Mater. Sci. Mater. Med. 25, 2445–2461, Copyright © The Authors.

augmentation, but is also widely used in spine surgery (Lewis, 2006). It is prepared by mixing calcium phosphate salts with a sodium phosphate buffer, thereby forming a putty that remains malleable for approximately 20 minutes. Bone Source fully crystallizes in HA and hardens within 24 hours; it tends to be absorbed very slowly over time and, if used for craniofacial reconstruction, is not indicated to fill defects with surface size over 25 $cm^2$.

Mimix Bone Void Filler (Biomet Microfixation, Jacksonville, FL, USA), like Bone Source, achieved FDA approval for use in filling burr hole and craniotomy defects and in smoothing facial skeletal contour abnormalities over a surface area with maximum size of 25 $cm^2$ (Pryor et al., 2009). Mimix putty is prepared by mixing dry cement powder with sodium citrate dehydrate and an anhydrous citric acid solution, which are both provided in the Mimix Quick Set by the producer. Mimix fully crystallizes in HA and can be prepared very rapidly as it remains malleable for 3–4 minutes and is completely set within 6 minutes, thus offering a potential advantage over other commercially available apatite-based cements that take longer time to harden and develop adequate mechanical strength for supporting the surrounding tissues (Goebel and Jacob, 2005).

Burstein et al. (2006) reviewed 150 patients who underwent orbito-cranial reconstruction using Bone Source and Mimix cements over a 7-year follow-up; a titanium mesh was also implanted in some patients who had large bone defects. Excellent results were reported, with 92% of patients having satisfactory functional and esthetic results over a minimum of 1-year follow-up. The overall complication rate was 9% but no cases of infection were reported. Other studies, however, reported a high rate of complications (10%–22%) including cement exposure, infection, and foreign body reaction (Baker et al., 2002; Gomez et al., 2005; Verret et al., 2005; Moreira-Gonzalez et al., 2003; Zins et al., 2007). The third complication was often associated with the postoperative microfragmentation of hardened HA cement (Baker et al., 2002; Zins et al., 2007). Losee et al. (2003) attributed this problem to brain pulsations in cranial reconstruction and suggested the implantation of a supporting titanium mesh along with the cement to mitigate this risk in large skull defects. Choice of cement may also affect the rate of microfragmentation, with Norian being the strongest and exhibiting the highest mean fracture force required to fracture a standardized test piece (Miller et al., 2005).

Zins et al. (2007) reviewed 121 patients undergoing craniofacial reconstructions using Norian and Bone Source with and without an additional supporting titanium mesh (depending on the defect size) and found an overall complication rate of 15%. However, in a subset of patients undergoing reconstructions for large defects (above 25 $cm^2$), major complications occurred in 63% of patients. In summary, the use of other biomaterials options, e.g., bone autografts, is recommended for the treatment of very large osseous defects.

Apart from calcium sulfate and calcium phosphate cements, an interesting injectable product for bone repair is Cortoss, a resin-based composite that can be safely used in load-bearing sites. Cortoss comprises a difunctional methacrylate matrix that forms a highly cross-linked 3D polymer reinforced with radiopaque and bioactive glass ceramic particles. Early clinical results in vertebroplasty for treating osteoporotic and metastatic vertebral compression fractures were promising (Palussiere et al., 2005).

Current research on bioceramic cements focuses on how to improve their ease of handling during surgery, their tissue-regenerative ability and their visualization under radiographic imaging: recent studies provide interesting inputs for the development of high-added-value commercial products.

Handling of calcium phosphate cements may be difficult as problems often arise during mixing, transferring to syringes, and subsequent injection. The risk of handling complications can be reduced via the use of premixed cements which, however, require a careful optimization of the setting time (Engstrand et al., 2013). Companies often provide surgeons with both the cement to be injected and the toolkit for surgery; an example is SynCage (Synthes, USA), an implant and instrument system for anterior lumbar interbody fusion which was successfully combined with ChronOs (β-TCP-based injectable granules; Synthes, USA) (Acharya et al., 2011).

A new bioceramic putty, marketed as SintLife and made of Mg-doped HA, aims at improving bone regeneration through the release of $Mg^{2+}$ ions which are known to stimulate osteoblast activity (Landi et al., 2008). Incorporation of growth factors in calcium phosphate-based composite cements enriched with mesoporous bioactive glass particles has also been recently reported to promote tissue regeneration (Schumacher et al., 2017).

A key requirement for cements used in vertebroplasty and kyphoplasty is the material radiopacity, which can be obtained by adding a radiopacifier (mainly $BaSO_4$) to the cement matrix. This strategy carries some drawbacks including barium-related toxicity issues and mechanical weakening of the cement (Lewis, 2006). Cortoss (described above) was developed in the attempt to overcome these limitations. A recent patent (Vitale-Brovarone et al., 2015) has also suggested the use of a composite cement containing Zr-doped mesoporous glass particles that exhibit the twofold function of radiopacifier and highly bioactive phase (Tallia et al., 2014).

## 7.8 Conclusions and outlook

Despite the significant advances in operative techniques and biomaterials used, bone substitution and repair persist as key challenges in surgery, and many alternatives are today available to patients and surgeons. There is an increasing need for bone substitutes and it has been estimated that over 2 million bone grafting procedures are performed worldwide per year (Campana et al., 2014). Autografts still represent the "gold standard" approach, albeit suffering from limitations such as limited availability and morbidity at the harvesting site. Banked bone (allografts) and xenografts are osteoconductive but still carry concerns about residual infective risks, and their resorption rate may be different from that desired. Ceramic-based bone substitutes allow the above-mentioned limitations of transplant materials to be overcome, and are highly versatile in terms of composition (calcium phosphates with different solubility rates, osteoinductive glasses and glass ceramics, bone-like composites), processing (monolithic devices, granules, scaffolds, moldable pastes), and functional properties. However, especially if produced in the form of rigid and porous structures, they suffer from inherent brittleness and are difficult to shape during surgery to fit the patient's anatomy.

Calcium phosphates and bioactive glasses have shown very promising results when manufactured as custom-made implants (Oka et al., 2010; Thompson, 2011; Suominen and Kinnunen, 1996; Kinnunen et al., 2000; Aitasalo et al., 2001; Peltola et al., 2008). This approach requires the acquisition of the patient's anatomy (e.g., by tomographic investigations) and a computer-aided design/computer-aided manufacture system to produce the devices; although it is expensive and time-consuming compared to using readily available commercial products of standard size and shape, some companies have become interested in this business since these high-added-value devices really help patients to achieve an excellent rehabilitation (Habraken et al., 2016).

Biomimetic collagen/bioceramic composites and injectable cements also represent an interesting evolution, and especially the latter ones enable minimally invasive surgical techniques.

Future research directions in the field of ceramics for bone repair mainly address to three objectives: (1) improvement of biomimicry, (2) multifunctionality, and (3) production of implants that are easy to shape intraoperatively.

As for the point (1), we have to consider that bioceramics are often designed to act as 3D scaffolds, i.e., porous templates for tissues that are then remodeled by the body to their natural form (Baino and Vitale-Brovarone, 2011). There is a general agreement on the fact that scaffolds mimicking the microarchitecture of bone promote osteogenic cell migration and reorganization along with better osteointegration after implantation in vivo (Wu et al., 2014). For this reason, it would be highly desirable to produce ceramic scaffolds exhibiting strong microarchitectural similarity to the bone tissue they have to replace, as well as to fabricate them easily and at a reasonable cost. In this regard, Nature is an invaluable laboratory from which we can take inspiration, as many natural structures of plants, flowers and fruits resemble closely the hierarchical microarchitecture of cancellous bone and can be then used as sacrificial templates for making bone-like ceramic scaffolds; this highly interesting research field has been recently reviewed elsewhere (Fan et al., 2009; Baino and Ferraris, 2017).

Point (2) aims at expanding the classical concept of bioactivity of ceramics for healthcare, i.e., the ability of bonding to bone and stimulating the growth of new healthy bone. Many surgical applications require a multifunctional implant providing some extra functionalities, such as antibacterial properties for the prevention of postoperative infections, or an anticancer action for a better treatment of osseous tumors (Vallet-Regi and Ruiz-Hernandez, 2011). These added values are typically provided by making use of biomolecules which can be directly entrapped in the material nanopores (e.g., in the case of sol-gel bioceramics (Wu and Chang, 2014; Baino et al., 2016; Owens et al., 2016)), incorporated in ceramic/polymer composites (Baino et al., 2017; Kargozar et al., 2017), or immobilized on the surface of the ceramic implant through functionalization strategies (Mourino and Boccaccini, 2010). A fascinating alternative to avoid the use of drugs is exploiting the therapeutic action of specific metal ions that have been deliberately introduced in the ceramic formulation (Cacciotti et al., 2009; Hoppe et al., 2011). Once released in vivo, drugs or ions can exert the desired therapeutic action. From commercial and clinical viewpoints, clearance of ceramic-based implants that comprise drugs is particularly long and laborious as these medical devices fall into class III according to current EU directives.

Finally, surgeons often want to use of materials which can not only fill the bone defect, but can also be shaped in an easy manner and not be prone to migration postoperatively (point 3); hence, rigid ceramic particles, and 3D brittle scaffolds are not the best choice. In order to meet this important challenge, biomaterials researchers are currently investigating two major types of moldable biomaterials for bone repair (apart from "classical" bone cements), i.e., bioceramic-reinforced polymeric hydrogels (Iviglia et al., 2016a) and organic–inorganic hybrid materials in which the components interact at the molecular level and are indistinguishable above the nanoscale (Baino et al., 2017). Hybrids allow cells to come into contact with both phases at one time, and the material may degrade at a single rate without having mismatched resorption kinetics of inorganic and organic phases (Valliant and Jones, 2011).

A comprehensive picture of novel ceramic-based tissue engineering approaches, including the use of cell-seeded biomaterial constructs, will be provided in the third part of this book.

## References

Acharya, S., Kumar, S., Srivastava, A., Tandon, E., 2011. Early results of one-level cervical discectomy and fusion with stand-alone cervical cage and bone marrow soaked tricalcium phosphate. Acta Orthop. Belg. 77, 218–223.

Aitasalo, K., Kinnunen, I., Palmgren, J., Varpula, M., 2001. Repair of orbital floor fractures with bioactive glass implants. J. Oral Maxillofac. Surg. 59, 1390–1396.

Araújo, M.G., Liljenberg, B., Lindhe, J., 2010. Dynamics of bio-Oss collagen incorporation in fresh extraction wounds: an experimental study in the dog. Clin. Oral Implants Res. 21, 55–64.

Ayers, R.A., Simske, S.J., Nunes, C.R., Wolford, L.M., 1998. Long-term bone ingrowth and residual microhardness of porous block hydroxyapatite implants in humans. J. Oral Maxillofac. Surg. 56, 1297–1302.

Bahmad Jr, F., Merchant, S.N., 2007. Histopathology of ossicular grafts and implants in chronic otitis media. Ann. Otol. Rhinol. Laryngol. 116, 181–191.

Baino, F., Ferraris, M., Bretcanu, O., Verné, E., Vitale-Brovarone, C., 2013. Optimization of composition, structure and mechanical strength of bioactive 3-D glass-ceramic scaffolds for bone substitution. J. Appl. Biomater. 27, 872–890.

Baino, F., Ferraris, M., 2017. Learning from Nature: using bioinspired approaches and natural materials to make porous bioceramics. Int. J. Appl. Ceram. Technol. http://dx.doi.org/10.1111/ijac.12677

Baino, F., Fiorilli, S., Vitale-Brovarone, C., 2016. Bioactive glass-based materials with hierarchical porosity for medical applications: review of recent advances. Acta Biomater. 42, 18–32.

Baino, F., Fiorilli, S., Vitale-Brovarone, C., 2017. Composite biomaterials based on sol-gel mesoporous silicate glasses: a review. Bioengineering. 3 (15), 1–18.

Baino, F., Novajra, G., Miguez-Pacheco, V., Boccaccini, A.R., Vitale-Brovarone, C., 2016. Bioactive glasses: special applications outside the skeletal system. J. Non-Cryst Solids. 432, 15–30.

Baino, F., Novajra, G., Vitale-Brovarone, C., 2015. Bioceramics and scaffolds: a winning combination for tissue engineering. Front Bioeng. Biotechnol. 3, 202.

Baino, F., Vitale-Brovarone, C., 2011. Three-dimensional glass-derived scaffolds for bone tissue engineering: current trends and forecasts for the future. J. Biomed. Mater. Res. A. 97, 514–535.

Baino, F., 2011. Biomaterials and implants for orbital floor repair. Acta Biomater. 7, 3248–3266.

Baino, F., 2015. How can bioactive glasses be useful in ocular surgery? J. Biomed. Mater. Res. A. 103, 1259–1275.

Baker, S.B., Weinzweig, J., Kirschner, R.E., Bartlett, S.P., 2002. Applications of a new carbonated calcium phosphate bone cement: early experience in pediatric and adult craniofacial reconstruction. Plast. Reconstr. Surg. 109, 1789–1796.
Banerjee, A., Hajatdoost-Sani, M., Farrell, S., Thompson, I., 2010. A clinical evaluation and comparison of bioactive glass and sodium bicarbonate air-polishing powders. J. Dent. 38, 475–479.
Barrere, F., Van Blitterswijk, C.A., De Groot, K., 2006. Bone regeneration: molecular and cellular interactions with calcium phosphate ceramics. Int. J. Nanomed. 1, 317–332.
Baumhauer, J., Pinzur, M.S., Donahue, R., Beasley, W., Digiovanni, C., 2014. Site selection and pain outcome after autologous bone graft harvest. Foot Ankle Int. 35, 104–107.
Benninger, E., Zingg, P.O., Kamath, A.F., Dora, C., 2014. Cost analysis of fresh-frozen femoral head allografts: is it worthwhile to run a bone bank? Bone Joint J. 96, 1307–1311.
Boskey, A.L., 2007. Mineralization of bones and teeth. Elements. 6, 385–392.
Burstein, F.D., Williams, J.K., Hudgins, R., Boydston, W., Reisner, A., Stevenson, K., et al., 2006. Hydroxyapatite cement in craniofacial reconstruction: experience in 150 patients. Plast Reconstr. Surg. 118, 484–489.
Cacciotti, I., Bianco, A., Lombardi, M., Montanaro, L., 2009. Mg-substituted hydroxyapatite nanopowders: synthesis, thermal stability and sintering behavior. J. Eur. Ceram. Soc. 29, 2969–2978.
Calvo, R., Figueroa, D., Dıaz-Ledezma, C., Vaisman, A., Figueroa, F., 2011. Bone allografts and the functions of bone banks. Rev. Med. Chil. 139, 660–666.
Campana, V., Milano, G., Pagano, E., Barba, M., Cicione, C., Salonna, G., et al., 2014. Bone substitutes in orthopaedic surgery: from basic science to clinical practice. J. Mater. Sci. Mater. Med. 25, 2445–2461.
Cao, W., Hench, L.L., 1996. Bioactive materials. Ceram. Int. 22, 493–507.
Carrel, J.P., Wiskott, A., Moussa, M., Rieder, P., Scherrer, S., Durual, S., 2016. A 3D printed TCP/HA structure as a new osteoconductive scaffold for vertical bone augmentation. Clin. Oral Implants Res. 27, 55–62.
Carrodeguas, R.G., De Aza, S., 2011. α-Tricalcium phosphate: synthesis, properties and biomedical applications. Acta Biomater. 7, 3536–3546.
Carroll, M., Lewis, G., Xu, J., Moseley, J., Cole, J., Haggard, W., 2004. Evaluation of a synthetic bone defect test model to aid in the selection of materials for use in vertebral body compression fracture repair. Orthopedics. 27 (Suppl.), S119–S122.
Charalambides, C., Beer, M., Cobb, A.G., 2005. Poor results after augmenting autograft with xenograft (Surgibone) in hip revision surgery: a report of 27 cases. Acta Orthop. 76, 544–549.
Chen, Q.Z., Thompson, I.D., Boccaccini, A.R., 2006. 45S5 Bioglass®-derived glass-ceramic scaffolds for bone tissue engineering. Biomaterials. 27, 2414–2425.
Chevalier, J., Gremillar, L., 2009. Ceramics for medical applications: a picture for the next 20 years. J. Eur. Ceram. Soc. 29, 1245–1255.
Constantz, B.R., Ison, I.C., Fulmer, M.T., Poser, R.D., Smith, S.T., Van Wagoner, M., et al., 1995. Skeletal repair by *in situ* formation of the mineral phase of bone. Science. 26, 1796–1799.
Cornell, C.N., Lane, J.M., Chapman, M., Merkow, R., Seligson, D., Henry, S., et al., 1991. Multicenter trial of collagraft as bone graft substitute. J. Orthop. Trauma. 5, 1–8.
Damien, E., Revell, P.A., 2004. Coralline hydroxyapatite bone graft substitute: a review of experimental studies and biomedical applications. J. Appl. Biomater. Biomech. 2, 65–73.
Dorozhkin, S.V., 2007. Calcium orthophosphates. J. Mater. Sci. 42, 1061–1095.

Dorozhkin, S.V., 2009. Calcium orthophosphate-based biocomposites and hybrid biomaterials. J. Mater. Sci. 44, 2343–2387.
Dorozhkin, S.V., 2010a. Calcium orthophosphates as bioceramics: state of the art. J. Funct. Mater. 1, 22–107.
Dorozhkin, S.V., 2010b. Amorphous calcium (ortho)phosphates. Acta Biomater. 6, 4457–4475.
Dorozhkin, S.V., 2012. Biphasic, triphasic and multiphasic calcium orthophosphates. Acta Biomater. 8, 963–977.
Dorozhkin, S.V., 2013a. A detailed history of calcium orthophosphates from 1770s till 1950. Mater. Sci. Eng. C. 33, 3085–3110.
Dorozhkin, S.V., 2013b. Calcium orthophosphate-based bioceramics. Materials. 6, 3840–3942.
Downing, M., Johansson, U., Carlsson, L., Walliker, J.R., Spraggs, P.D., Dodson, H., et al., 1997. A bone-anchored percutaneous connector system for neural prosthetic applications. Ear. Nose. Throat. J. 76, 328–332.
Dreesmann, H., 1892. Ueber knochenplombierung. Beitr. Klin. Chir. 9, 804–810.
Elmazar, H., Jackson, I.T., Degner, D., Miyawaki, T., Barakat, K., Andrus, L., et al., 2003. The efficacy of Gore-Tex vs hydroxyapatite and bone graft in reconstruction of orbital floor defects. Eur. J. Plast. Surg. 25, 362–368.
Elsinger, E.C., Leal, L., 1996. Coralline hydroxyapatite bone graft substitutes. J. Foot Ankle Surg. 35, 396–399.
Engstrand, J., Aberg, J., Engqvist, H., 2013. Influence of water content on hardening and handling of a premixed calcium phosphate cement. Mater. Sci. Eng. C. 33, 527–531.
Fan, T.X., Chow, S.K., Zhang, D., 2009. Biomorphic mineralization: from biology to materials. Prog. Mater. Sci. 54, 542–659.
Fu, Q., Rahaman, M.N., Bal, B.S., Brown, R.F., Day, D.E., 2008. Mechanical and *in vitro* performance of 13–93 bioactive glass scaffolds prepared by a polymer foam replication technique. Acta Biomater. 4, 1854–1864.
Fujikura, K., Karpukhina, N., Kasuga, T., Brauer, D.S., Hill, R.G., Law, R.V., 2012. Influence of strontium substitution on structure and crystallization of Bioglass® 45S5. J. Mater. Chem. 22, 7395–7402.
Gillam, D.G., Tang, J.Y., Mordan, N.J., Newman, H.N., 2002. The effects of a novel Bioglass® dentifrice on dentine sensitivity: a scanning electron microscopy investigation. J. Oral Rehabil. 29, 305–313.
Goebel, J.A., Jacob, A., 2005. Use of Mimix hydroxyapatite bone cement for difficult ossicular reconstruction. Otolaryngol. Head Neck Surg. 132, 727–734.
Gomez, E., Martın, M., Arias, J., Carceller, F., 2005. Clinical applications of Norian SRS (calcium phosphate cement) in craniofacial reconstruction in children: our experience at Hospital La Paz since 2001. J. Oral Maxillofac. Surg. 63, 8–14.
Habraken, W., Habibovic, P., Epple, M., Bohner, M., 2016. Calcium phosphates in biomedical applications: materials for the future? Mater. Today. 19, 69–87.
Hench, L.L., Day, D.E., Holand, W., Rheinberger, V.M., 2010. Glass in medicine. Int. J. Appl. Glass Sci. 1, 104–117.
Hench, L.L., Greenspan, D., 2013. Interactions between bioactive glass and collagen: a review and new perspectives. J. Aust. Ceram. Soc. 49, 1–40.
Hench, L.L., Hench, J.W., Greenspan, D.C., 2004. Bioglass: a short history and bibliography. J. Aust. Ceram. Soc. 40, 1–42.
Hench, L.L., 1991. Bioceramics: from concept to clinic. J. Am. Ceram. Soc. 74, 1487–1510.
Hench, L.L., 2006. The story of Bioglass®. J. Mater. Sci. Mater. Med. 17, 967–978.

Hill, R.G., Stevens, M.M., 2009. Bioactive glass. US patent no. US20090208428 A1.
Hing, K.A., Wilson, L.F., Buckland, T., 2007. Comparative performance of three ceramic bone graft substitutes. Spine J. 7, 475–490.
Hoppe, A., Guldal, N., Boccaccini, A.R., 2011. Biological response to ionic dissolution products from bioactive glass and glass-ceramics in the context of bone tissue engineering. Biomaterials. 32, 2757–2774.
Horch, H.H., Sader, R., Pautke, C., Neff, A., Deppe, H., Kolk, A., 2006. Synthetic, pure-phase beta-tricalcium phosphate ceramic granules (Cerasorb®) for bone regeneration in the reconstructive surgery of the jaws. Int. J. Oral Maxillofac. Surg. 35, 708–713.
Ilharreborde, B., Morel, E., Fitoussi, F., Presedo, A., Souchet, P., Pennecot, G.F., et al., 2008. Bioactive glass as a bone substitute for spinal fusion in adolescent idiopathic scoliosis a comparative study with iliac crest autograft. J. Pediatr. Orthop. 28, 347–351.
Irwin, R.B., Bernhard, M., Biddinger, A., 2001. Coralline hydroxyapatite as bone substitute in orthopedic oncology. Am. J. Orthop. 30, 544–550.
Iviglia, G., Cassinelli, C., Torre, E., Baino, F., Morra, M., Vitale-Brovarone, C., 2016a. Novel bioceramic-reinforced hydrogel for alveolar bone regeneration. Acta Biomater. 44, 97–109.
Iviglia, G., Cassinelli, C., Bollati, D., Baino, F., Torre, E., Morra, M., 2016b. Vitale-Brovarone C. Engineered porous scaffolds for periprosthetic infection prevention. Mater. Sci. Eng. C. 68, 701–715.
Jones, J.R., 2013. Review of bioactive glass: from Hench to hybrids. Acta Biomater. 9, 4457–4486.
Jones, J.R., Brauer, D.S., Hupa, L., Greenspan, D.C., 2016. Bioglass and bioactive glasses and their impact on healthcare. Int. J. Appl. Glass Sci. 7, 423–434.
Kargozar, S., Hashemian, S.J., Soleimani, M., Milan, P.B., Askari, M., Khalaj, V., et al., 2017. Acceleration of bone regeneration in bioactive glass/gelatin composite scaffolds seeded with bone marrow-derived mesenchymal stem cells over-expressing bone morphogenetic protein-7. Mater. Sci. Eng. C. 75, 688–698.
Kasten, P., Beyen, I., Niemeyer, P., Luginbuhl, R., Bohner, M., Richter, W., 2008. Porosity and pore size of b-tricalcium phosphate scaffold can influence protein production and osteogenic differentiation of human mesenchymal stem cells: an *in vitro* and *in vivo* study. Acta Biomater. 4, 1904–1915.
Kelly, C.M., Wilkins, R.M., 2004. Treatment of benign bone lesions with an injectable calcium sulfate-based bone graft substitute. Orthopedics. 27 (Suppl.), S123–S125.
Kenney, E.B., Lekovic, V., Han, T., Carranza Jr, F.A., Dimitrijevic, B., 1985. The use of a porous hydroxylapatite implant in periodontal defects. I. Clinical results after six months. J. Periodontol. 56, 82–88.
Khan, S.N., Cammisa, F.P.J., Sandhu, H.S., Diwan, A.D., Girardi, F.P., Lane, J.M., 2005. The biology of bone grafting. J. Am. Acad. Orthop. Surg. 13, 77–86.
Kinnunen, I., Aitasalo, K., Pollonen, M., Varpula, M., 2000. Reconstruction of orbital fractures using bioactive glass. J. Craniomaxollofac. Surg. 28, 229–234.
Kline Jr, R.M., Wolfe, S.A., 1995. Complications associated with the harvesting of cranial bone grafts. Plast. Reconstr. Surg. 95, 5–20.
Kunakornsawat, S., Kirinpanu, A., Piyaskulkaew, C., Sathira-Angkura, V., 2013. A comparative study of radiographic results using HEALOS collagen-hydroxyapatite sponge with bone marrow aspiration versus local bone graft in the same patients undergoing posterolateral lumbar fusion. J. Med. Assoc. Thai. 96, 929–935.

Landi, E., Logroscino, G., Proietti, L., Tampieri, A., Sandri, M., Sprio, S., 2008. Biomimetic Mg-substituted hydroxyapatite: from synthesis to in vivo behaviour. J Mater. Sci. Mater. Med. 19, 239–247.

Laurencin, C.T., El-Amin, S.F., 2008. Xenotransplantation in orthopaedic surgery. J. Am. Acad. Orthop. Surg. 16, 4–8.

Legeros, R.Z., Lin, S., Rohanizadeh, R., Mijares, D., LeGeros, J.P., 2003. Biphasic calcium phosphate bioceramics: preparation, properties and applications. J. Mater. Sci. Mater. Med. 14, 201–220.

LeGeros, R.Z., 2002. Properties of osteoconductive biomaterials: calcium phosphates. Clin. Orthop. Relat. Res. 395, 81–98.

Lewis, G., 2006. Injectable bone cements for use in vertebroplasty and kyphoplasty: state-of-the-art review. J. Biomed. Mater. Res. B. 76, 456–468.

Lewis, G., 2009. Properties of antibiotic-loaded acrylic bone cements for use in cemented arthroplasties: a state-of-the-art review. J. Biomed. Mater. Res. B. 89, 558–574.

Lindfors, N.C., Koski, I., Heikkila, J.T., Mattila, K., Aho, A.J., 2010. A prospective randomized 14-year follow-up study of bioactive glass and autogenous bone as bone graft substitutes in benign bone tumors. J. Biomed. Mater. Res. B. 94, 157–164.

Lofgren, H., Johannsson, V., Olsson, T., Ryd, L., Levander, B., 2000. Rigid fusion after cloward operation for cervical disc disease using autograft, allograft, or xenograft: a randomized study with radiostereometric and clinical follow-up assessment. Spine. 25, 1908–1916.

Lomas, R., Chandrasekar, A., Board, T.N., 2013. Bone allograft in the UK: perceptions and realities. Hip. Int. 23, 427–433.

Losee, J.E., Karmacharya, J., Gannon, F.H., Slemp, A.E., Ong, G., Hunenko, O., et al., 2003. Reconstruction of the immature craniofacial skeleton with a carbonated calcium phosphate bone cement: interaction with bioresorbable mesh. J. Craniofac. Surg. 14, 117–124.

Malca, S.A., Roche, P.H., Rosset, E., Pellet, W., 1996. Cervical interbody xenograft with plate fixation: evaluation of fusion after 7 years of use in post-traumatic discoligamentous instability. Spine. 21, 685–690.

Manyalich, M., Navarro, A., Koller, J., Loty, B., de Guerra, A., Cornu, O., et al., 2009. European quality system for tissue banking. Transplant. Proc. 41, 2035–2043.

Martinez, C., Krieke, G., Ločs, J., Berzina-Cimdina, L., Garrido, L., Gilabert, U., et al., 2015. Natural hydroxyapatite-Ti-dioxide bone substitutes. Proc. Mater. Sci. 8, 324–331.

Merwin, G.E., 1986. Bioglass middle ear prosthesis: preliminary report. Ann. Otol. Rhinol. Laryngol. 95, 78–82.

Miller, L., Guerra, A.B., Bidros, R.S., Trahan, C., Baratta, R., Metzinger, S.E., 2005. A comparison of resistance to fracture among four commercially available forms of hydroxyapatite cement. Ann. Plast. Surg. 55, 87–93.

Moreira-Gonzalez, A., Jackson, I.T., Miyawaki, T., Barakat, K., DiNick, V., 2003. Clinical outcome in cranioplasty: critical review in long-term follow-up. J. Craniofac. Surg. 14, 144–153.

Mourino, V., Boccaccini, A.R., 2010. Bone tissue engineering therapeutics: controlled drug delivery in three dimensional scaffolds. J. R. Soc. Interface. 7, 209–227.

Murugan, R., Ramakrishna, S., 2005. Development of nanocomposites for bone grafting. Compos. Sci. Technol. 65, 2385–2406.

Nam, S.B., Bae, Y.C., Moon, J.S., Kang, Y.S., 2006. Analysis of the postoperative outcome in 405 cases of orbital fracture using 2 synthetic orbital implants. Ann. Plast. Surg. 56, 263–267.

Ogose, A., Kondo, N., Umezu, H., Hotta, T., Kawashima, H., Tokunaga, K., et al., 2006. Histological assessment in grafts of highly purified beta-tricalcium phosphate (OSferion®) in human bones. Biomaterials. 27, 1542–1549.
Oka, K., Murase, T., Moritomo, H., Goto, A., Sugamoto, K., Yoshikawa, H., 2010. Corrective osteotomy using customized hydroxyapatite implants prepared by preoperative computer simulation. Int. J. Med. Robot. Comput. Assist. Surg. 6, 186–193.
Owens, G.J., Singh, R.K., Foroutan, F., Alqaysi, M., Han, C.M., Mahapatra, C., et al., 2016. Sol-gel based materials for biomedical applications. Prog. Mater. Sci. 77, 1–79.
Palussiere, J., Berge, J., Gangi, A., Cotten, A., Pasco, A., Bertagnoli, R., et al., 2005. Clinical results of an open prospective study of a bis-GMA composite in percutaneous vertebral augmentation. Eur. Spine J. 14, 982–991.
Pandey, A., Jan, E., Aswath, P.B., 2006. Physical and mechanical behavior of hot rolled HDPE/HA composites. J. Mater. Sci. 41, 3369–3376.
Pape, H.C., Evans, A., Kobbe, P., 2010. Autologous bone graft: properties and techniques. J. Orthop. Trauma. 24 (Suppl 1), S36–S40.
Peltier, L.F., 1961. The use of plaster of Paris to fill defects in bone. Clin. Orthop. 21, 1–31.
Peltola, M., Aitasalo, K., Suonpaa, J., Varpula, M., Yli-Urpo, A., 2006. Bioactive glass S53P4 in frontal sinus obliteration: a long-term clinical experience. Head Neck. 28, 834–841.
Peltola, M., Kinnunen, I., Aitasalo, K., 2008. Reconstruction of orbital wall defects with bioactive glass plates. J. Oral Maxillofac. Surg. 66, 639–646.
Piattelli, A., Podda, G., Scarano, A., 1997. Clinical and histological results in alveolar ridge enlargement using coralline calcium carbonate. Biomaterials. 18, 623–627.
Pradeep, A.R., Sharma, A., 2010. Comparison of clinical efficacy of a dentifrice containing calcium sodium phosphosilicate to a dentifrice containing potassium nitrate and to a placebo on dentinal hypersensitivity: a randomized clinical trial. J. Periodontol. 81, 1167–1173.
Pryor, L.S., Gage, E., Langevin, C.J., Herrera, F., Breithaupt, A.D., Gordon, C.R., et al., 2009. Review of bone substitutes. Craniomaxillofac. Trauma Reconstr. 2, 151–160.
Ramani, P.S., Kalbag, R.M., Sengupta, R.P., 1975. Cervical spinal interbody fusion with Kiel bone. Br. J. Surg. 62, 147–150.
Rea, S.M., Bonfield, W., 2004. Biocomposites for medical applications. J. Aust. Ceram. Soc. 40, 43–57.
Reck, R., Storkel, S., Meyer, A., 1988. Bioactive glass-ceramics in middle ear surgery: an 8-year review. Ann. NY Acad. Sci. 523, 100–106.
Reedy, B.K., Pan, F., Kim, W.S., Gannon, F.H., Krasinskas, A., Bartlett, S.P., 1999. Properties of coralline hydroxyapatite and expanded polytetrafluoroethylene membrane in the immature craniofacial skeleton. Plast. Reconstr. Surg. 103, 20–26.
Reznikov, R., Shahar, R., Weiner, S., 2014. Bone hierarchical structure in three dimensions. Acta Biomater. 10, 3815–3826.
Roy, D.M., Linnehan, S.K., 1974. Hydroxyapatite formed from coral skeletal carbonate by hydrothermal exchange. Nature. 247, 220–222.
Schlickewei, W., Schlickewei, C., 2007. The use of bone substitutes in the treatment of bone defects - the clinical view and history. Macromol. Symp. 253, 10–23.
Schumacher, M., Reither, L., Thomas, J., Kampschulte, M., Gbureck, U., Lode, A., et al., 2017. Calcium phosphate bone cement/mesoporous bioactive glass composites for controlled growth factor delivery. Biomater. Sci. 5, 578–588.
Shegarfi, H., Reikeras, O., 2009. Review article: bone transplantation and immune response. J. Orthop. Surg. (Hong Kong). 17, 206–211.

Silvola, J.T., 2012. Mastoidectomy cavity obliteration with bioactive glass: a pilot study. Otolaryngol. Head Neck Surg. 147, 119–126.

Siqueira, E.B., Kranzler, L.I., 1982. Cervical Interbody fusion using calf bone. Surg. Neurol. 18, 37–39.

Sousa, R.A., Reis, R.L., Cunha, A.M., Bevis, M.J., 2003. Processing and properties of bone-analogue biodegradable and bioinert polymeric composites. Compos. Sci. Technol. 63, 389–402.

Stanley, H.R., Hall, M.B., Clark, A.E., King, C.J., Hench, L.L., Berte, J.J., 1997. Using 45S5 bioglass cones as endosseous ridge maintenance implants to prevent alveolar ridge resorption: a 5-year evaluation. Int. J. Oral Maxillofac. Implants. 12, 95–105.

Stoor, P., Pulkkinen, J., Grenman, R., 2010. Bioactive glass S53P4 in the filling of cavities in the mastoid cell area in surgery for chronic otitis media. Ann. Otol. Rhinol. Laryngol. 119, 377–382.

Suchanek, W., Yoshimura, M., 1998. Processing and properties of hydroxyapatite-based biomaterials for use as hard tissue replacement implants. J. Mater. Res. 13, 94–117.

Suominen, E., Kinnunen, J., 1996. Bioactive glass granules and plates in the reconstruction of defects of the facial bones. Scand. J. Plast. Reconstr. Surg. Hand Surg. 30, 281–289.

Tadjoedin, E.S., De Lange, G.L., Lyaruu, D.M., Kuiper, L., Burger, E.H., 2002. High concentrations of bioactive glass material (BioGran) vs. autogenous bone for sinus floor elevation. Clin. Oral Implants Res. 13, 428–436.

Tai, B.J., Bian, Z., Jiang, H., Greenspan, D.C., Zhong, J., Clark, A.E., et al., 2006. Anti-gingivitis effect of a dentifrice containing bioactive glass (NovaMin®) particulate. J. Clin. Periodontol. 33, 86–91.

Tallia, F., Gallo, M., Pontiroli, L., Baino, F., Fiorilli, S., Onida, B., et al., 2014. Zirconia-containing radiopaque mesoporous bioactive glasses. Mater. Lett. 130, 281–284.

Tan, L., Yu, X., Wan, P., Yang, K., 2013. Biodegradable materials for bone repairs: a review. J. Mater. Sci. Technol. 29, 503–513.

Tanner, K.E., Downes, R.N., Bonfield, W., 1994. Clinical applications of hydroxyapatite reinforced polyethylene. Br. Ceram. Trans. 93, 104–107.

Tanner, K.E., 2010. Bioactive ceramic-reinforced composites for bone augmentation. J. R. Soc. Interface. 7, S541–S557.

Tay, B.K.B., Patel, V.V., Bradford, D.S., 1999. Calcium sulfate and calcium phosphate-based bone substitutes – mimicry of the mineral phase of bone. Orthop. Clin. North Am. 30, 615–662.

Thomas, M.V., Puleo, D.A., Al-Sabbagh, M., 2005. Calcium sulfate: a review. J. Long Term. Eff. Med. Implants. 15, 599–607.

Thomas, M.V., Puleo, D.A., 2009. Calcium sulfate: properties and clinical applications. J. Biomed. Mater. Res. B. 88, 597–610.

Thompson, I.D., 2011. Clinical applications of bioactive glasses for maxillofacial repair. In: Hench, L.L., Fenn, M.B., Jones, J.R. (Eds.), New Materials and Technologies for Healthcare. World Scientific, Singapore, pp. 77–96.

Toquet, J., Rohanizadeh, R., Guicheux, J., Couillaud, S., Passuti, N., Daculsi, G., et al., 1999. Osteogenic potential *in vitro* of human bone marrow cells cultured on macroporous biphasic calcium phosphate ceramic. J. Biomed. Mater. Res. 44, 98–108.

Vahid Golpayegani, M., Sohrabi, A., Biria, M., Ansari, G., 2012. Remineralization effect of topical NovaMin versus sodium fluoride (1.1%) on caries-like lesions in permanent teeth. J. Dent. (Tehran). 9, 68–75.

Vallet-Regi, M., Ruiz-Hernandez, E., 2011. Bioceramics: from bone regeneration to cancer nanomedicine. Adv. Mater. 23, 5177–5218.

Valliant, E.M., Jones, J.R., 2011. Softening bioactive glass for bone regeneration: sol-gel hybrid materials. Soft Matter. 7, 5083–5095.

Verret, D.J., Ducic, Y., Oxford, L., Smith, J., 2005. Hydroxyapatite cement in craniofacial reconstruction. Otolaryngol. Head Neck Surg. 133, 897–899.

Vitale-Brovarone, C., Verné, E., Bergui, M., Onida, B., Ferraris, S., Miola, M., et al., 2015. Injectable osteoinductive bone cements. EU patent no. EP2569025.

Walliker, J., Carson, H., Douek, E.E., Fourcin, A., Rosen, S., 1987. An extracochlear auditory prosthesis. In: Bansai, P. (Ed.), Proceedings of Cochlear Implant Symposium 90. Durer, Germany, p. 265.

Wang, M., Porter, D., Bonfield, W., 1994. Processing, characterisation, and evaluation of hydroxyapatite reinforced polyethylene. Br. Ceram. Trans. 93, 91–95.

Wang, M., 2003. Developing bioactive composite materials for tissue replacement. Biomaterials. 24, 2133–2151.

White, E.W., Webber, J.N., Roy, D.M., Owen, E.L., Chiroff, R.T., White, R.A., 1975. Replamineform porous biomaterials for hard tissue implant applications. J. Biomed. Mater. Res. Symp. 6, 23–27.

Wilson, J., Douek, E., Rust, K., 1995. Bioglass middle ear devices: ten year clinical results. In: Wilson, J., Hench, L.L., Greenspan, D. (Eds.), Bioceramics. Pergamon/Elsevier, Oxford, pp. 239–246.

Wu, C., Chang, J., 2014. Multifunctional mesoporous bioactive glasses for effective delivery of therapeutic ions and drug/growth factors. J. Controll Rel. 193, 282–295.

Wu, S., Liu, X., Yeung, K.W.K., Liu, C., Yang, X., 2014. Biomimetic porous scaffolds for bone tissue engineering. Mater. Sci. Eng. R. 80, 1–36.

Yukna, R.A., Yukna, C.N., 1998. A 5-year follow-up of 16 patients treated with coralline calcium carbonate (BIOCORAL) bone replacement grafts in infrabony defects. J. Clin. Periodontol. 25, 1036–1040.

Zamet, J.S., Darbar, U.R., Griffiths, G.S., Bulman, J.S., Bragger, U., Burgin, W., et al., 1997. Particulate bioglass as a grafting material in the treatment of periodontal intrabony defects. J. Clin. Periodontol. 24, 410–418.

Zhang, Y., Hao, L., Savalani, M.M., Harris, R.A., Tanner, K.E., 2008. Characterization and dynamic mechanical analysis of selective laser sintered hydroxyapatite-filled polymeric composites. J. Biomed. Mater. Res. A. 86, 606–616.

Zins, J.E., Moreira-Gonzalez, A., Papay, F.A., 2007. Use of calcium-based bone cements in the repair of large, full-thickness cranial defects: a caution. Plast. Reconstr. Surg. 120, 1332–1342.

# Ceramic devices for bone regeneration: Mechanical and clinical issues and new perspectives

**8**

*David Marchat*[1] *and Eric Champion*[2]
[1]University of Lyon, Saint-Etienne, France, [2]University of Limoges, Limoges, France

**Chapter Outline**

**8.1 Introduction 279**
**8.2 The origins of failure 280**
8.2.1 Biology of bone healing 280
8.2.2 Current biomaterials, osteogenic substances, and surgical procedures 281
8.2.3 Mechanical properties of CaP ceramics: a misconception? 282
**8.3 Rationale for the development of implant-based tissue engineering strategies 288**
8.3.1 From research to clinic: issues 289
8.3.2 BTE strategies 290
8.3.3 CaP bioceramics: choosing material features for specific clinical applications 291
**8.4 Concluding remarks 298**
**References 298**
**Further reading 311**

## 8.1 Introduction

When a bone is injured as a result of trauma, either surgical (e.g., for bone metastasis) or accidental (fracture), the spontaneous and natural phenomenon of healing begins. Healing consists of three independent consecutive phases that occur over time: inflammation, repair, and bone remodeling (Sela and Bab, 2012). Nevertheless, in some cases, especially when there is a loss of bone tissue, the natural regeneration process is not sufficient and a bone graft is required.

Currently, the repair of small bone defects is well handled and relatively easy and can be guided and enhanced with the use of bone-filling material of human, animal, natural, or synthetic origin (Campana et al., 2014; Lau et al., 2006). A bone autograft is still considered the gold standard in bone repair surgery because of the complete biocompatibility and on-site supply of osteogenic cells. However, these grafts are available in limited quantities and involve aggressive procedures, postsurgery complications, and additional cost (Henkel et al., 2013; Matassi et al.,

**Advances in Ceramic Biomaterials.**
**DOI: http://dx.doi.org/10.1016/B978-0-08-100881-2.00008-7**

2011; Meijer et al., 2007; Oryan et al., 2014). Allografts and xenografts eliminate the harvesting procedure but are associated with possible disease transmission and a high nonunion rate with host tissues. To overcome the difficulties encountered with biological grafts, grafts made of metallic (Alvarez and Nakajima, 2009), polymer (Puppi et al., 2010), or ceramic (Döbelin et al., 2010) materials have been developed. Calcium phosphates (CaP) ceramics are used most often because (1) the mineral constituent of natural bone is CaP so the degradation products of CaP bioceramics (calcium and phosphate ions) are naturally metabolized (Barrère et al., 2006), and (2) CaP bioceramics induce intimate and functional interfaces with the host bone (Habraken et al., 2016, Wang et al., 2014). Thus, because CaP scaffolds allow the growth of new bone tissue within their porous network, they have been used for many years.

When the defect to be repaired is too large, natural bone formation cannot fill the whole scaffold. There is a transition from small defects to large defects of critical size. Although there is no clear trend, some authors believe that natural physiological bone regeneration in humans cannot occur in a bone defect >10 mm (Reichert et al., 2012). In addition, autografts for bone defects >6 cm cannot adequately support bone regeneration (Marino and Ziran, 2010; Masquelet and Begue, 2010). The limitations of current grafts require the development of new synthetic implants based on tissue engineering (Henkel et al., 2013). In this context, Giannoudis et al. defined the "diamond concept" (Giannoudis et al., 2007, 2008), a model of bone healing based on interactions between an osteoconductive scaffold, growth factors, osteogenic cells, and an adapted mechanical environment (Fig. 8.1).

Before discussing the rationale for the development of ceramic implant-based tissue-engineering strategies, it is important to present an overview of why current ceramic devices fail with respect to bone regeneration.

## 8.2 The origins of failure

### *8.2.1 Biology of bone healing*

Although the absence of or limited natural bone regeneration in critical size defects has been studied, it still has not been clearly explained. The absence of "bone and vascular signals" and osteoprogenitor and endothelial cells within the defect may be the cause of deficient natural bone regeneration (Stegen et al., 2015); osteocompetent cells and biochemical signals remain near the native bone edges, mainly at the periosteal surface (Stegen et al., 2015; Zhang et al., 2005). Consequently, there could be a natural competition between bone regeneration, which proceeds at a slow rate, and the need for rapid restoration of the mechanical function of bone (even a partial restoration). This competition could lead to the replacement of intermediate scar tissue by fibrous tissue, which would prevent subsequent bone formation (Pelissier et al., 2004; Petite et al., 2000; Viateau et al., 2006).

Some studies have suggested that procedures for filling critical bone defects failed primarily because of a lack of vascularization within the implant (Petite

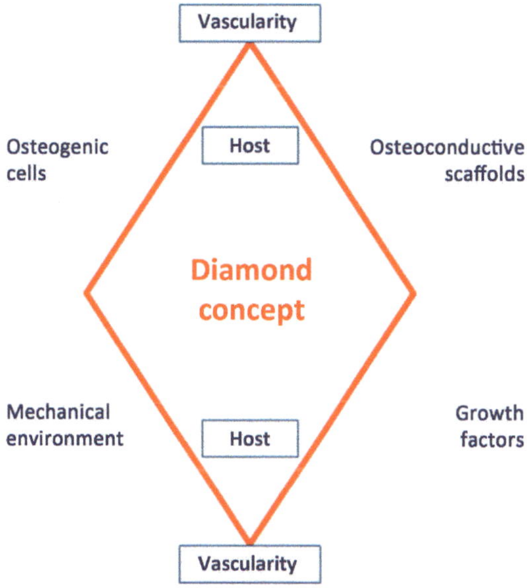


**Figure 8.1** The diamond model of bone fracture healing interactions.
*Source*: Reprinted from Giannoudis, P.V., Einhorn, T.A., Schmidmaier, G., Marsh, D., 2008. The diamond concept—open questions. Injury 39, S5—S8, copyright © 2008, with permission from Elsevier.

et al., 2000; Zhou et al., 2010). Indeed, the cells at the periphery of the filler material benefit from oxygen and nutrients via diffusion or local vascularization at the implant surface. However, cells more than 100—400 μm from those blood vessels or from the implant—host tissue interface die inexorably because of local ischemia (i.e., from hypoxia but, above all, from depletion of nutrients) (Petite et al., 2011; Deschepper et al., 2011; Schmitt et al., 2012; Pneumaticos et al., 2010; Das and Botchwey, 2011; Liu et al., 2015).

### 8.2.2 Current biomaterials, osteogenic substances, and surgical procedures

Few satisfactory treatments for large bone defects, especially critical size defects, are available today (Wiese and Pape, 2010). Of the ceramic materials capable of interacting with a living substance (i.e., bioactive materials) and promoting the formation of new bone tissue, only CaPs are an answer to this problem. Currently, the materials most commonly used to fill bone defects in the clinical setting are hydroxyapatite (HA, $Ca_{10}(PO_4)_6(OH)_2$) and beta-tricalcium phosphate (β-TCP, $Ca_3(PO_4)_2$) (Habraken et al., 2016). However, HA shows a limited ability to stimulate the development of new bone tissue, and has a limited and very low rate of biodegradation (Barralet et al., 2000a; Spence et al., 2009). Conversely, β-TCP ceramics degrade too rapidly because their in vivo solubility is about 10-times greater than that of HA (Barralet et al., 2000a). This rapid degradation proved to be detrimental to cells and newly formed bone (Yuan et al., 1998, 2001), although contradictory results were recently found (Zhanga et al., 2016).

A mixture of HA and β-TCP called biphasic calcium phosphate (BCP) was developed with the goal of having an optimum balance between the more stable phase of HA and the greater solubility of TCP for controlled gradual dissolution in the body (Daculsi, 1998). Commercialization of BCP bioceramics started in the 1990s (LeGeros, 2008). BCP blocks or granules are still used clinically as bone fillers for defects smaller than 3 cm, where osteoconduction is sufficient. Beyond 3 cm, the properties of these bone substitutes do not allow full regeneration of the bone without the addition of bioactive factors (Garrido et al., 2011).

To stimulate the repair and regeneration of bone, the use of osteogenic materials, including autologous bone marrow, peptide signaling molecules (fibroblast growth factor 2 and platelet-derived growth factors), and morphogenetic factors (bone morphogenetic proteins (BMPs)) (Einhorn and Gerstenfeld, 2015), is legally permitted (Dimitriou et al., 2011; Einhorn and Gerstenfeld, 2015; Pneumaticos et al., 2010; Schliephake, 2015). Unfortunately, in spite of interesting clinical results, public health authorities have limited the use of osteogenic materials and increasingly restricted the use of BMP2 (Hashimoto et al., 2012; Oryan et al., 2014). Serious adverse postoperative effects can occur because the optimal doses of growth factors released within the bone defect during the repair phase (i.e., release kinetics as a function of time) and burst release (i.e., fast and uncontrolled initial release) of high supraphysiological concentrations of BMP2, which occurs because the active factor is often included by adsorption to the surface of the biomaterial, are not known (Carragee et al., 2011).

The Ilizarov device (Demiralp et al., 2014) is a commonly used method for treating bone defects but the associated surgical procedure is very painful and can have serious consequences for the patient.

The Masquelet technique, which uses autologous bone-grafting material harvested by a Reamer–Irrigator–Aspirator (RIA) System, is a significant improvement for patients and surgeons. However, it still requires autologous bone (which causes chronic pain in the donor site) and several surgeries.

### 8.2.3 Mechanical properties of CaP ceramics: a misconception?

The mechanical properties of implants have always been considered of prime importance in the development of CaP ceramics as substitutes for bone. Habraken et al. showed that the first attempts at CaP ceramic development aimed at producing very dense materials strong enough for load-bearing applications (Habraken et al., 2016). The fracture strength of any CaP ceramic material depends on two main microstructural parameters: the grain size for dense ceramics and the amount of residual porosity for microporous (i.e., typical pore size $<10\,\mu m$) materials (Halouani et al., 1994; Raynaud et al., 1998). The denser the ceramic and the finer its grain size, the greater its strength. However, while CaP can be mechanically strong as cortical bone (Johnson and Herschler, 2011), the main limitation of these ceramics for load-bearing applications is their extreme brittleness (Habraken et al., 2016). The fracture toughness $K_c$ of dense CaP ceramics hardly reaches 1 MPa$\sqrt{m}$ (Halouani et al., 1994; Raynaud et al., 2002). Using this knowledge, research focused on the processing of scaffolds that include a network of macropores, typically 300–600 μm, which allow colonization by newly formed tissue via an osteoconduction mechanism. The idea was to promote bone formation. Ideally, the complete regeneration of damaged tissue could be expected with total degradation of the CaP scaffold (e.g., β-TCP), or at least a high percentage of regeneration with the use of a few highly porous degradable CaP scaffolds (e.g., HA). However, as illustrated in Fig. 8.2, increasing the porosity to >60–70 vol% (relative density

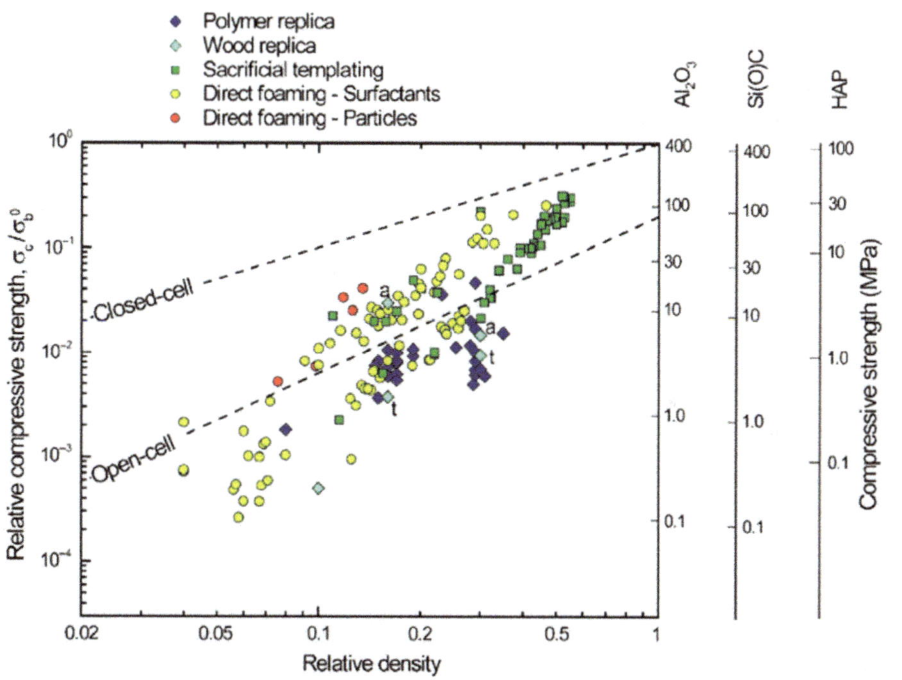


**Figure 8.2** Relative compressive strength as a function of the relative density of macroporous ceramics produced via replica, sacrificial template and direct-foaming methods. The relative strength was calculated from the ratio between the compressive strength of the porous structure (sc) and the bending strength of its dense counterpart ($\sigma_b^0$). The data were obtained from porous ceramics of different chemical compositions, assuming a bending strength of 400, 450, and 110 MPa for the alumina, silicon oxycarbide, and HA dense materials, respectively. The *y*-scales on the right hand side indicate the corresponding absolute compressive strength for alumina, silicon carbide/oxycarbide, and HA porous structures.
*Source*: Reprinted from Studart, A.R., Gonzenbach, U.T., Tervoort, E., Gauckler, L.J., 2006. Processing routes to macroporous ceramics: a review. J. Am. Ceram. Soc. 89:1771–1789, copyright ©2006, with permission from John Willey & Sons.

<0.4–0.3) induces a sharp decrease in the mechanical strength of cellular ceramics produced by different methods.

New ideas about mechanical properties have arisen with the development of porous ceramics for filling bone defects or scaffolds for engineering bone tissue. One by Bose et al. is as follows: "The mechanical properties of an ideal bone scaffold should match host bone properties and proper load transfer is important as well" (Bose et al., 2012). Two main approaches to the development of porous ceramics are related to the mechanical properties of the scaffold and the new forming bone.

### 8.2.3.1 Mechanical properties of scaffolds

Some authors investigated the possibility of mimicking the mechanical properties of bone by designing biomimetic materials at the macroscopic or microscopic level (Libonati and Vergani, 2016; Wu et al., 2016). One difficulty of such an approach is that the mechanical properties (i.e., compressive, flexural, and tensile strength, fracture toughness, elastic modulus) of bone vary greatly with the type of bone but also with the age and gender of the individual (Mirzaali et al., 2016; Reilly and Burstein, 1974). Another difficulty with designing biomimetic materials is that it requires the use of processing techniques that can produce highly complex shapes at either a microscopic or macroscopic multiscale level. Only computer-aided design and computer-aided manufacturing (CAD/CAM) can meet this requirement, but they currently suffer from limited resolution (see Chapter 14: Advanced processing techniques for customized ceramic medical devices), and, as illustrated in Fig. 8.3, the maximum macroporosity achievable using CAD/CAM is low because

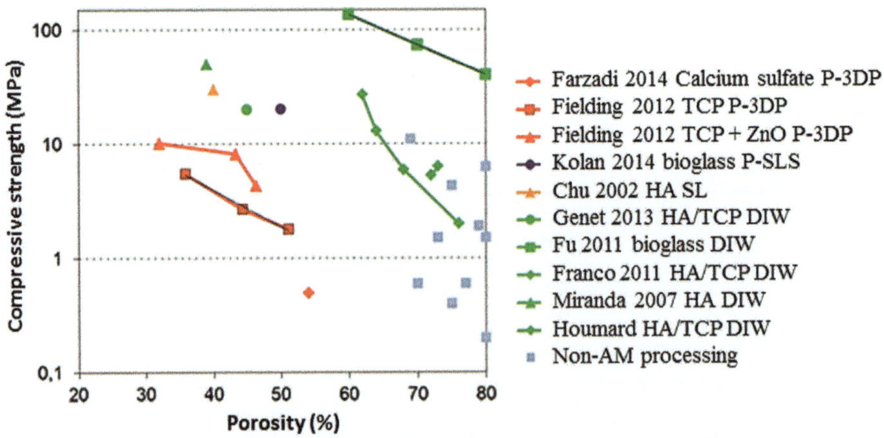


**Figure 8.3** Compressive strength versus porosity for porous bioceramic components fabricated using different additive manufacturing technologies.
*Source*: Reprinted from Zocca, A., Colombo, P., Gomes, C.M., Günster, J., 2015. Additive manufacturing of ceramics: issues, potentialities, and opportunities. J. Am. Ceram. Soc. 98:1983–2001, copyright ©2015, with permission from John Wiley & Sons.

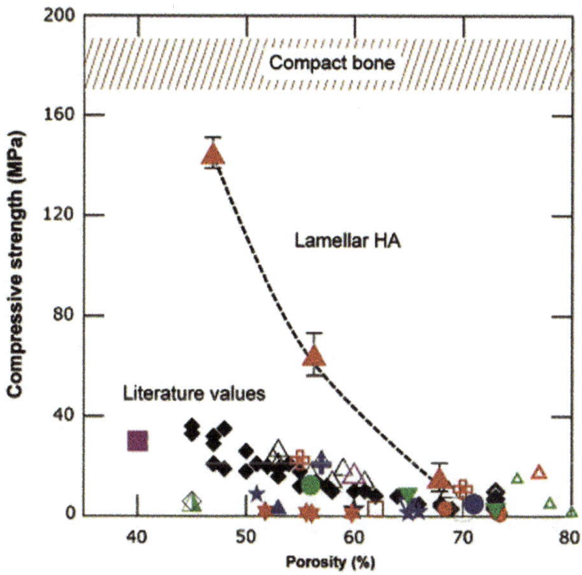


**Figure 8.4** Maximum compressive strength achieved by freeze-casting (cooling rate of 5°C/min) versus porosity. Comparison with compact bone and published values of porous hydroxyapatite (HA) for tissue engineering, conventional and computer-assisted processing techniques. Each point style represents a different publication.
*Source*: Reprinted from Deville, S., Saiz, E., Tomsia, A.P., 2006. Freeze casting of hydroxyapatite scaffolds for bone tissue engineering. Biomaterials 27:5480–5489, copyright © 2006, with permission from Elsevier.

of the minimum stiffness necessary for the stability of the construct (Zocca et al., 2015). Moreover, if mechanical strength is the target property, then that of CAD/CAM-engineered scaffolds is usually not superior to that of more porous scaffolds processed by conventional methods such as foam replica, sacrificial template, and direct foaming (Studart et al., 2006). Similarly, the use of freeze-casting, a direct-foaming technique, to produce scaffolds with lamellar interconnected pores (Deville et al., 2006) that are expected to be stronger has been investigated (Fig. 8.4). Additional improvements to this technique are required to allow adjustment of the size of the pores for effective cell colonization of scaffolds (see also Chapter 14: Advanced processing techniques for customized ceramic medical devices) (Fu et al., 2009; Meurice et al., 2016).

A recent trend that has arisen from the potentiality of CAD/CAM technologies is the theoretical modeling of the elastic modulus (Hollister and Lin, 2007; Hollister et al., 2002) or strength (Clausen et al., 2016; Entezari et al., 2016; Roohani-Esfahani et al., 2016; Wu et al., 2016) of the scaffold architecture to optimize its design. This approach focuses mainly on the development of scaffolds for load-bearing applications that mimic the natural structure of bone with a compact and stiff outer shell and an inner trabecular structure. An illustration is presented in Fig. 8.5.

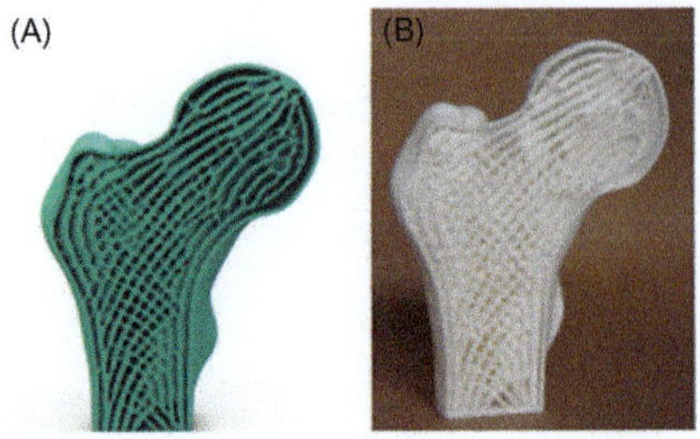


**Figure 8.5** (A) Cross-section of the optimized porous infill in a 3D bone model. (B) The 3D-printed bone model.
*Source*: Reprinted from Wu, J., Aage, N., Westermann, R., Sigmund, O., 2016. Infill Optimization for Additive Manufacturing--Approaching Bone-like Porous Structures. arXiv preprint arXiv:1608.04366, copyright with permission.

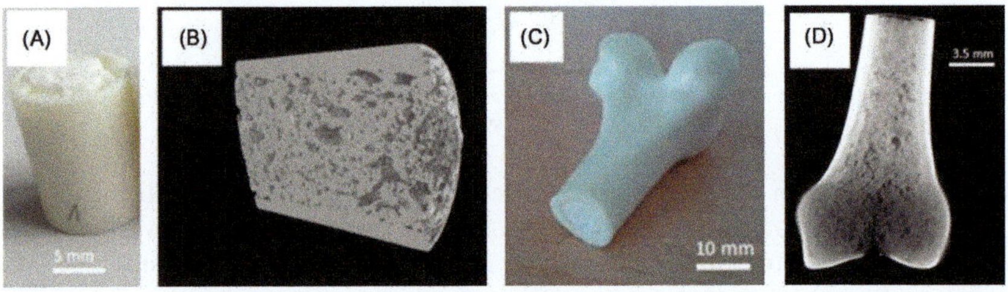


**Figure 8.6** (A) Comanufactured freeze foam-filled lithography-based ceramic manufacturing (LCM) specimen. (B) Reconstructed computed tomography (CT) image. (C) Femoral bone model: biocomposite of a dense LCM part and inner porous freeze foam. (D) Reconstructed CT image of the femoral bone model.
*Source*: Reprinted from Ahlhelm, M., Günther, P., Scheithauer, U., Schwarzer, E., Günther, A., Slawik, T., et al., 2016. Innovative and novel manufacturing methods of ceramics and metal-ceramic composites for biomedical applications. J. Eur. Ceram. Soc. 36:2883–2888, copyright ©2015, with permission from Elsevier.

Using a similar mimetic principle for the natural structure of bone, others have produced the architectural design of porous bulk and dense outer surface by combining several shaping processes (Fig. 8.6) (Ahlhelm et al., 2016).

The limitation of the concept of scaffolds based on the optimization or enhancement of their mechanical properties is that they can be composed of only inert ceramic materials such as alumina because bioactive materials such as CaPs are more or less degraded via chemical dissolution by body fluids and osteoclastic resorption. This biodegradation is necessary for the promotion of bone regeneration but is very detrimental to the mechanical properties of the ceramic substrate. Fig. 8.7A illustrates the effect of the chemical composition of CaP on the dissolution of a dense BCP ceramic caused by its liquid environment. While pure HA exhibited homogeneous surface dissolution except in the presence of residual microporosity, which might result in possible decohesion of HA grains located around residual pores, dense BCP exhibited nonhomogeneous degradation

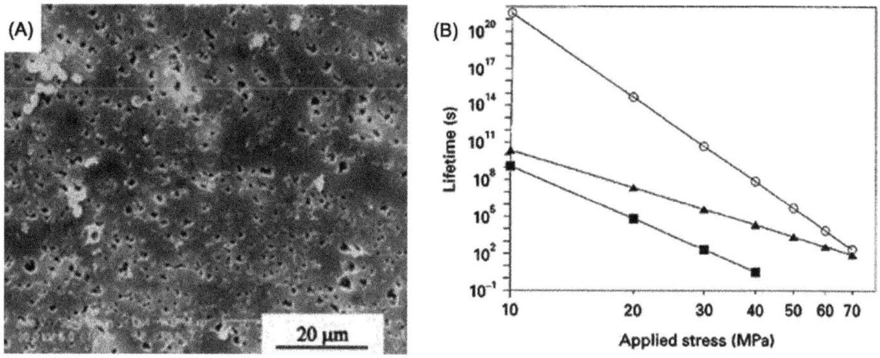


**Figure 8.7** (A) Surface of biphasic calcium phosphate (BCP) ceramic (88 wt% hydroxyapatite (HA)-12 wt% beta-tricalcium phosphate (β-TCP)) after 60 days in Ringer's solution, reprinted from (Raynaud et al., 2002), copyright © 2001, with permission from Elsevier. (B) Simulated plots of lifetime versus applied load: HA relative density 98% tested (O) in air and (▲) in Ringer's solution, (■) HA relative density 94% tested in air.
*Source*: Reprinted from Raynaud, S., Champion, E., Bernache-Assolant, D., Tetard, D., 1998. Dynamic fatigue and degradation in solution of hydroxyapatite ceramics. J. Mater. Sci. Mater. Med. 9:221–227, copyright 1998, with permission from Springer Science.

(Raynaud et al., 1998, 2002). Cavities resulting from the preferential dissolution of β-TCP grains formed at the surface of initially dense BCP. This showed that BCP ceramics do not really mediate the resorption between the less soluble HA (in vivo 60 $mg/m^2$ per day (Barralet et al., 2000a), $K_s = 10^{-116.8}$ (Rey et al., 2011)) and the much more soluble β-TCP (in vivo 520 $mg/m^2$ per day (Barralet et al., 2000a), $K_s = 10^{-28.9}$ (Rey et al., 2011)). At this point, the pertinent mechanical parameter of a scaffold is its resistance to mechanical fatigue in a physiological environment (i.e., the change in mechanical properties vs the time) rather than its "intrinsic" fracture strength measured in ambient air. However, this behavior has never been investigated. The work of Raynaud et al. showed that the lifetime of dense HA in air when the load is 45% of its intrinsic flexural strength is around 2 years but decreases to about 100 hours when the HA is in Ringer's solution and the load is only 30% of its intrinsic strength (Fig. 8.7B) (Raynaud et al., 1998).

### 8.2.3.2 Mechanical properties of new forming bone

From the approach described above, the mechanical properties of the scaffold made of bioactive or bioresorbable ceramics cannot be considered key parameters in its design.

Because it is impossible to promote bone regeneration with the use of biodegradable materials without altering the mechanical properties of the scaffold, load transfer from the scaffold to new forming tissues is being researched. The principle behind the research is that fast scaffold colonization and bone healing is promoted to transfer load from the bone defect to mature bone (Habraken et al., 2016). In this approach, the basic requirement is that the scaffold be stiff enough to be handled and not break or collapse before adequate bone ingrowth and sufficient load transfer have occurred (Henkel et al., 2013; Johnson and Herschler, 2011). Experimental studies on the changes in the compressive strength of porous CaP ceramics after implantation in rabbits showed a significant reinforcement due to bone ingrowth (Hing et al., 2004; Trecant et al., 1994, 1996). Other recent studies have aimed at developing numerical models that predict the increase in mechanical properties (Ren et al., 2012; Scheiner et al., 2016). Thus, Sheiner et al. showed that the design parameters of a scaffold influence its load-carrying capacity (Sheiner et al., 2007, 2008).

Finally, the main issue remaining in the development of a CaP scaffold for use in bone regeneration is the regulation of its degradation rate, which ideally should match the rate of new bone formation. Over the past few years, numerous studies have been devoted to acquiring better knowledge of the phenomena that occur at the material-living tissue interface. Both scaffold degradation and bone tissue formation rates greatly depend on the chemical composition of the CaP material and on the architecture of the scaffold. Efforts to understand the influential parameters and hypotheses used in the development of CaP scaffolds in the emerging field of bone tissue engineering (BTE) are presented below.

## 8.3 Rationale for the development of implant-based tissue engineering strategies

In tissue engineering, there are various definitions of an ideal scaffold for the regeneration of bone after large bone loss (Alghazali et al., 2015; Habraken et al., 2016; Henkel et al., 2013; Liu et al., 2015; Saiz et al., 2013). However, these scaffolds may be limited by the perception of what an ideal material should be rather than by the ability to manufacture it. As mentioned in the preceding section, the ideal implant is one whose mechanical properties can handle both macroscopic (defect scale/load-bearing) and microscopic (cell scale/stiffness) needs. Thus, the ideal material should be biomimetic, i.e., it should reproduce faithfully the characteristics of natural bone (e.g., mechanical, topographic, chemical analysis properties) (Fernandez-Yague et al., 2015; Moutos et al., 2007; Venugopal et al., 2010; Wegst et al., 2015). However, to our knowledge, this strategy does not work because the physiology of human bone tissue, unlike that of other vertebrates (Brockes and Gates, 2014; Kumar et al., 2007), is no longer able to regenerate bone after such bone loss; i.e., human bone tissue does not have the necessary intrinsic "tools" for regeneration. Therefore, tissue-engineered scaffolds must stimulate, accelerate, and/or amplify bone tissue regeneration by means of features, not necessarily bioinspired, that direct stem cell fate decisions.

This section discusses the different BTE strategies and their key elements, especially the scaffolds and the CaP ceramics used for these applications. The section begins with an attempt to explain the difficulties of transferring knowledge from research in this area to the clinic.

### 8.3.1 From research to clinic: issues

Except for in vitro three-dimensional (3D) bone tissue models (Bouët et al., 2014), the aim of BTE studies is to provide new therapeutic solutions for clinical use. However, as clearly emphasized in the comprehensive articles of Hollister (Hollister, 2009a,b), it remains a challenge to translate basic science to routine clinical application.

In addition to the substantial economic barrier, the main hurdle in transferring a concept to the clinic is the lack of a direct correspondence between the concept of scaffold-based tissue engineering and clinical applications. A meticulous assessment of clinical needs and the design of scaffold-based tissue engineering strategies is essential. Indeed, as stated by Henkel et al.: "the complexity and great variety of large bone defects require an individualized patient-specific approach with regards to surgical reconstruction in general and implant/tissue engineering selection in specific" (2013).

The problem of transferring a concept to the clinic reflects quite well the fundamental difference between a scientific invention (i.e., a laboratory concept) and an innovation (i.e., a socially adopted or utilized concept). If the invention does not respond to the needs of the patient, the surgeon, or society, it will not become an innovation, i.e., something not only clever but also useful. Therefore, clinical requirements must be considered early in the process of defining the BTE strategy and, in particular, the scaffold specifications. Scaffold features must be selected with respect to the characteristics of the bone to be repaired (i.e., its location, biology, biomechanics) and the surgical procedure to be used (e.g., minimally invasive). The latter includes the use of fixation devices with external or internal fixators that immobilize the fracture (Krishnakanth, 2012). Stability from fixation has a significant effect on bone healing, especially in challenging cases involving large bone defects (Dimitriou et al., 2011; Einhorn and Gerstenfeld, 2015). Nevertheless, this fundamental element of BTE is rarely discussed, and then just to state that the fixation is "stable," and is investigated even less. Fracture fixation devices should be designed in conjunction with the scaffold to provide a favorable mechanical and biological environment for healing (Glatt et al., 2016).

Of course, the effect of the main features of the tissue-engineered construct on new bone formation must first be investigated in clinically relevant animal models (Bigham-Sadegh and Oryan, 2015; Henkel et al., 2013; Li et al., 2015; von Rechenberg, 2014). Knowledge from these investigations will help to define more accurately the best BTE strategy (see Section 8.3.2) and CaP bioceramic scaffold features (see Section 8.3.3) with respect to clinical application.

Finally, the ability to get a tissue-engineered scaffold approved for targeted clinical applications is not related just to the success of the strategy at the laboratory or preclinical level, but to the ability to upscale the scaffold from laboratory use to industrial commercialization. This involves the use of good manufacturing practices to produce large implants (human vs animals) with the same specifications as those assessed in animal models. Henkel et al. (2013) and Hollister (2009a) suggest some key points that the scaffold should validate early in the process to facilitate its transfer from laboratory to patient.

### 8.3.2 BTE strategies

BTE entails the use of a three-dimensional scaffold structure (or construct) as an ephemeral carrier for bioactive molecules (Bose and Tarafder, 2012; Saiz et al., 2013) and cells (Bueno and Glowacki, 2009; Grayson et al., 2015; Liu et al., 2016; Meijer et al., 2007)

The success of a BTE strategy depends mainly on the ability of the implant to keep endogenous and exogenous cells alive and functional. The nutrient and oxygen supplies from blood vessels greatly affect the survival of any cell or tissue. However, the exchange of nutrients and oxygen between blood vessels and tissues is limited to a maximum range of 200 μm (Kumar et al., 2016; Liu et al., 2015). Therefore, the formation of new blood vessels from the host tissue to the core of the tissue-engineered construct is required.

A bone fracture disrupts the vascular tree that mainly supplies nutrients and oxygen and disposes of waste products. Thus, a bioceramic scaffold, biohybrid, or construct implanted in this defect causes abnormal ischemic conditions for cells, i.e., they experience not only hypoxia (severe depletion of oxygen, i.e., $pO_2$ <0.2%) but also a decrease in critical metabolic nutrients (e.g., glucose) and inadequate removal of potentially toxic metabolic waste (e.g., lactate) (Deschepper et al., 2011). However, this hypoxic condition has two benefits: (1) it seems to induce the mobilization of mesenchymal stem cells (MSCs), and (2) it provokes an upregulation by cells of various secretable factors, among which are important angiogenic factors such as vascular endothelial growth factor (Das et al., 2009; Ejtehadifar et al., 2015). In addition, MSCs preseeded in the CaP scaffold are most probably inducers (emitting signals) rather than effectors of bone formation (Gamblin et al., 2014; Grayson et al., 2015). Unfortunately, these benefits were found to be short-lived because under ischemic conditions, massive cell death occurs at about day 6 (Becquart et al., 2012; Deschepper et al., 2011). This may explain why the strategy of using MSCs as paracrine and host-derived factors to repair skeletal tissues stayed at the proof-of-concept stage (Caplan, 1991; Meijer et al., 2007).

Preconditioning MSCs via hypoxia (Das et al., 2009) or fetal bovine serum deprivation (Moya et al., 2017) can reduce hypoxia-induced cell death. More interesting is that exposing MSCs to severe and continuous hypoxia and an appropriate glucose supply not only doubled their survival time, but helped them maintain their functionality (e.g., morphology and in vivo osteogenic ability) (Deschepper et al., 2011; Moya et al., 2017). These findings are particularly relevant to the development of tissue-engineered constructs because they suggest that MSCs preconditioned and loaded into glucose-enriched scaffolds can delay their death and remain functional, resulting in an increase in the total amount of paracrine factors secreted. This is more important than the spontaneous growth of new blood vessels in mammals, which is however faster under inflammatory conditions, and is limited at a length of about 100 nm per day (Clark and Clark, 1939). To better adjust the formation of new blood vessels and MSC functions, Meijer et al. proposed postponing the injection of MSCs into the scaffold until after the chronic inflammation phase, i.e., when the new blood vessels are already invading the hematoma (Meijer et al., 2007).

Ultimately, without any endogenous or exogenous growth factors or bioactive substance (e.g., glucose or oxygen), the short-lived cellular survival in the construct and the slow extrinsic vascularization (neovascular bed originates from the periphery of the construct (Eweida et al., 2011)) result in the failure of bone regeneration. Fibrous tissue usually disrupts bone healing by invading the scaffold (Yuan et al., 2010), as observed by Petite et al. (2000).

Local and controlled delivery of exogenous growth factors (bone (Oryan et al., 2014) or vascular (Liu et al., 2015)) or a bioactive substance (oxygen (Farris et al., 2016) or glucose (Suhaimi and Bhusan Das, 2016; Zhu et al., 2016)) in the scaffold can accelerate the physiological process of new blood vessel formation (angiogenesis), reduce inflammation, enhance recruitment of progenitor cells, and stimulate osteogenic differentiation. The sustained release of these substances while they maintain their biological activity can be controlled by different methods such as the functionalization of the CaP surface through coprecipitation (Liu et al., 2004, 2017), covalent grafting (Chatzinikolaidou et al., 2010; Mercado et al., 2009), or encapsulation in hydrogel microspheres or a matrix (Alghazali et al., 2015; Watson et al., 2014).

To shorten the time needed to achieve effective vascularization of the tissue-engineered implant, some have proposed a coculture approach in which angiogenic cells are introduced into an osteogenic cell culture (Liu et al., 2015; Ma et al., 2014).

For the vascularization of a tissue-engineered construct and cell survival in a large bone defect, a tissue engineering strategy based on a prevascularized construct created in an in vivo bioreactor (e.g., intramuscularly within the latissimus dorsi) has been applied (Tatara et al., 2014). However, in addition to the multiple surgeries needed, this strategy results in significant donor site morbidity owing to the difficulty of harvesting while trying to preserve the vessels (Warnke et al., 2004). To avoid these drawbacks, another in vivo procedure that uses intrinsic axial vascularization *via* the arteriovenous (AV) loop was developed (Eweida et al., 2011) whereby the AV loop is introduced inside the scaffold to induce and sustain vascularization.

### 8.3.3 CaP bioceramics: choosing material features for specific clinical applications

The success of an implanted scaffold or construct is based on its capacity to be invaded, degraded, and replaced by host tissues (mainly bone and vascular tissues) as quickly as possible and with the right balance between ceramic scaffold degradation and new bone tissue formation. However, not all clinical and surgical applications are equivalent and the properties of the tissue-engineered scaffold, especially its degradation, should be modulated according to the function of the application.

A strategy in which only a scaffold is used to repair a large bone defect seems flawed. The bioceramic properties of the scaffold must be adjusted for instance: (1) to allow the seeding of implants with homogeneous cells, which affects the osteogenic activity of tissue-engineered bone grafts (Luo et al., 2013; Seebach et al.,

2010); (2) to facilitate the functionalization of the scaffold (see Section 8.3.2); (3) to place an AV loop into the scaffold or (4) to place a fixation device to stabilize the bone implant contact during healing (Eweida et al., 2011).

Scaffold properties are critical to the sustained success of scaffold-based tissue engineering strategies. The scaffold needs to be more than a support for tissue ingrowth; it must promote and stimulate it (Henkel et al., 2013; Zadpoor, 2015) or even regulate stem cell activity (Murphy et al., 2014). In other words, the inherent properties of bioceramic scaffolds must influence, or induce, lineage-specific stem cell differentiation (e.g., hematopoietic, mesenchymal) or direct and control cell activity (e.g., osteoclastic ceramic resorption, osteoblastic matrix deposition, blood vessel morphogenesis) (Murphy et al., 2014). Some authors call this type of biomaterial "smart" (Best et al., 2008; Camaioni et al., 2015; Meijer et al., 2007; Ripamonti et al., 2008, 2011) or "intelligent" (Henkel et al., 2013), but the adjective "bioinstructive" (Collinsa et al., 2016) seems to better characterize the potential function of the biomaterial. The physicochemical properties of CaP materials associated with new engineering processes that combine computational methods and additive manufacturing (AM) will yield such bioinstructive ceramics for large bone defect applications.

#### *8.3.3.1 Composition of CaP bioceramics*

Here, "composition" means all the physicochemical parameters, i.e., phase composition (amorphous or crystalline), crystalline structure, local order or crystallinity, chemical surface, and chemical composition, that can be separated from the architectural ones (detailed in Section 8.3.3.2). These physicochemical parameters are affected by the chemical, mechanical, and thermal treatment experienced by material during manufacturing. For instance, carbonated HA is always in equilibrium with the heat-treatment atmosphere (partial pressures of gas such as $CO_2$ and $H_2O$) (Lafon et al., 2008). Therefore, it is necessary to control effectively each step in the manufacture of bioceramics, from the chemical synthesis of the powder to the sterilization, including the accurate characterization of the final ceramic to ensure the chemical and structural standardization of the sample and the validity of the biological evaluation.

A striking feature of CaP, and particularly of the apatite group, is that the crystal structure can accommodate many different ions. Apatite can incorporate ions of half of the elements in the periodic table into its atomic structure (Elliott, 1994; Hughes and Rakovan, 2002). Some ions of biological interest, especially for bone repair, are those of zinc, selenium, silicate, strontium, and carbonate (Bose et al., 2013a; Elliott, 1994; Hughes and Rakovan, 2002; Ratnayake et al., 2016; Shepherd et al., 2012; Šupová, 2015). Thus, CaP bioceramics are considered delivery vehicles for bioinorganics (Habraken et al., 2016), also called by-products, that can affect cell fate decisions (Murphy et al., 2014). In addition, calcium and phosphate ions were proven to have a regulatory role in bone formation and osteoclastogenesis (Barrère et al., 2006; Chai et al., 2012; Danciu et al., 2003; Doi et al., 1998; Klar et al., 2013; Shih et al., 2014). However, for these ions to be active, they should be released into the microenvironment of the cell. Studies by Barralet et al. (2000a) and Spence et al. (2009, 2010) proved that the rate of degradation (i.e., chemical solubility and osteoclastic resorption) can be controlled by controlling the carbonate content of the HA lattice, an excellent way to adjust the rate of degradation of the HA ceramics with respect to the clinical target. This approach is of greater interest than the bioceramics made of carbonated HA degrade homogeneously since it is composed of a unique chemical phase (Spence et al., 2010), as opposed to the "shreds" degradation of a BCP ceramic (Weiss et al., 2007), which is a combination of highly soluble β-TCP and low biodegradable HA (Barralet et al., 2000b; Detsch et al., 2008; Doi et al., 1998; Spence et al., 2010). This homogeneous and medium-rate degradation, compared to that of HA and β-TCP, confers three interesting qualities to tissue-engineered scaffolds made of carbonated HA: (1) a moderate release of degradation by-products; (2) the development of a bone-like mineral layer containing organic compounds via a "surface precipitation" process (i.e., dissolution–precipitation process catalyzed by the CaP mineral surface) (Barrère et al., 2006; Henkel et al., 2013; Sposito, 2008), and (3) a relatively stable material–tissue interface, which is required for cell adhesion and de novo bone formation to occur (Barradas et al., 2011; Habraken et al., 2016). There must be a compromise between degradation capacity and interface stability; a rapid degradation of the scaffold impairs the regenerative capacity of the host bone (Hing et al., 2007; Yuan et al., 1998, 2001).

Many studies have shown that the bioactivity of carbonated HA is generally higher in vivo and in vitro than that of HA (e.g., higher bone ingrowth and coverage than HA in vivo) (Landi et al., 2003; Patel et al., 2002; Porter et al., 2005; Spence et al., 2008, 2009, 2010), but some studies have not (Habibovic et al., 2008, 2010; Melville et al., 2006). However, the purity of the carbonated HA bioceramics in the latter studies has been questioned.

Additionally, the cosubstitution of carbonate with bioinorganic ions, in particular, magnesium, strontium, and silicate ions, in the apatite lattice is possible (Shepherd et al., 2012; Sprio et al., 2008; Šupová, 2015). For instance, in vitro studies of cosubstitution have shown that controlled release of ions and improved biological response can be expected (Bang et al., 2015; Landi et al., 2010), although the purity of silicocarbonated HA bioceramics is in doubt (Bang et al., 2014, 2015).

From a wider point of view, ionic substitutions in the CaP lattice affect the chemical, physical, and mechanical characteristics (e.g., crystal structure, crystallinity, surface charge, solubility, wettability, stiffness, sinterability) of the mineral, but also the architectural features (e.g., grain size) discussed in Section 8.3.3.2. Apart from the ability of the substituted CaP bioceramics to release ions into the microenvironment of the cell, these physicochemical changes modify the inherent potential of the bioceramic to interact with proteins and cells. These dynamic exchanges at the cell-material interface were presented by Murphy et al. under the concept of "Give and Take" (Murphy et al., 2014). In summary, well-selected inherent material properties could dictate endogenous as well as exogenous stem cell fate decisions. Murphy et al. have even suggested an "autocatalytic process" in which cell-secreted signals, sequestered earlier at the cell–material interface, could regulate stem cell activity. Using material properties as stem cell regulators might become a reality, but the relationships between the bioceramic properties and stem cell fate will need to be identified before the material properties (e.g., composition) can be adjusted with respect to the clinical target. On the other hand, this material will be seemingly CaP because the vast majority of materials with osteoinductive properties contain this mineral (Barradas et al., 2011).

#### *8.3.3.2 Architectural features of the scaffold*

For large bone defects, a patient-specific approach is necessary. However, beyond the shape, morphology, and esthetic characteristics of the scaffold, many other architectural features are essential, especially from the perspective of the manufacture of the bioinstructive ceramic. Five features of the architecture of the scaffold influence the biological response: (1) macroscopic shape of the bioceramic, (2) porous network, (3) pore size and geometry, (4) surface microtopography, and (5) micro-, submicro-, and nanoporosity. Fig. 8.8 presents these different architectural features; features (2) and (3) are illustrated under the label "intern architecture."

The macroscopic shape of the implant must promote perfect contact between the construct and the adjacent host tissues to accelerate the exchange between the tissue-engineered scaffold and the host tissues and improve osseointegration (Nishimura, 2013; Novaes Jr et al., 2010; Vandamme et al., 2011); the slower the colonization of cells and tissues, the higher the risk of failure (Ferraro, 1979).

The macroscopic porous network corresponds to the distribution of macropores within the scaffold volume. It affects the mechanical properties of the scaffold (Entezari et al., 2016; Sabree et al., 2015); the degradation rate (Karageorgiou and Kaplan, 2005; Lam et al., 2008; Saito et al., 2012; Schaefer et al., 2011); mass transport (Melchels et al., 2010c; Jung et al., 2013; Grayson et al., 2012); cell seeding (Melchels et al., 2010a; Van Bael et al., 2012) cell response, cell-network formation, and tissue growth (Salerno et al., 2010; Di Luca et al., 2016; Karageorgiou and Kaplan, 2005; Van Bael et al., 2012; Zadpoor, 2015) and blood vessel guidance (Magnaudeix et al., 2016; Xiao et al., 2015). However, with respect to the porous network, it is not clear from the current data that cell behavior is independent of the other scaffold features (e.g., composition, microporosity) (Bohner et al., 2011). The confined areas created by this structural parameter are necessary for the intrinsic osteoinductive potential of the biomaterial (Barradas et al., 2011). The porous network is also an essential parameter for the strategy that releases bioactive proteins functionalized at the biomaterial surface (Alghazali et al., 2015).

The macroscopic porous network can be organized or randomized; graded; tortuous; heterogeneous or homogeneous; complex or basic; and open-, closed-, or blind-ended (Giannitelli et al., 2014b; Jun et al., 2007; Murr, 2016; Xiong et al., 2016; Yang et al., 2015; Yoo, 2012, 2013). The large class of periodic minimal surfaces is particularly interesting for BTE applications (Kapfer et al., 2011; Rajagopalan and Robb, 2006). For instance, the permeability of a scaffold with a gyroid network is more than 10-fold greater than that of a scaffold with

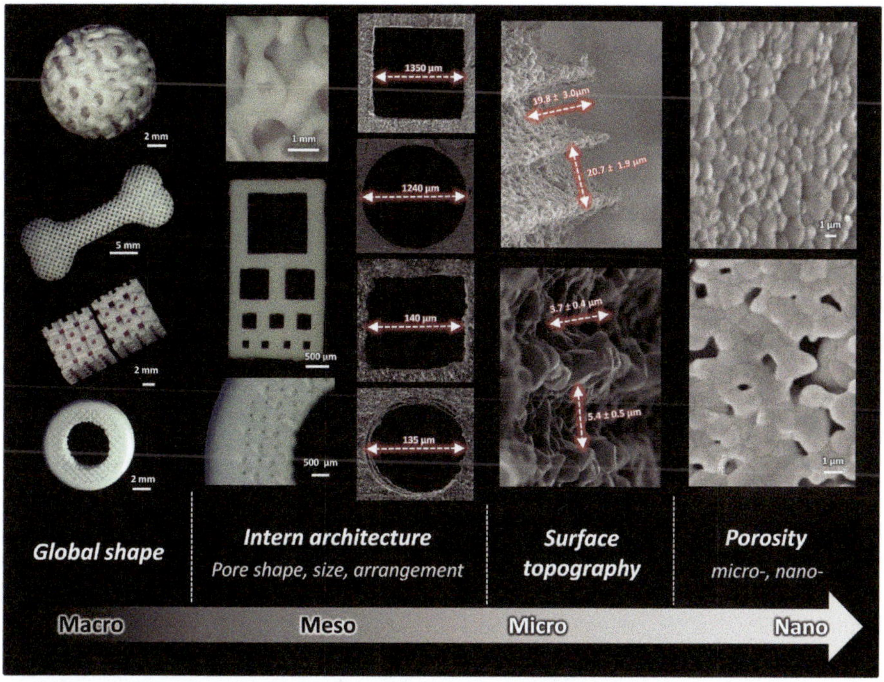


**Figure 8.8** Examples of porous HA bioceramics produced by impregnation of 3D-printed wax molds highlighting the five levels of architecture that influence the biological response: (1) macroscopic global bioceramic shape, (2) intern architecture, including the porous network, (3) pore size and geometry, (4) surface microtopography, and (5) micro-, submicro-, and nanoporosity. This standardized manufacturing process allows adjustment of the shape and the intern architecture by $\pm 20\ \mu m$ with respect to the CAD model. The smallest achievable frame or shape (i.e., circle or square) is 120 μm, the achievable surface microtopography corresponds to the cusp depth and width of 20–5 μm, and the micro- to nanopore density is controlled by the entire ceramic manufacturing process (e.g., powder synthesis, slurry formulation, sintering step).
*Source*: Reprinted from Charbonnier, B., Laurent, C., Blanc, G., Valfort, O., Marchat, D., 2016a. Porous bioceramics produced by impregnation of 3D-printed wax mold: ceramic architectural control and process limitations. Adv. Eng. Mater. 18:1728–1737 (Charbonnier et al., 2016a), copyright ©2016, with permission from John Wiley & Sons.

random-pore architecture of comparable porosity and pore size (Melchels et al., 2010a). Such triply periodic minimal surfaces are of great interest because they accelerate and improve mass transport as well as penetration of cells and tissues within the porous network. Thus, this type of porous structure can be used for homogeneous cell distribution after seeding in the case of cell-based BTE. Recent in vitro and in vivo evaluations confirmed the growing interest in such structures by the BTE community (Gorgin Karaji et al., 2017; Guillaume et al., 2017; Hara et al., 2016). Moreover, these periodic minimal surfaces can modulate the mechanical properties of scaffolds (Melchels et al., 2010b).

The scaffold is responsible for the temporal support of cells and tissues and must remain mechanically stable until the new bone has fully matured to avoid degeneration of blood vessels and newly formed bone tissue (Yuan et al., 2001). Unfortunately, what helps cell and tissue invasion, i.e., increased porosity, compromises the structural integrity of the biodegradable scaffold (Henkel et al., 2013). Additionally, the degradation rate of a scaffold is a function of its architectural features, or, more accurately, its porous network (including porosity and surface area-to-volume ratio). The higher the macropore surface area-to-volume ratio and permeability, the faster the chemical- and cell-induced degradation (Karageorgiou and Kaplan, 2005; Schaefer et al., 2011). In addition, this degradation rate depends on the implantation site. Thus, a "design strategy" is needed to match the macroporous network of the scaffold with the conflicting balance between support degradation and new bone tissue formation with respect to the bone defect site. One way to achieve scaffolds with specific target properties is to use computational tools to design their structure and AM processes for their production (Giannitelli et al., 2014a) (see below). This strategy has already been implemented to optimize scaffold design for mass transportation (Truscello et al., 2012), mechanical loading (Bormann et al., 2014; Wieding et al., 2014), or both (Hollister and Lin, 2007; Dias et al., 2014), as well as for scaffold degradation (Heljak et al., 2012; Bohner and Baumgart, 2004).

For many years, research has focused exclusively on the "optimal pore size," although this feature is insufficient for defining heterogeneous porosity (Bohner et al., 2011). In 2007, Rumpler et al. were the first to show that macropore geometry, i.e., "curvature," can modulate cell-network formation and tissue growth (Rumpler et al., 2007). The same team confirmed this fundamental discovery with in vitro and in silico experiments and proposed geometric models that explain the shape dependence of growth in terms of tension and local curvature (Bidan et al., 2012, 2013a,b, 2016; Dunlop et al., 2010; Gamsjäger et al., 2013; Guyot et al., 2014; Rumpler et al., 2008). In vitro studies proved that the substrate geometry promoted mineralization (Bianchi et al., 2014) and osteogenesis, whereas osteoblast differentiation is promoted by angular structures (Juignet et al., 2017). In Juignet et al., the substrate geometry is not defined in terms of the geometric concept of "curvature" but with the "macroscopic closure" of an angle. Indeed, curvature is inadequate to characterize angular designs as triangles. As with "pore size," one geometrical dimension is not enough for deciphering the link between the architectural features of the scaffold and cell response (Bohner et al., 2011); more geometrical dimensions are needed (Ashworth et al., 2014; Olson, 2011). In vivo tissue growth is considerably greater on concave surfaces than on convex and planar surfaces (Ripamonti et al., 2011, 2012), and pore geometry affects blood vessel guidance and angioconductive potential (Magnaudeix et al., 2016; Scarano et al., 2014). In conclusion, accurate control of macropore geometry (e.g., curvature, angle of closure) can positively affect the rate of bone tissue regeneration by promoting osteogenesis and angiogenesis.

Surface microtopography and micropores are both surface structures on a micrometer scale and are often mistaken for each other (see Fig. 8.8). Both can be randomized or ordered, but ordered ones are still difficult to obtain at the inner surface of a bioceramic scaffold.

In addition to its key role in protein adsorption and consequent cell adhesion (Samavedi et al., 2013), randomized surface microtopography can induce ectopic osteogenesis (Zhang et al., 2015). Controlling the implant at the submicrometer-scale topography level should permit the slowdown of osteoclastic resorption activity (Costa et al., 2013; Geblinger et al., 2011). However, equivalent in vitro studies performed on titanium (Nagasawa et al., 2016) and HA (Gomi et al., 1993) disks showed the opposite result. The study by Costa et al. (2013) raised the question: is the behavior of rat calvarial osteoblasts and osteoclasts isolated from long bone of rabbits, both seeded on polycaprolactone discs with various biomimetic HA coatings, induced by surface roughness or a change in surface chemistry?

Control of the microporosity levels is also important; they were shown to have a significant effect on osseointegration dynamics (Hing et al., 2005). This was recently confirmed in an orthotopic model and is attributed to micropore-induced capillarity (Rustom et al., 2016). However, the main value of this micrometer-scale surface structure to BTE strategies is its well-known "osteoinductive capacity" (Boyan and Schwartz, 2011; Habibovic and de Groot, 2007; Yuan et al., 2010). Indeed, it has been repeatedly proved that submicron pores promote osteoclastogenesis and trigger ectopic bone formation in macroporous β-TCP and BCP bioceramics (Davison et al., 2014a,b,c, 2015; Yuan et al., 1998, 2010; Zhang et al., 2014, 2017).

A patient-specific approach to CaP bioceramic scaffolds means the use of new developments in engineering that combine computational methods and AM technologies. There are various AM methods for manufacturing CaP bioceramics (see Chapter 14: Advanced processing techniques for customized ceramic medical devices) (Bose et al., 2013b; Do et al., 2015; Kumar et al., 2016; Trombetta et al., 2017; Zocca et al., 2015). Each method imposes its own technical limitations on the final architectural features of the ceramic, e.g., the arrangement of rods for robocasting (Carrel et al., 2016), deviations in architecture and composition for laser-based machines such as selective or cladding system (Colin et al., 2014; Comesaña et al., 2015; Shuai et al., 2013), or architectural limitations with respect to 3D printing (accuracy of deposition, depowdering (Butscher et al., 2013a,b; Kumar et al., 2016)). Combined AM approaches are also possible (Giannitelli et al., 2015). Just as there is no one scaffold material for the treatment of all pathologies that involve a large bone defect (see Section 8.3.1), there is no one AM process that applies to all proposals and scopes. With respect to the use of AM in BTE, the clear in vitro and in vivo differences in tissue growth, osteogenesis, and angiogenesis (Bidan et al., 2012; Juignet et al., 2017; Ripamonti et al., 2011) between concave and convex surfaces show that scaffolds composed of rods are not adequate for BTE applications (Gariboldi and Best, 2015). Therefore, manufacturing processes that use extrusion of pasty materials (e.g., robocasting) (Carrel et al., 2016; Do et al., 2015; Jakus et al., 2016; Rustom et al., 2016; Trombetta et al., 2017) or lattice structures developed for aerospace applications (Murr, 2016; Van Bael et al., 2012; Zhang et al., 2017) may not be very appropriate for ceramic-based tissue engineering strategies.

## 8.4 Concluding remarks

The first generation of inert ceramics, successfully used for more than 50 years in load-bearing applications, e.g., alumina in total hip prosthetics, led to the development of the second generation of bioactive CaP ceramics, which have been used since the late 1980s as a substitution for bone grafts in the repair or regeneration of small bone defects. However, the treatment of critical size defects, especially in load-bearing regions, currently remains without a satisfactory solution. Numerous issues must be overcome to successfully produce a new generation of bioceramic-based devices for the treatment of these pathologies. Implants that provide a real healthcare response are relevant to the BTE strategy and should be associated with a new paradigm for ceramic scaffolds. This implies that a personalized approach to a pathology is needed to help adjust the treatment. The important parameters of scaffold design include the physicochemical and architectural features of the scaffold at microscopic and macroscopic levels, and both features must be defined for the bone defect site where the cell mechanics and cell growth will occur. Thus, a biologically instructive design rather than a design based on mimicking bone tissue properties must be used. A combination of versatile AM technologies and CAD/CAM constitutes a powerful new way of fabricating ceramic devices, which is very important for the production of customized "bioinstructive" ceramic scaffolds.

## References

Ahlhelm, M., Günther, P., Scheithauer, U., Schwarzer, E., Günther, A., Slawik, T., et al., 2016. Innovative and novel manufacturing methods of ceramics and metal-ceramic composites for biomedical applications. J. Eur. Ceram. Soc. 36, 2883–2888.

Alghazali, K.M., Nima, Z.A., Hamzah, R.N., Dhar, M.S., Anderson, D.E., Biris, A.S., 2015. Bone-tissue engineering: complex tunable structural and biological responses to injury, drug delivery, and cell-based therapies. Drug. Metab. Rev. 47, 431–454.

Alvarez, K., Nakajima, H., 2009. Metallic scaffolds for bone regeneration. Materials. 2, 790–832.

Ashworth, J., Best, S., Cameron, R., 2014. Quantitative architectural description of tissue engineering scaffolds. Mater. Technol. 29, 281–295.

Bang, L., Long, B., Othman, R., 2014. Carbonate hydroxyapatite and silicon-substituted carbonate hydroxyapatite: synthesis, mechanical properties, and solubility evaluations. Sci. World J. 2014, Article ID 969876, 9 pages.

Bang, L., Ramesh, S., Purbolaksono, J., Ching, Y., Long, B., Chandran, H., et al., 2015. Effects of silicate and carbonate substitution on the properties of hydroxyapatite prepared by aqueous co-precipitation method. Mater. Des. 87, 788–796.

Barradas, A., Yuan, H., Blitterswijk, C.A., Habibovic, P., 2011. Osteoinductive biomaterials: current knowledge of properties, experimental models and biological mechanisms. Eur. Cell. Mater. 21, 407–429.

Barralet, J., Akao, M., Aoki, H., Aoki, H., 2000a. Dissolution of dense carbonate apatite subcutaneously implanted in Wistar rats. J. Biomed. Mater. Res. 49, 176–182.

Barralet, J.E., Best, S.M., Bonfield, W., 2000b. Effect of sintering parameters on the density and microstructure of carbonate hydroxyapatite. J. Mater. Sci. Mater. Med. 11, 719–724.

Barrère, F., Van Blitterswijk, C.A., De Groot, K., 2006. Bone regeneration: molecular and cellular interactions with calcium phosphate ceramics. Int. J. Nanomed. 1, 317.

Becquart, P., Cambon-Binder, A., Monfoulet, L.-E., Bourguignon, M., Vandamme, K., Bensidhoum, M., et al., 2012. Ischemia is the prime but not the only cause of human multipotent stromal cell death in tissue-engineered constructs in vivo. Tissue. Eng. Part. A. 18, 2084–2094.

Best, S.M., Porter, A.E., Thian, E.S., Huang, J., 2008. Bioceramics: past, present and for the future. J. Eur. Ceram. Soc. 28, 1319–1327.

Bianchi, M., Edreira, E.R.U., Wolke, J.G., Birgani, Z.T., Habibovic, P., Jansen, J.A., et al., 2014. Substrate geometry directs the in vitro mineralization of calcium phosphate ceramics. Acta. Biomater. 10, 661–669.

Bidan, C.M., Kollmannsberger, P., Gering, V., Ehrig, S., Joly, P., Petersen, A., et al., 2016. Gradual conversion of cellular stress patterns into pre-stressed matrix architecture during in vitro tissue growth. J. Royal Soc. Interface. 13, 20160136.

Bidan, C.M., Kommareddy, K.P., Rumpler, M., Kollmannsberger, P., Bréchet, Y.J.M., Fratzl, P., et al., 2012. How linear tension converts to curvature: geometric control of bone tissue growth. PLoS One. 7, e36336.

Bidan, C.M., Kommareddy, K.P., Rumpler, M., Kollmannsberger, P., Fratzl, P., Dunlop, J.W. C., 2013a. Geometry as a factor for tissue growth: towards shape optimization of tissue engineering scaffolds. Adv. Healthcare Mater. 2, 186–194.

Bidan, C.M., Wang, F.M., Dunlop, J.W., 2013b. A three-dimensional model for tissue deposition on complex surfaces. Comput. Methods. Biomech. Biomed. Engin. 16, 1056–1070.

Bigham-Sadegh, A., Oryan, A., 2015. Selection of animal models for pre-clinical strategies in evaluating the fracture healing, bone graft substitutes and bone tissue regeneration and engineering. Connect. Tissue. Res. 56, 175–194.

Bohner, M., Baumgart, F., 2004. Theoretical model to determine the effects of geometrical factors on the resorption of calcium phosphate bone substitutes. Biomaterials. 25, 3569–3582.

Bohner, M., Loosli, Y., Baroud, G., Lacroix, D., 2011. Commentary: deciphering the link between architecture and biological response of a bone graft substitute. Acta Biomater. 7, 478–484.

Bormann, T., Schulz, G., Deyhle, H., Beckmann, F., De Wild, M., Kuffer, J., et al., 2014. Combining micro computed tomography and three-dimensional registration to evaluate local strains in shape memory scaffolds. Acta Biomater. 10, 1024–1034.

Bose, S., Fielding, G., Tarafder, S., Bandyopadhyay, A., 2013a. Understanding of dopant-induced osteogenesis and angiogenesis in calcium phosphate ceramics. Trends Biotechnol. 31, 594–605.

Bose, S., Roy, M., Bandyopadhyay, A., 2012. Recent advances in bone tissue engineering scaffolds. Trends Biotechnol. 30, 546–554.

Bose, S., Tarafder, S., 2012. Calcium phosphate ceramic systems in growth factor and drug delivery for bone tissue engineering: a review. Acta Biomater. 8, 1401–1421.

Bose, S., Vahabzadeh, S., Bandyopadhyay, A., 2013b. Bone tissue engineering using 3D printing. Mater. Today. 16, 496–504.

Bouët, G., Marchat, D., Cruel, M., Malaval, L., Vico, L., 2014. In vitro three-dimensional bone tissue models: from cells to controlled and dynamic environment. Tissue Eng. Part B: Rev. 21, 133–156.

Boyan, B.D., Schwartz, Z., 2011. Regenerative medicine: are calcium phosphate ceramics' smart'biomaterials? Nat. Rev. Rheumatol. 7, 8–9.

Brockes, J.P., Gates, P.B., 2014. Mechanisms Underlying Vertebrate Limb Regeneration: lessons from the Salamander. Biochem. Soc. Trans. 42 (3), 625–630, Portland Press Limited.

Bueno, E.M., Glowacki, J., 2009. Cell-free and cell-based approaches for bone regeneration. Nat. Rev. Rheumatol. 5, 685–697.

Butscher, A., Bohner, M., Doebelin, N., Galea, L., Loeffel, O., Müller, R., 2013a. Moisture based three-dimensional printing of calcium phosphate structures for scaffold engineering. Acta Biomater. 9, 5369–5378.

Butscher, A., Bohner, M., Doebelin, N., Hofmann, S., Müller, R., 2013b. New depowdering-friendly designs for three-dimensional printing of calcium phosphate bone substitutes. Acta Biomater. 9, 9149–9158.

Camaioni, A., Cacciotti, I., Campagnolo, L., Bianco, A., 2015. Silicon substituted hydroxyapatite for biomedical applications. Hydroxyapatite for Biomedical Applications. Elsevier Ltd, United Kingdom, pp. 343–373.

Campana, V., Milano, G., Pagano, E., Barba, M., Cicione, C., Salonna, G., et al., 2014. Bone substitutes in orthopaedic surgery: from basic science to clinical practice. J. Mater. Sci. Mater. Med. 25, 2445–2461.

Caplan, A.I., 1991. Mesenchymal stem cells. J. Orthop. Res. 9, 641–650.

Carragee, E.J., Hurwitz, E.L., Weiner, B.K., 2011. A critical review of recombinant human bone morphogenetic protein-2 trials in spinal surgery: emerging safety concerns and lessons learned. Spine J. 11, 471–491.

Carrel, J.P., Wiskott, A., Moussa, M., Rieder, P., Scherrer, S., Durual, S., 2016. A 3D printed TCP/HA structure as a new osteoconductive scaffold for vertical bone augmentation. Clin. Oral. Implants. Res. 27, 55–62.

Chai, Y.C., Carlier, A., Bolander, J., Roberts, S.J., Geris, L., Schrooten, J., et al., 2012. Current views on calcium phosphate osteogenicity and the translation into effective bone regeneration strategies. Acta Biomater. 8, 3876–3887.

Charbonnier, B., Laurent, C., Blanc, G., Valfort, O., Marchat, D., 2016a. Porous bioceramics produced by impregnation of 3D-printed wax mold: ceramic architectural control and process limitations. Adv. Eng. Mater. 18, 1728–1737.

Chatzinikolaidou, M., Lichtinger, T., Müller, R., Jennissen, H., 2010. Peri-implant reactivity and osteoinductive potential of immobilized rhBMP-2 on titanium carriers. Acta. Biomater. 6, 4405–4421.

Clark, E.R., Clark, E.L., 1939. Microscopic observations on the growth of blood capillaries in the living mammal. Am. J. Anat. 64, 251–301.

Clausen, A., Aage, N., Sigmund, O., 2016. Exploiting additive manufacturing infill in topology optimization for improved buckling load. Engineering. 2, 250–257.

Colin, C., Bartout, J.-D., Shaker, E., Marchat, D., Nimal, D., 2014. Selective laser melting process. Google Patents.

Collins, K., Gates, E., Gilchrist, C., Hoffman, B., 2016. Bio-Instructive Cues. Scaffolds for Musculoskeletal Tissue Engineering and Regenerative Medicine1.

Comesaña, R., Lusquiños, F., Del Val, J., Quintero, F., Riveiro, A., Boutinguiza, M., et al., 2015. Toward smart implant synthesis: bonding bioceramics of different resorbability to match bone growth rates. Sci. Rep.5.

Costa, D.O., Prowse, P.D., Chrones, T., Sims, S.M., Hamilton, D.W., Rizkalla, A.S., et al., 2013. The differential regulation of osteoblast and osteoclast activity by surface topography of hydroxyapatite coatings. Biomaterials. 34, 7215–7226.

Daculsi, G., 1998. Biphasic calcium phosphate concept applied to artificial bone, implant coating and injectable bone substitute. Biomaterials. 19, 1473–1478.

Danciu, T.E., Adam, R.M., Naruse, K., Freeman, M.R., Hauschka, P.V., 2003. Calcium regulates the PI3K-Akt pathway in stretched osteoblasts. FEBS Lett. 536, 193–197.

Das, A., Botchwey, E., 2011. Evaluation of angiogenesis and osteogenesis. Tissue Eng. Part B: Rev. 17, 403–414.

Das, R., Jahr, H., Van Osch, G.J., Farrell, E., 2009. The role of hypoxia in bone marrow–derived mesenchymal stem cells: considerations for regenerative medicine approaches. Tissue Eng. Part B: Rev. 16, 159–168.

Davison, N., Luo, X., Schoenmaker, T., Everts, V., Yuan, H., Barrere-De Groot, F., et al., 2014a. Submicron-scale surface architecture of tricalcium phosphate directs osteogenesis in vitro and in vivo. Eur. Cell. Mater. 27, 281–297.

Davison, N., Su, J., Yuan, H., Van Den Beucken, J., De Bruijn, J., Barrere-De Groot, F., 2015. Influence of surface microstructure and chemistry on osteoinduction and osteoclastogenesis by biphasic calcium phosphate discs. Eur. Cell. Mater. 29, 314–329.

Davison, N.L., Gamblin, A.-L., Layrolle, P., Yuan, H., De Bruijn, J.D., Barrère-De Groot, F., 2014b. Liposomal clodronate inhibition of osteoclastogenesis and osteoinduction by submicrostructured beta-tricalcium phosphate. Biomaterials. 35, 5088–5097.

Davison, N.L., Ten Harkel, B., Schoenmaker, T., Luo, X., Yuan, H., Everts, V., et al., 2014c. Osteoclast resorption of beta-tricalcium phosphate controlled by surface architecture. Biomaterials. 35, 7441–7451.

Demiralp, B., Ege, T., Kose, O., Yurttas, Y., Basbozkurt, M., 2014. Reconstruction of intercalary bone defects following bone tumor resection with segmental bone transport using an Ilizarov circular external fixator. J. Orthop. Sci. 19, 1004–1011.

Deschepper, M., Oudina, K., David, B., Myrtil, V., Collet, C., Bensidhoum, M., et al., 2011. Survival and function of mesenchymal stem cells (MSCs) depend on glucose to overcome exposure to long-term, severe and continuous hypoxia. J. Cell. Mol. Med. 15, 1505–1514.

Detsch, R., Mayr, H., Ziegler, G., 2008. Formation of osteoclast-like cells on HA and TCP ceramics. Acta Biomater. 4, 139–148.

Deville, S., Saiz, E., Tomsia, A.P., 2006. Freeze casting of hydroxyapatite scaffolds for bone tissue engineering. Biomaterials. 27, 5480–5489.

Di Luca, A., Ostrowska, B., Lorenzo-Moldero, I., Lepedda, A., Swieszkowski, W., Van Blitterswijk, C., et al., 2016. Gradients in pore size enhance the osteogenic differentiation of human mesenchymal stromal cells in three-dimensional scaffolds. Sci. Rep.6.

Dias, M.R., Guedes, J.M., Flanagan, C.L., Hollister, S.J., Fernandes, P.R., 2014. Optimization of scaffold design for bone tissue engineering: a computational and experimental study. Med. Eng. Phys. 36, 448–457.

Dimitriou, R., Jones, E., Mcgonagle, D., Giannoudis, P.V., 2011. Bone regeneration: current concepts and future directions. BMC. Med. 9, 66.

Do, A.V., Khorsand, B., Geary, S.M., Salem, A.K., 2015. 3D printing of scaffolds for tissue regeneration applications. Adv. Healthcare Mater. 4, 1742–1762.

Döbelin, N., Luginbühl, R., Bohner, M., 2010. Synthetic calcium phosphate ceramics for treatment of bone fractures. CHIMIA Inter. J. Chem. 64, 723–729.

Doi, Y., Shibutani, T., Moriwaki, Y., Kajimoto, T., Iwayama, Y., 1998. Sintered carbonate apatites as bioresorbable bone substitutes. J. Biomed. Mater. Res. 39, 603–610.

Dunlop, J., Fischer, F., Gamsjäger, E., Fratzl, P., 2010. A theoretical model for tissue growth in confined geometries. J. Mech. Phys. Solids. 58, 1073–1087.

Einhorn, T.A., Gerstenfeld, L.C., 2015. Fracture healing: mechanisms and interventions. Nat. Rev. Rheumatol. 11, 45–54.

Ejtehadifar, M., Shamsasenjan, K., Movassaghpour, A., Akbarzadehlaleh, P., Dehdilani, N., Abbasi, P., et al., 2015. The effect of hypoxia on mesenchymal stem cell biology. Adv. Pharmaceut. Bull. 5, 141.

Elliott, J.C., 1994. Structure and Chemistry of the Apatites and Other Calcium Orthophosphates. Amsterdam, Elsevier, Studies in Organic Chemistry.

Entezari, A., Roohani-Esfahani, S.-I., Zhang, Z., Zreiqat, H., Dunstan, C.R., Li, Q., 2016. Fracture behaviors of ceramic tissue scaffolds for load bearing applications. Sci. Rep.6.

Eweida, A.M., Nabawi, A.S., Marei, M.K., Khalil, M.R., Elhammady, H.A., 2011. Mandibular reconstruction using an axially vascularized tissue-engineered construct. Ann. Surg. Innov. Res. 5, 2.

Farris, A.L., Rindone, A.N., Grayson, W.L., 2016. Oxygen delivering biomaterials for tissue engineering. J. Mater. Chem.. B. 4, 3422–3432.

Fernandez-Yague, M.A., Abbah, S.A., Mcnamara, L., Zeugolis, D.I., Pandit, A., Biggs, M.J., 2015. Biomimetic approaches in bone tissue engineering: integrating biological and physicomechanical strategies. Adv. Drug. Deliv. Rev. 84, 1–29.

Ferraro, J.W., 1979. Experimental evaluation of ceramic calcium phosphate as a substitute for bone grafts. Plast. Reconstr. Surg. 63, 634–640.

Fu, Q., Rahaman, M.N., Bal, B.S., Brown, R.F., 2009. Proliferation and function of MC3T3-E1 cells on freeze-cast hydroxyapatite scaffolds with oriented pore architectures. J. Mater. Sci. Mater. Med. 20, 1159–1165.

Gamblin, A.-L., Brennan, M.A., Renaud, A., Yagita, H., Lézot, F., Heymann, D., et al., 2014. Bone tissue formation with human mesenchymal stem cells and biphasic calcium phosphate ceramics: the local implication of osteoclasts and macrophages. Biomaterials. 35, 9660–9667.

Gamsjäger, E., Bidan, C., Fischer, F., Fratzl, P., Dunlop, J., 2013. Modelling the role of surface stress on the kinetics of tissue growth in confined geometries. Acta Biomater. 9, 5531–5543.

Gariboldi, M.I., Best, S.M., 2015. Effect of ceramic scaffold architectural parameters on biological response. Front. Bioeng. Biotechnol. 3, 151.

Garrido, C.A., Lobo, S.E., Turíbio, F.M., Legeros, R.Z., 2011. Biphasic calcium phosphate bioceramics for orthopaedic reconstructions: clinical outcomes. Inter. J. Biomater. 2011, 129727.

Geblinger, D., Zink, C., Spencer, N.D., Addadi, L., Geiger, B., 2011. Effects of surface microtopography on the assembly of the osteoclast resorption apparatus. J. Royal Soc. Interface. Available from: http://dx.doi.org/10.1098/rsif20110659.

Giannitelli, S., Accoto, D., Trombetta, M., Rainer, A., 2014a. Current trends in the design of scaffolds for computer-aided tissue engineering. Acta Biomater. 10, 580–594.

Giannitelli, S., Mozetic, P., Trombetta, M., Rainer, A., 2015. Combined additive manufacturing approaches in tissue engineering. Acta Biomater. 24, 1–11.

Giannitelli, S.M., Accoto, D., Trombetta, M., Rainer, A., 2014b. Current trends in the design of scaffolds for computer-aided tissue engineering. Acta Biomater. 10, 580–594.

Giannoudis, P.V., Einhorn, T.A., Marsh, D., 2007. Fracture healing: the diamond concept. Injury. 38, S3–S6.

Giannoudis, P.V., Einhorn, T.A., Schmidmaier, G., Marsh, D., 2008. The diamond concept—open questions. Injury. 39, S5–S8.

Glatt, V.G., Evans, C., Tetsworth, K., 2016. A concert between biology and biomechanics: the influence of the mechanical environment on bone healing. Front. Physiol. 7, 678.

Gomi, K., Lowenberg, B., Shapiro, G., Davies, J., 1993. Resorption of sintered synthetic hydroxyapatite by osteoclasts in vitro. Biomaterials. 14, 91–96.
Gorgin Karaji, Z., Speirs, M., Dadbakhsh, S., Kruth, J.-P., Weinans, H., Zadpoor, A.A., et al., 2017. Additively Manufactured and Surface Biofunctionalized Porous Nitinol. ACS Appl. Mater. Interfaces. 9, 1293–1304.
Grayson, W.L., Bunnell, B.A., Martin, E., Frazier, T., Hung, B.P., Gimble, J.M., 2015. Stromal cells and stem cells in clinical bone regeneration. Nat. Rev. Endocrinol. 11, 140–150.
Grayson, W.L., Vunjak-Novakovic, G., Obradovic, B., 2012. Bioreactors in tissue engineering. In: Obradović, B. (Ed.), Cell and Tissue Engineering. Springer Berlin Heidelberg, Belgrade, Serbia, p. 217.
Guillaume, O., Geven, M., Sprecher, C., Stadelmann, V., Grijpma, D., Tang, T., et al., 2017. Surface-enrichment with hydroxyapatite nanoparticles in stereolithography-fabricated composite polymer scaffolds promotes bone repair. Acta Biomater. 54, 386–398.
Guyot, Y., Papantoniou, I., Chai, Y.C., Van Bael, S., Schrooten, J., Geris, L., 2014. A computational model for cell/ECM growth on 3D surfaces using the level set method: a bone tissue engineering case study. Biomech. Model. Mechanobiol. 13, 1361–1371.
Habibovic, P., De Groot, K., 2007. Osteoinductive biomaterials—properties and relevance in bone repair. J. Tissue. Eng. Regen. Med. 1, 25–32.
Habibovic, P., Juhl, M.V., Clyens, S., Martinetti, R., Dolcini, L., Theilgaard, N., et al., 2010. Comparison of two carbonated apatite ceramics in vivo. Acta Biomater. 6, 2219–2226.
Habibovic, P., Kruyt, M.C., Juhl, M.V., Clyens, S., Martinetti, R., Dolcini, L., et al., 2008. Comparative in vivo study of six hydroxyapatite-based bone graft substitutes. J. Orthop. Res. 26, 1363–1370.
Habraken, W., Habibovic, P., Epple, M., Bohner, M., 2016. Calcium phosphates in biomedical applications: materials for the future? Mater. Today. 19, 69–87.
Halouani, R., Bernache-Assolant, D., Champion, E., Ababou, A., 1994. Microstructure and related mechanical properties of hot pressed hydroxyapatite ceramics. J. Mater. Sci. Mater. Med. 5, 563–568.
Hara, D., Nakashima, Y., Sato, T., Hirata, M., Kanazawa, M., Kohno, Y., et al., 2016. Bone bonding strength of diamond-structured porous titanium-alloy implants manufactured using the electron beam-melting technique. Mater. Sci. Eng. C. 59, 1047–1052.
Hashimoto, R., Raich, A., Yoder, E., Mcmullen, K., Dettori, J., 2012. On-and Off-Label Uses of rhBMP-2 or rhBMP-7 for Spinal Fusion. Washington State Health Care Authority, Olympia, WA.
Heljak, M.K., Swieszkowski, W., Lam, C.X.F., Hutmacher, D.W., Kurzydlowski, K.J., 2012. Evolutionary design of bone scaffolds with reference to material selection. Int. J. Num. Methods Biomed. Eng. 28, 789–800.
Henkel, J., Woodruff, M.A., Epari, D.R., Steck, R., Glatt, V., Dickinson, I.C., et al., 2013. Bone regeneration based on tissue engineering conceptions—a 21st century perspective. Bone Res. 1, 216–248.
Hing, K.A., Annaz, B., Saeed, S., Revell, P.A., Buckland, T., 2005. Microporosity enhances bioactivity of synthetic bone graft substitutes. J. Mater. Sci. Mater. Med. 16, 467–475.
Hing, K.A., Best, S.M., Tanner, K.E., Bonfield, W., Revell, P.A., 2004. Mediation of bone ingrowth in porous hydroxyapatite bone graft substitutes. J. Biomed. Mater. Res. A. 68, 187–200.
Hing, K.A., Wilson, L.F., Buckland, T., 2007. Comparative performance of three ceramic bone graft substitutes. Spine J. 7, 475–490.
Hollister, S.J., 2009a. Scaffold design and manufacturing: from concept to clinic. Adv. Mater. 21, 3330–3342.

Hollister, S.J., 2009b. Scaffold engineering: a bridge to where? Biofabrication. 1, 012001.

Hollister, S.J., Lin, C.Y., 2007. Computational design of tissue engineering scaffolds. Comp. Methods Appl. Mech. Eng. 196, 2991–2998.

Hollister, S.J., Maddox, R., Taboas, J.M., 2002. Optimal design and fabrication of scaffolds to mimic tissue properties and satisfy biological constraints. Biomaterials. 23, 4095–4103.

Hughes, J.M., Rakovan, J., 2002. The crystal structure of apatite, Ca5 (PO4) 3 (F, OH, Cl). Rev. Mineral. Geochem. 48, 1–12.

Jakus, A.E., Rutz, A.L., Jordan, S.W., Kannan, A., Mitchell, S.M., Yun, C., et al., 2016. Hyperelastic "bone": a highly versatile, growth factor–free, osteoregenerative, scalable, and surgically friendly biomaterial. Sci. Transl. Med. 8, 358ra127.

Johnson, A.J.W., Herschler, B.A., 2011. A review of the mechanical behavior of CaP and CaP/polymer composites for applications in bone replacement and repair. Acta Biomater. 7, 16–30.

Juignet, L., Charbonnier, B., Dumas, V., Bouleftour, W., Thomas, M., Laurent, C., et al., 2017. Macrotopographic closure promotes tissue growth and osteogenesis in vitro. Acta Biomater. 53, 536–548.

Jun, I.-K., Koh, Y.-H., Lee, S.-H., Kim, H.-E., 2007. Novel hydroxyapatite (HA) dual-scaffold with ultra-high porosity, high surface area, and compressive strength. J. Mater. Sci. Mater. Med. 18, 1071–1077.

Jung, J.W., Yi, H.-G., Kang, T.-Y., Yong, W.-J., Jin, S., Yun, W.-S., et al., 2013. Evaluation of the effective diffusivity of a freeform fabricated scaffold using computational simulation. J. Biomech. Eng. 135, 084501.

Kapfer, S.C., Hyde, S.T., Mecke, K., Arns, C.H., Schröder-Turk, G.E., 2011. Minimal surface scaffold designs for tissue engineering. Biomaterials. 32, 6875–6882.

Karageorgiou, V., Kaplan, D., 2005. Porosity of 3D biomaterial scaffolds and osteogenesis. Biomaterials. 26, 5474–5491.

Klar, R.M., Duarte, R., Dix-Peek, T., Dickens, C., Ferretti, C., Ripamonti, U., 2013. Calcium ions and osteoclastogenesis initiate the induction of bone formation by coral-derived macroporous constructs. J. Cell. Mol. Med. 17, 1444–1457.

Krishnakanth, P., 2012. Mechanical Considerations in Fracture Fixation. Queensland University of Technology, Brisbane.

Kumar, A., Godwin, J.W., Gates, P.B., Garza-Garcia, A.A., Brockes, J.P., 2007. Molecular basis for the nerve dependence of limb regeneration in an adult vertebrate. Science. 318, 772–777.

Kumar, A., Mandal, S., Barui, S., Vasireddi, R., Gbureck, U., Gelinsky, M., et al., 2016. Low temperature additive manufacturing of three dimensional scaffolds for bone-tissue engineering applications: processing related challenges and property assessment. Mater. Sci. Eng. R: Rep. 103, 1–39.

Lafon, J.P., Champion, E., Bernache-Assollant, D., 2008. Processing of AB-type carbonated hydroxyapatite Ca10-x(PO4)6-x(CO3)x(OH)2-x-2y(CO3)y ceramics with controlled composition. J. Eur. Ceram. Soc. 28, 139–147.

Lam, C.X., Savalani, M.M., Teoh, S.-H., Hutmacher, D.W., 2008. Dynamics of in vitro polymer degradation of polycaprolactone-based scaffolds: accelerated versus simulated physiological conditions. Biomed. Mater. 3, 034108.

Landi, E., Celotti, G., Logroscino, G., Tampieri, A., 2003. Carbonated hydroxyapatite as bone substitute. J. Eur. Ceram. Soc. 23, 2931–2937.

Landi, E., Uggeri, J., Sprio, S., Tampieri, A., Guizzardi, S., 2010. Human osteoblast behavior on as-synthesized SiO4 and B-CO3 co-substituted apatite. J. Biomed. Mater. Res. A. 94A, 59–70.

Lau, K.H., Kapur, S., Kesavan, C., Baylink, D.J., 2006. Up-regulation of the Wnt, estrogen receptor, insulin-like growth factor-I, and bone morphogenetic protein pathways in C57BL/6J osteoblasts as opposed to C3H/HeJ osteoblasts in part contributes to the differential anabolic response to fluid shear. J. Biol. Chem. 281, 9576–9588.

Legeros, R.Z., 2008. Calcium phosphate-based osteoinductive materials. Chem. Rev. 108, 4742–4753.

Li, Y., Chen, S.-K., Li, L., Qin, L., Wang, X.-L., Lai, Y.-X., 2015. Bone defect animal models for testing efficacy of bone substitute biomaterials. J. Orthop. Transl. 3, 95–104.

Libonati, F., Vergani, L., 2016. Understanding the structure–property relationship in cortical bone to design a biomimetic composite. Compos. Struct. 139, 188–198.

Liu, S., Zhou, J., Zhang, X., Liu, Y., Chen, J., Hu, B., et al., 2016. Strategies to optimize adult stem cell therapy for tissue regeneration. Int. J. Mol. Sci. 17, 982.

Liu, T., Zheng, Y., Wu, G., Wismeijer, D., Pathak, J.L., Liu, Y., 2017. BMP2-coprecipitated calcium phosphate granules enhance osteoinductivity of deproteinized bovine bone, and bone formation during critical-sized bone defect healing. Sci. Rep.7.

Liu, Y., Chan, J.K., Teoh, S.H., 2015. Review of vascularised bone tissue-engineering strategies with a focus on co-culture systems. J. Tissue. Eng. Regen. Med. 9, 85–105.

Liu, Y., Hunziker, E.B., Layrolle, P., De Bruijn, J.D., De Groot, K., 2004. Bone morphogenetic protein 2 incorporated into biomimetic coatings retains its biological activity. Tiss. Eng. 10, 101–108.

Luo, F., Hou, T.-Y., Zhang, Z.-H., Xie, Z., Wu, X.-H., Xu, J.-Z., 2013. Effects of initial cell density and hydrodynamic culture on osteogenic activity of tissue-engineered bone grafts. PLoS One. 8, e53697.

Ma, J., Both, S.K., Yang, F., Cui, F.-Z., Pan, J., Meijer, G.J., et al., 2014. Concise review: cell-based strategies in bone tissue engineering and regenerative medicine. Stem Cells Transl. Med. 3, 98–107.

Magnaudeix, A., Usseglio, J., Lasgorceix, M., Lalloue, F., Damia, C., Brie, J., et al., 2016. Quantitative analysis of vascular colonisation and angio-conduction in porous silicon-substituted hydroxyapatite with various pore shapes in a chick chorioallantoic membrane (CAM) model. Acta Biomater. 38, 179–189.

Marino, J.T., Ziran, B.H., 2010. Use of solid and cancellous autologous bone graft for fractures and nonunions. Orthop. Clin. North Am. 41, 15–26.

Masquelet, A.C., Begue, T., 2010. The concept of induced membrane for reconstruction of long bone defects. Orthop. Clin. North Am. 41, 27–37.

Matassi, F., Nistri, L., Paez, D.C., Innocenti, M., 2011. New biomaterials for bone regeneration. Clin. Cases Mineral Bone Metabol. 8, 21–24.

Meijer, G.J., De Bruijn, J.D., Koole, R., Van Blitterswijk, C.A., 2007. Cell-based bone tissue engineering. PLoS Med. 4, e9.

Melchels, F.P., Barradas, A.M., Van Blitterswijk, C.A., De Boer, J., Feijen, J., Grijpma, D. W., 2010a. Effects of the architecture of tissue engineering scaffolds on cell seeding and culturing. Acta Biomater. 6, 4208–4217.

Melchels, F.P., Bertoldi, K., Gabbrielli, R., Velders, A.H., Feijen, J., Grijpma, D.W., 2010b. Mathematically defined tissue engineering scaffold architectures prepared by stereolithography. Biomaterials. 31, 6909–6916.

Melchels, F.P.W., Barradas, A.M.C., Van Blitterswijk, C.A., De Boer, J., Feijen, J., Grijpma, D.W., 2010c. Effects of the architecture of tissue engineering scaffolds on cell seeding and culturing. Acta Biomater. 6, 4208–4217.

Melville, A.J., Harrison, J., Gross, K.A., Forsythe, J.S., Trounson, A.O., Mollard, R., 2006. Mouse embryonic stem cell colonisation of carbonated apatite surfaces. Biomaterials. 27, 615–622.

Mercado, A.E., Ma, J., He, X., Jabbari, E., 2009. Release characteristics and osteogenic activity of recombinant human bone morphogenetic protein-2 grafted to novel self-assembled poly (lactide-co-glycolide fumarate) nanoparticles. J. Control. Release. 140, 148–156.

Meurice, E., Bouchart, F., Hornez, J., Leriche, A., Hautcoeur, D., Lardot, V., et al., 2016. Osteoblastic cells colonization inside beta-TCP macroporous structures obtained by ice-templating. J. Eur. Ceram. Soc. 36, 2895–2901.

Mirzaali, M.J., Schwiedrzik, J.J., Thaiwichai, S., Best, J.P., Michler, J., Zysset, P.K., et al., 2016. Mechanical properties of cortical bone and their relationships with age, gender, composition and microindentation properties in the elderly. Bone. 93, 196–211.

Moutos, F.T., Freed, L.E., Guilak, F., 2007. A biomimetic three-dimensional woven composite scaffold for functional tissue engineering of cartilage. Nat. Mater. 6, 162–167.

Moya, A., Larochette, N., Paquet, J., Deschepper, M., Bensidhoum, M., Izzo, V., et al., 2017. Quiescence Preconditioned Human Multipotent Stromal Cells Adopt a Metabolic Profile Favorable for Enhanced Survival under Ischemia. Stem Cells. 35, 181–196.

Murphy, W.L., Mcdevitt, T.C., Engler, A.J., 2014. Materials as stem cell regulators. Nat. Mater. 13, 547–557.

Murr, L.E., 2016. Frontiers of 3D printing/additive manufacturing: from human organs to aircraft fabrication. J. Mater. Sci. Technol. 32, 987–995.

Nagasawa, M., Cooper, L.F., Ogino, Y., Mendonca, D., Liang, R., Yang, S., et al., 2016. Topography influences adherent cell regulation of osteoclastogenesis. J. Dent. Res. 95, 319–326.

Nishimura, I., 2013. Genetic networks in osseointegration. J. Dent. Res. 92, 109S–118S.

Novaes JR, A.B., Souza, S.L.S.D., Barros, R.R.M.D., Pereira, K.K.Y., Iezzi, G., Piattelli, A., 2010. Influence of implant surfaces on osseointegration. Braz. Dent. J. 21, 471–481.

Olson, E., 2011. Particle shape factors and their use in image analysis-part 1: theory. J. GXP Compl. 15, 85.

Oryan, A., Alidadi, S., Moshiri, A., Bigham-Sadegh, A., 2014. Bone morphogenetic proteins: a powerful osteoinductive compound with non-negligible side effects and limitations. Biofactors. 40, 459–481.

Patel, N., Gibson, I.R., Hing, K.A., Best, S.M., Damien, E., Revell, P.A., et al., 2002. The *in vivo* response of phase pure hydroxyapatite and carbonate substituted hydroxyapaite granules of varying size ranges. Key Eng. Mater. 218-220, 383–386.

Pelissier, P., Masquelet, A., Bareille, R., Pelissier, S.M., Amedee, J., 2004. Induced membranes secrete growth factors including vascular and osteoinductive factors and could stimulate bone regeneration. J. Orthop. Res. 22, 73–79.

Petite, H., Vandamme, K., Monfoulet, L., Logeart-Avramoglou, D., 2011. Strategies for improving the efficacy of bioengineered bone constructs: a perspective. Osteop. Int. 22, 2017–2021.

Petite, H., Viateau, V., Bensaid, W., Meunier, A., De Pollak, C., Bourguignon, M., et al., 2000. Tissue-engineered bone regeneration. Nat. Biotechnol. 18, 959–963.

Pneumaticos, S.G., Triantafyllopoulos, G.K., Basdra, E.K., Papavassiliou, A.G., 2010. Segmental bone defects: from cellular and molecular pathways to the development of novel biological treatments. J. Cell. Mol. Med. 14, 2561–2569.

Porter, A., Patel, N., Brooks, R., Best, S., Rushton, N., Bonfield, W., 2005. Effect of carbonate substitution on the ultrastructural characteristics of hydroxyapatite implants. J. Mater. Sci. Mater. Med. 16, 899–907.

Puppi, D., Chiellini, F., Piras, A., Chiellini, E., 2010. Polymeric materials for bone and cartilage repair. Prog. Polymer Sci. 35, 403–440.

Rajagopalan, S., Robb, R.A., 2006. Schwarz meets Schwann: design and fabrication of biomorphic and durataxic tissue engineering scaffolds. Med. Image. Anal. 10, 693–712.

Ratnayake, J.T., Mucalo, M., Dias, G.J., 2016. Substituted hydroxyapatites for bone regeneration: a review of current trends. J. Biomed. Mater. Res. Part B Appl. Biomater. 20, 7821–7828.

Raynaud, S., Champion, E., Bernache-Assolant, D., Tetard, D., 1998. Dynamic fatigue and degradation in solution of hydroxyapatite ceramics. J. Mater. Sci. Mater. Med. 9, 221–227.

Raynaud, S., Champion, E., Lafon, J.P., Bernache-Assollant, D., 2002. Calcium phosphate apatites with variable Ca/P atomic ratio III. Mechanical properties and degradation in solution of hot pressed ceramics. Biomaterials. 23, 1081–1089.

Reichert, J.C., Cipitria, A., Epari, D.R., Saifzadeh, S., Krishnakanth, P., Berner, A., et al., 2012. A tissue engineering solution for segmental defect regeneration in load-bearing long bones. Sci. Transl. Med. 4, 141ra93.

Reilly, D.T., Burstein, A.H., 1974. The mechanical properties of cortical bone. JBJS. 56, 1001–1022.

Ren, L.-M., Arahira, T., Todo, M., Yoshikawa, H., Myoui, A., 2012. Biomechanical evaluation of porous bioactive ceramics after implantation: micro CT-based three-dimensional finite element analysis. J. Mater. Sci. Mater. Med. 23, 463–472.

Rey, C., Combes, C., Drouet, C., Grossin, D., 2011. Bioactive ceramics: physical chemistry. Comprehen. Biomater. 1, 187–221.

Ripamonti, U., Richter, P., Nilen, R., Renton, L., 2008. The induction of bone formation by smart biphasic hydroxyapatite tricalcium phosphate biomimetic matrices in the non-human primate Papio ursinus. J. Cell. Mol. Med. 12, 2609–2621.

Ripamonti, U., Roden, L.C., Ferretti, C., Klar, R.M., 2011. Biomimetic matrices self-initiating the induction of bone formation. J. Craniof. Surg. 22, 1859–1870.

Ripamonti, U., Roden, L.C., Renton, L.F., 2012. Osteoinductive hydroxyapatite-coated titanium implants. Biomaterials. 33, 3813–3823.

Roohani-Esfahani, S.-I., Newman, P., Zreiqat, H., 2016. Design and fabrication of 3D printed scaffolds with a mechanical strength comparable to cortical bone to repair large bone defects. Sci. Rep.6.

Rumpler, M., Woesz, A., Dunlop, J.W.C., Van Dongen, J.T., Fratzl, P., 2008. The effect of geometry on three-dimensional tissue growth. J. Royal Soc. Interface. 5, 1173–1180.

Rumpler, M., Woesz, A., Varga, F., Manjubala, I., Klaushofer, K., Fratzl, P., 2007. Three-dimensional growth behavior of osteoblasts on biomimetic hydroxylapatite scaffolds. J. Biomed. Mater. Res. A. 81, 40–50.

Rustom, L.E., Boudou, T., Lou, S., Pignot-Paintrand, I., Nemke, B.W., Lu, Y., et al., 2016. Micropore-induced capillarity enhances bone distribution in vivo in biphasic calcium phosphate scaffolds. Acta Biomater. 44, 144–154.

Sabree, I., Gough, J., Derby, B., 2015. Mechanical properties of porous ceramic scaffolds: influence of internal dimensions. Ceram. Int. 41, 8425–8432.

Saito, E., Liu, Y., Migneco, F., Hollister, S.J., 2012. Strut size and surface area effects on long-term in vivo degradation in computer designed poly (L-lactic acid) three-dimensional porous scaffolds. Acta Biomater. 8, 2568–2577.

Saiz, E., Zimmermann, E.A., Lee, J.S., Wegst, U.G., Tomsia, A.P., 2013. Perspectives on the role of nanotechnology in bone tissue engineering. Dent. Mater. 29, 103–115.

Salerno, A., Guarnieri, D., Iannone, M., Zeppetelli, S., Netti, P.A., 2010. Effect of micro- and macroporosity of bone tissue three-dimensional-poly(ε-caprolactone) scaffold on human mesenchymal stem cells invasion, proliferation, and differentiation in vitro. Tissue. Eng. Part. A. 16, 2661–2673.

Samavedi, S., Whittington, A.R., Goldstein, A.S., 2013. Calcium phosphate ceramics in bone tissue engineering: a review of properties and their influence on cell behavior. Acta Biomater. 9, 8037–8045.

Scarano, A., Perrotti, V., Artese, L., Degidi, M., Degidi, D., Piattelli, A., et al., 2014. Blood vessels are concentrated within the implant surface concavities: a histologic study in rabbit tibia. Odontology. 102, 259–266.

Schaefer, S., Detsch, R., Uhl, F., Deisinger, U., Ziegler, G., 2011. How degradation of calcium phosphate bone substitute materials is influenced by phase composition and porosity. Adv. Eng. Mater. 13, 342–350.

Scheiner, S., Komlev, V.S., Hellmich, C., 2016. Strength increase during ceramic biomaterial-induced bone regeneration: a micromechanical study. Int. J. Fract. 202, 217–235.

Schliephake, H., 2015. Clinical efficacy of growth factors to enhance tissue repair in oral and maxillofacial reconstruction: a systematic review. Clin. Implant. Dent. Relat. Res. 17, 247–273.

Schmitt, A., Van Griensven, M., Imhoff, A.B., Buchmann, S., 2012. Application of stem cells in orthopedics. Stem Cells International. 2012, Article ID 394962, 11 pages.

Seebach, C., Schultheiss, J., Wilhelm, K., Frank, J., Henrich, D., 2010. Comparison of six bone-graft substitutes regarding to cell seeding efficiency, metabolism and growth behaviour of human mesenchymal stem cells (MSC) in vitro. Injury. 41, 731–738.

Sela, J.J., Bab, I.A., 2012. Principles of Bone Regeneration. Springer Science & Business Media, Berlin.

Shepherd, J.H., Shepherd, D.V., Best, S.M., 2012. Substituted hydroxyapatites for bone repair. J. Mater. Sci. Mater. Med. 23, 2335–2347.

Shih, Y.-R.V., Hwang, Y., Phadke, A., Kang, H., Hwang, N.S., Caro, E.J., et al., 2014. Calcium phosphate-bearing matrices induce osteogenic differentiation of stem cells through adenosine signaling. Proc. Natl. Acad. Sci. 111, 990–995.

Shuai, C., Li, P., Liu, J., Peng, S., 2013. Optimization of TCP/HAP ratio for better properties of calcium phosphate scaffold via selective laser sintering. Mater. Charact. 77, 23–31.

Spence, G., Patel, N., Brooks, R., Bonfield, W., Rushton, N., 2010. Osteoclastogenesis on hydroxyapatite ceramics: the effect of carbonate substitution. J. Biomed. Mater. Res. A. 92, 1292–1300.

Spence, G., Patel, N., Brooks, R., Rushton, N., 2009. Carbonate substituted hydroxyapatite: resorption by osteoclasts modifies the osteoblastic response. J. Biomed. Mater. Res. A. 90, 217–224.

Spence, G., Phillips, S., Campion, C., Brooks, R., Rushton, N., 2008. Bone formation in a carbonate-substituted hydroxyapatite implant is inhibited by zoledronate: the importance of bioresorption to osteoconduction. J. Bone. Joint. Surg. Br. 90, 1635–1640.

Sposito, G., 2008. The Chemistry of Soils. Oxford University Press, New York, NY.

Sprio, S., Tampieri, A., Landi, E., Sandri, M., Martorana, S., Celotti, G., et al., 2008. Physico-chemical properties and solubility behaviour of multi-substituted hydroxyapatite powders containing silicon. Mater. Sci. Eng. C. 28, 179–187.

Stegen, S., Van Gastel, N., Carmeliet, G., 2015. Bringing new life to damaged bone: the importance of angiogenesis in bone repair and regeneration. Bone. 70, 19–27.

Studart, A.R., Gonzenbach, U.T., Tervoort, E., Gauckler, L.J., 2006. Processing routes to macroporous ceramics: a review. J. Am. Ceram. Soc. 89, 1771–1789.

Suhaimi, H., Bhusan Das, D., 2016. Glucose diffusion in tissue engineering membranes and scaffolds. Rev. Chem. Eng. 32, 629–650.

Šupová, M., 2015. Substituted hydroxyapatites for biomedical applications: a review. Ceram. Int. 41, 9203–9231.

Tatara, A., Wong, M., Mikos, A., 2014. In vivo bioreactors for mandibular reconstruction. J. Dent. Res. 93, 1196–1202.

Trecant, M., Delecrin, J., Nguyen, J., Royer, J., Passuti, N., Daculsi, G., 1996. Influence of post-implantation physico-chemical changes in a macroporous ceramic on its mechanical strength. J. Mater. Sci. Mater. Med. 7, 227–229.

Trecant, M., Delecrin, J., Royer, J., Goyenvalle, E., Daculsi, G., 1994. Mechanical changes in macro-porous calcium phosphate ceramics after implantation in bone. Clin. Mater. 15, 233–240.

Trombetta, R., Inzana, J.A., Schwarz, E.M., Kates, S.L., Awad, H.A., 2017. 3D printing of calcium phosphate ceramics for bone tissue engineering and drug delivery. Ann. Biomed. Eng. 45, 23–44.

Truscello, S., Kerckhofs, G., Van Bael, S., Pyka, G., Schrooten, J., Van Oosterwyck, H., 2012. Prediction of permeability of regular scaffolds for skeletal tissue engineering: a combined computational and experimental study. Acta Biomater. 8, 1648–1658.

Van Bael, S., Chai, Y.C., Truscello, S., Moesen, M., Kerckhofs, G., Van Oosterwyck, H., et al., 2012. The effect of pore geometry on the in vitro biological behavior of human periosteum-derived cells seeded on selective laser-melted Ti6Al4V bone scaffolds. Acta Biomater. 8, 2824–2834.

Vandamme, K., Holy, X., Bensidhoum, M., Logeart-Avramoglou, D., Naert, I.E., Duyck, J. A., et al., 2011. In vivo molecular evidence of delayed titanium implant osseointegration in compromised bone. Biomatcrials. 32, 3547–3554.

Venugopal, J., Prabhakaran, M.P., Zhang, Y., Low, S., Choon, A.T., Ramakrishna, S., 2010. Biomimetic hydroxyapatite-containing composite nanofibrous substrates for bone tissue engineering. Philos. Trans. Royal Soc.London A: Math. Phys. Eng. Sci. 368, 2065–2081.

Viateau, V., Guillemin, G., Calando, Y., Logeart, D., Oudina, K., Sedel, L., et al., 2006. Induction of a barrier membrane to facilitate reconstruction of massive segmental diaphyseal bone defects: an ovine model. Vet. Surg. 35, 445–452.

Von Rechenberg, B., 2014. Animal models in bone repair. Drug Discov. Today: Dis. Models. 13, 23–27.

Wang, P., Zhao, L., Liu, J., Weir, M.D., Zhou, X., Xu, H.H., 2014. Bone tissue engineering via nanostructured calcium phosphate biomaterials and stem cells. Bone Res. 2, 14017.

Warnke, P., Springer, I., Wiltfang, J., Acil, Y., Eufinger, H., Wehmöller, M., et al., 2004. Growth and transplantation of a custom vascularised bone graft in a man. Lancet. 364, 766–770.

Watson, B.M., Kasper, F.K., Engel, P.S., Mikos, A.G., 2014. Synthesis and characterization of injectable, biodegradable, phosphate-containing, chemically cross-linkable, thermoresponsive macromers for bone tissue engineering. Biomacromolecules. 15, 1788–1796.

Wegst, U.G., Bai, H., Saiz, E., Tomsia, A.P., Ritchie, R.O., 2015. Bioinspired structural materials. Nat. Mater. 14, 23–36.

Weiss, P., Layrolle, P., Clergeau, L.P., Enckel, B., Pilet, P., Amouriq, Y., et al., 2007. The safety and efficacy of an injectable bone substitute in dental sockets demonstrated in a human clinical trial. Biomaterials. 28, 3295–3305.

Wieding, J., Wolf, A., Bader, R., 2014. Numerical optimization of open-porous bone scaffold structures to match the elastic properties of human cortical bone. J. Mech. Behav. Biomed. Mater. 37, 56–68.

Wiese, A., Pape, H.C., 2010. Bone defects caused by high-energy injuries, bone loss, infected nonunions, and nonunions. Orthop. Clin. North Am. 41, 1–4.

Wu, J., Aage, N., Westermann, R., Sigmund, O., 2016. Infill Optimization for Additive Manufacturing--Approaching Bone-like Porous Structures. *arXiv preprint arXiv:1608.04366.*

Xiao, X., Wang, W., Liu, D., Zhang, H., Gao, P., Geng, L., et al., 2015. The promotion of angiogenesis induced by three-dimensional porous beta-tricalcium phosphate scaffold with different interconnection sizes via activation of PI3K/Akt pathways. Sci. Rep. 5, 9409.

Xiong, Q., Baychev, T.G., Jivkov, A.P., 2016. Review of pore network modelling of porous media: experimental characterisations, network constructions and applications to reactive transport. J. Contam. Hydrol. 192, 101–117.

Yang, N., Tian, Y., Zhang, D., 2015. Novel real function based method to construct heterogeneous porous scaffolds and additive manufacturing for use in medical engineering. Med. Eng. Phys. 37, 1037–1046.

Yoo, D.-J., 2012. Heterogeneous porous scaffold design for tissue engineering using triply periodic minimal surfaces. Inte. J. Precision Eng. Manufact. 13, 527–537.

Yoo, D., 2013. New paradigms in hierarchical porous scaffold design for tissue engineering. Mater. Sci. Eng. C. 33, 1759–1772.

Yuan, H., De Bruijn, J., Li, Y., Feng, J., Yang, Z., De Groot, K., et al., 2001. Bone formation induced by calcium phosphate ceramics in soft tissue of dogs: a comparative study between porous α-TCP and β-TCP. J. Mater. Sci. Mater. Med. 12, 7–13.

Yuan, H., Fernandes, H., Habibovic, P., De Boer, J., Barradas, A.M., De Ruiter, A., et al., 2010. Osteoinductive ceramics as a synthetic alternative to autologous bone grafting. Proc. Natl. Acad. Sci. 107, 13614–13619.

Yuan, H., Yang, Z., Li, Y., Zhang, X., De Bruijn, J., De Groot, K., 1998. Osteoinduction by calcium phosphate biomaterials. J. Mater. Sci. Mater. Med. 9, 723–726.

Zadpoor, A.A., 2015. Bone tissue regeneration: the role of scaffold geometry. Biomater. Sci. 3, 231–245.

Zhang, J., Barbieri, D., Ten Hoopen, H., De Bruijn, J.D., Van Blitterswijk, C.A., Yuan, H., 2015. Microporous calcium phosphate ceramics driving osteogenesis through surface architecture. J. Biomed. Mater. Res. A. 103, 1188–1199.

Zhang, J., Luo, X., Barbieri, D., Barradas, A.M., De Bruijn, J.D., Van Blitterswijk, C.A., et al., 2014. The size of surface microstructures as an osteogenic factor in calcium phosphate ceramics. Acta. Biomater. 10, 3254–3263.

Zhang, X.-Y., Fang, G., Zhou, J., 2017. Additively manufactured scaffolds for bone tissue engineering and the prediction of their mechanical behavior: a review. Materials. 10, 50.

Zhang, X., Xie, C., Lin, A.S., Ito, H., Awad, H., Lieberman, J.R., et al., 2005. Periosteal progenitor cell fate in segmental cortical bone graft transplantations: implications for functional tissue engineering. J. Bone Mineral Res. 20, 2124–2137.

Zhanga, J., Sunc, L., Luod, X., Barbierid, D., De Bruijnd, J.D., Van Blitterswijka, C.A., et al., 2016. Cells responding to surface structure of calcium phosphate ceramics for bone regeneration. Instructive Function of Surface Structure of Calcium Phosphate Ceramics in Bone Regeneration, 99.

Zhou, J., Lin, H., Fang, T., Li, X., Dai, W., Uemura, T., et al., 2010. The repair of large segmental bone defects in the rabbit with vascularized tissue engineered bone. Biomaterials. 31, 1171–1179.

Zhu, Y., Song, K., Jiang, S., Chen, J., Tang, L., Li, S., et al., 2017. Numerical simulation of mass transfer and three-dimensional fabrication of tissue-engineered cartilages based on

chitosan/gelatin hybrid hydrogel scaffold in a rotating bioreactor. Appl. Biochem. Biotechnol. 181, 250–266.
Zocca, A., Colombo, P., Gomes, C.M., Günster, J., 2015. Additive manufacturing of ceramics: issues, potentialities, and opportunities. J. Am. Ceram. Soc. 98, 1983–2001.

## Further reading

Charbonnier, B., Laurent, C., Marchat, D., 2016b. Porous hydroxyapatite bioceramics produced by impregnation of 3D-printed wax mold: slurry feature optimization. J. Eur. Ceram. Soc. 36, 4269–4279.

# Clinical issues of ceramic devices used in total hip arthroplasty

# 9

*Jonathan S. De Mattia*[1], *Emanuela Castiello*[2] *and Saverio Affatato*[1]
[1]Rizzoli Orthopaedic Institute, Bologna, Italy, [2]Ospedale "S.M.della Scaletta" Imola, Bologna, Italy

**Chapter Outline**

**Abbreviations 313**
**9.1 Introduction 314**
9.1.1 Alumina ceramics 314
9.1.2 Zirconia ceramics 315
9.1.3 ZTA ceramics 316
**9.2 Ceramics as orthopedic medical devices: advantages and disadvantages 317**
**9.3 Technical issues and surgical aspects 320**
**9.4 In vitro performance and in vivo failure analysis 321**
**9.5 Challenges and future trends 323**
**9.6 Conclusions 324**
**Acknowledgments 324**
**References 324**
**Further Reading 328**

## Abbreviations

| | |
|---|---|
| **CoC** | ceramic-on-ceramic |
| **CoCHR** | ceramic-on-ceramic hip resurfacing |
| **CoP** | ceramic-on-polymer |
| **HIP** | hot isostatic pressing |
| **HR** | hip resourfacing |
| **Mg-PSZ** | magnesia-partially stabilized zirconia |
| **MoM** | metal-on-metal |
| **MoP** | metal-on-polymer |
| **THA** | total hip arthroplasty |
| **THR** | total hip replacement |
| **UHMWPE** | ultra-high-molecular-weight polyethylene |
| **XLPE** | highly cross-linked polyethylene |
| **Y-TZP** | yttria-stabilized tetragonal zirconia polycrystals |
| **ZTA** | zirconia toughened alumina |

**Advances in Ceramic Biomaterials.**
**DOI: http://dx.doi.org/10.1016/B978-0-08-100881-2.00009-9**

# 9.1 Introduction

Ceramics have been successfully used for more than 40 years for orthopedic prostheses, as articulating bearing surfaces against ceramic or polymer components. In fact, ceramics are characterized by low friction coefficient and low wear rate, compared to metallic materials (stainless steels, titanium and chromium-cobalt alloys) (Rieu and Goeuriot, 1993). Ceramic is a class of engineering materials, showing wear-resistant characteristics under severe environments (Affatato et al., 1999). Alumina and zirconia-toughened alumina (ZTA) are currently used as constituents of prosthetic components for total hip replacement (THR), due to their high strength, wear resistance, stability, nontoxicity and biocompatibility in vivo (Willman et al., 1996). The technical characteristics of the biomedical-grade ceramics (alumina, zirconia and ZTA) which have been or are currently used in total hip arthroplasty (THA) are here described. For sake of clarity, THA (also called Total Hip Replacement (THR)) is the reconstructing surgical procedure which consists on the removal of the head of the thighbone (femoral head) and the damaged socket (acetabulum) and their replacement with prostheses (femoral and acetabular components).

## 9.1.1 *Alumina ceramics*

Despite the development of various ceramics for sliding surfaces in THA, alumina (aluminum oxide, $Al_2O_3$), used in clinical practice since the 1970s, shows unique physical and mechanical properties mainly due to the ionic/covalent nature of its chemical bonds (Piconi et al., 2003). Alumina is stable against oxidation, meaning that further oxidative processes as well as consequent corrosion and ion release in a physiological environment are not physically possible. Furthermore, the binding energy makes the material extremely hard, wear-resistant, and nondeformable under load because of its high Young's modulus. In addition, the spatial structure of the alumina molecule allows the adhesion of thin films of polar liquids. This characteristic, called wettability, constitutes a considerable advantage compared to metal components since it allows the formation of a thin layer of liquid at the interface of the alumina joint couplings, acting as a lubricant and thus reducing the friction of the prosthetic joint (Piconi, 2011).

The choice of alumina as a biomaterial was based on its unsurpassed biological safety and stability in the human body. However, the first generation of alumina showed relatively low density, scarce purity, large grain size, and uncontrolled microstructure, which reduced the mechanical properties and reliability of the alumina devices. In the following years, the continuous advances in manufacturing techniques allowed the production of a biomaterial with full density, controlled and fine microstructure and therefore improved performance (Affatato et al., 2012). As a consequence, during more than 40 years of clinical use, we can estimate that today more than 12 million alumina components have been implanted worldwide (Walter, 2017). Alumina performs very well under compression, but is brittle under tension. Like many ceramics, alumina does not show (at room temperature) plastic deformation before fracture (e.g., no yield point in the stress–strain curve before fracture) and once started, fractures progress very rapidly (due to alumina low fracture toughness, $K_{IC}$). In general terms, the strength of alumina improves with higher density and smaller grain size. Alumina manufacturers carefully select raw materials and control the production process to optimize the mechanical properties (Heart, 2016). Continuous efforts to improve the properties of alumina bioceramics are being made, e.g., by the introduction of high-purity raw materials, hot isostatic pressing after pressureless sintering, proof testing on 100% of manufactured components. The use of hot isostatic pressing in bioceramics production minimizes the residual stresses within ceramic pieces and produces ceramics with density close to the theoretical ones, improving the strength and reliability of the product (Heart, 2016). More details are provided in Chapter 5, Ceramics for joint replacement: design and application of commercial bearings.

A further process improvement is the introduction of the proof testing of components. This test consists of the application of internal pressure to the ball head (or to the inlay) inducing a stress close to the maximum load-bearing capability of the component. When applied to 100% of the parts manufactured, defective products can be eliminated before final inspection (Richter and Willman, 1999).

In clinical practice, alumina heads may be coupled both to ultra-high-molecular-weight polyethylene (UHMWPE) acetabular sockets, and to alumina inlays. The favorable wear behavior of these joints is dependent upon the hardness of alumina, that makes it extremely resistant to third-body wear. In addition, this feature is also facilitated by the wettability of the material (Heart, 2016).

## 9.1.2 Zirconia ceramics

The first reports on the use of zirconia (zirconium dioxide, $ZrO_2$) as a biomaterial derive from Helmer and Driskell (1969) and Monticelli et al. (1981). However, the real development of zirconia ceramics as a biomaterial started in the mid-eighties, introduced in orthopedics for the manufacturing of ball heads able to overcome the mechanical limits of the first alumina ceramics (Christel et al., 1988).

The early developments were focused on magnesia-partially stabilized zirconia (Mg-PSZ), but this material never reached large-scale clinical applications. The rapid shift towards yttria-stabilized tetragonal zirconia polycrystals (Y-TZP) was due to its much better strength, finer grain size, and better wear properties. Among the zirconia materials, Y-TZP is today the benchmark material for clinical applications (ISO, 2015). Use of zirconia ball heads began in 1985, but their performance has been both confusing and controversial (Clarke et al., 2003). Zirconia is a complex ceramic material and its process includes proprietary methods unique to each manufacturer. For this reason, it cannot be assumed that all types of zirconia balls are identical in quality, regardless of existing manufacturing standards (ISO, 2015). However, thanks to the high bending strength and toughness of Y-TZP ceramics, it is possible to manufacture small-diameter Y-TZP ball heads (22 or 26 mm diameter) and long necks. Smaller heads may constitute an advantage for THA design, making it possible to increase UHMWPE inlay thickness for a given socket diameter. Mechanical properties of Y-TZP ceramics depend on some microstructural parameters and specifically on the equilibrium between them (see Chapter 2: Types of ceramics: material class and Chapter 3: Assessment of mechanical properties of ceramic materials).

### 9.1.3 ZTA ceramics

One of the primary restrictions on clinical use of bioceramics is the uncertain lifetime under the complex stress states, slow crack growth, and cyclic fatigue that arise in many clinical applications (Hench, 1993). While, over the years, efforts were made to improve many of the mechanical properties of the alumina, one of the limitations of this material remained its low resistance to fracture, due to its intrinsic brittleness. To overcome this limit, around 1985, zirconia ceramics were introduced in orthopedic technology, but their use has always been the subject of debate, because of the contradictory clinical results obtained from the THA that made use of zirconia femoral heads (Piconi et al., 2007). Furthermore, the hardness of zirconia, lower than that of alumina, coupled with its low thermal conductivity, does not allow its clinical use in articular ceramic–ceramic pairs. A further disadvantage is the technology used for zirconia manufacturing, particularly critical and therefore relatively expensive. The fractures reported by two series of heads due to incorrect process control (Maccauro et al., 2004), and the resulting global withdrawal of the product have resulted in the abandonment of the zirconia heads in orthopedics.

Advances in technology have reduced the risk of fracture of ceramic THA implants. However, the real turning point derived from the introduction into orthopedics of ceramic composite materials based on alumina and zirconia, called ZTA composites. Today, such composites dominate the THA heads and inserts market (Piconi et al., 2005), since they offer an even wider range of applications as compared to bulk alumina, because of their significantly enhanced mechanical properties (Stewart et al., 2003). The idea of combining the tribological properties of alumina and the mechanical characteristics of Y-TZP allows the production of a new class of ceramic materials with overall outstanding properties (Affatato et al., 2015). The most well-known and representative commercial product of this class of materials is undoubtedly the Biolox delta, introduced in 2002 by the *CeramTec Medical Products Division* (Plochingen, Germany), whose success has pushed other ceramic manufacturers to develop competitive products for the composite market. Fig. 9.1 shows the three major types of ceramics used in THA: zirconia, alumina (Biolox forte) and ZTA (Biolox delta) ceramics.

The matrix of the Biolox delta is constituted by a fine-grained, high-purity alumina, reinforced by a homogeneous dispersion (about 17% of the volume) of zirconia grains having submicrometer dimensions (average diameter approximately 0.27 μm). Moreover, Biolox delta ceramic also contains strontium oxide, added to generate platelets and to limit cracking propagation (Massin et al., 2014). In situ formation of strontium hexa-aluminate, while representing only 3% of the volume, provides an effective reinforcement action and an increase in fracture resistance. The presence in solid solution of chromium oxide with the alumina compensates for the loss of hardness due to the addition of zirconia to the alumina matrix, and gives the material the characteristic pink coloring (Burger and Richter, 2001;

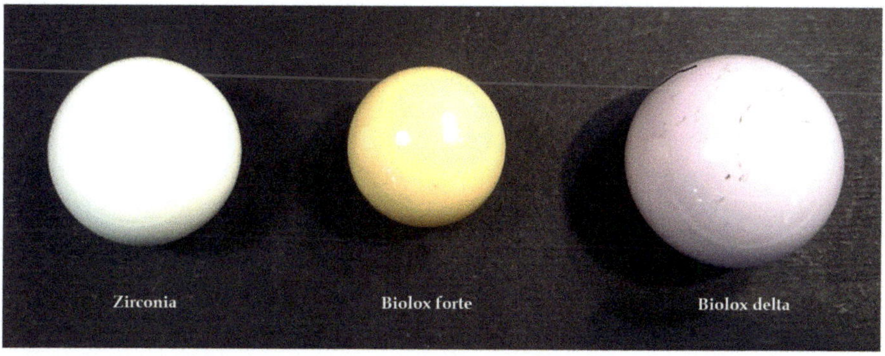


**Figure 9.1** Major types of ceramics for total hip arthroplasty: zirconia, alumina (Biolox forte) and ZTA (Biolox delta).

Magnani and Brillante, 2005; Piconi et al., 2005; Affatato et al., 2015). More details are provided in Chapter 3, Assessment of mechanical properties of ceramic materials and Chapter 5, Ceramics for joint replacement: design and application of commercial bearings.

The reinforcing elements significantly increase the fracture resistance: the microstructure has been adapted in order to provide an optimum resistance to crack propagation. In cases where overload conditions occur with sufficient energy to generate a microtrauma to the microstructure of the material, this ceramic has the ability to stop the propagation of the crack. The mechanism is the result of the transition from tetragonal to monoclinic phase of zirconia particles, which occurs with volume expansion, thus generating compression forces at the tip of the propagating crack (Hannink et al., 2000).

## 9.2 Ceramics as orthopedic medical devices: Advantages and disadvantages

Despite the fact that early generations of ceramics coupled to primitive designs yielded mixed clinical results (Hannouche et al., 2005; Sharkey, 2009; Castillo et al., 2014; Le and Murphy, 2014), modern generations of ceramic bearings show excellent performance with long-term survivoral and low complication rates (Kim et al., 2010; Kang et al., 2015). Several material properties of ceramics make them the ideal bearing surface for THA. Ceramic is biocompatible with low risk for local adverse soft tissue reactions unlike metal bearings (Greenwald et al., 2001; Roualdes et al., 2010).

Among the different materials which can be used for orthopedic medical devices, ceramics offer a number of beneficial mechanical properties, such as high hardness, good chemical resistance, high strength, and a good fracture toughness (Affatato et al., 2001). The use of ceramic-on-ceramic (CoC) as bearing surfaces for hip joint prostheses ensures high wettability, and consequently its lubrication properties are improved (Skinner, 1999). Friction can be reduced by lubrication, while the low friction coefficient of ceramic biomaterial leads to an improvement in the tribological behavior of the coupling. Throughout recent years, a trend towards increasing femoral head size in THA, to improve stability and range of motion, has been observed (Cross et al., 2012). Moreover, a femoral head with a large diameter contributes to decrease the risk of fracture (Lee and Garino, 2011). The advantage of choosing a bigger femoral head (≥36 mm) is the significant decrease in the dislocation rate and the increase in range of motion of the coupling (Cross et al., 2012). Therefore, disadvantages of a larger femoral head size include more volumetric wear.

While improvements in materials and design have led to a dramatic reduction in ceramic fractures, technical factors such as acetabular component malposition, incomplete seating of ceramic liner, and femoral taper mismatch can still result in modern ceramic component failures. Consequently, despite ceramic's excellent material and wear properties, concerns remain about the risk of ceramic fractures, noise, and squeaking. A further problem is the still very high production cost. Early fractures during clinical use were due to a combination of material impurities, poor implant design, and sterilization procedures, such as autoclaving and rapid cooling leading to changes in the material properties of ceramics and fractures (Le and Murphy, 2014; Castillo et al., 2014; Kim et al., 2009).

Ceramic bearing fractures usually occur during normal daily activities, above all in obese patients (Ms et al., 2013), rarely as a result of trauma (Mclean et al., 2002).

In the literature, it has been demonstrated that a small femoral head (28 mm) and a short neck size are considered the main risk factors of ceramic head fracture; on the other hand, an acetabular component malposition (more vertical and more anteversion cups) and misalignment of the liner during insertion represent two relevant and mechanical risk factors associated with ceramic liner fracture as a result of neck-to-cup impingement with head subluxation and increased edge loading on the liner rim (Toni et al., 2006). Table 9.1 summarizes the main risks of ceramic fracture.

Other critical issues leading to ceramic fractures include edge loading and component impingement (Traina et al., 2012). Figs. 9.2 and 9.3 show the X-ray of an elderly man and the explanted fractured ceramic femoral head.

Noise and squeaking following CoC THA remains poorly understood, despite the efforts that the scientific community is putting into understanding the causes (Abdel et al., 2014; Walter et al., 2007, 2010). Squeaking is defined as an audible

**Table 9.1 Main risks of ceramic fracture**

| Implant and surgery factors | |
|---|---|
| Risk of ceramic head fracture | • Short neck 28-mm heads |
| Risk of liner fractures | • Malposition of the cup on the axial plane<br>• Misalignment of the liner during insertion |
| Patient risk factors | • Excessive weight<br>• Advanced age |

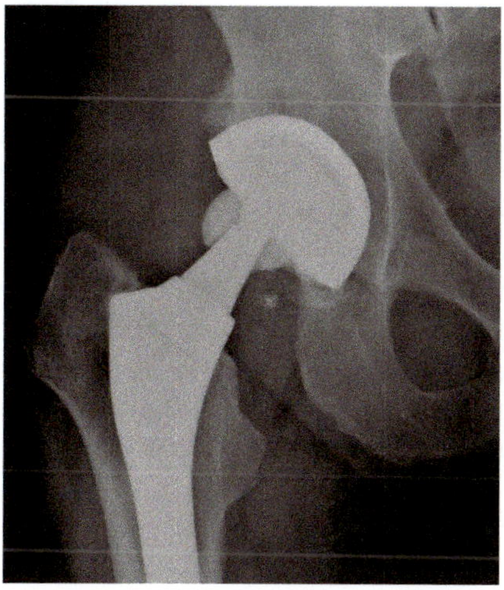

**Figure 9.2** Antero-posterior radiograph showing ceramic head fracture.

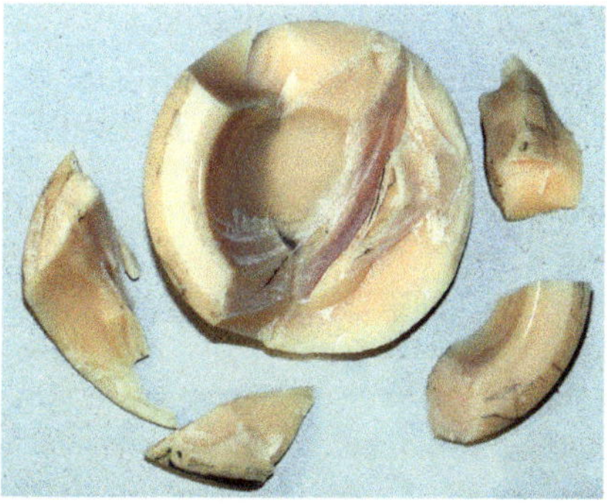

**Figure 9.3** Photograph of retrieved ceramic head fragments.

sound that occurs during movement of the hip joint. Clinically, squeaking may manifest in extreme hip flexion or during the normal gait cycle, however it is rarely associated with pain. Baruffaldi et al. (2017) identified and classified noise by duration, intensity, and frequency of three noise types: squeaking, clicking, and popping. The sounds generated were assessed in correlation with the gait cycle and with the CoC bearing surface. They observed that noise appeared during walking, followed by squating, and squeaking showed the longest duration and the highest amplitude.

Several factors have been implicated in the etiology leading to noise production including component malposition, edge loading, fluid film breakdown, metal transfer to the femoral head, and frequencies produced by specific implants leading to audible noise. The role of component position and squeaking continues to be debated (Jarrett et al., 2009). Studies to define the contributions of material, prosthetic, patient, and surgical factors to squeaking are needed to improve understanding and to prevent this complication postoperatively. Moreover, recent studies (Elpers et al., 2014; Taddei et al., 2012, 2016; Affatato et al., 2016; Merola et al., 2016) highlighted the harmful effects of metal debris transfer from the metal surface of an acetabular cup on ceramic femoral heads. The adherence of these third-body metallic particles to the alumina femoral head increases its surface roughness (Chang et al., 2008). This inevitably leads to an increase in wear, due to a worsening of the coupling tribological behavior: metal transfer induces an important surface modification of the femoral heads, which could strongly modify the fluid dynamic behavior of the synovial fluid and favor a fluid film rupture, causing localized contacts of the prosthetic surfaces. A recent investigation (Affatato et al., 2016) has also shown that the metal transfer phenomenon leads to a deterioration of the properties of the material subsurface layer, confirming that this problem is not marginal.

## 9.3 Technical issues and surgical aspects

In order to minimize or avoid the risks of failure of THA ceramic bearings, such as noise and ceramic fracture, surgeons should take care regarding the proper association between bearing and patient. In fact, ceramic bearings are indicated in the younger and more active patients with correct muscle tension, avoiding hip dislocation of the implant and initial microseparation and a damage of the liner rim (Ceroni et al., 2006). Furthermore, an accurate surgical technique is mandatory to reduce catastrophic failure.

Care should be taken to obtain implant stability, checking acetabular and femoral component orientation (avoiding antiversion cup position) with a good soft tissue balancing. It is useful to remove osteophytes and acetabular wall, preventing impingement between femoral neck and cup rim, especially in external rotation and in flexion internal rotation preventing edge loading. Surgeons should take care not to damage the metal back during implantation of components and pay attention to the exact placement of ceramic liners. For this last operation, a simple running of the finger around the rim is suggested. In case of patient presenting hip arthroplasty pain or noise, X-ray and computerized tomography (CT) scan are requested in order to analyze acetabular component position and to recognize huge ceramic head fragments in the articular space; conversely, the clinical and radiological signs of ceramic liner fractures are usually underestimated. Therefore, although synovial fluid analysis through joint aspiration is not mandatory, it is strongly suggested to determine the presence of ceramic particles and their dimension (Toni et al., 2006). It has been suggested that the presence of ceramic particles $>2$ μm indicate an early-stage liner fractures while ceramic particles $>5$ μm indicate a macroscopic liner fracture (Stea et al., 2012).

Once the diagnosis of ceramic component fracture is complete, revision surgery should be carried out urgently in order to reduce the risk that ceramic particles further damage the metal taper. In addition, rest and no load bearing until revision surgery are advisable for the patient, with the aim of reducing the spread of the ceramic particles in the soft tissue and abrasive damage to the acetabular component and/or the femoral taper (Traina et al., 2011). It is well known that THA revision for fractured ceramic bearings is still difficult with high rates of repeated revisions and with poor clinical outcomes. Revision surgery should be carried out and it is based on an accurate intraoperative evaluation of cup malposition and morse taper damage; a complete synovectomy and thorough complete debridement of the fractured ceramic fragments are needed with the purpose of avoiding third-body wear, thus increasing the survival rate of the new implant (Rambani et al., 2017).

In order to have a low rate of complications, it is recommended to revise the ceramic hip with new CoC or ceramic-on-polymer (CoP) implants, while the use of metal-on-polymers (MoPs) couples for revision has to be avoided. In fact, MoP couplings that have a lower hardness with respect to the ceramics used in the primary surgery, can undergo abrasive wear from remaining ceramic particles, thus inducing metallosis (Sharma et al., 2013). In addition, metal components (cobalt–chrome alloys) should be avoided, due to cobalt toxicity as reported by Zywiel and Turgeon, 2013.

In order to avoid catastrophic ceramic fracture, early diagnosis of ceramic component failure is mandatory. This is also required for updated management strategies.

THA noise is considered a potential predictor and a clinical sign of prosthetic failure and it is an ongoing concern for hard-on-hard bearings, such as CoC, while it is generally not reported in hard-on-soft bearings such as ceramic-on-polyethylene (CoP type) (Tai et al., 2015; Wyatt et al., 2014). Hip noise also represents a significant psychological awkwardness to the patients who may be anxious and embarrassed by the noise.

In order to reduce hip prosthesis noise, the correct position of the ceramic insert within the acetabular cup can be checked by running a finger along its rim. In this way it is possible to prevent excessive cup deformation at the moment of implanting the device, put in a proper cup position and properly adjust the soft-tissue tension, and finally, check the presence of impingement of components intraoperatively.

## 9.4 In vitro performance and in vivo failure analysis

The optimal type of bearing for THA represents a challenge and remains a matter of debate. Wear and osteolysis are the major reasons for revision surgery in THA. Therefore, improvements in materials, surgical technique, and implant design have improved the reliability of ceramic components over the years (Lee and Garino, 2011). Consequently, nowadays modern CoC bearings are ideally suited for the young, active patient undergoing primary THA. The low wear rates associated with ceramic hip articulations have made them an increasingly popular bearing choice in THA (Shafafy et al., 2016). Fig. 9.4 shows the wear behavior of different pairs after in vivo use.

As shown in Fig. 9.4, CoC pairs have the lowest in vitro wear rates compared with all other bearing surface options (Fisher et al., 2006). By comparing metal heads and ceramic heads, both articulating against conventional polyethylene, CoC

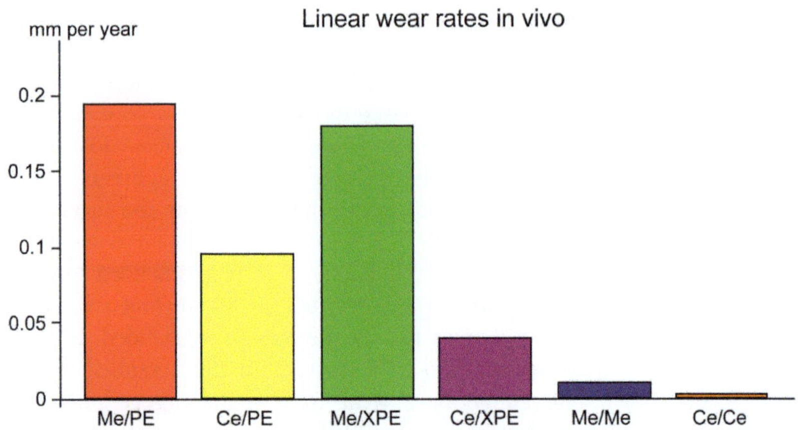


**Figure 9.4** In vivo linear wear rate for several femoral head/acetabular component pairs. Me/PE, Metal on Polyethylene; Ce/PE, Ceramic on Polyethylene; Me/XLPE, Metal on CrosslinkedPE; Ce/XLPE, Ceramic on CrosslinkedPE; Ce/Ce, Ceramic on Ceramic.

bearings lower wear by the order of over 1000 and 400 times in vitro. Even though highly cross-linked polyethylene (XLPE) has reduced wear rates of 40% compared to conventional polyethylene, CoC bearing surfaces still significantly outperform these new polymer materials in vitro (Callaghan et al., 2008).

In vivo data analysis shows that CoC bearings have better survival than metal-on-metal (MoM) bearings at the 10-year follow-up; the difference is significant when revision for aseptic loosening was defined as a failure (Milošev et al., 2012).

However, neither the CoC nor the MoM alternative bearings provided improved midterm results when compared with the results of the conventional MoP bearings. For older, less active patients, traditional metal-on-polyethylene bearings are still the appropriate choice (Milošev et al., 2012).

Despite the stunning wear performance, ceramic brittleness remains an unresolved question and it contributes significantly to lowering the average useful life of these prosthetic implants (Traina et al., 2013). Ceramic head fracture is a catastrophic event and several cases of fractured heads are reported in scientific databases (Lee et al., 2010; Aldrian et al., 2009; Koo et al., 2008; Fayard et al., 2006; Park et al., 2006; Yoo et al., 2005, 2006; Hamadouche et al., 2002).

CoCs were introduced as alternative bearings to MoM prostheses, to improve the long-term performance of hip prostheses and overcome the problem of the release of metal ions (McMinn et al., 2011; Hing et al., 2007; Holland et al., 2012; Dickinson et al., 2011). However, it should be noted that some cases of early failure of CoC have been reported in the scientific literature (Kawano et al., 2013; Matharu et al., 2015; Traina et al., 2013).

In a case of hip resurfacing (HR), a new CoC hip resurfacing (CoCHR) design was offered to young patients showing metal allergies (Matharu et al., 2015). HR is an alternative form of hip arthroplasty, in which the femoral head is not removed, but is trimmed and capped with a smooth metal covering. On the contrary, the damaged bone and cartilage within the socket is removed and replaced with a metal shell, just as in a traditional THA. HR has some advantages with respect to THA, such as a greater range of motion of the hip joint after surgery, a lower rate of dislocation, less prosthetic bearing wear, and easier revision surgery. For this reason, HR is particularly suitable for young and active patients. Matharu et al. (2015) discussed the clinical outcomes of the implantation of a new CoCHR device, consisting of a cemented femoral head with a metallic base made of cobalt−chrome alloy and a solid ceramic coating. This articulated with an acetabular liner, made by a novel ceramic-composite: two-thirds polyurethane and one-third alumina ceramic. All five patients showed excellent early results, including low systemic metal ion concentrations. However, after 3 years, all patients developed symptoms and progressively increased systemic metal ion concentrations, showing metallosis and requiring revision surgery (Matharu et al., 2015).

A prospective study (Kawano et al., 2013) reports the outcome of THA performed in a consecutive series of patients using an alumina ceramic on a ceramic-layered component (Alumina-Bearing-Surface system), highlighting the risk factors of implant failure such as preoperative range of motion of the hip joint and postoperative dislocation.

## 9.5 Challenges and future trends

The failure mechanism of joint replacements are multifactorial and not related to the materials used and/or design features exclusively. Ceramic brittleness remains a major concern (Traina et al., 2013). Due to the increased number of CoC implants, more revision surgeries and reports on ceramic components failure are expected in the future. Although Biolox delta ceramic is more resistant to fractures than alumina ceramic, it can be fractured under suboptimal implantation conditions including edge loading. Its use requires the same precautions as other hard-on-hard bearings and requires special attention to cup position, insertion on or in morse tapers, and adjustment of leg length (Massin et al., 2014).

In addition, there are uncertainties about the fracture-resistance and wear-resistance of the materials under in vivo loading conditions (Matharu et al., 2015).

Attempts to obtain an alumina ceramic composite reinforced with carbon nanotubes (CNT) with high wear resistance are the subject of many researches (Dai, 2002; Sun et al., 2002; Raravikar et al., 2005; Affatato et al., 2015). However, many difficulties are encountered or found to disperse the CNT inside the ceramic matrix due to an agglomeration effect. A possible solution to these unwanted results is the use of in situ synthesis of CNTs within the oxide powder. An alternative solution consists of an in situ synthesis of $ZrO_2$ nanoparticles on the surfaces of CNTs by liquid phase reactions and a proper heat treatment process. Subsequently, the $ZrO_2$/CNTs product was mechanically mixed with or blended in liquid alumina suspensions. The mixtures were then sintered under vacuum (Zhu et al., 2008). The combined effect of $ZrO_2$ particles and CNTs allowed the production of sintered materials with very good mechanical properties (bending strength of 505 MPa and 7.8 MPa$\sqrt{m}$), significantly higher than those of monolithic alumina ceramics.

Clinical concerns of using ceramic bearings include impingement, squeaking, and fracture. A very precise surgical technique, modifications to implant design, and material manufacturing processes have been implemented to reduce these complications.

## 9.6 Conclusions

Bearings made of last-generation alumina ceramics and of ZTA composites have been shown to possess extremely low wear properties that make them both suitable for THA. Any technology that can reduce bearing wear rates in THA can potentially decrease the morbidity and risks associated with premature revision surgery related to wear. Extensive specialized knowledge in development and production together with uncompromising quality management make Biolox advanced ceramic implants the successful, clinically proven standard for medical professionals worldwide. Improved wear resistance also allows the use of large-diameter femoral heads in THA, leading to increased arc of movement and less risk of prosthesis dislocation. Despite the theoretical improvement in ceramic biomaterials, a relatively high rate of catastrophic ceramic bearing surface failure is still observed. Furthermore, the use of these bearings requires an accurate surgical procedure based on correct positioning of the all components. Thanks to all these properties and a detailed surgical technique, ceramic bearings represent an excellent choice even for the young active patient requiring THA.

## Acknowledgments

The authors would like to thank Luigi Lena (Rizzoli Orthopaedic Institute) for his help with the original images.

## References

Abdel, M.P., et al., 2014. Ceramic liner fractures presenting as squeaking after primary total hip arthroplasty. J. Bone. Joint. Surg. Am. 96 (1), 27–31. Available at: http://www.ncbi.nlm.nih.gov/pubmed/24382721 [Accessed April 18, 2014].

Affatato, S., et al., 2016. Does metal transfer affect the tribological behaviour of femoral heads? Roughness and phase transformation analyses on retrieved zirconia and Biolox® delta composites. Composites Part B: Engineering 92, 290–298.

Affatato, S., et al., 1999. Mixed oxides prosthetic ceramic ball heads. Part 2: effect of the $ZrO_2$ fraction on the wear of ceramic on ceramic joints. Biomaterials 20, 971–975.

Affatato, S., et al., 2001. Mixed oxides prosthetic ceramic ball heads. Part 3: effect of the $ZrO_2$ fraction on the wear of ceramic on ceramic hip joint prostheses. A long-term in vitro study. Biomaterials 22, 717–723.

Affatato, S., et al., 2012. Retrieval analysis of three generations of Biolox® femoral heads: spectroscopic and SEM characterization. J. Mech. Behav. Biomed. Mater. 13, 118–128. Available at: http://www.ncbi.nlm.nih.gov/pubmed/22842282 [Accessed April 8, 2014].

Affatato, S., Ruggiero, A., Merola, M., 2015. Advanced biomaterials in hip joint arthroplasty. A review on polymer and ceramics composites as alternative bearings. Comp. Part B Eng. 83, 276–283. Available at: http://www.sciencedirect.com/science/article/pii/S1359836815004473 [Accessed September 25, 2015].

Aldrian, S., et al., 2009. Medium-term analysis of modern ceramic-on-ceramic bearing in THA. HIP Int. 19 (1), 36–40.

Greenwald, A.S., Garino, J.P., American Academy of Orthopaedic Surgeons. Committee on Biomedical Engineering, American Academy of Orthopaedic Surgeons. Committee on Hip and Knee Arthritis, 2001. Alternative bearing surfaces: the good, the bad, and the ugly. J. Bone Joint Surg. 83 (Suppl. 2), S68–S72.

Baruffaldi, F., et al., 2017. Characterisation of noise on ceramic-on-ceramic total hip arthroplasty. Bone Joint J. 99-B (Suppl. 2), 66.

Burger, W., Richter, H.G., 2001. High strength and toughness alumina matrix composites by transformation toughening and "in situ" platelet reinforcement (ZPTA) – The new generation of bioceramics. Key Eng. Mater. 192–195, 545–548. Available at: http://www.scientific.net/KEM.192-195.545 [Accessed June 27, 2016].

Callaghan, J.J., et al., 2008. How have alternative bearings (such as metal-on-metal, highly cross-linked polyethylene, and ceramic-on-ceramic) affected the prevention and treatment of osteolysis. J. Am. Acad. Orthop. Surg. 16 (Suppl. 1), S33–S38.

Castillo, T.N., Kaufman, D., Maloney, W.J., 2014. Ceramic-on-ceramic total hip arthroplasty: a new standard-Opposes. Semin. Arthroplasty 25 (2), 116–119.

Ceroni, R.G., et al., 2006. Tricks and tips in every day utilization of ceramic on ceramic coupling. Bioceram. Alt. Bearing Joint Arthroplasty 219–223.

Chang, C., et al., 2008. Transfer of metallic debris from the metal surface of an acetabular cup to artificial femoral heads by scraping: comparison between alumina and cobalt-chrome heads. J. Biomed. Mater. Res. 85 (1), 204–209. Available at: http://www.ncbi.nlm.nih.gov/pubmed/17854069 [Accessed March 30, 2016].

Christel, P., et al., 1988. Biomechanical compatibility and design of ceramic implants for orthopedic surgery. Ann. N. Y. Acad. Sci. 523, 234–256.

Clarke, I., et al., 2003. Current status of zirconia used in total hip implants. J. Bone Joint Surgery. Am. Vol. 85–A (Suppl.), 73–84. Available at: http://www.ncbi.nlm.nih.gov/pubmed/14652396 [Accessed September 17, 2015].

Cross, M.B., Nam, D., Mayman, D.J., 2012. Ideal femoral head size in total hip arthroplasty balances stability and volumetric wear HHS J. 8 270–274

Dai, H., 2002. Carbon nanotubes: synthesis, integration, and properties. Acc. Chem. Res. 35 (12), 1035–1044.

Dickinson, A.S., et al., 2011. Pre-clinical evaluation of ceramic femoral head resurfacing prostheses using computational models and mechanical testing. Proc. Instit. Mech. Eng. Part H J. Eng. Med. 225 (9), 866–876.

Elpers, M., et al., 2014. Zirconia phase transformation, metal transfer, and surface roughness in retrieved ceramic composite femoral heads in total hip arthroplasty. J. Arthroplasty 29 (11), 2219–2223. Available at: http://linkinghub.elsevier.com/retrieve/pii/S0883540314005877.

Fayard, J.P., et al., 2006. Ten-year results of ALIZE acetabular cup with hydroxyapatite coating and AURA hydroxyapatite-coated stem in total hip arthroplasty. J. Arthroplasty 21 (7), 1021–1025.

Fisher, J., et al., 2006. Tribology of alternative bearings. Clin. Orthop. Relat. Res. 453 (453), 25–34.

Hamadouche, M., et al., 2002. Alumina-on-alumina total hip arthroplasty: a minimum 18.5-year follow-up study. J. Bone Joint Surg. Am. 84–A (1), 69–77.
Hannink, R.H.J., Kelly, P.M., Muddle, B.C., 2000. Transformation toughening in zirconia-containing ceramics. J. Am. Ceram. Soc. 83 (3), 461–487.
Hannouche, D., et al., 2005. Ceramics in total hip replacement. Clin. Orthop. Relat. Res. 430, 62–71. Available at: http://www.ncbi.nlm.nih.gov/entrez/query.fcgi?cmd = Retrieve&db = PubMed&dopt = Citation&list_uids = 15662305.
Heart, S., 2016. Alumina and zirconia ceramics in joint replacements. J. Appl. Biomater. Biomech. JABB Appl. Biomater. April, 19–32.
Helmer, J.D., Driskell, T.D., 1969. Research on bioceramics. Symposium on Use of Ceramics as Surgical Implants. Clemson University, Clemson, SC.
Hench, L.L., 1993. Bioceramics – from concept to clinic. Am. Ceram. Soc. Bull. 74 (7), 1487–1510.
Hing, C., Back, D., Shimmin, A., 2007. Hip resurfacing: indications, results, and conclusions. Instr. Course. Lect. 56, 171–178.
Holland, J.P., et al., 2012. Ten-year clinical, radiological and metal ion analysis of the Birmingham Hip Resurfacing from a single, non-designer surgeon. J. Bone Joint Surg. Br. 9494 (4), 471–476.
ISO, 2015. ISO 13356: 2015: implants for surgery – ceramic materials based on yttria-stabilized tetragonal zirconia (Y-TZP).
Jarrett, C.A., et al., 2009. The squeaking hip: a phenomenon of ceramic-on-ceramic total hip arthroplasty. J. Bone Joint Surg. 91 (6), 1344–1349.
Kang, B.J., et al., 2015. Third-generation alumina-on-alumina total hip arthroplasty: 14- to 16-year follow-up study. J. Arthroplasty 30 (3), 411–415.
Kawano, S., et al., 2013. Failure analysis of alumina on alumina total hip arthroplasty with a layered acetabular component. Minimum ten-year follow-up study. J. Arthroplasty 28 (10), 1822–1827.
Kim, H.T., et al., 2009. The effect of low temperature aging on the mechanical property & phase stability of Y-TZP ceramics. J. Adv. Prosthodont. 1 (3), 113–117.
Kim, Y.H., Choi, Y., Kim, J.S., 2010. Cementless total hip arthroplasty with ceramic-on-ceramic bearing in patients younger than 45 years with femoral-head osteonecrosis. Int. Orthop. 34 (8), 1123–1127.
Koo, K.-H., et al., 2008. Isolated fracture of the ceramic head after third-generation alumina-on-alumina total hip arthroplasty. J. Bone. Joint. Surg. Am. 90 (2), 329–336.
Le, D.T., Murphy, S.B., 2014. Ceramic-on-ceramic total hip arthroplasty: a new standard-Affirms. Semin. Arthroplasty 25 (2), 107–115.
Lee, G.C., Garino, J.P., 2011. Reliability of ceramic components. Semin. Arthroplasty 22 (4), 271–275.
Lee, Y.-K., et al., 2010. Alumina-on-alumina total hip arthroplasty: a concise follow-up, at a minimum of ten years, of a previous report. J. Bone. Joint. Surg. Am. 92 (8), 1715–1719.
Maccauro, G., et al., 2004. Fracture of a Y-TZP ceramic femoral head. J. Bone. Joint. Surg. 86 (8), 1192–1196. Available at: http://www.bjj.boneandjoint.org.uk/cgi/doi/10.1302/0301-620X.86B8.15012 [Accessed April 8, 2014].
Magnani, G., Brillante, A., 2005. Effect of the composition and sintering process on mechanical properties and residual stresses in zirconia–alumina composites. J. Eur. Ceram. Soc. 25 (15), 3383–3392.
Massin, P., et al., 2014. Does Biolox® Delta ceramic reduce the rate of component fractures in total hip replacement? Orthop. Traumatol. Surg. Res. 100 (6), S317–S321.
Matharu, G.S., et al., 2015. Failure of a novel ceramic-on-ceramic hip resurfacing prosthesis. J. Arthroplasty 30 (3), 416–418.

McLean, C.R., et al., 2002. Delayed fracture of the ceramic femoral head after trauma. J. Arthoplasty 17 (4), 503–504.
McMinn, D.J.W., et al., 2011. Indications and results of hip resurfacing. Int. Orthop. 35 (2), 231–237.
Merola, M., et al., 2016. On the tribological behavior of retrieved hip femoral heads affected by metallic debris. A comparative investigation by stylus and optical profilometer for a new roughness measurement protocol. Measurement 90, 365–371. Available at: http://linkinghub.elsevier.com/retrieve/pii/S0263224116301439.
Milošev, I., et al., 2012. Comparison of ten-year survivorship of hip prostheses with use of conventional polyethylene, metal-on-metal, or ceramic-on-ceramic bearings. J. Bone Joint Surg. Am. 94 (19), 1756–1763.
Monticelli, G. et al., 1981. First consideration on the use of $ZrO_2$ in hip prosthesis stem coating. In *Ann Meeting ESAO*. Copenhagen, Denmark.
Ms, J.M.E., et al., 2013. Do obesity and / or stripe wear increase ceramic liner fracture risk? An XFEM analysis. Clin. Orthop. Relat. Res. 471 (2), 527–536.
Park, Y.S., et al., 2006. Ceramic failure after total hip arthroplasty with an alumina-on-alumina bearing. J. Bone Joint Surg. Am. 88 (4), 780–787. Available at: http://www.ncbi.nlm.nih.gov/entrez/query.fcgi?cmd=Retrieve&db=PubMed&dopt=Citation&list_uids=16595468.
Piconi, C., 2011. Alumina. In: Paul, D. (Ed.), Comprehensive Biomaterials. Elsevier, Oxford, pp. 73–94.
Piconi, C., et al., 2003. Alumina and zirconia ceramics in joint. J. Appl. Biomater. Biomech. 1 (1), 19–32.
Piconi, C., et al., 2007. Zirconia heads in perspective: a survey of zirconia outcomes in total hip replacement. Hip. Int. 17 (3), 119–130.
Piconi, C., Maccauro, G., Muratori, F., 2005. Alumina matrix composites in arthroplasty. Key Eng. Mater. 284–286, 979–982.
Rambani, R., et al., 2017. Revision total hip arthroplasty for fractured ceramic bearings: a review of best practices for revision cases. J. Arthroplasty 1–6.
Raravikar, N.R., et al., 2005. Synthesis and characterization of thickness-aligned carbon nanotube-polymer composite films. Chem. Mater. 17 (5), 974–983.
Richter, H.G., Willman, G., 1999. Reliability of ceramic components for total hip endoprostheses. Br. Ceram. Trans. 98 (1), 29–34.
Rieu, J., Goeuriot, P., 1993. Ceramic composites for biomedical applications. Clin. Mater. 12, 211–217.
Roualdes, O., et al., 2010. *In vitro* and *in vivo* evaluation of an alumina–zirconia composite for arthroplasty applications. Biomaterials 31 (8), 2043–2054.
Shafafy, R., Foote, J., Hargrove, R., 2016. A novel technique for identification of fractured ceramic acetabular liner in total hip arthroplasty: a case report. Hip Int. 25 (5), 492–494.
Sharkey, P.F., 2009. Ceramic-on-ceramic bearings in total hip arthroplasty. Surgical Treatment of Hip Arthritis: Reconstruction, Replacement, and Revision 478–484.
Sharma, O.P., et al., 2013. Severe metallosis leading to femoral head perforation. Orthopedics 36 (2), 241–243.
Skinner, H.B., 1999. Ceramic bearing surfaces. Clin. Orthop. Relat. Res. 369, 83–91. Available at: http://www.ncbi.nlm.nih.gov/entrez/query.fcgi?cmd = Retrieve&db = PubMed&dopt = Citation&list_uids=10611863.
Stea, S., et al., 2012. Synovial fluid microanalysis allows early diagnosis of ceramic hip prosthesis damage. J. Orthop. Res. 30 (8), 1312–1320.
Stewart, T.D., et al., 2003. Long-term wear of ceramic matrix composite materials for hip prostheses under severe swing phase microseparation. J. Biomed. Mater. Res. B. Appl.

Biomater. 66 (2), 567–573. Available at: http://www.ncbi.nlm.nih.gov/entrez/query.fcgi?cmd=Retrieve&db=PubMed&dopt=Citation&list_uids=12861609.
Sun, J., Gao, L., Li, W., 2002. Colloidal processing of carbon nanotube / alumina composites. Chem. Mater. 14 (16), 5169–5172.
Taddei, P., et al., 2012. Raman and fluorescence investigations on retrieved Biolox delta femoral heads. J. Raman Spectroscopy 43 (12), 1868–1876.
Taddei, P., et al., 2016. Transfer of metallic debris after in vitro ceramic-on-metal simulation: wear and degradation in Biolox ® Delta composite femoral heads *. Composites Part B1–11.
Tai, S.M., et al., 2015. Squeaking in large diameter ceramic-on-ceramic bearings in total hip arthroplasty. J. Arthroplasty 30 (2), 282–285. Available at: http://dx.doi.org/10.1016/j.arth.2014.09.010.
Toni, A., et al., 2006. Early diagnosis of ceramic liner fracture. Guidelines based on a twelve-year clinical experience. J. Bone. Joint. Surg. Am. 88 (Suppl 4), 55–63. Available at: http://www.ncbi.nlm.nih.gov/pubmed/17142435 [Accessed April 8, 2014].
Traina, F., et al., 2013. Fracture of ceramic bearing surfaces following total hip replacement: a systematic review. BioMed. Res. Int. 2013, 157247.
Traina, F., et al., 2011. Revision of ceramic hip replacements for fracture of a ceramic component: AAOS exhibit selection. J. Bone Joint Surg. [Am]. 93 (24), e147.
Traina, F., et al., 2012. Risk factors for ceramic liner fracture after total hip arthroplasty. HIP Int. 22 (6), 607–614.
Walter, W., 2017. Longevity, biocompatibility and wear resistance practical guide for handling noises in hard-on-hard bearings. CeramTec Ceram. Expert3. Available at: https://www.ceramtec.com/biolox/?redirect = biolox.com.
Walter, W.L., et al., 2007. Squeaking in ceramic-on-ceramic hips. The importance of acetabular component orientation. J. Arthroplasty 22 (4), 496–503.
Walter, W.L., Yeung, E., Esposito, C., 2010. A review of squeaking hips. J. Am. Acad. Orthop. Surg. 18 (6), 319–326.
Willman, G., Fruh, H.J., Pfaff, H.G., 1996. Wear characteristics of sliding pairs of zirconia (Y-TZP) for hip endoprostheses. Biomaterials 17 (22), 2157–2162.
Wyatt, M.C., et al., 2014. Noise from total hip replacements. Bone Joint Res. 3 (6), 183–186.
Yoo, J.J., et al., 2005. Alumina-on-alumina total hip arthroplasty. A five-year minimum follow-up study. J. Bone joint Surgery. Am. Volume. 87 (3), 530–535. Available at: http://www.ncbi.nlm.nih.gov/pubmed/15741618 [Accessed April 18, 2014].
Yoo, J.J., et al., 2006. Contemporary alumina-on-alumina total hip arthroplasty performed in patients younger than forty years: a 5-year minimum follow-up study. J. Biomed. Mater. Res. 78 (1), 70–75.
Zhu, Y.-F.F., et al., 2008. Synthesis of zirconia nanoparticles on carbon nanotubes and their potential for enhancing the fracture toughness of alumina ceramics. Comp. Part B Eng. 39 (7–8), 1136–1141. Available at: http://www.sciencedirect.com/science/article/pii/S1359836808000553 [Accessed September 25, 2015].
Zywiel, M.G., Turgeon, T.R., 2013. Fatal cardiomyopathy after revision total hip replacement for fracture of a ceramic liner. Bone Joint J. 95 (1), 31–37.

## Further Reading

Gührs, J., et al., 2015. The influence of stem taper re-use upon the failure load of ceramic heads. Med. Eng. Phys. 37 (6), 545–552.

# Part III

# Engineering and Challenges of New Ceramics for Medical Devices

# Design of ceramic materials for orthopedic devices

# 10

*Frank Kern*[1], *Anke Bernstein*[2] *and Andreas Killinger*[1]
[1]University of Stuttgart, Stuttgart, Germany, [2]University of Freiburg, Freiburg, Germany

**Chapter Outline**

**10.1 Bulk ceramics 331**
10.1.1 From a retrospect to the current state-of-the-art 331
10.1.2 New developments: oxides 334
10.1.3 New developments: nonoxides 340
**10.2 Coatings 341**
10.2.1 Coatings with biocompatible ceramics 341
10.2.2 Carbon based coatings 344
10.2.3 Carbide and nitride thin films and surfaces 345
**10.3 Conclusions and perspectives 346**
**References 348**

## 10.1 Bulk ceramics

### *10.1.1 From a retrospect to the current state-of-the-art*

Currently the market for hip implants (ceramic knee-, shoulder-, and other joint replacements are widespread yet) is to a large extent covered by two materials: alumina and zirconia-toughened alumina (ZTA), where the latter is the dominant product in the market. Although a certain number of patients still have yttria-stabilized zirconia (Y-TZP) implants, the importance of Y-TZP is negligible for the new components. For a comprehensive overview of the state-of-the-art in hip and knee arthroplasty the review papers by Rahaman and by McEntire are recommended (Rahaman et al., 2007; McEntire et al., 2015).

Alumina was the first ceramic material applied in orthopedic bearing devices. Advantages of alumina are its high hardness and abrasion resistance (which also enable using ceramic–ceramic couples), its moderate price and a practically unlimited availability. Due to the limited strength and fracture resistance, alumina to date is only applied in femoral balls and cups operating under moderate loading conditions. Developments in the past have emphasized the improvement of reliability of the brittle components by reducing the defect sizes over the whole production cycle (Willmann, 1996). The first generation of alumina balls had a hardness of 18 GPa, a strength of 400 MPa, and a fracture resistance of 4 $MPa\sqrt{m}$, the grain size was 4.5 μm, and they were 99.5% dense. In the following two stages, the strength and

Advances in Ceramic Biomaterials.
DOI: http://dx.doi.org/10.1016/B978-0-08-100881-2.00011-7

hardness were increased to 580 MPa and 19.5 GPa, respectively, at unchanged fracture resistance. The introduction of a hot isostatic pressing operation after pressureless sintering allowed full densification and reduction of the grain size below 2 μm (Willmann, 1996). At present, a high stage of maturity has been achieved and the potential to further improve the material is limited. Further reduction of sintering temperature, time and thus grain size may improve strength but would reduce fracture resistance by eliminating any R-curve behavior (see Chapter 3: Assessment of mechanical properties of ceramic materials on this regard).

The next material to follow alumina in the late 1980s was yttria stabilized zirconia polycrystals (Y-TZP). Y-TZP, having considerably higher strength (> 1000 MPa) and fracture resistance (5–6 MPa$\sqrt{m}$) than alumina, seemed the ultimate solution for hip joints and also potentially applicable for knee implants (Tsukuma et al., 1983). Due to its lower hardness, Y-TZP has to be applied with a polymer counterpart (Willmann, 2001). Low-temperature degradation (LTD) of the tetragonal phase, i.e., the nonstress-induced transformation of metastable tetragonal to stable monoclinic under the influence of moisture at elevated temperature, an effect first shown by Kobayashi, was initially considered irrelevant in the application scenario at body temperature (Kobayashi et al., 1981). In 1999, 12 suppliers produced Y-TZP balls and Y-TZP reached a >50% market share of ceramic balls in France, Japan, and the United States (Piconi et al., 2006). In 2001, 600,000 hip joints were implanted, among them 2/3 supplied by the market leader SGCA Desmarquest. After a change in the manufacturing cycle at SGCA to boost productivity, sudden in vivo failures were observed, among them more than 100 from the same production batch. Balls were bursting in vivo without application of extreme external stress. Studies of failed and explanted balls showed that the catastrophic failure was initiated by LTD, but not as initially suspected, from the side of the tribological pairing, but from the backside. It was postulated that moisture had penetrated into the gap between the stem and the femoral ball, initiating LTD coupled with volume expansion, which put the ball under tensile stress from the inside (Chevalier et al., 2009). This was promoted by pressing defects in the center of the CIPed balls which laid open when machining the conical cavity for the stem. This episode put an abrupt end to the use of Y-TZP materials in hip joints. Unfortunately, it also finished some promising developments in Y-TZP materials with drastically higher aging resistance (Burger et al., 1997; Piconi et al., 1998). While Y-TZP was de facto banned for hip joints, the material has recently seen a renaissance in dental applications (Denry and Kelly, 2008). Chevalier et al. (2007, 2009) have published some excellent reviews about LTD of Y-TZP and its consequences.

As a result of this drawback, implant manufacturers shifted back to alumina, which had drastically lost market share during the Y-TZP boom. In the following period, CeramTec were first to develop, before all other companies, a material which promised to bring together the advantages of alumina (hardness, abrasion resistance, LTD stability) and Y-TZP (strength, toughness) and allowed the implantation of all-ceramic joints. This was BIOLOX delta, a product originally developed for cutting tools under the tradename DC25, having a ZTA composition, with a zirconia content close to the percolation limit. The material has a strength of up to 1250 MPa, a fracture toughness of 5.7 MPa$\sqrt{m}$ and a hardness of 17 GPa (Burger and Richter 2001; Kuntz, 2006). Due to its favorable properties and patented composition (it contains chromia to enhance hardness and strontia to form a hexa-aluminate platelet reinforcement in situ), BIOLOX delta has nowadays a market share of ~90% in ceramic hip implants with ~1 million pieces manufactured every year. Meanwhile other producers, such as CoorsTek medical, have also developed ZTA materials with very similar properties. Fig. 10.1 shows the microstructure of a fine-grain ZTA with 17 vol% zirconia comparable to the material commercially applied. It is clearly visible that the material is fully densified and has a good dispersion of the second phase. Zirconia grains located at the four junctions of alumina block the grain growth of the matrix efficiently and ensure a fine grain microstructure.

Alumina-toughened Y-TZP (ATZ) has also been identified as a suitable material for joint replacement. An ATZ material is currently sold by Mathys under the brand name Ceramys. With a typical alumina content of 20–30 vol%, ATZ shows superior aging resistance (Schneider et al., 2008) compared to 3Y-TZP. Fracture toughness of ATZ is comparable (~5 MPa$\sqrt{m}$) and fracture strength (up to 2000 MPa) is superior to medical-grade 3Y-TZP (Tsukuma et al., 1985; Kern and Gadow, 2012). The higher strength of ATZ is attributed to a lower defect size. At identical $K_{I0}/K_{IC}$ ratio as in Y-TZP (see Chapter 2: Types of ceramics: material class), the excellent bending strength offers also higher fatigue strength in ATZ.

Nonoxides such as liquid-phase sintered silicon nitride and silicon carbide have been proposed for joint replacements. While their mechanical properties (strength, hardness, toughness) are definitely sufficient, there is some controversy regarding the biocompatibility issues. As both nonoxides are covered with a silica layer, which is expected to grow further by corrosion processes, spallation of this silica layer was feared as this would lead to third-body wear. For silicon nitride applied in spinal implants, successful short-term compatibility results are available (Bal and Rahaman, 2012).

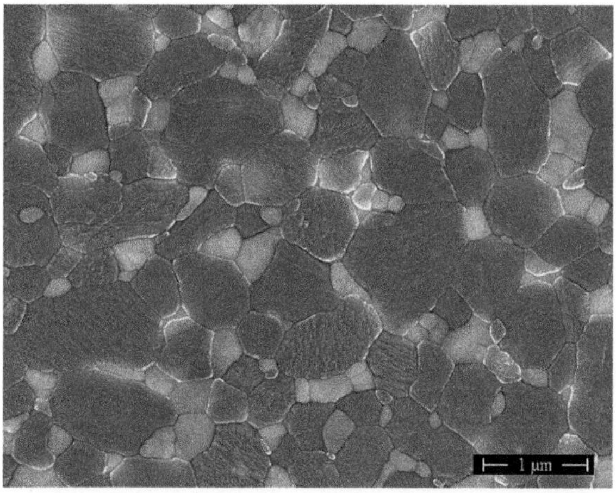


**Figure 10.1** Microstructure of zirconia-toughened alumina (ZTA); scanning electron microscopic image, thermally etched sample unpublished data from (Kern et al., 2016).

### 10.1.2 New developments: oxides

Hip- and knee implants are medical products classified as class 3 Medical Devices, with a high risk potential. Therefore regulations are strict, demanding extensive procedures to validate the conformity and guarantee the product safety and service capability of a newly developed product. Keeping this in mind and considering the high performance of existing solutions, the development of a new material for implants is not only a scientific and technical challenge, but the development of new materials, thus represents a high economic risk and a lengthy procedure with an uncertain outcome.

It is therefore not surprising that many scientific developments, despite showing great potential and technical advantage, never reached clinical testing or were implemented in new products. Manufacturers with established products were reluctant to launch 'new' products, instead focussing their efforts to adapt the component designs or to apply the established materials with a proven track record in new applications such as for knee, shoulder, or spinal implants.

Most implant manufacturers have now focused on ZTA. According to the current ISO standard 6474-2, ZTA (ISO, 2012) biomedical applications may contain:

- 60–90 wt% alumina;
- 10–30 wt% $ZrO_2$ (<5% $HfO_2$);
- < 10 wt% projected additives;
- 0.2 wt% Impurities such as, e.g., $SiO_2$, CaO, $Na_2O$.

Assuming 16–17 vol% (~25 wt%) zirconia as the percolation threshold in a composite with equal grain sizes of both matrix and dispersion, the standard covers materials with zirconia contents well below (6.5 vol%) to slightly above the percolation threshold.

The high threshold, of up to 10 wt% "projected additives", (besides, e.g., yttria required to stabilize the zirconia and chromia and strontia in the product of the market leader) provides quite a high degree of freedom for the creation of new materials. However, there is little evidence that this compositional range is actually being exploited.

It has emerged, however, that playing with different dopants with the sole aim of improving the mechanical properties or the aging resistance has to be carried out with extreme care. Puppulin et al. (2014) have recently highlighted the role of dopants in the alteration of surface chemistry and the resulting implications on chemical and tribochemical resistance of alumina, Y-TZP and ZTA materials. Contrary to the orthodox belief that these oxides are entirely bioinert, recent studies have shown that even alumina does interact with the in vivo environment. Consequently, after long time exposure in the range of the typical implant lifetime of ~10 years, these changes in surface chemistry, i.e., creation of vacancies and take up of aliovalent cations such as $Ca^{2+}$ and $Mg^{2+}$, may lead to roughening of the surface and, in extreme cases, even to a spallation of the grains in the top layer, due to formation of chemically induced stresses (Pezzotti, 2014). For zirconia, it is known that take-up of oxygen-containing species leads to elimination of oxygen vacancies, which were introduced by yttria doping, and to a destabilization of the tetragonal phase resulting in surface roughening or even complete failure (Chevalier et al., 2007).

With reference to the regulatory framework for ZTA (ISO, 2012) it has to be said that the requirements for mechanical properties in the ISO standard are relatively moderate. A strength of 600 MPa, a fracture toughness of 4 MPa$\sqrt{m}$, together with a Young's modulus of 320 GPa and a hardness of >16 GPa are required. Average grain sizes have to be kept below 1.5 μm for alumina and below 0.6 μm for zirconia. The more challenging requirements are those of fatigue resistances of 400 MPa (as received) and 320 MPa (hydrothermally aged) up to 10 million cycles. Wear of aged components should not be increased by more than 20% compared to the as-processed state.

With respect to fatigue resistance, these minimum requirements can be translated into values for resistance to subcritical crack growth/threshold toughness $K_{I0} = K_{IC}$ *320/600 = 2.1 MPa$\sqrt{m}$, a value well below the $K_{I0}$ value for alumina (DeAza et al., 2003a). Threshold toughness values published for ZTA strongly depend on the method used. Stable indentation crack growth in bending showed values between 2.5 MPa$\sqrt{m}$ in the composite alumina/15 wt% zirconia (Kern et al., 2015) and 3.2 MPa$\sqrt{m}$ in alumina/32 wt% zirconia (Kern, 2013a). Double torsion tests show values between 4 and 5 MPa$\sqrt{m}$ for alumina/15 wt% zirconia (Gutknecht et al., 2007).

Literature on fatigue resistance values of biomedical ZTA materials are rare: Ramalingam et al. (2011) measured a fatigue strength of 360 MPa in a ZTA material containing 25 wt% zirconia and hexa-aluminate platelets and a $K_{IC}/K_{IO}$ value of 0.78 at 100% relative humidity. Kirsten et al. (2010) published slow crack growth data on the four typical oxide ceramics for implants (ZTA, ATZ, alumina, and 3Y-TZP) and found the lowest failure probabilities for ATZ after 6 months (42%) and 5 years (48%) at a load of 815 MPa. Alumina and 3Y-TZP showed much steeper failure probability versus service time curves. It has to be considered, however, that these tests did not take into account the effect of the tribological stress and chemical environment in the human body.

Among ZTA materials, we may subdivide between materials with different amounts of unstabilized zirconia and materials in which the zirconia is stabilized by, e.g., yttria.

ZTA with unstabilized zirconia dispersion tends to be more stable in hydrothermal environments as long as the dispersion is homogeneously distributed and has a narrow grain size distribution (Gutknecht et al., 2007). Intergranular zirconia grains depending on shape and location stay tetragonal under the influence of the rigid alumina matrix if they have grain sizes below ~0.4 μm (Heuer et al., 1982). However, the percolation limit (~16%) is a theoretical upper limitation for addition of unstabilized zirconia. Depending on the manufacturing process and the quality of the starting powders used, the practical limit is somewhat lower (~10–12 vol%) (Lange, 1982; Messing and Kumagai, 1989).

Studies in this field have been carried out over the last 30 years by different authors. The lowest zirconia content in ZTA mandatory to suppress abnormal grain growth can be located somewhere between 5 and 7 vol%, depending on sintering conditions and zirconia grain size (Lange, 1982). It is necessary to block the four junctions between alumina grains. In plain ZTA, if using sufficiently fine starting powders and assuming proper processing to distribute the zirconia and alumina homogeneously, it is not necessary to stabilize with yttria up to zirconia contents of 10–12 vol%, even if mixing and milling technologies are applied (Kern, 2011). Application of coating technologies to deposit the zirconia on the alumina starting powder ensure a homogeneous zirconia distribution and can be seen as an innovative approach to improve and efficiently control the dispersion of the second phase (Palmero et al., 2009, 2014). Fig. 10.2 shows the improved and refined microstructure of ZTA made from coated powder.

Due to the limited fraction of zirconia that can be added, ZTA materials containing unstabilized zirconia as a predominantly tetragonal dispersion have a limited fracture toughness and strength, but such values are still more than sufficient to fulfill the ISO 6474-2 standard (Kern, 2011; Gutknecht et al., 2007).

In the field of ZTA materials with partially stabilized zirconia, systematic studies are rare, probably due to the fact that only 3Y-TZP and unstabilized zirconia are readily available in the market. So, many studies with stabilized zirconia use 3Y-TZP and do not selectively adjust the stabilizer content (Douillard et al., 2012). Such materials containing the TZP as a fine dispersion are, however, relatively brittle, since the zirconia dispersion is untransformable. In spite of this, examples of tough materials of this kind are known, in which the mechanism of their toughening is, however, based on relatively large 3Y-TZP dispersoids and residual stress, rather than transformation toughening (Langlois and Konsztowicz, 1992).

Exare et al. recently published a comprehensive paper on the phase relations in alumina/zirconia composites, with different stabilizer contents and covering a very

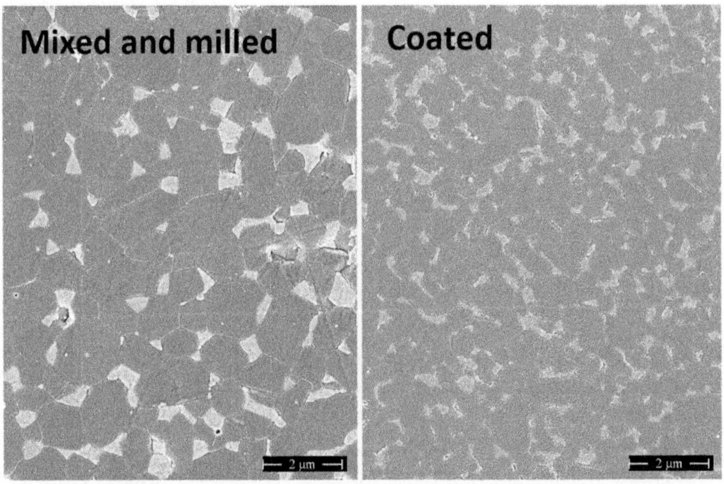


**Figure 10.2** Microstructure of ZTA containing 10 vol% unstabilized zirconia sintered at 1500°C for 3 h in air, left (compounding by mixing and milling of alumina and zirconia), right (zirconia coated on alumina starting powder); unpublished data from previous study (Kern et al., 2015).

wide range of compositions; the grid was, however, too coarse to obtain detailed information in the range relevant for biomedical-grade ZTA (Exare et al., 2015). Even though the basic mechanism of toughening and the influence of microstructural issues are well known, producing a strong and tough ZTA material from alumina and stabilized zirconia is still challenging. Sommer et al. (2012a,b) have demonstrated in a $3 \times 3 \times 3$ experimental plan—varying zirconia content from 10 to 24 vol%, sintering time at 1475°C from 1 to 3 hours and yttria content from 1 to 2 mol%—that the parameter range for best results is very narrow. Starting from the compositional optimum found by Sommer et al. (1 mol% yttria, 17 vol% zirconia), a more detailed study on variation of stabilizer content was carried out, by using the same raw materials (Kern et al., 2016). The study clearly showed an exponential rise in toughness with decreasing yttria content, a very steep toughness optimum at 0.8–1 mol% yttria (depending on testing protocol) and a strength maximum between 1.0 and 1.6 mol% yttria. Two main statements may thus be made: (1) in the system studied it is impossible to optimize strength and toughness at the same time; (2) ZTA materials offered by CeramTec and CoorsTek (besides further addition of chromia and strontia in the commercial products) have a composition in the optimum range, where a good compromise between strength and toughness is achieved.

The basic challenge in the field of ZTA-based materials is the balance between the microstructure, phase composition, and LTD resistance, on the one hand, and strength and fracture toughness on the other. Those requirements are somewhat contradictory and a compromise has to be found to safely fulfill all requirements. Changes in raw material selection and processing technology may slightly increase the absolute values measured, but it seems, however, that in the absence of further phases/additives, the ZTA system has reached a high maturity and offers little room for further improvement.

Within the EU-Project BIOKER, an entirely different material concept was pursued. ZTA with a very low amount of zirconia addition was developed, featuring a new intratype micro-nanostructure, in which almost all zirconia grains are very small, globular, and incorporated into the relatively large and nonisometric alumina grains (Chevalier et al., 2005; Chevalier and Gremillard, 2009). In this material, a different toughening effect was exploited, associated to the presence of large compressive residual stress in the alumina particles, $ZrO_2$ inclusions. On the other hand, $ZrO_2$ particles located at the alumina grain boundaries—like in conventional ZTA—do not give rise to such high residual stresses. This leads to materials with moderate strength of ~600 MPa a relatively high toughness of 6 $MPa\sqrt{m}$ and a very favorable $K_{I0}$ of 5 $MPa\sqrt{m}$. The inclusions are untransformable under stress and no LTD is observed. The material is, however, off-specification due to its low zirconia content and has never been commercially applied.

Recently, the Panasonic Electric Works has produced a nano-nano-type zirconia–alumina composite, commercialized under the tradename of NANOZR for the dental market. This material shows excellent properties, in terms of bending strength (1290 MPa), fracture toughness (8.62 $MPa\sqrt{m}$) and crack propagation threshold ($K_{I0}$ of 4.6 $MPa\sqrt{m}$, as determined by Chevalier and Gremillard, 2009).

As $K_{I0}$ represents the safe range for using ceramics in hip joints, the high values determined in both micro-nano- and nano-nanocomposites further explain the interest in these kinds of structures. The slow crack growth behavior of these materials has been already reported and discussed in Chapter 2, Types of ceramics: material class and Chapter 3, Assessment of mechanical properties of ceramic materials, and compared to those of monolithic alumina, zirconia, and conventional ZTA.

Addition of further "projected additives" seems to open up new possibilities to further improve the oxide-based systems.

In 2015, a patent application was filed by Burger and Kiefer (Oximatec GmbH, Hochdorf, Germany), describing a ZTA material with a Y-Ce cotabilized zirconia dispersion and a platelet reinforcement by lanthanum hexaluminate. Additionally, 0.2–0.5 mol% praseodymium oxide were added, which due to its mixed valence may be incorporated into zirconia as a stabilizer or form a mixed hexa-aluminate together with lanthana and alumina. Materials reach 4-pt bending strength values between 900 MPa (pressureless sintered) and 1250 MPa (post HIPed). Fracture resistance values range from 6 to 7.8 $MPa\sqrt{m}$, suggesting high damage tolerance. No studies have been published yet about resistance to subcritical crack growth and LTD resistance. Due to the Y-Ce mixed stabilizer system, it can however be hypothesized that the material has higher aging resistance as the state-of-the-art yttria stabilized ZTA (Burger and Kiefer, 2015).

Kyocera Medical Co. introduced a new ZTA material KM AZ209 containing 14% of unstabilized zirconia and 2 vol% other additives such as $TiO_2$, SrO, MgO, and $SiO_2$. The materials, up to now, have only been marketed in Japan. KM AZ209 contains a very fine-grained zirconia dispersion and also contains a strontium hexa-aluminate platelet reinforcement. Bending strength in as received and aged condition is high (>1200 MPa) and constant over 300 hours of autoclave aging. A degradation of the tetragonal phase was not observed after the same aging treatment, and the monoclinic content stayed constant at ~17% (Pezzotti, 2014). However, as the alumina matrix at the surface is under tensile stress, the wear resistance is not superior to alumina. This surprising behavior was attributed to the influence of the titania dopant which favors formation of vacancies (Pezzotti, 2014). In spite of the widespread use of hexa-aluminates platelets in ZTA ceramics, systematic investigations related to the role of their morphology and aspect ratio on their toughening/reinforcing effects are still lacking in literature. A deepening of such features could lead to even further improvements in the use of this approach.

In the case of zirconia materials, some efforts were made to either further improve Y-TZP or develop TZP or TZP/alumina composites materials using different stabilizers. In the case of Y-TZP, it was known that materials derived from yttria-coated monoclinic zirconia rather than coprecipitated 3Y-TZP powders lead to superior aging resistance (Burger et al., 1997) (Piconi et al., 1998). Moreover, "coated" Y-TZPs show finer microstructure and considerably higher fracture resistance. These studies have recently been revived by different groups. Zhang et al. have recently shown that the concept leads to ultrafine microstructures in 3Y-TZP, fair toughness and, dealing with the major concern against Y-TZP, a significantly improved LTD resistance (Zhang et al., 2014, 2015). Moreover, it has been shown that in order to boost toughness, the stabilizer content in these "coated" Y-TZP systems can be reduced while maintaining a comparable aging resistance as in state of the art biomedical 3Y-TZP (Kern and Gadow, 2013). At the current state-of-the-art, these materials would be well suited for hip and knee joints. However, considering the bad experience in the past, it may be doubted whether Y-TZP will ever be used again in arthroplasty.

Mixed trivalent rare earth stabilizer systems in TZP (e.g., 1Y-2Nd-TZP) offer improved LTD resistance compared to 3Y-TZP (Salehi et al., 2010). As this higher aging resistance comes along with improved fracture toughness, resistance to subcritical crack growth (Kern, 2013b) and high strength, such materials could be attractive for applications especially in the knee, where the counterpart will be polymer anyway. A zirconia may be more suitable here than the alumina-based composites, due to the lower elastic modulus and the resulting lower Hertzian stress at identical load.

Shifting from yttria to ceria stabilizers in TZP drastically improves toughness and LTD resistance. In particular, in the high toughness formulations, the tetragonal-to-monoclinic transformation can be autocatalytic (Hannink et al., 2000). The drawback of Ce-TZP compared to Y-TZP is that the strength is drastically reduced, due to a significant grain growth of ceria-doped zirconia during sintering. Therefore, addition of fine alumina grains, able to retain zirconia grain growth, boosts strength of Ce-TZP but limits zirconia transformability and hence fracture toughness. Thus, addition of second-phase particles with elongated morphology, like the hexa-aluminates, able to exert further toughening by additional crack deflection mechanism, partially restores the high toughness, without losing strength (Cutler et al., 1991). Ce-TZP/alumina nanocomposites also offer a favorable combination of strength, toughness, and LTD resistance (Nawa et al., 1998), even if the extremely high toughness values determined by direct crack length measurement were not confirmed by more conservative methods (Benzaid et al., 2008). Apel et al. (2012) presented Ce-TZP/spinel nanocomposites with outstanding fracture resistance and resistance to subcritical crack growth.

Mixed stabilizer systems, such as Y-Ce-TZP, could also be interesting materials. By the codoping, material characteristics between Y-TZP and Ce-TZP can be achieved resulting in higher strength than Ce-TZP and higher toughness and aging resistance than Y-TZP. A broad range of Y-Ce-costabilized TZP materials has been tested by Lin (Lin and Duh, 2002). Due to the reasons explained above, it is more likely that Ce-TZP-based nanocomposites or Y-Ce-TZP will be employed in dental implants rather than in arthroplasty, due to the regulatory concerns and inherent conservatism with the use of zirconia materials in this field.

Regarding zirconia codoping, a further strategy exploited in literature (Pitek et al., 2007; Lee et al., 1998) for the production of zirconia that are free from LTD, implies the combination of equimolar ratios of trivalent (such as $Y^{3+}$) and pentavalent (such as $Nb^{5+}$ or $Ta^{5+}$) ions. This system seems very promising, since it allows the retention of the tetragonal zirconia phase at room temperature, without producing oxygen vacancies, which make the material susceptible to LTD.

With respect to the high quality and reliability of the existing materials and the significant financial committment and risk to develop and qualify a completely new material system for ceramic joint replacements, the current activities are directed towards fine adjustment of the existing systems, improvements in manufacturing processes, and implementation of existing materials in new applications.

Besides sufficient mechanical properties in as-received state, the main concerns are based on the LTD behavior of the materials and the fatigue resistance.

Monitoring the recent developments in the ZTA materials of the market leader, a clear tendency can be observed to manufacture ZTA materials with lower amounts of monoclinic zirconia in as-received state. It is quite straightforward that the phase composition of the zirconia dispersion controls the state of residual stress in the alumina matrix (Gregori et al., 1999). Without phase transformation, the matrix is under compressive stress. If zirconia grains are too large or do contain insufficient amount of stabilizer, they transform during cooling forming the monoclinic phase. Phase transformation is associated with volume expansion and puts the matrix under tensile stress. The stress neutral state is reached at approximately 20% monoclinic (relative to total zirconia content and further additives). Larger fractions set the matrix under tensile stress. The consequence to mechanical properties has recently been demonstrated (Kern et al., 2016). Boffelli has recently reported results from retrieved ball heads of BIOLOX delta, produced in the years 2009, 2011, and 2014 (Boffelli et al., 2016). Materials with earlier production data have a higher monoclinic content in as-manufactured state. Zirconia dispersions in materials produced in 2009 had average monoclinic contents of 27 vol%, this was reduced to 21 vol% in 2011 and further to 17 vol% in 2014. According to the calibration curve published by Gregori, this means that the earliest materials contained a matrix under tensile stress, in 2011 parts were stress neutral and in the latest generation the alumina matrix is under compression. This indicates that the manufacturer has slightly altered the recipe and/or processing to obtain a lower initial monoclinic content, probably aiming at improved hydrothermal stability (Gregori et al., 1999). However, we may suppose, with respect to the latest results, that some fracture resistance (required only to offset risk of overload resulting in of catastrophic failure) was sacrificed for the sake of higher fatigue resistance (Kern et al., 2016).

## 10.1.3 New developments: nonoxides

Liquid-phase sintered silicon nitride is a material well known for its excellent strength and fracture resistance. Depending on starting powders, type of liquid phase, and processing conditions, materials with a broad variety of properties can be produced ranging from materials with equiaxed grains and relatively low toughness to materials with nodular silicon nitride grains exhibiting high fracture resistance (Riley, 2000). Moreover silicon nitride and silicon carbide show a much more favorable $K_{I0}/K_{IC}$ ratio (>0.8) than oxides (0.5–0.6) and should thus be excellent in applications exposed to cyclic fatigue (Chevalier et al., 2005). The excellent mechanical properties with strength up to 1000 MPa and a fracture toughness between 5 and 9 $\text{MPa}\sqrt{\text{m}}$ allows this ceramic material to be used in highly loaded components such as bearing balls or ceramic springs. Moreover, the material is being used in high-temperature applications such as glow plugs and turbine blades.

As silicon nitride is biocompatible and partially radiolucent (Neumann et al., 2004), the idea to implement it in endoprosthesis is obvious. Today the first encouraging short-term results concerning silicon carbide in cervical spacers and spinal fusion devices are available (Taylor et al., 2010). These are, however, parts which do not suffer from tribological loading. Bal and Rahaman (2012) have given an excellent overview on the potential of silicon nitride in orthopedic applications. Encouraging comments have recently been given by Pezzotti (2014). The formation of a silica scale on the surface of silicon nitride and its partial hydrolysis, which in the past has often been seen as an adverse indication, may be very beneficial in tribocouples such as hip joints due to inducing a self-lubricating effect (Muratov et al., 1998; Dante and Kajdas, 2012).

Amedica (Salt Lake City, USA) introduced silicon nitride components in spinal reconstruction and plans to use silicon nitride in endoprosthetics. Besides the tribological properties, antiinfective and osseointegrative properties were recently shown (Gorth et al., 2012; Webster et al., 2012). Some concerns have been expressed by Pezzotti with respect to the fracture mechanics in the specific application. As the high fracture resistance of silicon nitride is due to the self-reinforcing effect and which finally comes down to a low grain boundary strength, it is unclear how the material will behave under contact damage environment (swing and microseparation) (Pezzotti, 2014). These problems will have to be thoroughly investigated. If such future studies provide a positive outcome, it may well be that nonoxide hip and knee implants will be introduced in the future.

## 10.2 Coatings

### *10.2.1 Coatings with biocompatible ceramics*

In general, prostheses should ideally restore the joint function immediately and completely. This normally requires the use of mechanically and chemically stable materials such as metals and metal alloys. The coating of an implant with bioactive materials containing important bone minerals facilitates the ingrowth of tissue and thus a firmer bond between tissue and prosthesis. These chemical and biological requirements are fulfilled excellently by ceramic materials based on calcium orthophosphates and by the bioactive glasses (Sumenev et al., 2014; Xuereb et al., 2015). Unfortunately, these substances lack the necessary mechanical qualities, whereas metals fail to fulfill the chemical and biological requirements. To compensate for these disadvantages, load-bearing metal implants are coated with ceramic materials (Kay, 1990). Such materials can reduce the time between primary stabilization (the force-fit conjunction between bone and implant achieved during surgery) and secondary stabilization (definitive bone integration). To achieve durable chemical-biological stability of weight-bearing implants with ceramic coatings in osseous bedding, currently two oppositional paths are pursued: (1) development of long-lasting ceramic coatings ensuring biological stimulation throughout complete implantation period; (2) development of biodegradable ceramics that show controlled resorption rates in sync to bone regeneration, limiting the use of their stimulating effect to the duration of the healing process. Newly formed bone compensates for coating material erosion in the interface and the metal implant is firmly anchored in the bone via contact osteogenesis.

Coatings are affected by some disadvantages, such as disintegration of the ceramic layer and detached ceramic fragments. This limitation depends on adhesion of ceramic layer to the substrate, which is directly related to the chemical bonds between ceramic and bulk material as well as the elastic properties of both substances.

Hydroxyapatite (HA) ceramic is the most commonly used and best-studied coating material (Dorozhkin, 2015; Brown et al., 2013; Ducheyne and Qiu, 1999; DeAza et al., 2003b; Voigt and Mosier, 2011). Although many alternative coating technologies exist to form HA on metal surfaces, like physical vapor deposition (PVD; sputter deposition, laser ablation), sol-gel, electrophoretic deposition, it should be noted that at present, atmospheric and vacuum plasma spraying represent the most commonly used commercial techniques to manufacture HA coatings on metal implants on the industrial scale. Some implant manufacturers apply vacuum plasma sprayed Ti coating with a rough and open-porous structure on the upper part of a hip joint prosthesis, either with no post treatment or in combination with calcium phosphate- (CaP) or HA-based top-coating applied (either by vaccuum plasma spraying (VPS) or electrochemically) (Fink, 1996). The advantage of HA is its shortening of the implant healing phase. In common with all other combinations of materials, however, HA suffers from a number of problems, ranging from material properties to biological effects. Sudden uncontrollable inflammatory reactions (Ducheyne and Cuckler, 1992) often lead to loosening and the need for implant replacement. Problems can also occur as a result of surface defects in the coating, production faults, and errors in implantation. Such factors may lead to abrasion, fissuring, coating detachment, and fragmentation, which also require exchange of the prosthesis (Ducheyne and Qiu, 1999; DeAza et al., 2003b).

Calcium phosphate ceramic coatings are bioactive coatings that have been shown to conduct bone apposition by direct bone bonding. Their rate of degradation should ideally be synchronized with bone regeneration. The in vivo performance of such coatings depends on a large variety of factors such as chemical composition, crystallinity, phase purity, and resorption behavior.

In recent work, it was shown that supersonic flame spray technologies using HA-containing suspensions as a feedstock (high-velocity suspension flame spraying, HVSFS) are capable of forming thin, dense, and well adherent coatings on metal surfaces. Therefore, HVSFS could be an interesting alternative to atmospheric and vacuum plasma spray techniques (Stiegler et al., 2012), as the coatings exhibit better mechanical properties compared to plasma sprayed ones. It is shown that the ratio of amorphous to crystal phase within the coating can be adjusted by spray process parameters, making it possible to tailor the grade of resorbability to a desired level. Moreover, using HVSFS, bioresorbable bioglasses can be successfully sprayed, offering new possibilities by introducing an entire new material family of bioresorbable coating materials. Suspension spraying in general offers many new opportunities in terms of new material design and material modification. Fig. 10.3 shows the morphology of HA-layers deposited by three different thermal spray technologies. Coating structures can be tailored ranging from lamellar (atmospheric plasma spraying, APS) via dense with particular inclusions (high velocity oxyfuel spraying, HVOF) to fully dense (HVSFS).

The authors have shown, in a recently published work, that thin Ca/P-containing layers (HA and tricalcium phosphate (TCP)) without doping can be prepared with the aid of the HVSFS coating process. With the help of such coatings, a faster ingrowth and significantly improved mechanical stability after operation is expected. We have succeeded in establishing the necessary process for the HVSFS suspensions and in obtaining very finely structured, thin homogeneous layers. With the help of such coatings, a faster ingrowth and significantly improved mechanical stability after operation is to be achieved. The colonization of biomaterials with bacteria represents the main cause of implant-associated infections. Both an antibiotic prophylaxis and a faster osteointegration can be obtained by incorporation of bactericidal active metals in degradable CaP coatings. It is possible to get thin homogeneous layers containing silver, copper, and bismuth in bacteriostatic/bactericidal concentrations. These layers do not change the biocompatibility of the applied raw materials and enable continuous release kinetics of metal ions.

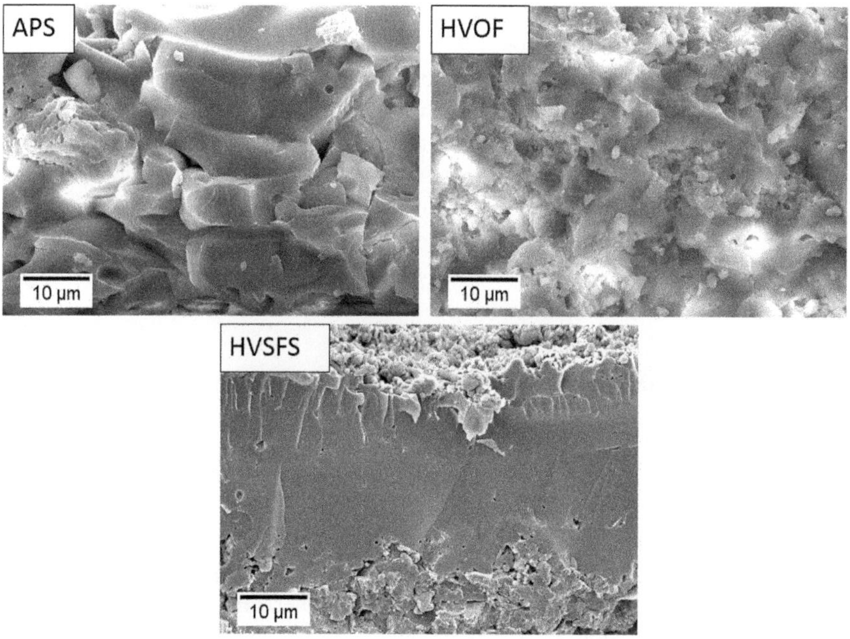


**Figure 10.3** Structure of hydroxyapatite coatings deposited by conventional atmospheric plasma spraying (APS) technology, high velocity oxyfuel spraying (HVOF), and high-velocity suspension flame spraying (HVSFS), coatings made at IFKB University of Stuttgart, Germany; images courtesy G. Bolelli, UNIMORE, Modena, Italy.

Immediately after implantation, dynamic processes occur at the boundary layer between ceramic and bone involving the release of calcium- and phosphate-ions. Increased ceramic solubility means more material reactivity in order to boost the stimulation of bone regeneration (Dorozhkin, 2015; Brown et al., 2013; Ducheyne and Qiu, 1999; DeAza et al., 2003b; Voigt and Mosier, 2011).

Modified after Heimann (2004), the reactions in the interface can be characterized as follows:

1. Release of calcium- and phosphate-ions (Doi et al., 1997), stimulation of osteoblasts.
2. Precipitation of biological apatite (= biomimetic apatite, = BCA (Biologic Carbonated Apatite), = amorphous HA, = calcium-depleted defect-apatite) on the ceramic surface (Ducheyne and Cuckler, 1992; Porter et al., 2003; Cazalbou et al., 2004).
3. Adsorption of serum proteins to the apatite structure (Ducheyne and Cuckler, 1992).
4. Biologic binding of collagen to the modified surface, mineralization of the collagen matrix (Chen et al., 2004).

Direct binding of bone to the ceramic surface is the most important precondition for a durable and persistent osteointegration. Bone regeneration was observed on the immediate surface of the calcium phosphate ceramics (Hing et al., 1998). First, the aim was to evaluate the biocompatibility of these coatings in vivo. MG63 cell line is a validated model to test the biocompatibility and was used in several previous works on such a substrate.

Coatings can also be used to affect a wide range of changes to surface properties without changing the bulk material. For example, they could act as an ion barrier to minimize the release of ions due to tribocorrosion (Sonntag et al., 2012). For load-bearing implant biomaterials, tribocorrosion is the main degradation mechanism, resulting from the combined action of wear and corrosion. Therefore surface modification techniques, such as ion implantation, anodization, plasma nitriding are used to convert metal surfaces to form oxide and nonoxide surfaces. Traditional vacuum deposition techniques like physical vapor deposition (PVD) and chemical vapor deposition (CVD) are widely used in biomedical applications to form nonoxide ceramic layers.

## 10.2.2 Carbon based coatings

### 10.2.2.1 Diamond-like carbon films

Amorphous carbon films, also known as diamond-like carbon (DLC) coatings are manufactured using PVD or combined PVD/CVD processes and appear as a promising class of coatings in order to improve the surface degradation resistance of metal implants (i.e., wear and corrosion). DLC coatings represent a whole family of carbon- and hydrocarbon-containing amorphous films, exhibiting either a more diamond like character (mainly $sp^3$ hybridization) or a more graphite like character ($sp^2$ hybridization), thus covering a wide range of mechanical properties like microhardness and elastic modulus. By adding hydrogen during deposition, the films can even shift to polymer-like structures showing an increasing grade of amorphous phase with increasing hydrogen concentration. Doping with metals like Cr, Ti, or W can further influence chemical behavior of the coatings like surface wetting, friction behavior, and much more. Basically, most DLC coatings are regarded as biocompatible, and that makes them attractive as they combine many of the unique properties of natural diamond like low friction, high hardness, and high corrosion resistance. Poor adhesion of the DLC coatings on the substrate was reported in vivo, and this is still a major concern for its application at least in load-bearing applications to date (Antilla et al., 1999).

#### *10.2.2.2 Nano-crystalline diamond*

Nano-crystalline diamond (NCD) is another type of diamond-based material. NCD is a thin film of diamond with nanometer-size crystals and can be grown on many substrates such as metals, quartz and other transparent glasses, piezoelectrics. NCD has most of the properties of diamond. Its low friction and wear properties make it an advanced tribological coating. Hardness, surface smoothness (Amaral et al., 2008a) and corrosion resistance (Grabarczyk et al., 2007) were found to be suitable for endoprosthesis application (Amaral et al., 2008b). However, high levels of compressive stress in the NCD coatings due to impurities at the grain borders directly affected their adhesion and may still cause them to delaminate (Vila et al., 2006). So far, no clinical studies have been performed on NCD.

#### *10.2.2.3 Pyrolytic carbon*

Pyrolytic carbon (PyC) is a material similar to graphite. This material is deposited from gaseous hydrocarbon compounds on suitable underlying substrates (carbon materials, metals, ceramics) at temperatures ranging from 1000K to 2500K (chemical vapor deposition). A wide range of microstructures and a varied content of remaining hydrogen, can occur in PyCs, depending on the deposition conditions (temperature, type, concentration and flow rate of the source gas, surface area of the underlying substrate, etc.).

PyC offers good fatigue resistance (Ma and Sines, 2000), wettability, and wear properties (More et al., 2004; Stanley et al., 2008), as well as a modulus of elasticity very similar to that of cortical bone (Kawalec et al., 1998). In addition to its use in a large number of mechanical heart valves, PyC has been applied in smaller joints, such as the proximal interphalangeal (Wijk et al., 2010) and metacarpophalangeal joint (Cook et al., 1999), for which a survival rate of 81.4% has been reported after 10 years. To date, little literature on load-bearing applications has been published.

### **10.2.3 Carbide and nitride thin films and surfaces**

In the 1980s, titanium nitride (TiN) was considered as the first ceramic coating for the functional surfaces in total hip and knee replacements (Röstlund et al., 1989). TiN, as well as titanium niobium nitride (TiNbN), titanium carbide (TiC) and titanium carbonitride (TiCN), are deposited using PVD. These types of PVD coatings are well known in engineering applications especially from coated cemented carbide cutting tools. They are easily identifiable through their golden color and, compared with the metal substrate, exhibit a substantial increase in hardness (Stone et al., 1991) and a decrease in metal-ion release from the substrate (Heide and Schultze, 1993). These coatings show very high hardness, whereas their adhesion resistance on the softer metal is apparently a major limitation. In contrast to a coating, which does not alter the underlying bulk material, a surface modification is defined as a treatment that chemically transforms the outer layers of an existing bulk material at the surface. For instance, titanium and steel alloy surfaces can be nitrided using the ion implantation techniques.

#### *10.2.3.1 Surface oxidized zirconium*

More than a decade ago, Smith & Nephew introduced OXINIUM-Oxidized Zirconium (Bourne et al., 2005). Its metallic surface transformed by oxidation into ceramic oxide, oxidized zirconium. This metal has proven to be a good metal for use in hip and knee implants due to its reduced friction and increased resistance to scratching and abrasion (Bourne et al., 2005; Tan et al., 2016).

#### *10.2.3.2 Oxidized titanium*

Early clinical experiences revealed the poor tribological performance of bulk titanium and its alloys (Budinski, 1991). Titanium oxide ($TiO_2$), which is naturally formed on the surface as a protective layer at ambient conditions, has a ceramic-like nature similar to TiN. Its thickness is only in the range of several nanometers. This has been shown to provide considerable corrosion resistance (Kumar et al., 2010), even after severe surface damage (Komotori et al., 2001). However, for dental implants, anodized titanium, carrying a titanium oxide conversion layer, formed by an electrochemical process has been used for decades. The layer exhibits a typical micro or nanoporous surface structure and shows excellent ingrowth behavior in dental implant surgery practise with very low failure rates. One major concern of theses implants is more related to cosmetic restrictions, as the dark coloring of the titanium does not fit to the natural light teeth surface.

## 10.3 Conclusions and perspectives

The field of bulk ceramics for orthopedic devices is nowadays dominated by alumina and alumina-based composites (ZTA), while zirconia and zirconia-matrix composite ceramics play a minor role. Nonoxides are currently not commercially available yet. The current trend goes towards a progressive replacement of alumina by ZTA due to the much better properties of the latter material. Especially in knee implants, which are exposed to more complex and drastic loading conditions than the hip joints, the strength and fracture toughness of alumina is not sufficient. ZTA is provided by one big supplier, which manufactures platelet-reinforced ZTA, with high strength and toughness. However, as the patent protection has now expired, more suppliers are entering this field offering materials with similar characteristics.

The question of LTD has been—based on traumatic experience in the past with Y-TZP—intensively studied and from the view of the authors probably a bit overstressed in case of the composites ceramics, in which Y-TZP grains are dispersed into the alumina matrix. In fact, the standard tests by X-ray diffraction and Raman reveal only moderate aging of ZTA materials, if any.

However, some new results from spectroscopic tests show that the LTD behavior is not as simple as previously considered and that improvements may be achieved by adding different dopants to the ZTA materials. This consideration has to be kept in mind for the design of materials for orthopedic devices having long-term stability, besides outstanding mechanical properties. Some main key parameters related to composition and microstructure, to be considered in the design of new materials, are summarized below.

1. Compositional design
   a. Codoping of $ZrO_2$ powders seems to be an effective strategy. The main successful attempts relate to the use of a mixture of trivalent ions (such as $Y^{3+}/Nd^{3+}$), a mixture of tri and tetravalent ions (such as $Y^{3+}/Ce^{4+}$, to simultaneously exploit the beneficial effect from both dopants) and a mixture of tri and pentavalent ions (such as $Y^{3+}/Nb^{5+}$, to avoid the creation of oxygen vacancies which could favor the LDT). These approaches, exploited for zirconia materials, deserve further investigation in ZTA composites.
   b. Addition of proper additives. In fact, according to the current ISO standard 6474-2, biomedical-grade ZTA may contain up to 10 wt% of "projected additives," which provides a high degree of freedom for the design of new materials. Example are provided by some key manufactures, such of CeramTec GmbH (Germany), Oximatec GmbH (Germany) and Kyocera Medical Co. (Japan) which added small amounts of various oxides (e.g., SrO, $Cr_2O_3$, $TiO_2$, MgO, $SiO_2$, $Pr_6O_{11}$) for generating platelet-reinforced ceramics and for improving specific properties, such as fracture toughness and hardness. In spite of such successful examples, there is still room for further materials optimization, based on proper compositional design.
2. Microstructural design
   a. Addition of hexa-aluminate platelets. This approach is nowadays widely exploited in different ZTA commercial products, even if the role of their morphology (length, aspect ratio) on the toughening/reinforcing effects is still not clearly reported in literature. A deeper understanding of this aspect could lead to even further optimization in the materials microstructure and related properties.
   b. Amount, type, size, and distribution of second phases. Besides the specific properties exerted by the matrix and each second-phase, the residual stresses generated during cooling from the sintering temperature could affect the overall behavior of the composites and has to be carefully controlled and optimized.
   c. Innovative microstructures, such as nano-nano or micro-nano intragranular types of composites, deserve deeper investigations. With nanostructured materials we can expect higher hardness and better wear behavior, besides specific toughening mechanisms. While the wear resistance of the current devices in more than sufficient, improving the mechanical properties and particularly the crack resistance (e.g., higher $K_{I0}$ values, which represent the safety threshold to use materials for joint replacement) is desiderable and could give access to new implant designs.

A new development in the field of materials for orthopedics is provided by non-oxide ceramics. These materials were already proposed decades ago and it seems that at least in the case of silicon nitride there is reason to believe that the material fulfills the necessary criteria. In addition, these materials are almost insensitive to slow crack growth, which leads to a better reliability of the implants. Tests are underway, and it may well be that for the next generation of endoprothetic devices the silicon nitride materials will be considered.

Concerning the coatings applied to the stem and acetabular cup to provide biocompatibility, VPS-sprayed titanium and APS sprayed HA are the accepted standard materials. New thermal spray technologies (either suspension flame or suspension plasma spraying) may provide a larger variety of coating morphologies. Together with "new" coating materials such as bioglass or calcium phosphates, this may open up new opportunities for optimized bone ingrowth. The latest trends in surface functionalization go far beyond the field of ceramic technology and include biofunctionalization of surfaces.

Currently, the regulatory framework for bulk ceramic materials and coatings applied in the field of prosthetic devices are efficiently protecting the patient by demanding very sophisticated and comprehensive procedures for the homologization of new materials and components. At the same time, this strict regulatory process including high expense in time and money is an obstacle for new developments. New products/materials will only come to market if significant new progress is foreseeable, if there is a threat to lose market share, or if completely new components are developed which justify this expense.

## References

Amaral, M., Gomes, P., Lopes, M., Santos, J., Silva, F., Fernandes, M., 2008a. Nanocrystalline diamond as a coating for joint implants: cytotoxicity and biocompatibility assessment. J. Nanomater. 2008, 1–9.

Amaral, M., Abreu, C.S., Oliveira, F., Gomes, J., Silva, R., 2008b. Tribological characterization of NCD in physiological fluids. Diamond Relat. Mater. 17, 848–852.

Antilla, A., Lappalainen, R., Heinonen, H., Santavirta, S., Konttinen, Y., 1999. Superiority of diamondlike carbon coating on articulating surfaces of artificial hip joints. New Diamond Front. Carbon Technol. 9, 283–288.

Apel, E., Ritzberger, C., Courtois, N., Reveron, H., Chevalier, J., Schweiger, M., et al., 2012. Introduction to a tough, strong and stable Ce-TZP/MgAl2O4 composite for biomedical applications. J. Eur. Ceram. Soc. 32 (11), 2697–2703.

Bal, B.S., Rahaman, M.H., 2012. Orthopedic applications of silicon nitride ceramics. Acta. Biomater. 8 (8), 2889–2898.

Benzaid, R., Chevalier, J., Saâdaoui, M., Fantozzi, G., Nawa, M., Diaz, L.A., et al., 2008. Fracture toughness, strength and slow crack growth in a ceria stabilized zirconia–alumina nanocomposite for medical applications. Biomaterials. 29, 3636–3641.

Brown, T., Harper, B., Bjorgul, K., 2013. Comparison of cemented and uncemented fixation in total knee arthroplasty. Orthopedics. 36, 380–387.

Boffelli, M., Doimo, A., Marin, E., Puppulin, L., Zhu, W., Sugano, N., et al., 2016. Chemically driven tetragonal-to-monoclinic polymorphic transformation in retrieved ZTA femoral heads from dual mobility hip implants. J. Mater. Sci. Mater. Med. 56, 195–204.

Bourne, R., Barrack, R., Rorabeck, C., Salehi, A., Good, V., 2005. Arthroplasty options for the young patient: oxinium on cross-linked polyethylene. Clin. Orthop. Relat. Res. 441, 159–167.

Budinski, K., 1991. Tribological properties of titanium-alloys. Wear. 151, 203–217.

Burger, W., Richter, H.G., Piconi, C., Vatteroni, R., Cittadini, A., Boccalari, M., 1997. New Y-TZP powders for medical grade zirconia. J. Mater. Sci. Mater. Med. 8, 113–118.

Burger, W., Richter, H.G., 2001. High strength and toughness alumina matrix composites by transformation toughening and 'in situ' platelet reinforcement (ZPTA) – the new generation of bioceramics. Key Eng. Mater. 192-195, 545–548.

Burger, W., Kiefer, G., 2015. Patent application Keramikwerkstoff, WO 2015/074921.

Cazalbou, S., Combes, C., Eichert, D., Rey, C., Glimcher, M., 2004. Poorly crystalline apatites: evolution and maturation in vitro and in vivo. J. Bone. Miner. Metab. 22, 310–317.

Chen, Q., Wong, C., Lu, W., Cheung, K., Leong, J., Luk, K., 2004. Strengthening mechanisms of bone bonding to crystalline hydroxyapatite in vivo. Biomaterials. 25, 4243–4254.

Chevalier, J., Fantozzi, G., Bartolomé, J.F., Pecharroman, C., Moya, J.S., Diaz, L.A., et al., 2005. Nanostructured ceramic oxides with a slow crack growth resistance close to covalent materials. Nanoletters. 5 (7), 1297–1301.

Chevalier, J., Gremillard, L., Deville, S., 2007. Low temperature degradation of zirconia and implications for biomedical implants. Ann. Rev. Mater. Res. 37, 1–32.

Chevalier, J., Gremillard, 2009. Ceramics for medical applications: a picture for the next 20 years. J. Eur. Ceram. Soc. 29, 1245–1255.

Chevalier, J., Gremillard, L., Virkar, A.V., Clarke, D.R., 2009. The tetragonal-monoclinic transformation in zirconia: lessons learned and future trends. J. Am. Ceram. Soc. 92 (9), 1901–1920.

Cook, S., Beckenbaugh, R., Redondo, J., Popich, L., Klawitter, J., Linscheid, R., 1999. Long-term follow-up of pyrolytic carbon metacarpophalangeal implants. J. Bone. Joint. Surg. Am. 81, 635–648.

Cutler, R.A., Mayhew, R.J., Prettiman, K.M., Virkar, A., 1991. High-toughness Ce-TZP/Al2O3 ceramics with improved hardness and strength. J. Am. Ceram. Soc. 74 (1), 179–186.

Dante, R.C., Kajdas, C.K., 2012. A review and a fundamental theory of silicon nitride tribochemistry. Wear. 288, 27–38.

DeAza, A., Chevalier, J., Fantozzi, G., Torrecillas, R., Schehl, M., 2003a. Slow-crack-growth behavior of zirconia-toughened alumina ceramics processed by different methods. J. Am. Ceram. Soc. 86 (1), 115–120.

DeAza, P., Luklinska, Z., Santos, C., Guitian, F., DeAza, S., 2003b. Mechanism of bone like formation on a bioactive implant in vivo. Biomaterials. 24, 1437–1445.

Denry, I., Kelly, J.R., 2008. State of the art of zirconia for dental applications. Dental Mater. 24, 299–307.

Doi, Y., Shibutani, T., Moriwake, J., Kajimoto, T., Iwayama, Y., 1997. Sintered carbonate apatites as bioresorbable bone substitutes. J. Biomed. Mater. Res. 39, 603–610.

Dorozhkin, S., 2015. Calcium orthophosphate deposits: preparation, properties and biomedical applications. Mater. Sci. Eng. C Mater. Biol. Appl. 55, 272–326.

Douillard, T., Chevalier, J., Descamps-Mandine, A., Warner, I., Galais, Y., Whitaker, P., et al., 2012. Comparative ageing behaviour of commercial, unworn and worn 3Y-TZP and zirconia-toughened alumina hip joint heads. J. European Ceram. Soc. 32 (8), 1529–1540.

Ducheyne, P., Cuckler, J., 1992. Bioactive prosthetic coatings. Clin. Orthop. 276, 102–114.
Ducheyne, P., Qiu, Q., 1999. Bioactive ceramics: the effect of surface reactivity on bone formation and bone cell function. Biomaterials. 20, 2287–2303.
Exare, C., Kiat, J.-M., Guiblin, N., Porcher, F., Petricek, V., 2015. Structural evolution of ZTA composites during synthesis and processing. J. Eur. Ceram. Soc. 35, 1273–1283.
Fink, U., 1996. Plasmapore: a plasma-sprayed microporous titanium coating to improve the long term stability. In: Mainard, D. (Ed.), Actualités en Biomatériaux, Vol. III. Romillat Edit., Paris, pp. 97–104.
Gorth, D.J., Puckett, S., Ercan, B., Webster, T.J., Rahaman, M., Bal, S.B., 2012. Decreased bacteria activity on Si3N4 surfaces compared with PEEK or titanium. Int. J. Nanomed. 7, 4829–4840.
Grabarczyk, J., Batory, D., Louda, P., Couvrat, P., Kotela, I., 2007. Carbon coatings for medical implants. JAMME. 20, 107–110.
Gregori, G., Burger, W., Sergo, V., 1999. Piezo-spectroscopic analysis of the residual stresses in zirconia-toughened alumina ceramics: the influence of the tetragonal-to-monoclinic transformation. Mater. Sci. Eng. A. 271, 401–406.
Gutknecht, D., Chevalier, J., Garnier, V., Fantozzi, G., 2007. Key role of processing to avoid low temperature ageing in alumina zirconia composites for orthopaedic application. J. Eur. Ceram. Soc. 27, 1547–1552.
Hannink, R.H.J., Kelly, P.M., Muddle, B.C., 2000. Transformation toughening in zirconia-containing ceramics. J. Am. Ceram. Soc. 83 (3), 461–487.
Heide, N., Schultze, J., 1993. Corrosion stability of TiN prepared by ion implantation and PVD. Nucl. Instrum. Methods Phys. Res., Sect. B. 80–81, 467–471.
Heimann, R., 2004. Entwicklung biokeramischer Beschichtungen für Hüft-Endoprothesen Teil 1. Zeitschrift der TU Clausthal-Zellerfeld. 15, 44–47.
Heuer, A.H., Claussen, N., Kriven, W.M., Rühle, W., 1982. Stability of tetragonal $ZrO_2$ particles in ceramic matrices. J. Am. Ceram. Soc. 65 (12), 642–650.
Hing, K., Best, S., Tanner, K., Revell, P., Bonfield, W., 1998. Histomorphological and biomechanical characterisation of calcium phosphates in the osseous environment. Proc. Inst. Mech. Eng. 212, 437–451.
ISO 6474-2, 2012. Implants for surgery – Ceramic materials – Part 2: Composite materials based on a high-purity alumina matrix with zirconia reinforcement.
Kawalec, J., Hetherington, V., Melillo, T., Corbin, N., 1998. Evaluation of fibrocartilage regeneration and bone response at full-thickness cartilage defects in articulation with pyrolytic carbon or cobalt–chromium alloy hemiarthroplasties. J. Biomed. Mater. Res. B. 41, 534–540.
Kay, J., 1990. Bioactive surface coatings for hard tissue biomaterials. In: Yamamuro T, Hench LL, Wilsch J, editors. CRC Handbook of Bioactive Ceramics 2, pp. 111–112.
Kern, F., 2011. Sintering conditions, microstructure and properties of alumina 10 vol% zirconia nanocomposites. J. Ceram. Sci. Technol. 3 (1), 1–8.
Kern, F., Gadow, R., 2012. Alumina toughened zirconia from yttria coated powders. J. Eur. Ceram. Soc. 32, 3911–3918.
Kern, F., 2013a. Effect of ceriumhexaaluminate precipitates on properties of alumina -24 vol-% zirconia (1.4Y) composites. J. Ceram. Sci. Technol. 4 (4), 177–186.
Kern, F., 2013b. Ytterbia–neodymia–costabilized TZP—Breaking the limits of strength–toughness correlations for zirconia? J. Eur. Ceram. Soc. 33, 965–973.
Kern, F., Gadow, R., 2013. Mechanical properties and low temperature degradation resistance of 2.5Y-TZP – alumina composites. Ceram. Mater./Mater. Ceramiczne. 65 (3), 258–266.

Kern, F., Palmero, P., Garcia Marro, F., Mestra, A., 2015. Processing of alumina zirconia composites by surface modification route with enhanced hardness and wear resistance. Ceram. Int. 41, 889–898.

Kern, F., Koummarasy, S., Gadow, R., 2016. The influence of stabilizer concentration on the mechanical properties of alumina – 17 vol% zirconia (0.6Y-2Y) composites. J. Ceram. Sci. Technol. 7 (3), 295–300.

Kirsten, A., Begand, S., Oberbach, T., Telle, R., Fischer, H., 2010. Subcritical crack growth behavior of dispersion oxide ceramics. J. Biomed. Mater. Res. Part B Appl. Biomater. 95B (1), 202–206.

Komotori, J., Lee, B., Dong, H., Dearnley, P., 2001. Corrosion response of surface engineered titanium alloys damaged by prior abrasion. Wear. 251, 1239–1249.

Kuntz, M., 2006. Validation of a new high performance alumina matrix composite for use in total joint replacement. Semin. Arthroplasty. 17, 141–145.

Kobayashi, K., Kuwajima, H., Masaki, T., 1981. Phase change and mechanical properties of ZrO2-Y2O3 solid electrolyte after ageing. Solid State Ionics. 3 (4), 489–493.

Kumar, S., Narayanan, T., Raman, S., Seshadri, S., 2010. Thermal oxidation of CP Ti—an electrochemical and structural characterization. Mater. Charact. 61, 589–597.

Lange, F.F., 1982. Transformation toughening – Part 4: fabrication, fracture toughness and strength of $Al_2O_3$ - $ZrO_2$ composites. J. Mater. Sci. 17, 247–254.

Lee, D.Y., et al., 1998. Low-temperature phase stability and mechanical properties of $Y_2O_3$- and $Nb_2O_5$- co-doped tetragonal zirconia polycrystal ceramics. J. Mater. Sci. Lett. 17, 185–187.

Lin, J.D., Duh, J.G., 2002. Correlation of mechanical properties and composition in tetragonal $CeO_2-Y_2O_3-ZrO_2$ ceramic system. Mater. Chem. Phys. 78, 246–252.

Langlois, R., Konsztowicz, K.J., 1992. Toughening in zirconia-toughened alumina composites with non-transforming zirconia. J. Mater. Sci. Lett. 11, 1454–1456.

Ma, L., Sines, G., 2000. Fatigue behavior of a pyrolytic carbon. J. Biomed. Mater. Res. 51, 61–68.

McEntire, B.J., Bal, B.S., Rahaman, M.N., Chevalier, J., Pezzotti, G., 2015. Ceramics and ceramic coatings in orthopaedics. J. Eur. Ceram. Soc. 35 (16), 4327–4369.

Messing, G., Kumagai, M., 1989. Low-temperature sintering of seeded sol-gel-derived, $ZrO_2$-toughened $Al_2O_3$ composites. J. Am. Ceram. Soc. 72 (1), 40–44.

More, R., Haubold, A., Bokros, J., 2004. Pyrolytic carbon for long-term medical implants. In: Ratner, B.D., Hoffman, A.S., Schoen, F.J., Lemons, J.E. (Eds.), Biomaterials Science: An Introduction to Materials in Medicine. Elsevier Academic Press, London, pp. 170–181.

Muratov, V.A., Luangvaranunt, T., Fischer, T.E., 1998. The tribochemistry of silicon nitride: effects of friction, temperature and sliding velocity. Tribol. Int. 31, 601–611.

Nawa, M., Nakamoto, S., Sekino, T., Niihara, K., 1998. Tough and strong Ce-TZP/Alumina nanocomposites doped with titania. Ceram. Int. 24, 497–506.

Neumann, A., Jahnke, K., Maier, H.R., Ragoß, C., 2004. Biocompatibility of silicon nitride ceramic in vitro. A comparative fluorescence-microscopic and scanning electron-microscopic study. Laryngorhinootologie. 83, 845–851.

Palmero, P., Naglieri, V., Chevalier, J., Fantozzi, G., Montanaro, L., 2009. Alumina based nanocomposites obtained by doping with inorganic salt solutions: application to immiscible and reactive systems. J. Eur. Ceram. Soc. 29, 59–66.

Palmero, P., Montanaro, L., Reveron, H., Chevalier, J., 2014. Surface coating of oxide powders: a new synthesis method to process biomedical grade nano-comp. Materials. 7, 5012–5037.

Pezzotti, G., 2014. Bioceramics for hip joints: the physical chemistry viewpoint. Materials. 7, 4367–4410.

Piconi, C., Burger, W., Cittadini, A., Maccauro, G., Covacci, V., Bruzzese, N., et al., 1998. Y-TZP ceramics for artificial joint replacements. Biomaterials. 19, 1489–1494.

Piconi, C., Maccauro, G., Pilloni, L., Burger, W., Muratori, F., Richter, H.G., 2006. On the fracture of a zirconia ball head. J. Mater. Sci. Mater. Med. 17 (3), 289–300.

Pitek, F.M., et al., 2007. Opportunities for TBCs in the $ZrO_2$-$YO_{1.5}$-$TaO_{2.5}$ system. Surface Coating Technol. 201, 6044–6050.

Porter, A., Patel, N., Skepper, J., Best, S., Bonfield, W., 2003. Comparison of in vivo dissolution processes in hydroxyapatite and silicon-substituted hydroxyapatite bioceramics. Biomaterials. 24, 4609–4620.

Puppulin, L., Leto, A., Zhu, W., Sugano, N., Pezzotti, G., 2014. Innovative tribometer for in situ spectroscopic analyses of wear mechanisms and phase transformation in ceramic femoral heads. J. Mech. Behav. Biomed. Mater. 31, 45–54.

Rahaman, M.N., Yao, A., Bal, B.S., Garino, J.P., Ries, M.D., 2007. Ceramics for prosthetic hip and knee joint replacement. J. Am. Ceram. Soc. 90 (7), 1965–1988.

Ramalingam, S., Reimanis, I.E., Fuller, E.R., Haftel, J.D., 2011. Slow Crack Growth Behavior of zirconia-toughened alumina and alumina using the dynamic fatigue indentation technique. J. Am. Ceram. Soc. 94, 576–583.

Riley, F.L., 2000. Silicon nitride and related materials. J. Am. Ceram. Soc. 83, 245–265.

Röstlund, T., Albrektsson, B., Albrektsson, T., McKellop, H., 1989. Wear of ion-implanted pure titanium against UHMWPE. Biomaterials. 10, 176–181.

Salehi, S.A., Vanmeensel, K., Swarnakar, A.K., Van der Biest, O., Vleugels, J., 2010. Hydrothermal stability of mixed stabilised tetragonal (Y, Nd)-$ZrO_2$ ceramics. J. Alloys Compounds. 495, 556–560.

Schneider, J., Begand, S., Kriegel, R., Kaps, C., Glien, W., Oberbach, T., 2008. Low-temperature aging behavior of alumina-toughened zirconia. J. Am. Ceram. Soc. 91 (11), 9613–9619.

Sommer, F., Landfried, R., Kern, F., Gadow, R., 2012a. Mechanical properties of zirconia toughened alumina with 10–24 vol.% 1.5 mol% Y-TZP reinforcement. J. Eur. Ceram. Soc. 32 (15), 3905–3910.

Sommer, F., Landfried, R., Kern, F., Gadow, R., 2012b. Mechanical properties of zirconia toughened alumina with 10–24 vol.% 1Y-TZP reinforcement. J. Eur. Ceram. Soc. 32 (16), 4177–4184.

Sonntag, R., Reinders, J., Kretzer, J., 2012. What's next? Alternative materials for articulation in total joint replacement. Acta. Biomater. 8, 2434–2441.

Stanley, J., Klawitter, J., More, R., 2008. Replacing joints with pyrolytic carbon. In: Revell, P.A. (Ed.), Joint Replacement Technology. Woodhead Publishing Ltd, London, pp. 631–656.

Stiegler, N., Bellucci, D., Bolelli, G., Cannillo, V., Gadow, R., Killinger, A., et al., 2012. High-velocity suspension flame sprayed (HVSFS) hydroxyapatite coatings for biomedical applications. Surf. Coat. Techn. 21, 275–287.

Stone, D., Yoder, K., Sproul, W., 1991. Hardness and elastic modulus of TiN based on continuous indentation technique and new correlation. J. Vac. Sci. Technol. A. 9, 2543–2547.

Surmenev, R., Surmeneva, M., Ivanova, A., 2014. Significance of calcium phosphate coatings for the enhancement of new bone osteogenesis—a review. Acta. Biomater. 10, 557–579.

Tan, S., Lau, A., Del Balso, C., Howard, J., Lanting, B., Teeter, M., 2016. Tribocorrosion: ceramic and oxidized zirconium vs cobalt-chromium heads in total hip arthroplasty. J. Arthroplasty. 31, 2064–2071.

Taylor, R.M., Bernero, J.P., Patel, A.A., Brodke, D.S., Khandkar, A.C., 2010. Silicon nitride: a new material for spinal implants. J. Bone Joint Surg. Br. 92 (Suppl. 1), 133.

Tsukuma, K., Kubota, Y., Tsukidate, T., 1983. Thermal and mechanical properties of Y2O3-stabilized tetragonal zirconia polycrystals. Science and technology of zirconia II. American Ceramic Society, Inc, United States, pp. 382–390.

Tsukuma, K., Ueda, K., Shimada, K., 1985. Strength and fracture toughness of isostatically hot pressed composites of $Al_2O_3$ and $Y_2O_3$-partially-stabilized $ZrO_2$. J. Am. Ceram. Soc. 68 (1), C4–C5.

Vila, M., Amaral, M., Oliveira, F., Silva, R., Fernandes, A., Soares, M., 2006. Residual stress minimum in nanocrystalline diamond films. Appl. Phys. Lett. 89, 93–109.

Voigt, J., Mosier, M., 2011. Hydroxyapatite (HA) coating appears to be of benefit for implant durability of tibial components in primary total knee arthroplasty. Acta. Orthop. 82, 448–459.

Webster, T.J., Patel, A.A., Rahaman, M.N., Bal, S.B., 2012. Anti-infective and osteointegration properties of silicon nitride, poly(etheretherketone), and titanium implants. Acta. Biomater. 8, 4447–4454.

Wijk, U., Wollmark, M., Kopylov, P., Tägil, M., 2010. Outcomes of proximal interphalangeal joint pyrocarbon implants. J. Hand. Surg. 35, 38–43.

Willmann, G., 1996. Developments in medical grade alumina over the last two decades. J. Mater. Proc. Technol. 56, 168–176.

Willmann, G., 2001. Improving bearing surfaces of artificial joints. Adv. Eng. Mater. 3 (3), 135–141.

Xuereb, M., Camilleri, J., Attard, N., 2015. Systematic review of current dental implant coating materials and novel coating techniques. Int. J. Prosthodont. 28, 51–59.

Zhang, F., Vanmeensel, K., Inokoshi, M., Batuk, M., Hadermann, J., Van Meerbeek, J., et al., 2014. 3Y-TZP ceramics with improved hydrothermal degradation resistance and fracture toughness. J. Eur. Ceram. Soc. 34, 2453–2463.

Zhang, F., Inokoshi, M., Vanmeensel, K., Van Meerbeek, J., Naert, I., Vleugels, J., 2015. Lifetime estimation of zirconia ceramics by linear ageing kinetics. Acta. Mater. 92, 290–298.

# Design and development of dental ceramics: Examples of current innovations and future concepts

11

*Marta Fornabaio*[1,2], *Helen Reveron*[3], *Erik Adolfsson*[4], *Laura Montanaro*[1], *Jerome Chevalier*[3] *and Paola Palmero*[1]
[1]Politecnico di Torino, Turin, Italy, [2]École Polytechnique Fédérale de Lausanne (EPFL), Lausanne, Switzerland, [3]Université de Lyon-INSA Lyon, Villeurbanne, France, [4]Swerea, IVF AB, Mölndal, Sweden

**Chapter Outline**

**11.1 Introduction 355**
**11.2 Requirements for dental ceramic materials 357**
**11.3 The use and key advantages of zirconia as a dental material 361**
**11.4 Design and development of strong, tough, and stable $ZrO_2$-based dental materials 365**
**11.5 Bio-inspired design of dental ceramics 374**
**11.6 Dental tissue regeneration: advanced materials and technologies 379**
**11.7 Conclusions 383**
**Acknowledgments 384**
**References 384**
**Further Reading 389**

## 11.1 Introduction

Understanding the structure–properties relationship of a human tooth is the indispensable starting point for the design and development of dental restorative materials. The unique hierarchical architecture of the human tooth gives rise to the extraordinary mechanical properties required during mastication processes.

The structural parts of a human tooth can be classified as enamel, dentin, and dentin–enamel junction (DEJ) as shown in Fig. 11.1.

Enamel forms the outer layer of a tooth, it is made of 92–96 wt% apatite crystals, 1%–2% organic material and 3%–4% water. Its microstructure is schematically reported in Fig. 11.1: hydroxyapatite crystals form large rods (~5 μm diameter) arranged parallel in a perpendicular direction from the DEJ toward the tooth surface and held together by the organic phase (a protein/peptide

Advances in Ceramic Biomaterials.
DOI: http://dx.doi.org/10.1016/B978-0-08-100881-2.00025-7

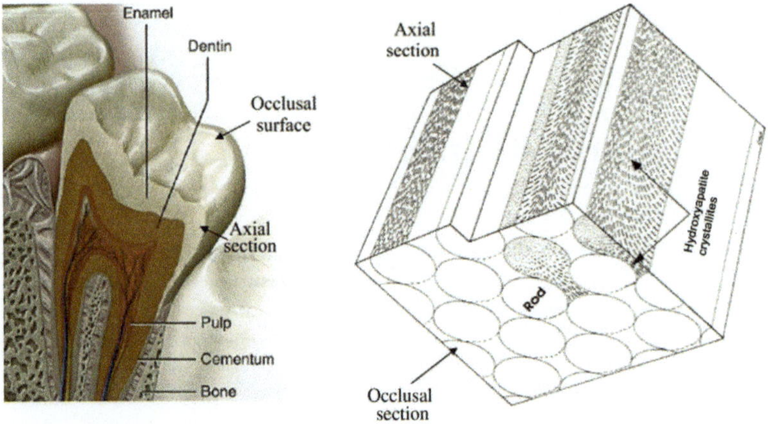


**Figure 11.1** Impression of the tooth structure (left) and the enamel structure (right).
*Source*: From Xie, Z.H., Swain, M.V., Swadener, G., Munroe, P., Hoffman, M., 2009. Effect of microstructure upon elastic behaviour of human tooth enamel. J. Biomech. 42, 1075–1080, with the permission of Elsevier, under license no. 4115230248460.

mixture). In the central part of each rod, hydroxyapatite crystals are parallel to the rod axis while near its edge they form an angle of 15–45 degrees with respect to the longitudinal axis (Madfa and Yue, 2016). Its intrinsic anisotropy (i.e., rod orientation) and the presence of organics is known for being the reason for excellent mechanical properties. Enamel must resist high contact stress (of ~2.5 GPa considering a direct contact with opposite teeth and external objects, under normal oral conditions) meanwhile retaining its shape over a lifetime scale (Xie et al., 2009). Therefore, high hardness and stiffness are essential for dental function along with sufficient toughness to minimize cracking and fracture. Enamel can be represented as a composite of mineral apatite platelets reinforcing a minor, softer protein matrix: under an applied tensile stress, while platelets carry the load, the matrix transfers it among crystals via shear (Madfa and Yue, 2016; Ji and Gao, 2004).

Dentin consists of dentinal tubules (65–70 wt%) wrapped with peritubular dentin embedded in a collagen matrix containing hydroxyapatite prisms. In Fig. 11.2A the scanning electron micrograph image depicts the dentinal tubules as dark cavities.

Between the harder, brittle enamel and the softer, durable dentin, a functionally graded junction (DEJ) is present allowing a smooth transition of the mechanical properties (Fig. 11.2B) (i.e., hardness decreases from the outside enamel region toward the dentin meanwhile toughness increases). Such an interface inhibits the propagation of cracks from the enamel to the dentin thus supporting the tooth integrity during masticatory actions. The complex mechanism behind this extraordinary crack-arrest capability has not been completely understood yet (Imbeni et al., 2005; Chan et al., 2011; Madfa and Yue, 2016; Marshall et al., 2003). According to Imbeni et al., first the cracks penetrate the DEJ then, when entering the tougher

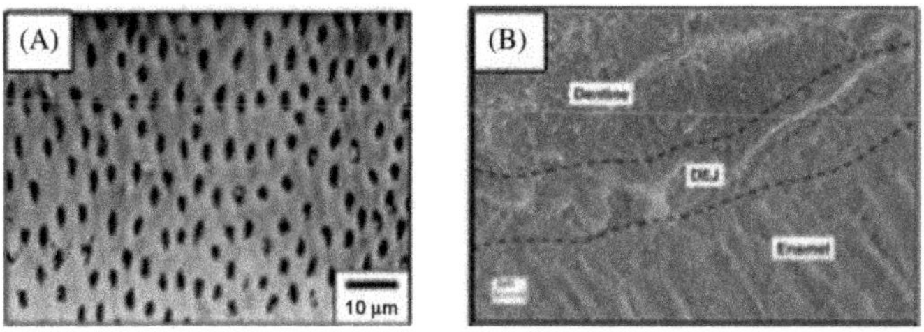


**Figure 11.2** Scanning electron micrographs of (A) dentinal tubules embedded in a mineralized matrix. (B) An acid-etched human permanent molar microstructure near the DEJ.
*Source*: (A) Reprinted from Roy, S., Basu, B., 2008. Mechanical and tribological characterization of human tooth. Mater. Characterization 59, 747–756, with the permission of Elsevier, under license no. 4115230928115. (B) Reprinted from Chan, Y.L., Ngan, A.H.W., King, N.M., 2011. Nano-scale structure and mechanical properties of the human dentine–enamel junction. J. Mech. Behav. Biomed. Mater. 4, 785–795, with the permission of Elsevier, under license no. 4115260173357).

dentin adjacent to the junction, they arrest, thanks to bridging by uncracked ligaments (Imbeni et al., 2005).

Fathoming the teeth's mechanical properties is essential when designing a restorative material. Among the available appropriate techniques to characterize the tooth structure, the nano-indentation is the most widely used, as it allows the measurement of hardness and elastic modulus in the nanoscale range. However, due to the influence of several factors (i.e., shape of indenter, applied load, sample nature, and preparation) results can vary strongly. The review of Zhang et al. collects some of the main results regarding enamel and dentin structures: on the one hand, hardness and modulus values of enamel are in the range 3–7 and 60–100 GPa, respectively (Zhang et al., 2014b). On the other hand, dentin hardness values of 0.3–4 GPa and modulus of 13–45 GPa have been reported. Evaluation of fracture toughness reveals values in the range 0.7–4 and 1–2 $MPa\sqrt{m}$ for the enamel and dentin, respectively (Zhang et al., 2014b; Imbeni et al., 2005).

## 11.2 Requirements for dental ceramic materials

It is possible to state that the progress in dentistry stems not only from the development of therapeutic procedures and dental techniques but also from the progress of new materials, achievable thanks to the current state of tooth knowledge and capabilities.

Onlays, inlays, crowns, bridges, dentures, and veneers treatments belong to the so-called indirect restoration, since they are fabricated outside the mouth using the dental impressions of the tooth (Nakonieczny et al., 2017). Magnets, clips, hooks, and implants used to attach removable prosthetics to natural teeth can also

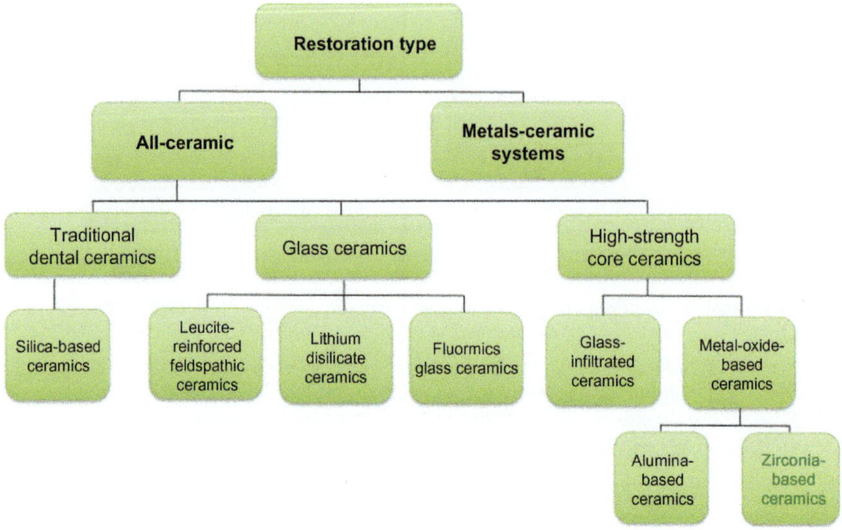


**Figure 11.3** Classification diagram by the type of restoration.
*Source*: Adapted from Ho, G.W., Matinlinna, J.P., 2011. Insights on ceramics as dental materials. Part I: Ceramic material types in dentistry. Silicon 3, 109–115.

be classified as a form of dental restoration. Both the increasing patient demand for an esthetic restoration and the potential biological risk (i.e., allergy and toxicity) of metal-based dental materials, have greatly encouraged the development of ceramic-based materials.

*All-ceramic* restorations often have the same design of a metal–ceramic restoration consisting of a core material with improved mechanical properties and a veneer glass ceramic with enhanced esthetic features. Many ceramics such as spinel, alumina, zirconia, and lithium disilicate glass ceramics, are nowadays employed depending on the clinical use, as illustrated in Fig. 11.3.

While such a matter has been extensively presented in Chapter 6—Ceramics for Dentistry: Commercial Devices and Their Clinical Analysis—here the focus is on the new directions researchers have been taking in order to enhance the performances of a ceramic dental restoration and to design new materials with graded and heterogeneous architectures, inspired by the knowledge of natural tooth features (i.e., microstructure and mechanical response).

Researchers tasks are guided by the requirements of (1) mechanical performances, (2) biocompatibility, and (3) esthetical properties that a dental prosthesis and restoration have to fulfill in order to be clinically approved as dental materials. The International Organization for Standardization (ISO) addresses some of them, as is the case for mechanical properties and biocompatibility.

1. *Mechanical performance*: when it comes to mechanical and physical requirements, researchers can address the standard ISO 13356:2008(E), that specifies characteristics—and the corresponding testing methods—of chemical composition, microstructure,

**Table 11.1 Minimum flexural strength for dental ceramics**

| Clinical indications | Flexural strength minimum (mean[a]) (MPa) |
|---|---|
| Monolithic ceramic for single-unit anterior prostheses, veneers, inlays, or onlays adhesively cemented | 50 |
| Monolithic ceramic for single-unit anterior or posterior prostheses adhesively cemented | 100 |
| Partially or fully covered substructure ceramic for single-unit anterior or posterior prostheses adhesively cemented | 100 |
| Monolithic ceramic for single-unit anterior or posterior prostheses and for three-unit prostheses not involving molar restoration adhesively or nonadhesively cemented | 300 |
| Partially or fully covered substructure ceramic for single-unit anterior or posterior prostheses and for three-unit prostheses not involving molar restoration adhesively or nonadhesively cemented | 300 |
| Monolithic ceramic for three-unit prostheses involving molar restoration | 500 |
| Partially or fully covered substructure for three-unit prostheses involving molar restoration | 500 |
| Monolithic ceramic for prostheses involving partially or fully covered substructure for four or more units | 800 |

[a]At least 10 and preferably 30 specimens should be tested.

strength, cyclic fatigue, radioactivity, and accelerated aging test for surgical implants. Notwithstanding the range of properties considered by the standard, it should be noticed that it refers only to ceramic materials based on yttria-stabilized tetragonal zirconia polycrystals (Y-TZP). A second standard, ISO 14801:2016, specifies a method of fatigue testing of single post endosseous dental implants, useful for comparing endosseous dental implants of different designs or sizes. More generally, the standard ISO 6872:2015, provides the recommended values of flexural strength for ceramic dental prostheses and restorations with respect to the intended clinical use, as recalled in Table 11.1. Three flexural test methods are acceptable by the standard meaning: (1) three-point bending, (2) four-point bending, and (3) biaxial flexure (piston-on-three-ball). However, in the dental field, a notable preference for the last one is observed, probably as it is easier to perform (simplified fixture and sample preparation). Suitable test and sample preparation for the evaluation of fracture toughness (namely, the SEVNB method) are also considered in the same standard and in the recent review of Cesar et al. (2017).

2. *Biocompatibility*: In order to assess the biocompatibility of materials in an ethical and economical manner, researchers have to first conduct in vitro experiments where a test material is immersed in physiological fluid containing cell cultures or constituents. For better mimicking the in vivo conditions, nowadays enamel and/or dentin discs have been incorporated in the test methodologies. One successful protocol envisages the use of the so-called artificial pulp chamber (APC) where the pulpal surface of the disk is kept in

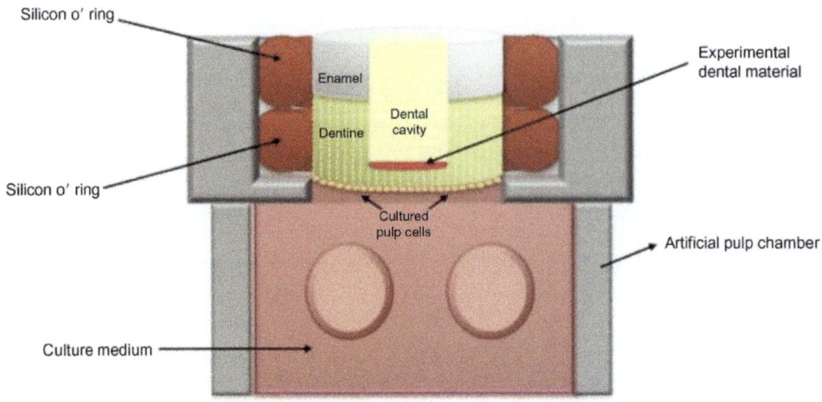


**Figure 11.4** Schematic representation of an APC.
*Source*: Reprinted from De Souza Costa, C.A., Hebling, J., Scheffel, D.L, Soares, D.G., Basso, F.G., Ribeiro, A.P., 2014. Methods to evaluate and strategies to improve the biocompatibility of dental materials and operative techniques. Dent. Mater. 30, 769–784, with the permission of Elsevier, under license no. 4115240166147.

contact with the culture medium and the occlusal surface remains exposed, thus allowing materials evaluation (Fig. 11.4).

Responses of cytotoxicity, inflammatory events, bio-stimulation, or cell differentiation capacity can be obtained (De Souza Costa et al., 2014). Scanning electron microscopy can be also performed in order to evaluate the effect of dental material on cell cultures, such as morphological changes.

In vivo tests involve the implementation of a test material in a living animal body with the scope of investigating its interaction with the living tissues. However, various events that might simultaneously occur as well as the challenging statistical analysis make their application still controversial and the interpretation of the results very complex. The further step in assessing biocompatibility is conducting clinical studies where human volunteers experiment with the restorative material.

The reader is referred to the standard ISO 7405:2009, in order to deepen their knowledge of tests, sample preparation, results analysis suitable for assessing the biocompatibility of dental materials.

3. *Esthetic requirements* are strongly related to the ability of the human eye and to the individual's perception of color. Defining the specifications is certainly the most challenging aspect, requiring the selection of a proper reference value as well as appropriate materials and techniques able to reproduce it. Regarding the definition of a shade guide, two systems are commonly used: CIE*Lab** and HSB/HSV. In the former, color is expressed by three coordinates, $L^*$, $a^*$, and $b^*$, which represent the degree of lightness, redness/greenness, and yellowness/blueness, respectively. In the latter system, H (hue) and S (saturation or chroma) are defined as the radial component of the cylindrical coordinates CIEC*Lab** and related to the $a^*$ and $b^*$ parameters according to two different mathematical formulae. The L value (lightness or brightness or value) corresponds directly to the $L^*$ parameter of the CIEC*Lab** system and it represents the lightness–darkness of a color. Nowadays instruments like colorimeters and spectrophotometers can be routinely applied in clinical dentistry allowing the evaluation of these parameters and, consecutively,

of the $\Delta E_{ab}$ parameter defined as the color differences between two materials (i.e., natural and restorative tooth). In 2004 the Commission Internationale de l'Eclairage (CIE) updated the formula in $\Delta E_{00}$ including also weighting functions and parametric factors (such as geometric attributes, texture, gloss, opacity, transparency) with the aim of improving the correlation between the calculated values and the visual perception of color (CIE, 2004). However, the relative complexity of the $\Delta E_{00}$ formula is hindering its exploitation and still most papers in this field refer to $\Delta E_{ab}$. Whatever the applied $\Delta E$ formula, the following step is to define a threshold value below which this difference can be considered clinically accepted. Although underling that the ability of the human eye to appreciate differences in color differs among individuals, Vichi et al. (2011) suggested $\Delta E = 3.3$ units as threshold value: $\Delta E$ values $<1$ unit cannot be appreciated by the human eye while values higher than 3.3 units can be perceived by untrained observers. Therefore, values in the range 1–3.3 units are considered appreciable by skilled operators but clinically acceptable. Despite this suggestion, the identification of a $\Delta E$ threshold value is still debatable and dentists and technicians are only guided by instructions supplied by ceramic manufacturers.

## 11.3 The use and key advantages of zirconia as a dental material

With reference to the above-mentioned requirements related to mechanical properties, biocompatibility and esthetics, zirconia represents certainly the favorite candidate for a dental application, as the increasing use of Y-TZP in restorative dentistry shows. It displays an excellent combination of mechanical properties, wear resistance, natural tooth appearance, chemical durability, and biocompatibility. Zirconia is a polymorphic material that occurs in three phases: monoclinic (from room temperature to 1170°C), tetragonal (in the range 1170–2370°C), and cubic (from 2370°C up to the melting point 2680°C). Upon cooling the martensitic lattice transformation from the tetragonal to the monoclinic phase is responsible for a substantial increase in volume of $\sim 5\%$. Pure zirconia cannot be processed without fracture because all the grains would transform upon cooling after sintering. By alloying pure zirconia with metal oxides, such as MgO, $CeO_2$, CaO, and $Y_2O_3$, it is possible to retain a metastable tetragonal phase (TZP) at room temperature that can transform into a monoclinic phase if mechanical or chemical energy is provided. In particular, when a crack develops in the metastable tetragonal phase, the presence of tensile stresses in the vicinity of the crack triggers locally the transformation into the monoclinic phase inducing compressive stresses (due to the volume expansion) that hinder the crack propagation. This local transformation of zirconia grains to the monoclinic symmetry is highly beneficial and leads to increased toughness when compared to nontransforming ceramics. This process is known as transformation toughening and has a great importance in the engineering of zirconia materials, significantly extending their use as technical advanced ceramics. Comprehensive reviews on zirconia crystallography and phase transformation can be found by Chevalier et al. (2009), Kelly and Denry (2008), and Hannink et al. (2000).

Among the stabilizing oxides, $Y_2O_3$ and $CeO_2$ represent the most attractive ones: zirconia doped with 3 mol% $Y_2O_3$ (3Y-TZP) shows exceptional fracture strength (above 1200 MPa) and moderate fracture toughness (<6 $MPa\sqrt{m}$) depending on grain size (Mitov et al., 2011; Zhang et al., 2014a; Fischer and Stawarczyk, 2007). Notwithstanding its excellent mechanical properties, 3Y-TZP presents a major drawback due to the spontaneous phase transformation in moist atmosphere. Such a phenomenon called low-temperature degradation (LTD) or aging, causes a loss of strength and generation of micro-cracking in the presence of water in a range of temperature close to clinical applications (from room temperature up to 400°C). A reduction of 30% of Young's modulus and hardness of 3Y-TZP (Lava, 3M-ESPE) ceramics exposed to water steam at 140°C for 7 days was attested by Cattani-Lorente et al. (2011). It has been largely reported that LTD is strongly related to grain size, residual stress, surface defects, temperature, and processing techniques (Lughi and Sergo, 2010). However, its mechanisms have not been fully clarified despite the vast number of studies on this topic. Among the most cited and discussed models, Chevalier et al. and Lawson proposed a degradation mechanism trigged by the $OH^-$ groups: the chemically adsorbed water reacts with the $O^{2-}$ group on the zirconia surface thus forming $OH^-$ ions. Such ions can penetrate into the inner part through grain boundary diffusion, fill the oxygen vacancies of the zirconia lattice, and generate a proton defect. When the oxygen vacancy concentration is reduced to a certain extent, the tetragonal phase is no longer stable and transforms into monoclinic (Chevalier, 2006; Lawson, 1995).

According to this model, one of the most significant impacts on the susceptibility to degradation is the choice of the stabilizing oxide: by doping $ZrO_2$ with a $Me^{4+}$ cation, no additional $O^{2-}$ vacancies are introduced into the lattice thus strongly hindering the aging mechanism. For this reason, research focus on $Ce^{4+}$ is currently gaining a lot of interest: ceria possesses a very high solubility in zirconia and up to 12 mol% it is able to stabilize the tetragonal zirconia phase. The most investigated compositions vary in the range 8–12 mol% $CeO_2$. Ceria-doped zirconia ceramics (Ce-TZP) exhibit reduced aging sensitivity and superior toughness (>15 $MPa\sqrt{m}$) with a pronounced pseudo-plastic behavior depending on the amount of ceria (Tsukuma and Shimada, 1985; El Attaoui et al., 2007; Deville et al., 2005). The significant greater stability of Ce-TZP over Y-TZP is illustrated in Fig. 11.5 depicting the amount of monoclinic content as a function of the aging time. It is possible to note that Ce-TZP does not show degradation in the timeframe of biomedical applications.

However, with respect to 3Y-TZP, Ce-TZP presents lower fracture strength (~600 MPa, Tsukuma and Shimada, 1985) and esthetic issues due to its yellowish color and the lack of translucency. Both aspects are related to the difficulty of producing Ce-TZP with a reduced grain size (<0.5 μm as for 3Y-TZP ceramic). Nowadays, the approach used to achieve satisfactory esthetical results is to cover the zirconia restoration with veneering porcelain. Despite the esthetic improvements, this approach often leads to chipping or cracking of the veneer ceramic to such an extent that it is considered to be the most common cause of failure of

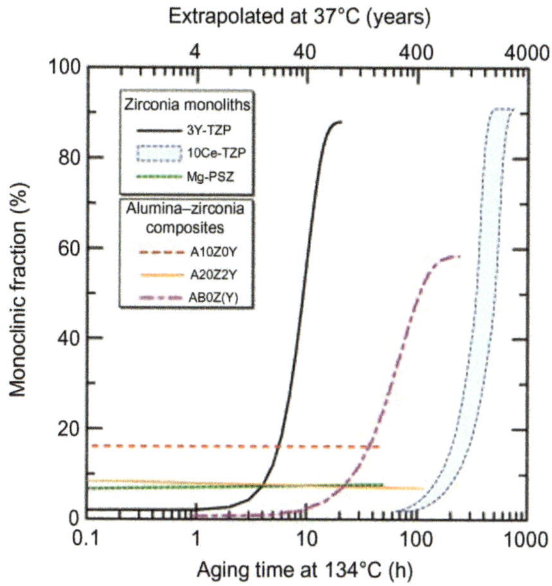


**Figure 11.5** Aging resistance of pure zirconia stabilized with Y (3Y-TZP), Ce (Ce-TZP), and Mg (Mg-TZP), and for alumina–zirconia composites.
*Source*: Reprinted from Chevalier, J., Gremmilard, L., Virkar, A.V., Clarke, D.R., 2009. The tetragonal-monoclinic transformation in zirconia: lessons learned and future trends. J. Am. Ceram. Soc. 92, 1901–1920, with the permission of Elsevier, under license no. 4115220979873.

zirconia restoration. Numerous possible reasons for chipping fractures have been indicated in literature. Among them, the mismatch of the coefficient of thermal expansion between the zirconia and the veneering porcelain, surface defects, overloading and fatigue, low fracture toughness of the veneering layer and, the most accepted, the development of residual stresses within the veneering porcelain. Such residual stresses can be compressive or tensile depending on the mismatch of the coefficient of thermal expansion, the cooling rates and the thickness of the veneering porcelain and they can be only partially reduced by performing slow cooling programs after firing (Al-Amleh et al., 2014).

In order to overcome the issue of chipping, the use of monolithic zirconia has been recently proposed. Besides its excellent mechanical properties, this material offers the advantage of a computer-aided manufacturing technology. Esthetics, namely its opaque-whitish appearance, can be improved by applying a coloring liquid to the zirconia before the sintering process, thus creating a natural tooth appearance without using a veneering porcelain, therefore minimizing fracture and/or chipping events. Surface treatments such as polishing and glazing can further improve the esthetic characteristics (Kim et al., 2016). However, since hardness of Y-TZP is much higher than that of porcelain, wear of the enamel of the opposing tooth can take place. Recent in vitro and in vivo studies showed that such a wear phenomenon is less pronounced on polished zirconia rather than on glazed zirconia (Malkondu et al., 2016). In addition, since monolithic crowns are exposed directly to the oral environment, the phenomenon of LTD should be kept in mind (Adabo et al., 2015). If, on the one hand, surface treatments may have a positive effect in bone apposition, on the other hand, they can facilitate the water penetration into the bulk, thus accelerating the degradation. Long-term results and standardized protocols to assess the effect of aging on mechanical properties, depending on the kind of surface treatment, are still lacking. In fact, it should be noted that the standard ISO 13356:2008 refers only to polished medical-grade zirconia. Recently, Sanon et al. (2015) proposed a protocol to validate the functionality and safety of zirconia implants, mainly in terms of phase transformation. By highlighting the limit of the current standard, they proposed to perform, along with X-ray diffraction analyses, aging kinetics directly on the implant surface, direct observations of the transformation zone and mechanical tests, in terms of load to failure, under realistic conditions, for a given clinical application.

If implants and restorations share some requirements, they also have specific ones. Implants do not need to be translucent and highly esthetic (except for some anterior teeth and thin gingiva). Conversely, the direct contact with bone necessitates steps further in understanding and improving bone-tissue response. Regarding biocompatibility features, many tests have been conducted in vitro and in vivo on zirconia ceramics, proving neither adverse tissue response nor cytotoxic and degradation effects (El-Ghani and Sherief, 2016; Mai et al., 2012). Moreover, compared to titanium specimens, zirconia surfaces positively show a significant reduction in bacterial adhesion (Scarano et al., 2004). However, when it comes to implants, zirconia has no direct bone bonding properties or osteoconduction behavior and biological tissues interact with only the outermost atomic layers of the implant (El-Ghani and Sherief, 2016). Surface modification methods such as roughening, acid-etching, laser treatment, and bioactive coating have been proposed so far, with the aim of improving the biological response. According to Payer et al., the surface roughness of zirconia improves initial bone healing and resistance to removal torque, enhancing osteoblast and fibroblast cell adhesion on zirconia implants (Payer et al., 2010). One of the most promising methods, recently proposed by Wu et al., is based on a polishing (or sandblasting) treatment of the zirconia surface followed by oxygen plasma irradiation. Oxygen plasma irradiation improves the zirconia wettability, retaining a stable hydrophilic surface, without changing the surface topography, thus promoting cell proliferation and differentiation (Wu et al., 2015).

On the grounds of the above-cited limitations of zirconia ceramics, different strategies can be envisaged with the aim of approaching the zirconia performances with those of a human tooth.

One strategy stems from the design and development of zirconia-based composite materials where additional phases, such as alumina or spinel, aid in refining the microstructure, thus improving fracture strength. Thanks to advanced processing methods, a high degree of microstructural control (grain refinement, zirconia stabilizing content, secondary phase positioning, composition, etc.) can be achieved, as it will be described in detail in Section 11.4. Inspired by the human tooth architecture, a parallel strategy is the design of functionally graded materials (FGM) with enhanced esthetical performances (Section 11.5). Finally, in Section 11.6, the most innovative results on tissue engineering devoted to the improvement of cell adhesion and proliferation on zirconia implants will be presented.

## 11.4 Design and development of strong, tough, and stable $ZrO_2$-based dental materials

Current research in dental materials is expected to develop *all-ceramic* implants and restorations. In particular, research is focusing on strong, tough, and stable ceramics, needed in the posterior part of the mouth where crowns, bridges, and abutments are subjected to the highest stresses. These ceramic materials are equally necessary for implants, which are always subjected to challenging mechanical conditions (Geng et al., 2001).

Thus, materials and implants development is taking advantage of (1) zirconia properties (excellent chemical durability, biocompatibility, wear and mechanical resistance, environmental friendliness, esthetics, etc.) and (2) the possibility of processing through advanced techniques such as computer-aided design/computer-aided manufacturing (CAD/CAM).

As pointed out earlier, Y-TZP shows higher mechanical strength than other conventional pure dental ceramics but it suffers from LTD and presents relatively low toughness. Therefore, on the one hand the strategy has been focusing on avoiding LTD of Y-TZP (Ross et al., 2001); on the other hand, it has focused on the development of alternative zirconia-based systems showing at the same time outstanding mechanical properties and a perfect stability in vivo, as is the case of Ce-TZP and its composites. It should be noted that both pure Y-TZP and Ce-TZP-based composites are currently available as alternatives to metals for dental prostheses and restorations. Dental implants are still largely made of titanium and titanium alloys but the market will probably shift more and more toward zirconia-based composites (especially Ce-TZP-based materials), as better mechanical resistance, machinability, and a perfect stability become possible today. In the context of this section, only innovative Ce-TZP-based composites will be considered.

Since 1985, Ce-TZP has been extensively studied due to its ability to undergo a large amount of stress-induced phase transformation, which leads to very high fracture toughness values (transformation toughening effect).

Transformation toughening in ceramics refers to the increase in fracture toughness that is the direct result of a phase transformation occurring at the tip of an advancing crack as it happens in partially stabilized zirconia (PSZ). As proposed by Swain and Rose (1986), the strength of PSZ is governed by the critical stress necessary to induce the tetragonal to monoclinic phase transformation and by the inherent R-curve behavior of these materials. Therefore, as a certain amount of crack extension is needed to develop the steady-state toughness, $K_{IC}$,

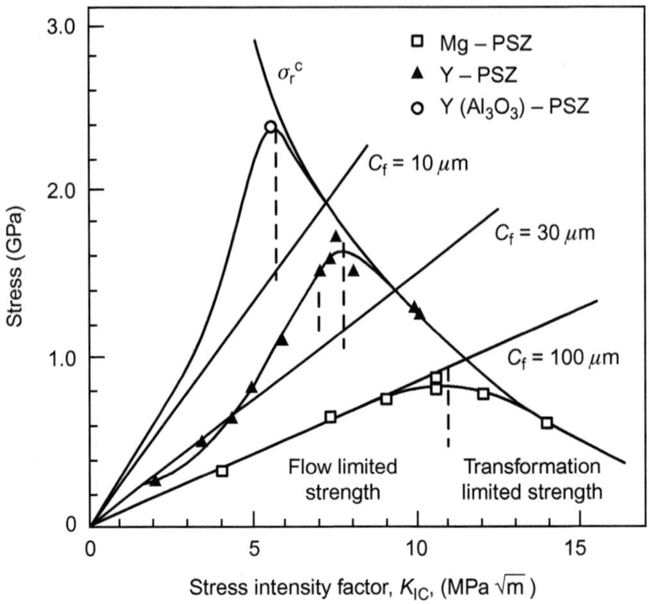


**Figure 11.6** Toughness/strength relationship for Mg PSZ and Y-PSZ materials of different compositions. The hyperbolic curve represents critical stress to initiate the transformation as a function of $K_{IC}$. Straight lines from the origin are the Griffith estimation for various critical flaw sizes $c_f$.
*Source*: From Swain, M.V., 1985. Inelastic deformation of Mg-PSZ and its significance for strength–toughness relationship of zirconia toughened ceramics. Acta Metall. 33, 11, 2083–2091, with the permission of Elsevier, under license no. 4115251020872.

the toughness vs strength curve passes through a maximum value. As shown in Fig. 11.6, in the case of zirconia-toughened ceramics, measured strengths increase with increasing $K_{IC}$, reaching a maximum before decreasing for higher toughness values. This maximum is located at ~8 MPa$\sqrt{}$m and 780 MPa for Ce-TZP (Swain and Rose, 1986).

The significance of this behavior is that two regimes on the toughness/strength relationship appear:

1. Below a given $K_{IC}$ value (e.g., ~8 MPa$\sqrt{}$m and 780 MPa for Ce-TZP) the maximum strength is flaw-size-dependent and follows the Griffith theory, i.e.,

$$\sigma f = \frac{K_{IC}}{Y\sqrt{c_f}} \tag{11.1}$$

where $\sigma_f$ is the strength for brittle failure, $K_{IC}$ is the toughness, $Y$ is a geometrical factor (usually $Y = \sqrt{\pi}$), and $c_f$ is the size of the most critical flaw. In the example of Fig. 11.6, for Mg PSZ strength can be predicted by assuming a critical flaw size of 100 μm (straight line).

2. Once the toughening influence becomes dominant, the critical transformation stress decreases and limits the maximum strength of the material (hyperbolic curve). Thus, above a given $K_{IC}$ value (on the right side of the maximum), the strength is controlled by the critical stress to initiate the tetragonal to monoclinic phase transformation, as follows:

$$\sigma^{c}_{t-m} = \beta^2 \sigma^{T} \left[ \frac{K_{I0}}{(K_{IC} - K_{I0})} \right] \tag{11.2}$$

where the constant $\beta$ depends on the transformed zone shape and $K_{I0}$ is the toughness of the material containing pre-transformed precipitates. For Ce-TZP ceramics with $K_{IC} = 12$ MPa$\sqrt{m}$, $K_{I0} = 3$ MPa$\sqrt{m}$ and $\beta^2\sigma^T = 1.4$ GPa, the calculated critical stress is 467 MPa (Swain and Rose, 1986).

Another interesting result of these observations is the influence of the critical transformation stress on maximum strength. For Ce-TZP and other transformable zirconia systems, even if fitting the experimental strength points to a universal $\sigma^{c}_{t-m}$ has not been achieved, it has been observed that data tend to form a hyperbolic function similar to that predicted by the $\sigma^{c}_{t-m}$ expression.

The zirconia grain size and/or stabilization degree can also play an important role in the transformability. Their influence is nowadays well known. As shown in Fig. 11.7A, fracture toughness decreases with the stabilization degree and increases with the grain size. Instead, the optimum fracture strength was observed for ceramics containing ~10–12 mol% ceria (Fig. 11.7B): out of this range, the strength decreases. For lower ceria amounts, the material is too unstable and the strength is limited by the low critical stress to induce transformation; for higher ceria amounts, the transformation is hindered and the strength is mainly limited by the critical flaw size (Tsukuma and Shimada, 1985).

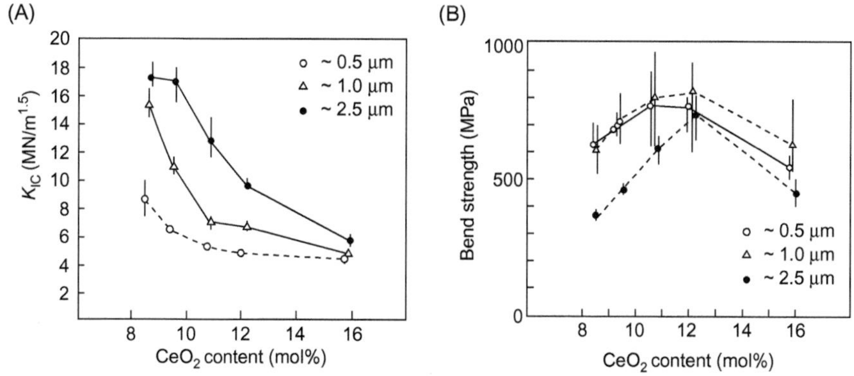


**Figure 11.7** Ce-TZP fracture toughness (A) and bending strength (B) containing different amounts of ceria and exhibiting different mean grain sizes.
*Source*: From Tsukuma, K., Shimada, M., 1985. Strength, fracture toughness and Vickers hardness of CeO2-stabilized tetragonal ZrO2 polycrystals (Ce-TZP). J. Mater. Sci. 20, 1178–1184.

As discussed above, the main drawback of using pure Ce-TZP in the dental field is related to its low mechanical resistance (flexural strength of ~600 MPa for Ce-TZP ceramics as compared to more than 1 GPa for Y-TZP), which is due to the significant grain growth experienced by Ce-TZP during sintering.

Therefore, from the late 1980s, many studies have been devoted to decreasing the Ce-TZP grain size by hindering its growth during sintering; in other words, by adding second phases to the matrix and developing Ce-TZP-based composites (Sato et al., 1989; Tsai et al., 1990; Yu et al., 1992; Schmid et al., 1992; Miura et al., 1994; Cutler et al., 1994; Nawa et al., 1998; Maschio et al., 1998; Yamaguchi et al., 1998; Benzaid et al., 2008; Apel et al., 2012; Ori et al., 2012; Kern, 2014; Palmero et al., 2015).

Among the several oxides added to Ce-TZP composites, $Al_2O_3$ has certainly been one of the most employed. The first work belongs to Sato et al. (1989) who reported a refinement of zirconia grains (from 3.5 to 1.5 μm) moving from Ce-TZP to Ce-TZP/20 vol% $Al_2O_3$ composite. Due to matrix refinement and in agreement with the rule of mixture, an increase in the hardness and Young's modulus was also recorded. In the following years, several authors developed Ce-TZP/$Al_2O_3$ composites characterized by zirconia grains of ~1 μm in size (Tsai et al., 1990; Yu et al., 1992; Schmid et al., 1992) and enhanced strength. Recently, very high fracture toughness (15 $MPa\sqrt{m}$) and excellent flexural strength (900 MPa) were reported by Apel et al. on 10Ce-TZP/16 vol% $MgAl_2O_4$ composites (zirconia and magnesium spinel grain size of 500 and 300 nm, respectively) (Apel et al., 2012).

In 1998 Nawa et al. (1998) developed a Ce-TZP-based composite (10 mol% $CeO_2$, zirconia grain size of 1 μm) containing 30 vol% $Al_2O_3$ particles, characterized by fracture toughness values of 9.8 $MPa\sqrt{m}$ and bending strength of 950 MPa. This composite shows a dual-phase interpenetrating microstructure, with several $Al_2O_3$ particles (10–100 nm in size) entrapped within the zirconia grains and 30- to 50-nm-sized $ZrO_2$ particles trapped within the $Al_2O_3$ grains. The $ZrO_2$ matrix consisted primarily of the tetragonal phase, with only a small fraction of the monoclinic phase. In this material, the strengthening achieved upon addition of $Al_2O_3$ grains was imputed to a decrease in flaw size, due to the overall ultrafine microstructure. It was also proposed that the $Al_2O_3$ and $ZrO_2$ nano-dispersions have a role in dividing each grain into even finer-sized particles, by forming sub-grain boundaries (Nawa et al., 1998). As a reduction of the grain size was predicted to increase the critical stress that induces the tetragonal-monoclinic transformation, an improvement in the strength was obtained in such ultrafine composites.

Thanks to the strict control of many microstructural and compositional parameters, the mechanical properties were further optimized (bending strength of 1290 MPa and fracture toughness of 8.6 $MPa\sqrt{m}$), giving rise to the commercial product named NANOZR (Panasonic Electric Works, Japan). In Fig. 11.9A, a schematic illustration of the intergranular-type Ce-TZP/alumina composite is depicted, while in Fig. 11.9B, the microstructure of the developed commercial product is shown.

From the above, a reduction in grain size—as achieved in Ce-TZP-based composites—is mandatory to increase the strength. However, the presence of (stiff) second phases inevitably decreases the effectiveness of phase transformation toughening and these new composites still remain brittle (flaw-sensitive) with Weibull moduli of ~20 (Lambrigger, 1997).

Therefore, a second strategy to simultaneously increase fracture strength and toughness was also explored. Ce-TZP-based (nano)-composites were developed through the addition of both round-shaped and elongated second phases, the former to decrease grain size and increase the strength (as previously discussed), the latter to increase the toughness by additional crack deflection/bridging mechanisms. The first investigations on Ce-TZP reinforced by in situ formed strontium hexa-aluminate ($SrAl_{12}O_{19}$) were carried out by Cutler et al. (1994), who developed three-phasic composites with the addition of 15–30 vol% $Al_2O_3$ and 0.5–8 wt% $SrZrO_3$ to a 12 mol% Ce-TZP matrix. Depending on the composition, fracture strength in the range 500–700 MPa, fracture toughness of 10–15 MPa$\sqrt{m}$ (by double cantilever beam) and hardness values of 10–14 GPa were obtained. In particular, the hardness and strength increased within the alumina content, whereas the toughness showed the opposite trend.

Based on these results, innovative Ce-TZP-based triphasic composites were recently developed in the frame of an EU Project (LONGLIFE, *Advanced multifunctional zirconia ceramics for long-lasting implants*, grant agreement no. 280741). The strategy envisages, along with the addition of both rounded and elongated second phases, the fine-tuning of the ceria amount inside zirconia grains, thus preserving the transformation toughening mechanism. In fact, as pointed out earlier (Fig. 11.7), the latter strongly depends on the amount of stabilizing oxide and it needs to be tuned on the grounds of the final microstructure. This approach is schematically represented in Fig. 11.8. With respect to benchmark Y-TZP, Ce-TZP shows a less fine microstructure, a lower strength, but a higher fracture toughness and stability against LTD. Biphasic composites are effective in decreasing the grain size and improving the strength, but only innovative triphasic composites seem able to meet all the requirements for strength, toughness, and stability.

Following this approach, Ce-TZP/8 vol%$Al_2O_3$/8 vol%$SrAl_{12}O_{19}$ composites (referred to as ZA8Sr8) were recently developed. Due to the complex composition and microstructure of this triphasic material, the elaboration of the composite powders was carried out following a recently developed *surface-coating* route (Schehl et al., 2002; Palmero et al., 2009). Starting from a commercial zirconia powder, its surface is coated (or graft) by precursors of the second phases, which then crystallize in situ under proper thermal treatment. With respect to the traditional mixing and milling powder route, this method allows a highly homogeneous distribution of the second phases in the zirconia matrix, a perfect tailoring of grain size and morphology, a close control of the stoichiometry and purity of all the phases. Moreover, the innovative surface-coating elaboration method allows a fine-tuning of the $CeO_2$ stabilizer content (performed in the range 10–11.5 mol%) inside the zirconia matrix, thus allowing the control and optimization of the mechanical properties, as discussed later (Fig. 11.10). The microstructure of ZA8Sr8 is depicted

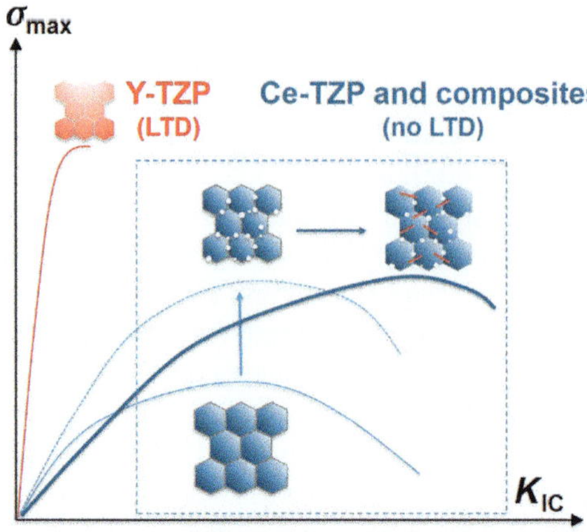


**Figure 11.8** Schematic representation of the innovative approach toward the development of strong, tough, and stable zirconia-based materials. The purple line and respective microstructure relate to Y-TZP, which undergoes LTD. The blue lines relate to the LTD-free Ce-TZP materials: monolithic Ce-TZP (light-blue, solid line); Ce-TZP-based biphasic composites, containing only fine rounded second-phase grains to increase the strength (light-blue, dotted line) and to Ce-TZP-based triphasic composites, containing both rounded and elongated second-phase grains (dark blue, solid line), to increase the strength and the toughness at the same time.

in Fig. 11.9D, showing that all the microstructural features match very closely the material design (Fig. 11.9C). The composite structure is made by a fine $ZrO_2$ matrix (average particle size of $0.6 \pm 0.2\ \mu m$), ultrafine $Al_2O_3$ grains (average size of $0.3 \pm 0.1\ \mu m$), and rod-like strontium hexa-aluminate grains, characterized by mean length of $0.6 \pm 0.2\ \mu m$ and aspect ratio of $5 \pm 2$.

Table 11.2 summarizes the main mechanical properties of commercially available ceramics (3Y-TZP and Ce-TZP/alumina composites) and of materials under development (Ce-TZP-based) potentially available in the market within 3–5 years.

Compared to NANOZR, higher fracture toughness ($15\ MPa\sqrt{m}$) but lower flexural strength (930 MPa) were reported by Apel et al. (2012) on 10Ce-TZP/16 vol% $MgAl_2O_4$ composites. Exceptional mechanical properties were shown by the triphasic composite ZA8Sr8, as recently reported by Reveron et al. (2017). As shown in Fig. 11.10, ZA8Sr8-based materials exhibited relatively high biaxial flexural strength (up to 1100 MPa) with the maximum located at 10.5 mol% ceria (toughness $>10.2\ MPa\sqrt{m}$, critical transformation stress near 500 MPa). Monoclinic transformed zones can be easily observed on the tensile side of biaxial specimens (failure stresses of 680 and 756 MPa for 10.0 and 11.5 mol% ceria, respectively) even on the most stabilized system.

As expected, zirconia transformability decreased with the ceria content. In less-stabilized materials (10.0 and 10.5 mol% ceria; higher toughness), zirconia phase transformation started well before crack propagation and the maximum strength was driven by the transformation. Moreover, these ceramics exhibited a certain

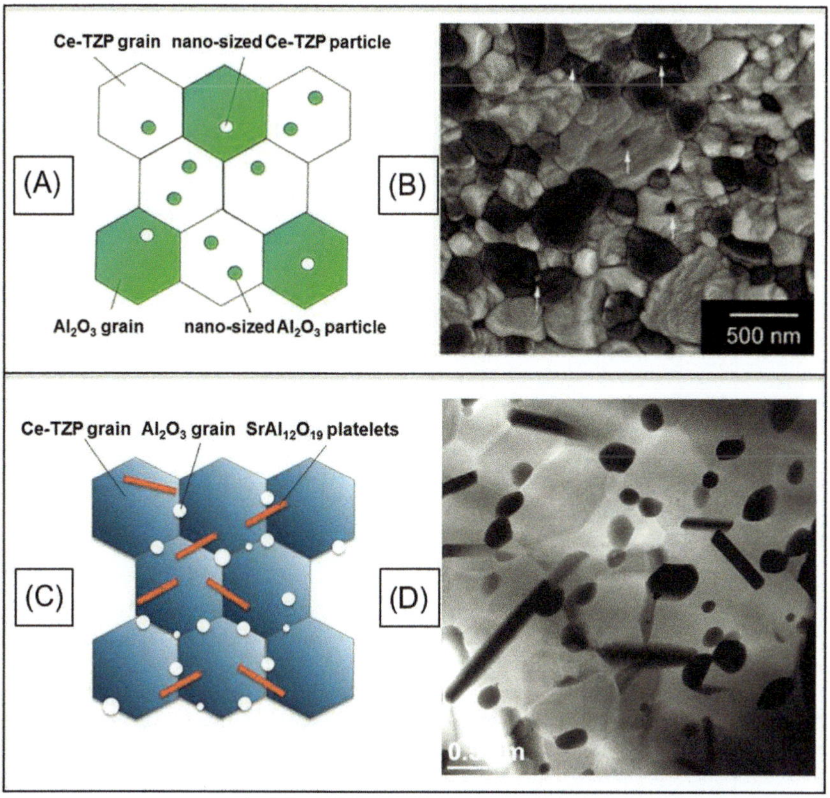


**Figure 11.9** Schematic illustration (A) and corresponding microstructure (B) of 10Ce-TZP/30 vol%$Al_2O_3$ interpenetrated intergranular-type composite (NANOZR). Design (C) and corresponding microstructure (D) of 10.5Ce-TZP/8 vol%$Al_2O_3$/8 vol%$SrAl_{12}O_{19}$ (ZrA8Sr8).

*Source*: (A) and (B) Adapted from Ban, S., Sato, H., Suehiro, Y., Nakanishi, H., Nawa, M., 2008. Biaxial flexure strength and low temperature degradation of Ce-TZP/$Al_2O_3$ nanocomposite and Y-TZP as dental restoratives. J. Biomed. Mater. Res. B Appl. Biomater. 87, 492–498, under the creative common license. (C) and (D) Reprinted from Palmero, P., Fornabaio, M., Montanaro, L., Reveron, H., Esnouf, C., Chevalier, J., 2015. Towards long lasting zirconia-based composites for dental implants. Part I: Innovative synthesis, microstructural characterization and in vitro stability. Biomaterials 50, 38–46, with the permission of Elsevier, under license no. 4095250242904).

degree of transformation-induced ductility. For instance, composites with 10.0 mol % ceria showed a region of plastic deformation and the strain to failure reached 0.5% (Fig. 11.11). It is observed that all load–unload curves ran parallel even for large strain, demonstrating that plasticity occurs without damage. More surprisingly, for these two compositions, measuring toughness by the SEVNB method was impossible since samples remained unbroken even when loads of 1 kN were applied, corroborating the "ductile-like" behavior of such composites. On the left

## Table 11.2 Mechanical properties of different dental zirconia ceramics

| Material | Composition (vol%) | Grain size (μm) | Toughness ($K_{IC}$, MPa$\sqrt{m}$) | Biaxial strength* (MPa) | Vickers hardness (MPa) | Weibull modulus (m) |
|---|---|---|---|---|---|---|
| 3Y-TZP[a,b]<br>TZ-3YB-E<br>*Tosoh* | 3 mol% $Y_2O_3-ZrO_2$: 100 | 0.32 ± 0.10 | 5.17 (Vickers indentation) | 1046 ± 112<br>892 ± 101 (aged) | ~1100–1250 | 9.5 |
| Ce-TZP-alumina[a,c]<br>NANOZR<br>*Matsushita Electric Works* | 10 mol% $CeO_2-ZrO_2$: 70<br>$Al_2O_3$: 30 | 0.59 ± 0.09<br>0.42 ± 0.08 | 8.62 (SEVNB) | 1422 ± 60<br>1386 ± 50 (aged) | 1150 | 23 |
| Ce-TZP-Mg spinel[d] | 10 mol% $CeO_2-ZrO_2$: 84<br>$MgAl_2O_4$: 16 | 0.50 ± 0.25<br>0.01–0.20 | > 15 (double torsion) | 930 ± 110 | 1040 | 10.1 |
| Ce-TZP-alumina-Sr aluminate<br>ZA8Sr8-Ce10.5[e]*LONGLIFE* | 10.5 mol% $CeO_2-ZrO_2$: 84<br>$Al_2O_3$: 8<br>$SrAl_{12}O_{19}$: 8 | 0.6 ± 0.2<br>0.3 ± 0.1<br>0.6 ± 0.2 | > 10.2 (*SEVNB*) | 1197 ± 23 | 985 | 60 |

In NANOZR composites several 10- to 100-nm-sized $Al_2O_3$ particles are trapped within the $ZrO_2$ grains and several 10-nm-sized $ZrO_2$ particles are trapped within the $Al_2O_3$ grains; microstructures of other composites are mainly intergranular-type. SEVNB, single edge V-notched beam method in a four-point-bending fixture.

*Biaxial strength determined by piston-on-three-ball method.

[a]Ban, S., Sato, H., Suehiro, Y., Nakanishi, H., Nawa, M., 2008. Biaxial flexure strength and low temperature degradation of Ce-TZP/$Al_2O_3$ nanocomposite and Y-TZP as dental restoratives. J. Biomed. Mater. Res. B Appl. Biomater. 87, 492–498.

[b]Trunec M., 2008. Effect of grain size on mechanical properties of 3Y-TZP ceramics. Ceram. Silikaty 52, 165–171.

[c]NANOZR Brochure—Panasonic Healthcare.

[d]Apel, E., Ritzberger, C., Courtois, N., Reveron, H., Chevalier, J.C., Schweiger, M., et al., 2012. Introduction to a tough, strong and stable Ce-TZP/$MgAl_2O_4$ composite for biomedical applications. J. Eur. Ceram. Soc. 32, 2697–2703.

[e]Reveron, H., Fornabaio, M., Palmero, P., Fürderer, T., Adolfsson, E., Lughi, V., et al., 2017. Towards long lasting zirconia-based composites for dental implants: transformation induced plasticity and its consequence on ceramic reliability. Acta. Biomater. 48, 423–432.

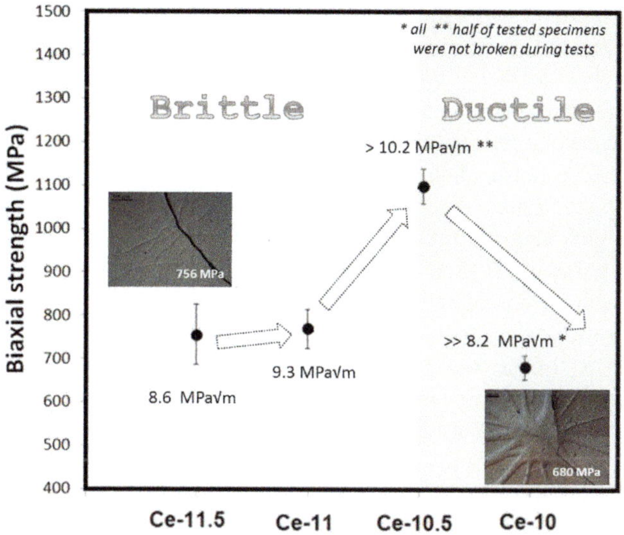


**Figure 11.10** Toughness and biaxial flexural strength for ZA8Sr8-based ceramics containing different amounts of ceria. Transformed zones after failure were observed by optical microscopy using Nomarski interference.
*Source*: Adapted from Reveron, H., Fornabaio, M., Palmero, P., Fürderer, T., Adolfsson, E., Lughi, V., et al., 2017. Towards long lasting zirconia-based composites for dental implants: transformation induced plasticity and its consequence on ceramic reliability. Acta. Biomater. 48, 423–432, with the permission of Elsevier, under license no. 4115241075685.

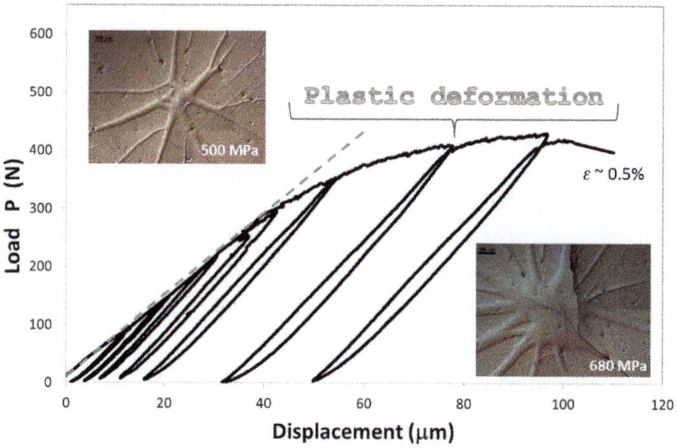


**Figure 11.11** Load–displacement curves recorded during biaxial bending for a ZA8Sr8–10Ce ceramic composite. Optical characterization of tensile side after 500 MPa and failure are also displayed here.
*Source*: Adapted from Reveron, H., Fornabaio, M., Palmero, P., Fürderer, T., Adolfsson, E., Lughi, V., et al., 2017. Towards long lasting zirconia-based composites for dental implants: transformation induced plasticity and its consequence on ceramic reliability. Acta. Biomater. 48, 423–432, with the permission of Elsevier, under license no. 4115241075685.

side of the maximum, for higher ceria contents (11.0 and 11.5 mol%; lower toughness), as the zirconia became more stable, the phase transformation was hindered and occurred when a crack propagated from a preexisting processing flaw.

From this recent work it can be seen that composites based on 84 vol% Ce-TZP containing two second phases (8 vol% alumina and 8 vol% strontium hexa-aluminate) are able to develop outstanding high strength, toughness, and ductility if the content of ceria and the sintering conditions are both accurately controlled. Moreover, these ceramics exhibited almost no dispersion in the strength values, and were biocompatible and safe against LTD (Schienle et al., 2016; Palmero et al., 2015). As a consequence, they can be considered as very promising candidates for innovative dental implants and restorations. Specifically, composites containing 10.5 mol% ceria (flexural strength >1.1 GPa and fracture toughness >10.2 MPa$\sqrt{}$m) exceed all ISO 6872:2015 standard requirements (see Table 11.1). The fact that the transformation occurs well before failure leads to an extraordinary high flaw tolerance which is reflected by a Weibull modulus never before reported for a ceramic ($m$=60), enhancing machinability (Reveron et al., 2017). Such excellent mechanical properties as compared to pure Ce-TZP monolithic ceramics corroborate the positive effect of refining zirconia grains by adding two second phases and of preserving transformation toughening by adapting ceria content in a very precise manner.

Finally, it should be noted that strength values can vary greatly depending on the type of mechanical test (four-point bending or biaxial piston-on-three-ball) as recently reported for 10Ce-TZP/$Al_2O_3$/$La_2AlO_3$ composite (Touahier et al., 2016). The mean strength obtained for the uniaxial tests was of 596 MPa and that of the biaxial tests of 1470 MPa, i.e., four-point-bending strength was ~2.5 times lower than the biaxial one. Such variation is attributed to different transformation behaviors characterizing these two bending configurations independently from the effect of the sample volume on strength, generally predicted by the standard Weibull analysis. The importance of this finding is that the significant influence of the loading configuration on the strength should be integrated when designing a component from a highly transformable ceramic. Therefore, standards in the dental field should also be revised because, as presented before, three flexural test methods are acceptable by ISO 6872:2015 (three-point bending, four-point bending, and biaxial piston-on-three-ball), without taking into consideration that the last one can really overestimate strength data of highly transformable zirconia-based composites and generally speaking materials deviating from a simple linear-elastic behavior.

## 11.5 Bio-inspired design of dental ceramics

Ceramic dental crown restorations are normally used to replace the damaged tooth structure. However, in spite of continuous advances in materials and technologies, their failure rate is still high, ~1%–3% each year (Burke et al., 2002). The major clinical failure mode is the subsurface radial crack in the ceramic, induced by the tensile stress concentration at the interface between the crown (dental ceramic) and the cement (Huang et al., 2007), which plays the role of joining the crown to the dentin. As pointed out in Section 11.1, the Young's modulus of the ceramic crown material varies typically between 70 and 380 GPa (Dong and Darvell, 2003; Rekow et al., 2006; Petrini et al., 2013), whereas for the cement it ranges between 2 and 13 GPa (O'Brien, 1997). Such a difference in stiffness is responsible for high interface stress concentration. Furthermore, stiff and hard ceramics are abrasive to the opposing dentation, producing sensitivity and occlusal imbalance (Petrini et al., 2013; Jacobi et al., 1991). On the other hand, the natural tooth (dentin) is characterized by an elastic modulus of ~20 GPa (Marshall et al., 2001) and the DEJ provides a graded interface between these two layers, thus reducing the stress in the enamel or crown parts (Marshall et al., 2001).

Therefore, inspired by the structure of the DEJ, many efforts today are focusing on the development of FGM layers, to be placed between the ceramic core and the dental cement, with the aim of grading the stiffness from the exterior to the inner part. Finite-element simulation shows that the presence of an FGM layer can significantly reduce the interfacial stress (up to 30%) and increase the critical crack length (Huang et al., 2007), with the result of improved durability of the ceramic prosthesis. Rahbar and Soboyevo (2011) also suggested that the reduced stress concentrations associated with FGM can be used to engineer significant reductions in pop-in loads. Because pop-in can occur by subcritical crack growth mechanisms in the top ceramic layers (Lawn et al., 2002), this should result in improved resistance to subcritical fatigue crack growth.

A further issue of high-strength ceramic cores, like alumina and zirconia, is their quite opaque appearance (and this is even more important for composites). Therefore, a thick porcelain veneer is needed, that is able to induce a gradual change in translucency to mask the ceramic core and to achieve a better esthetic outcome. New FGM materials have been successfully designed and developed recently, in order to combine an esthetic, low-elastic-modulus and low-hardness glass veneer with a high-strength ceramic core, without a sharp interface between the materials. The lack of interface due to grading improves interfacial bond strengths, reduces residual stresses, and eliminates delamination. Recently, Zhang et al. (2012) have produced elastically graded materials, with different elastic modulus profiles and bulk-to-surface modulus ratios. In particular, two core ceramic materials were exploited, alumina and Y-TZP. Accordingly, two silicate glasses were developed to infiltrate alumina and zirconia substrates, by tuning the glass compositions in order to have the same thermal expansion coefficient (CTE) in the veneer and the core and to avoid long-range residual thermal stress introduced by glass infiltration. In such a way, only elastic gradient effects were induced into the system, as an ideal condition to evaluate its effect on the critical load for flexural fracture. Fully sintered and polished ceramics were then infiltrated with the glass slurries under thermal treatment. As an example, the microstructure of the glass-infiltrated zirconia material is depicted in Fig. 11.12A: the high glass content present at the surface gradually decreases as the distance from the surface increases. In spite of a significant growth of the zirconia grains at the surface, the glass-infiltrated Y-TZP was composed of only the

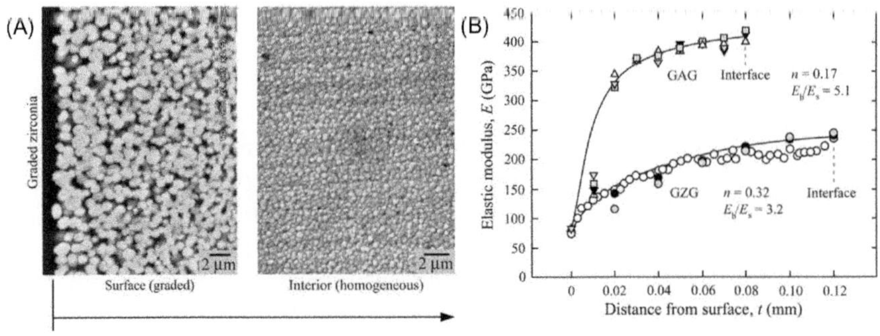


**Figure 11.12** (A) Backscattered electron (BSE) image showing cross-sectional view of a graded glass–zirconia structure. Note that the glass content (dark phase) gradually decreases as it proceeds toward the interior. (B) Evolution of elastic modulus as a function of the distance from the surface. The individual points are the Young's modulus data obtained from nano-indentation. The solid curves are semiempirically fit to the Young's modulus data, according to Zhang et al. (2010).
*Source*: Adapted from Zhang, Y., Chai, H., Lawn, B.R., 2010. Graded structures for all-ceramic restorations. J. Dent. Res. 89, 417–421, with the permission of Elsevier under license no. 4114710977578.

tetragonal zirconia phase. As shown in Fig. 11.12B, the infiltrating glass at the external surfaces of both materials had a modulus of ~67 GPa, similar to that of dental porcelains. The graded glass ceramic surface possessed a modulus of ~80 and ~75 GPa for glass-infiltrated alumina (GAG) and glass-infiltrated zirconia (GZG), respectively. Both materials exhibited superior load-bearing capacity, 20%–50% higher than conventional homogeneous materials.

Similar results were achieved by Fabris et al. (2017), who investigated the thermal residual stresses generated inside "traditional" ceramic restorations, made by a strong ceramic framework and an external esthetic veneer. In fact, in the processing of all-ceramic restorations, the porcelain is fired onto the framework at high temperature, creating high thermal residual stresses upon cooling to room temperature, due to the CTE mismatch between the two ceramic parts. Three different multilayer designs were simulated: (1) a conventional bilayer (core-veneer) design; (2) a trilayer design, with an intermediate composite layer with constant composition; (3) a graded design, with an intermediate layer with gradation of properties. It was shown that both homogeneous and graded interlayers yielded the lowest thermal stress, significantly lower compared to the bilayer system. These results indicate that, by proper design, it is thus possible to reduce the risk of failure for all-ceramic dental materials and to develop more reliable restorative systems.

Driven by the demand for designing restorations with real tooth functions, a novel composite system, polymer-infiltrated-ceramic-network material (PICN) has emerged in recent years (He and Swain, 2011), inspired by the glass-infiltrated ceramic structure. Different from conventional filler-reinforced resin composites, PICN is composed primarily of a porous ceramic structure with an interpenetrating resin phase, thus meeting both mechanical and esthetic requirements. Up until now, commercial products like Vita Enamic have mainly focused on polymer-infiltrated feldspar ceramics for esthetic purposes, but this product shows a relatively low flexural strength ($\sim$100–160 MPa) and toughness (0.4–1.7 MPa$\sqrt{m}$) (Li et al., 2017; He and Swain, 2011; Coldea et al., 2013). Therefore, to simulate the mechanical properties of the natural teeth, a composite made by a zirconia (3Y-TZP) network was infiltrated with a blend of TEGDMA (tri(ethyl-englycol) dimethacrylate), BPO (benzoyl peroxide), and Bis-GMA (bisphenol A glycidyl dimethacrylate). By tuning the pre-sintering temperature of zirconia ceramic precursors, it was possible to obtain different porosities and polymer contents. Optimal mechanical properties, in terms of flexural strength, fracture toughness, hardness, and elastic modulus (240 MPa, 3.7 MPa$\sqrt{m}$, 3.1 GPa, and 58.8 GPa, respectively) were achieved. Thanks to the high strength of the zirconia ceramic network, the toughening mechanism by crack bridging and the controlled amount of polymer phase, the material shows tooth-like mechanical properties and feasible application as a restorative material in dental clinics.

However, such innovative polymer–ceramic composites are isotropic and are unable to mimic the aligned tissue structure of the dentin and enamel (see Fig. 11.1). Based on this observation, a further bio-inspired design was recently proposed by Petrini et al. (2013) who developed a new composite characterized by a multilevel hierarchical structure of its inorganic components. The freeze-casting technique was used to obtain the hierarchically structured architecture of the ceramic preforms, which were then infiltrated with epoxy resin. An aligned and graded structure has been obtained in the ceramic phase with lamellae-like morphology, similarly to that of natural dentin.

A very innovative approach, in terms of both design and technology, was recently proposed by Le Ferrand et al. (2015), dealing with the development of heterogeneous/graded materials produced by magnetically assisted slip casting. Inspired by the layer-by-layer approach used by living cells to fabricate complex architectures, a new additive manufacturing route was proposed to create lamellar composites, with locally controlled texture. This was achieved by combining the slip-casting technology with a recently developed approach able to control the orientation and distribution of anisotropic particles, contained in the slurry, by applying magnetic fields. To this aim, the anisotropic particles were coated with superparamagnetic iron oxide nanoparticles, to become magnetically responsive (Erb et al., 2012). During slip casting, a cake formed on the surface of the porous mold. The application of an external magnetic field was able to orient the anisotropic particles throughout the thickness of the cake. Changing the direction of the magnetic field, heterogeneous composites with any desired orientation of anisotropic particles throughout the thickness of the material were obtained. This approach was successfully used to reproduce the complex architecture of a biological tooth, as shown in Fig. 11.13. To this end, a porous plaster mold was first prepared as an imprint of an actual human molar (see Fig. 11.13C). A bilayer structure that mimics the dentin–enamel layers of a natural tooth was then fabricated by sequentially casting two different aqueous suspensions into the porous mold (Fig. 11.13A).

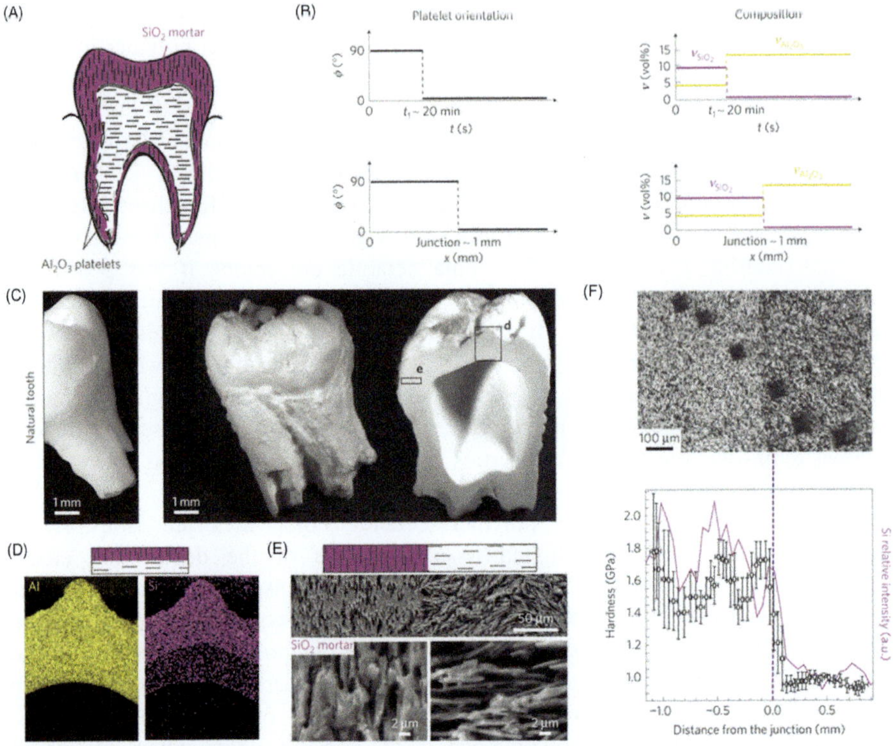


**Figure 11.13** Design and fabrication of bio-inspired composite through magnetically assisted slip casting: (A) Schematic representation of the target complex-shaped part comprising a bilayer with locally distinct platelet orientation and chemical composition. (B) Top: programed temporal pattern of the magnetic field angle ($\phi = f(t)$) and volume fraction of chemical constituents ($\nu = f(t)$); bottom: target local orientation of platelets and chemical composition as a function of the thickness of the cast layer ($\phi = f(x)$) and ($\nu = f(x)$, respectively). (C) Left: natural tooth used as a positive template for the fabrication of the complex-shaped porous mold; right: synthetic tooth-like part obtained using magnetically assisted slip casting, including cross-sectional cut to reveal its internal bilayer structure. (D) Elemental analysis of a part of the bilayer (box d in C), confirming the higher concentration of Si in the outer enamel-like layer. (E) Scanning electron micrograph image of the synthetic DEJ, highlighting the distinct platelet orientation in each of the two adjacent layers (box e in C). (F) Micro-indentation across the synthetic DEJ, indicating the hardness gradient achieved by tuning the local platelet orientation and chemical composition within the composite. Error bars indicate standard deviation over three measurements.
*Source*: Reproduced from Le Ferrand, H., Bouville, F., Niebel, T.P., Studard, A.R., 2015. Magnetically assisted slip casting of bioinspired heterogeneous composites. Nat. Mater. 14, 1172–1181, with the permission of Nature Publishing Group under license no. 4111531502105.

While both suspensions consisted mainly of 20 vol% alumina platelets, the one used to mimic the dentin-like layer also contained 13 vol% isotropic alumina nanoparticles, whereas in the suspension used to mimic the denser and harder material enamel-like layer, 4 vol% alumina nanoparticles were replaced by nanometric silica particles (see Fig. 11.13B). Silica forms a liquid phase during sintering that increases the bonding strength between platelets. The casting procedure was carried out in the presence of a rotating magnetic field, so as to replicate the orientation of reinforcing elements found in natural teeth. Such reinforcing building blocks are typically aligned perpendicular to the cusp surface within the enamel layer and parallel to the surface in the underlying dentin layer Fig. 11.13E, matching the targeted texture. After sintering, the bilayer structure was polymer-infiltrated to create a tooth-like complex-shaped composite with 50 and 64 vol% inorganic phase in dentin-like and enamel-like layers, respectively. In addition, as shown by the electron diffraction X-ray mapping, Si atoms are exclusively present in the outer enamel-like layer (Fig. 11.13D). Micro-hardness measurements of the material across the boundary between the enamel- and dentin-like layers showed a continuous decrease in the hardness from the enamel-like layer to the bilayer interface, before reaching a lower plateau value at the dentin-like side, similar to the DEJ of natural tooth. This gradual transition was imputed to the change in platelets orientation and density across the bilayer interface.

This technology appears as an effective approach to generate multilayered composites with mechanical properties that can potentially outperform the most state-of-the-art dental materials.

## 11.6 Dental tissue regeneration: advanced materials and technologies

Modern dental therapies for the replacement of missing teeth largely utilize restorative ceramics as well as titanium implants capped with prosthetic crowns. Although these prostheses are effective, they are not equivalent, neither in function nor in esthetics to natural teeth. The most recent advances in restorative dentistry therefore also involve the development of materials and technologies to regenerate the *whole-tooth* complex in a biological manner. This implies the successful formation of a heterogeneous and dynamic array of tissues, including roots, the periodontal ligament, nerve, and vascular tissue, as well as the essential dentine-pump system. Following this approach and considering the limited regeneration capability of dental tissues, the combination of stem cells and proper scaffold material is necessary to facilitate the regeneration of enamel, cement, and dentin. The former is the most difficult to regenerate, owing to the fact that ameloblasts cells are no longer present in the adult dental tissue (Moradian-Oldak et al., 2006; Yen and Yelick, 2011; Xavier et al., 2015; Ono et al., 2017).

To apply this strategy, it is first important to understand the tooth development (odontogenesis) process and the chemical and physical properties of the natural dental tissues. Teeth are complex structures consisting of the crown, neck, and root. Tooth development can broadly be divided into five major stages: dental lamina, initiation, bud stage, cap stage, bell stage, and eruption. Initially, ameloblast and odontoblast cells differentiate at the junction between epithelium and mesenchyme to form enamel and dentin, which are the tooth-specific hard tissues. Root formation is then initiated by differentiation of cementoblasts from dental follicle mesenchyme to form cement, which is the third hard tissue of the tooth (Thesleff and Tummers, 2009). Besides these hard tissues, cells are the other most important components of dental tissue. Cells present in dental tissue include osteoclasts and osteoblasts located on the face of the alveolar bone, cementoblasts on the surface of the root canal, and mesenchymal tissue in the ligament tissue that is essential for the long-term survival of these dental tissues. Molecular signals initiated by these cells trigger a set of events that regulate tissue morphogenesis, regeneration, and differentiation. However, human teeth do not have the capacity to regenerate after eruption. Therefore, the use of nondental cells is seen today as a potential alternative for bioengineered human teeth.

It is evident that odontogenesis is a complex process involving a series of reciprocal epithelial–mesenchymal interactions and coordination between the crown and the root with its associated periodontium. Accordingly, cells dissociated from epithelium and mesenchymal tissues of prenatal or postnatal tooth germ were used to reconstitute a "bioengineered tooth germ" in vitro (Ono et al., 2017). Ono et al. attempted to produce a whole tooth by transplantation of such bioengineered tooth germ into the oral environment or an organ culture and demonstrated that functional tooth restoration—through the autologous transplantation of the germ—is possible today not only in the mouse model, but even in a postnatal large-animal (canine) model. A scheme of this challenging process is illustrated in Fig. 11.14. Tooth germs of mandibular premolars were dissected from 30-day-old beagle dogs, to generate the bioengineered tooth germ using an organ-germ culture method (Nakao et al., 2017). Next, canine bioengineered tooth germs were reconstructed using epithelial tissue and mesenchymal single cells derived from permanent premolar tooth germs of 30-day postnatal dogs. Both a bioengineered and a reference natural (not-dissected) tooth germ were autologously transplanted into the alveolar bone socket in the mandible after 2 days of organ culture (Fig. 11.14A). The photograph in Fig. 11.14B shows the extracted deciduous molar, with permanent premolar tooth germ (red arrowhead), while in Fig. 11.14C a photograph and a histological image of the isolated permanent premolar tooth germ are respectively shown. In Fig. 11.14D, an image of the reconstituted canine tooth germ is depicted, while in Fig. 11.14E the transplanted bioengineered tooth germ (red arrowhead) into canine lower jawbone is shown. At 180 days after transplantation, a successful tooth eruption into the oral cavity was observed (Fig. 11.14F). The developmental process of the bioengineered tooth after transplantation was practically identical to that of a natural tooth, as it showed the correct tooth tissue structure and a single root shape composed of enamel, dentin, cement, and periodontal ligament, with the same architecture and components as the natural tooth.

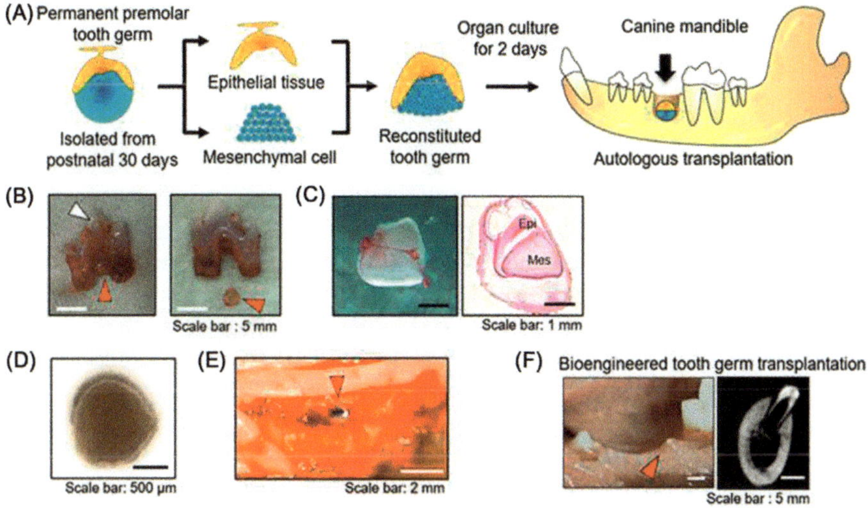


**Figure 11.14** (A) Schematic representation of autologous transplantation methods for the bioengineered tooth using postnatal canine-derived tissue. (B) Photograph of the extracted deciduous molar with permanent premolar tooth germ (left) and isolation of the permanent premolar tooth germ (right). White arrowhead, extracted deciduous molar; red arrowheads, permanent premolar tooth germs. (C) Photograph (left) and histological image by hematoxylin and eosin (HE) staining (right) of the isolated permanent premolar tooth germ. Epi, epithelial tissue; Mes, mesenchymal tissue. (D) Phase contrast image of the reconstituted canine tooth germ using epithelial tissue and mesenchymal cells derived from permanent premolar tooth germ after 2 days in organ culture; (E) Photograph of the autologous transplantation of bioengineered tooth germ into canine lower jawbone; red arrowhead, bioengineered tooth germ. (F) Oral photographs and computerized tomography (CT) images of the erupted bioengineered tooth at 180 days after transplantation; red arrowhead, erupted tooth.
*Source*: Adapted from Ono, M., Oshimal, M., Ogawa, M., Sonoyama, W., Satoshi Hara, E., Oida, Y., et al., 2017. Practical whole-tooth restoration utilizing autologous bioengineered tooth germ transplantation in a postnatal canine model. Sci. Rep. 7, 44522, doi:10.1038/srep44522, under the creative common license.

A further challenging procedure in dental surgery consists of *guided bone regeneration* (GBR) (Liu and Kerns, 2014), which is a technique used for the treatment of periodontal bone defects. It consists of creating a space between the bone and its surrounding tissues, using a barrier that allows new bone to migrate into the space, while preventing other cell types from interfering. Dahlin et al. demonstrated in fact that if a barrier membrane is placed in direct contact with the surrounding bone surface and a space was created, only cells from the neighboring bone or bone marrow can migrate into this bone defect, without in-growth of competing soft tissue cells from the overlying mucosa (Dahlin, 1994). There may be additional benefits of the use of a membrane, such as protection of the wound from mechanical disruption and salivary contamination.

The membrane material should satisfy the following requirements: biocompatibility, ability to integrate with the surrounding tissues, suitable occlusive properties to prevent invasion of fibrous connective tissue, protection from bacteria if exposed to the oral environment and physical stability with reduced displacement as respect to the living tissue, thus not to alter bone formation.

A wide range of barrier membranes have been used, both nonresorbable (e.g., expanded polytetrafluoroethylene (e-PTFE), high-density PTFE (d-PTFE), titanium mesh, titanium-reinforced PTFE), and resorbable membranes (such as collagen, synthetic polyesters, polyglycolides, polylactides, or copolymers) (Hämmerle and Jung, 2003; Liu and Kerns, 2014).

The most commonly used membranes are e-PTFE, collagen, and titanium mesh. However, the first two materials do not present sufficient mechanical strength; the latter offers superior mechanical properties but can penetrate the oral mucosa, which could lead to an esthetically unsuccessful result (von Arx and Kurt, 1998).

Therefore, inert high-strength ceramics such as $ZrO_2$, are nowadays attracting much attention as alternative membrane materials for GBR. This class of materials is expected to solve the major clinical dilemmas, like exposure of the materials and lack of stability in terms of larger GBR treatments. Due to the inert character of $ZrO_2$, a thin fibrous layer will be formed at the surface (Hench, 1998). The thickness of this layer is influenced by the surrounding tissue; however, some material features, such as surface morphology and chemical composition, also play an important role in the tissue response.

Malmström et al. (2016) have recently demonstrated the effectiveness of $ZrO_2$ membranes in the GBR process, describing a new method to achieve a perfect bone regeneration and to facilitate the subsequent installation of dental implants. First, a digital model of the initial shape of the bone structure (of three different patients) was obtained from computed tomography data, showing in all cases inadequate bone volume to allow dental implants to be installed. Then, starting from the digital models, $ZrO_2$ membranes with a thickness of $\sim 0.7$ mm and customized shape were fabricated. In particular, the shape of the ceramic membrane is defined by the desired bone height and the initial bone shape; the inner surface corresponds to the desired bone surface while the edge of the sheet should follow the surface of the initial bone shape (Fig. 11.15A). Each customized ceramic membrane was

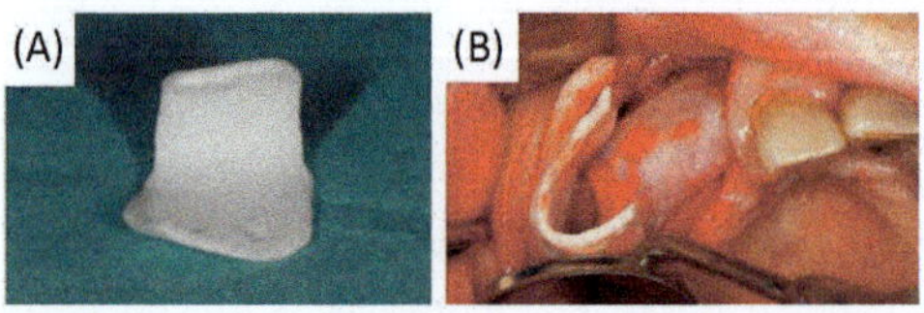


**Figure 11.15** Customized zirconia sheet (A) and its removal of a zirconia after healing (B). *Source*: Reprinted from Malmström, J., Anderud, J., Abrahamsson, P., Wälivaara, DÅ., Isaksson, SG., Adolfsson E., 2016. Guided bone regeneration using individualized ceramic sheets. Int. J. Oral. Maxillofac. Surg. 45, 1246–1252, with the permission of Elsevier under license no. 4119390987033.

prepared by conventional machining of cold isostatically pressed and pre-sintered compacts, followed by sintering at 1450°C.

The surgery was then performed by fixing the sheet to the bone by using a single screw and allowing the healing process. The close contact between the edge of the ceramic membrane and the initial bone surface made it possible to avoid undesired ingrowth of soft tissue into the cavity between the bone and the inner surface of the zirconia membrane. Conversely, an optimal bone formation was achieved, which proceeds from the initial bone surface toward the inner surface of the zirconia membrane. Bone regeneration follows a specific sequence of events (Dahlin et al., 1988). Briefly, within the first 24 h after fixation of the membrane, the created space is filled with the blood clot, which releases growth factors and cytokines, to attract neutrophils and macrophages. The clot is absorbed and replaced with granulation tissue, which is rich in newly formed blood vessels. Through these blood vessels, nutrients and mesenchymal stem cells capable of osteogenic differentiation can be transported and contribute to osteoid formation. Mineralization of osteoid forms woven bone (Schenk et al., 1994), which later serves as a template for the apposition of lamellar bone (Javed et al., 2010). This transformation of primary sponge would eventually constitute both compact and reticular bone with mature bone marrow. These events occur normally 3–4 months postoperatively (Buser, 2009).

In this work, after 7 months of healing, the zirconia membranes were removed (Fig. 11.15B), showing that bone had regenerated in the entire interior volume of the ceramic sheets, for all three patients. The stiffness of $ZrO_2$ in combination with the customized shape of the sheets ensured completely stable fixation, facilitating bone formation. Bone biopsies revealed newly formed trabecular bone, with a lamellar structure, while soft tissue biopsies showed connected tissue with no sign of inflammatory response or adverse reaction.

The use of $ZrO_2$ membranes for GBR has not been previously used for the treatment of patients. However, the successful outcomes of this study suggest the potential of $ZrO_2$ in GBR procedures, demonstrate the feasibility to design the new bone in a customized and predicable manner, and open new opportunities for more complicated and large grafting areas in the region of planned oral implants.

## 11.7 Conclusions

Ceramics play a pivotal role in dentistry, owing to their natural esthetics and excellent biocompatibility, good mechanical properties, with no known adverse reactions. They are currently applied to two categories of restorative dentistry: all--ceramic fixed-partial dentures and implantable components (covering implants, abutments, and ancillaries). While the former category aims at balancing mechanical properties with esthetical appearance, the latter aims at maximizing mechanical performance, reliability, and lifetime.

By keeping in mind such main applications and related requirements, this chapter provides some guidelines for the design and development of innovative ceramics for next-generation dental products and discusses the direction for future developments.

Three main strategies are here illustrated concerning the design of new dental restorative materials.

The first strategy focuses on strong, tough, and stable ceramics, needed for implants and in the posterior part of the mouth where crowns, bridges, and abutments are subjected to the highest stresses. Such requirements are fully satisfied by innovative zirconia-based composites, in which a proper design associated with a controlled processing and fine-tuning of microstructural and compositional parameters allows the fabrication of ceramics with outstanding properties, which are reliable and long-lasting.

The second parallel strategy is related to the biomimetic approach, in which the design of dental ceramics is inspired by the human tooth architecture. FGM, used to grade mechanical properties as in the DEJ structures and to approach the esthetic appearance of the natural tooth, are attracting much attention. Besides, starting from the polymer-infiltrated ceramics approach, innovative mineralized tissue-based hierarchical structures have been recently developed, also proving the feasibility of smart additive manufacturing routes for the fabrication of heterogeneous systems, designed to match the demands of specific target applications.

The third ambitious approach relates to tissue engineering in dentistry. Some examples of the most recent advances for regenerating the whole-tooth complex in a biological manner as well as the new challenging approaches, in terms of biomaterials and technologies, applied to the GBR process are illustrated.

Research on ceramic materials, ceramic implant designs, and processing technologies has increased in the past few years and is expected to expand in the future, opening new opportunities for using innovative ceramics in dentistry and, most relevantly, increasing patients' quality life (less invasive procedures, shorter recovery times, no revision surgeries, etc.).

## Acknowledgments

Some of the results presented in this work were achieved in the framework of the LongLife project (Advanced multifunctional zirconia ceramics for long-lasting implants) funded by the European Community's Seventh Framework Programme (FP7/2007–2013) under the grant agreement no. 280741.

## References

Adabo, G.L., Mariscal, E.M., Hatanaka, G.R., 2015. Flexural strength and microstructure of anterior/monolithic zirconia after low-temperature aging. Dent. Mater. 31, 48–49.

Al-Amleh, B., Waddel, J.N., Lyons, K., Swain, M.V., 2014. Influence of veneering porcelain thickness and cooling rate on residual stresses in zirconia molar crowns. Dent. Mater. 30, 271–280.

Apel, E., Ritzberger, C., Courtois, N., Reveron, H., Chevalier, J.C., Schweiger, M., et al., 2012. Introduction to a tough, strong and stable Ce-TZP/$MgAl_2O_4$ composite for biomedical applications. J. Eur. Ceram. Soc. 32, 2697−2703.

Ban, S., Sato, H., Suehiro, Y., Nakanishi, H., Nawa, M., 2008. Biaxial flexure strength and low temperature degradation of Ce-TZP/$Al_2O_3$ nanocomposite and Y-TZP as dental restoratives. J. Biomed. Mater. Res. B Appl. Biomater. 87, 492−498.

Benzaid, R., Chevalier, J., Saâdaoui, M., Fantozzi, G., Nawa, M., Diaz, L.A., et al., 2008. Fracture toughness, strength and slow crack growth in a ceria stabilized zirconia−alumina nanocomposite for medical applications. Biomaterials. 29, 3636−3641.

Burke, F.J., Fleming, G.J., Nathanson, D., Marquis, P.M., 2002. Are adhesive technologies needed to support ceramics? An assessment of the current evidence. J. Adhes. Dent. 4, 7−22.

Buser, D., 2009. 20 Years of Guided Bone Regeneration in Implant Dentistry. second ed. Quintessence Pub. Co., Chicago, IL.

Cattani-Lorente, M., Scherrer, S.S., Ammann, P., Jobin, M., Wiskott, H.W. A., 2011. Low temperature degradation of a Y-TZP dental ceramic. Acta. Biomater. 7, 858−865.

Cesar, P.M., Della Bona, A., Scherrer, S.S., Tholey, M., Van Noort, R., Vichi, A., et al., 2017. ADM guidance-ceramics: fracture toughness testing and method selection. Dent. Mater. 33, 575−584.

Chan, Y.L., Ngan, A.H.W., King, N.M., 2011. Nano-scale structure and mechanical properties of the human dentine−enamel junction. J. Mech. Behav. Biomed. Mater. 4, 785−795.

Chevalier, J., 2006. What future for zirconia as a biomaterial? Biomaterials. 27, 535−543.

Chevalier, J., Gremmilard, L., Virkar, A.V., Clarke, D.R., 2009. The tetragonal-monoclinic transformation in zirconia: lessons learned and future trends. J. Am. Ceram. Soc. 92, 1901−1920.

CIE (Commision Internationale de l'Eclairage), 2004. Colorimetry technical report. CIE 15, p. 18.

Coldea, A., Swain, M.V., Thiel, N., 2013. Mechanical properties of polymer-infiltrated-ceramic-network materials. Dent. Mater. 29, 419−426.

Cutler, R.A., Lindemann, J.M., Ulvensøen, J.H., Lange, H.I., 1994. Damage-resistant SrO-doped Ce-TZP/$Al_2O_3$ composites. Mater. Des. 15, 123−133.

Dahlin, C., 1994. Scientific background of guided bone regeneration. In: Buser, D., Dahlin, C., Schenk, R. (Eds.), Guided Bone Regeneration in Implant Dentistry. Quintessence Pub. Co., Chicago, IL.

Dahlin, C., Linde, A., Gottlow, J., et al., 1988. Healing of bone defects by guided tissue regeneration. Plast. Reconstruct. Surg. 81, 672−676.

De Souza Costa, C.A., Hebling, J., Scheffel, D.L., Soares, D.G., Basso, F.G., Ribeiro, A.P., 2014. Methods to evaluate and strategies to improve the biocompatibility of dental materials and operative techniques. Dent. Mater. 30, 769−784.

Deville, S., El Attaoui, H., Chevalier, J., 2005. Atomic force microscopy of transformation toughening in ceria-stabilized zirconia. J. Eur. Ceram. Soc. 25, 3089−3096.

Dong, X.D., Darvell, B.W., 2003. Stress distribution and failure mode of dental ceramic structures under Hertzian indentation. Dent. Mater. 19, 542−551.

El Attaoui, H., Saâdaoui, M., Chevalier, J., Fantozzi, G., 2007. Static and cyclic propagation in Ce-TZP ceramics with different amounts of transformation toughening. J. Eur. Ceram. Soc. 27, 483−486.

El-Ghani, O.S.A., Sherief, A.H., 2016. Zirconia based ceramics, some clinical and biological aspects: Review. Future Dent. J. 2, 55−64.

Erb, R.M., Libanori, R., Rothfuchs, N., Studart, A.R., 2012. Composites reinforced in three dimensions by using low magnetic fields. Science. 335, 199–204.

Fabris, D., Souz, J.C.M., Silva, F.S., Fredel, M., Mesquita-Guimarães, J., Zhang, Y., et al., 2017. Thermal residual stresses in bilayered, trilayered and graded dental ceramics. Ceram. Int. 43, 3670–3678.

Fischer, J., Stawarczyk, B., 2007. Compatibility of machined Ce-TZP/$Al_2O_3$ nanocomposite and a veneering ceramic. Dent. Mater. 23, 1500–1505.

Geng, J., Tan, K.B.C., Liu, G., 2001. Application of finite element analysis in implant dentistry: a review of the literature. J. Prosthet. Dent. 85, 585–598.

Hämmerle, C.H.F., Jung, R.E., 2003. Bone augmentation by means of barrier membranes. Periodontology 2000. 33 (1), 36–53.

Hannink, R.H.J., Kelly, P.M., Muddle, B.C., 2000. Transformation toughening in zirconia-containing ceramics. J. Am. Ceram. Soc. 83, 461–487.

He, L.-H., Swain, M., 2011. A novel polymer infiltrated ceramic dental material. Dent. Mater. 27, 527–534.

Hench, L.L., 1998. Biomaterials: a forecast of the future. Biomaterials. 19, 1419–1423.

Ho, G.W., Matinlinna, J.P., 2011. Insights on ceramics as dental materials. Part I: Ceramic material types in dentistry. Silicon. 3, 109–115.

Huang, M., Rahbar, N., Wang, R., Thompson, V., Rekow, D., Soboyejo, W.O., 2007. Bioinspired design of dental multilayers. Mater. Sci. Eng. A. 464, 315–320.

Imbeni, V., Kruzic, J.J., Marshall, G.W., Marshall, S.J., Ritchie, R.O., 2005. The dentin–enamel junction and the fracture of human teeth. Nat. Mater. 4, 229–232.

Jacobi, R., Shillingburg, H.T., Duncanson, M.G., 1991. A comparison of the abrasiveness of six ceramic surfaces and gold. J. Prosthet. Dent. 66, 303–309.

Javed, A., Chen, H., Ghori, F.Y., 2010. Genetic and transcriptional control of bone formation. Oral. Maxillofac. Surg. Clin. North. Am. 22, 283–293.

Ji, B., Gao, H., 2004. Mechanical properties of nanostructure of biological materials. J. Mech. Phys. Solids. 52, 1963–1990.

Kelly, J.R., Denry, I., 2008. Stabilized zirconia as structural ceramic: an overview. Dent. Mater. 24, 289–298.

Kern, F., 2014. A comparison of microstructure and mechanical properties of 12Ce-TZP reinforced with alumina and in situ formed strontium- or lanthanum hexaaluminate precipitates. J. Eur. Ceram. Soc. 34, 413–423.

Kim, H.-K., Kim, S.-H., Lee, J.-B., Ha, S.-R., 2016. Effects of surface treatments on the translucency, opalescence, and surface texture of dental monolithic zirconia ceramics. J. Prosthet. Dent. 115, 773–779.

Lambrigger, M., 1997. Evaluation of Weibull master curves of zirconia ceramics and zirconia/alumina composites. J. Mater. Sci. Lett. 16, 924–926.

Lawn, B.R., Deng, Y., Lloyd, I.K., Janal, M.N., Rekow, E.D., Thompson, V.P., 2002. Material design of ceramic-based layer structure for crown. J. Dent. Res. 81, 433–438.

Lawson, S., 1995. Environmental degradation of zirconia ceramics. J. Eur. Ceram. Soc. 15, 485–502.

Le Ferrand, H., Bouville, F., Niebel, T.P., Studard, A.R., 2015. Magnetically assisted slip casting of bioinspired heterogeneous composites. Nat. Mater. 14, 1172–1181.

Li, J., Zhang, X.-H., Cui, B.-C., Lin, Y.-H., Deng, X.-L., Li, M., et al., 2017. Mechanical performance of polymer-infiltrated zirconia ceramics. J. Dent. 58, 60–66.

Liu, J., Kerns, D.D., 2014. Mechanisms of guided bone regeneration: a review. Open Dent. J. 16 (8), 56–65.

Lughi, V., Sergo, V., 2010. Low temperature degradation—aging—of zirconia: a critical review of the relevant aspects in dentistry. Dent. Mater. 26 (8), 807–820.

Madfa, A.A., Yue, X.-G., 2016. Dental prostheses mimic the natural enamel behavior under functional loading: a review article. Jpn. Dent. Sci. Rev. 52, 2–13.

Mai, R., Kunert-Keil, C., Grafe, A., Gedrange, T., Lauer, G., Dominiak, M., et al., 2012. Histological behaviour of zirconia implants: an experiment in rats. Ann. Anat. 194, 561–566.

Malkondu, O., Tinastepe, N., Akan, E., Kazazoglu, E., 2016. An overview of monolithic zirconia in dentistry. Biotechnol. Biotechnol. Equip. 30, 644–652.

Malmström, J., Anderud, J., Abrahamsson, P., Wälivaara, D.Å., Isaksson, S.G., Adolfsson, E., 2016. Guided bone regeneration using individualized ceramic sheets. Int. J. Oral. Maxillofac. Surg. 45, 1246–1252.

Marshall, S.J., Balooch, M., Habelitz, S., Balooch, G., Gallagher, R., Marshall, G.W., 2003. The dentin–enamel junction—a natural, multilevel interface. J. Eur. Ceram. Soc. 23, 2897–2904.

Maschio, S., Pezzotti, G., Sbaizero, O., 1998. Effect of $LaNbO_4$ addition on the mechanical properties of ceria-tetragonal zirconia polycrystal matrices. J. Eur. Ceram. Soc. 18, 1779–1785.

Mitov, G., Gessner, J., Lohbauer, U., Woll, K., Muecklich, F., Pospiech, P., 2011. Subcritical crack growth behavior and life data analysis of two types of dental Y-TZP ceramics. Dent. Mater. 27, 684–691.

Miura, M., Hongoh, H., Yogo, T., Hirano, S., Fujll, T., 1994. Formation of plate-like lanthanum-β-aluminate crystal in Ce-TZP matrix. J. Mater. Sci. 29, 262–268.

Moradian-Oldak, J., Bo Wen, H., Schneider, G.B., Stanford, C.M., 2006. Tissue engineering strategies for the future generation of dental implants. Periodontology. 41, 157–176.

Nakonieczny, D.S., Ziebowicz, A., Paszenda, Z.K., Krawczyk, C., 2017. Trends and perspectives in modification of zirconium oxide for a dental prosthetic applications—a review. Biocybernet. Biomed. Eng. 37, 229–245.

Nawa, M., Nakamoto, S., Sekino, T., Niihara, K., 1998. Tough and strong Ce-TZP/alumina nanocomposites doped with titania. Ceram. Int. 10, 381–392.

O'Brien, W.J., 1997. Dental Materials and Their Selection. 2nd ed. Quintessence Publishing Co, Chicago, IL.

Ono, M., Oshimal, M., Ogawa, M., Sonoyama, W., Satoshi Hara, E., Oida, Y., et al., 2017. Practical whole-tooth restoration utilizing autologous bioengineered tooth germ transplantation in a postnatal canine model. Sci. Rep. 7, 44522. Available from: http://dx.doi.org/10.1038/srep44522.

Ori, S., Kojima, T., Hara, T., Uekawa, N., Kakegawa, K., 2012. Fabrication of Ce-TZP/β hexaaluminate composites using amorphous precursor of the second phase. J. Ceram. Soc. Jpn. 120, 111–115.

Palmero, P., Naglieri, V., Chevalier, J., Fantozzi, G., Montanaro, L., 2009. Alumina-based nanocomposites obtained by doping with inorganic salt solutions: application to immiscible and reactive systems. J. Eur. Ceram. Soc. 29, 59–66.

Palmero, P., Fornabaio, M., Montanaro, L., Reveron, H., Esnouf, C., Chevalier, J., 2015. Towards long lasting zirconia-based composites for dental implants. Part I: Innovative synthesis, microstructural characterization and in vitro stability. Biomaterials. 50, 38–46.

Payer, M., Lorenzoni, M., Jakse, N., Kirmeier, R., Dohr, G., Stopper, M., et al., 2010. Cell growth on different zirconia and titanium surface textures: a morphologic in vitro study. Implants. 26, 20–33.

Petrini, M., Ferrante, M., Su, B., 2013. Fabrication and characterization of biomimetic ceramic/polymer composite materials for dental restoration. Dent. Mater. 29, 375–381.

Rahbar, N., Soboyejo, W.O., 2011. Design of functionally graded dental multilayers. Fatigue Fract. Eng. Mater. Struct. 34, 887–897.

Rekow, E.D., Harsono, M., Janal, M., Thompson, V.P., Zhang, G., 2006. Factorial analysis of variables influencing stress in all-ceramic crowns. Dent. Mater. 22, 125–132.

Reveron, H., Fornabaio, M., Palmero, P., Fürderer, T., Adolfsson, E., Lughi, V., et al., 2017. Towards long lasting zirconia-based composites for dental implants: transformation induced plasticity and its consequence on ceramic reliability. Acta. Biomater. 48, 423–432.

Ross, I.M., Rainforth, W.M., McComb, D.W., Scott, A.J., Brydson, R., 2001. The role of trace additions of alumina to yttria-tetragonal zirconia polycrystals (Y-TZP). Scripta Mater. 45, 653–660.

Roy, S., Basu, B., 2008. Mechanical and tribological characterization of human tooth. Mater. Characterization. 59, 747–756.

Sanon, C., Chevalier, J., Douillard, T., Cattani-Lorente, M., Scherrer, S.S., Gremillard, L., 2015. A new testing protocol for zirconia implants. Dent. Mater. 31, 15–25.

Sato, T., Endo, T., Shimada, M., 1989. Post-sintering hot isostatic pressing of ceria-doped tetragonal zirconia/alumina composites in an argon–oxygen gas atmosphere. J. Am. Ceram. Soc. 72, 761–764.

Scarano, A., Piattelli, M., Caputi, S., Favero, G.A., Piattelli, A., 2004. Bacterial adhesion on commercially titanium and zirconium oxide disks: an in vivo human study. J. Periodontol. 75, 292–296.

Schehl, M., Díaz, M.A., Torrecillas, R., 2002. Alumina nanocomposites from powder–alkoxide mixtures. Acta. Mater. 50, 1125–1139.

Schenk, R.K., Buser, D., Hardwick, W.R., et al., 1994. Healing pattern of bone regeneration in membrane-protected defects: a histologic study in the canine mandible. Int. J. Oral Maxillofacial Impl. 9, 13–29.

Schienle, S., Al-Ahmad, A., Kohal, R.J., Bernsmann, F., Adolfsson, E., Montanaro, L., et al., 2016. Microbial adhesion on novel yttria-stabilized tetragonal zirconia (Y-TZP) implant surfaces with nitrogen-doped hydrogenated amorphous carbon (a-C:H:N) coatings. Clin. Oral. Investig. 20, 1719–1732.

Schmid, H.K., Pennefather, R., Meriani, S., Schmid, C., 1992. Redistribution of Ce and La during processing of Ce(La)–TZP/$Al_2O_3$ composites. J. Eur. Ceram. Soc. 72, 761–764.

Swain, M.V., 1985. Inelastic deformation of Mg-PSZ and its significance for strength–toughness relationship of zirconia toughened ceramics. Acta Metall. 33 (11), 2083–2091.

Swain, M.V., Rose, L.R.F., 1986. Strength limitations of transformation-toughened zirconia alloys. J. Am. Ceram. Soc. 69, 511–518.

Thesleff, I., Tummers, M., 2009. Tooth Organogenesis and Regeneration. StemBook. Harvard Stem Cell Institute, Cambridge, UK.

Touaiher, I., Saâdaoui, M., Chevalier, J., Reveron, H., 2016. Effect of loading configuration on strength values in a highly transformable zirconia-based composite. Dent. Mater. 32, e211–e219.

Trunec, M., 2008. Effect of grain size on mechanical properties of 3Y-TZP ceramics. Ceram. Silikaty. 52, 165–171.

Tsai, J.F., Yu, C.S., Shetty, D.K., 1990. Fatigue crack propagation in ceria-partially stabilized zirconia (Ce-TZP)-alumina composites. J. Am. Ceram. Soc. 73, 2292–3001.

Tsukuma, K., Shimada, M., 1985. Strength, fracture toughness and Vickers hardness of $CeO_2$-stabilized tetragonal $ZrO_2$ polycrystals (Ce-TZP). J. Mater. Sci. 20, 1178–1184.

Vichi, A., Louca, C., Corciolani, G., Ferrari, M., 2011. Color related to ceramic and zirconia restorations: a review. Dent. Mater. 27, 97–108.
von Arx, T., Kurt, B., 1998. Implant placement and simultaneous peri-implant bone grafting using a micro titanium mesh for graft stabilization. Int. J. Periodont. Restor. Dent. 18 (2), 117–127.
Wu, C.-C., Wei, C.-K., Ho, C.-C., Ding, S.-J., 2015. Enhanced hydrophilicity and biocompatibility of dental zirconia ceramics by oxygen plasma treatment. Materials. 8, 684–699.
Xavier, J.R., Desai, P., Gopal Varanasi, V., Al-Hashimi, I., Gaharwar A.K., 2015. Advanced nanomaterials: promises for improved dental tissue regeneration. In: Nanotechnology in Endodontics: Current and Potential Clinical Applications, pp. 5–22 (Chapter 2).
Xie, Z.H., Swain, M.V., Swadener, G., Munroe, P., Hoffman, M., 2009. Effect of microstructure upon elastic behaviour of human tooth enamel. J. Biomech. 42, 1075–1080.
Yen, A.-H., Yelick, P.C., 2011. Dental tissue regeneration—a mini-review. Gerontology. 57, 85–94.
Yu, C.S., Shetty, D.K., Shaw, M.C., Marshall, D.B., 1992. Transformation zone shape effects on crack shielding in ceria-partially-stabilized zirconia (Ce-TZP)-alumina composites. J. Am. Ceram. Soc. 75, 2991–2994.
Zhang, F., Vanmeensel, K., Inokoshi, M., Batuk, M., Hadremann, J., Van Meerbeek, B., et al., 2014a. 3Y-TZP ceramics with improve hydrothermal degradation resistance and fracture toughness. J. Eur. Ceram. Soc. 34, 2453–2463.
Zhang, Y.-R., Du, W., Zhou, X.-D., Yu, H.-Y., 2014b. Review of research on the mechanical properties of the human tooth. Int. J. Oral Sci. 6, 61–69.
Zhang, Y., Chai, H., Lawn, B.R., 2010. Graded structures for all-ceramic restorations. J. Dent. Res. 89, 417–421.
Zhang, Y., Sun, M.-J., Zhang, D., 2012. Designing functionally graded materials with superior load-bearing properties. Acta. Biomater. 8, 1101–1108.

## Further reading

Anderud, J., Abrahamsson, P., Jimbo, R., Isaksson, S., Adolfsson, E., Malmström, J., et al., 2015. Guided bone augmentation using ceramic space-maintaining devices: the impact of chemistry. Clin. Cosmet. Invest. Dent. 7, 45–53.
Bartolomé, J.F., Montero, I., Díaz, M., López-Esteban, S., Moya, J.S., Deville, S., et al., 2004. Accelerated aging in 3-mol%-yttria-stabilized tetragonal zirconia ceramics sintered in reducing conditions. J. Am. Ceram. Soc. 87, 2282–2285.
Chevalier, J., Gremillard, L., 2009. Ceramics for medical applications: a picture for the next 20 years. J. Eur. Ceram. Soc. 29, 1245–1255.
Fornabaio, M., Palmero, P., Traverso, R., Esnouf, C., Reveron, H., Chevalier, J., et al., 2015. Zirconia-based composites for biomedical applications: Role of second phases on composition, microstructure and zirconia transformability. J. Eur. Ceram. Soc. 34, 4039–4049.
Nakao, K., Morita, R., Saji, Y., Ishida, K., Tomita, Y., Ogawa, M., et al., 2007. The development of a bioengineered organ germ method. Nat. Method.. 4, 227–230.
Sato, T., Shimada, M., 1985. Transformation of yttria-doped tetragonal $ZrO_2$ polycrystals by annealing in water. J. Am. Ceram. Soc. 68, 356–356.
Yamaguchi, T., Sakamoto, W., Yogo, T., Fujii, T., Hirano, S., 1999. In situ formation of Ce-TZP/Ba-hexaaluminate composites. J. Ceram. Soc. Jpn. 107, 814–916.

# Patient-specific design of tissue engineering scaffolds, based on mathematical modeling

**12**

*Stefan Scheiner and Christian Hellmich*
Vienna University of Technology, Vienna, Austria

**Chapter Outline**

**12.1 Introduction 391**
12.1.1 Patient-specific design—definition and implied requirements 391
12.1.2 Measurements and observations are not enough 392
12.1.3 Integration of experimental, clinical, and computational approaches 393
**12.2 Overview of mathematical models in bone tissue engineering 393**
**12.3 Utilization of mathematical models for patient-specific scaffold design 396**
12.3.1 X-ray physics-based analysis of CT data 396
12.3.2 Prediction of bone regeneration based on mathematical modeling 400
**12.4 Conclusions and outlook 402**
**References 402**

## 12.1 Introduction

### *12.1.1 Patient-specific design—definition and implied requirements*

Tissue engineering is the field dealing with provision of a substrate which is supposed to facilitate the regeneration of biological tissues. If the regenerating tissue is bone tissue, the strategy usually consists in implanting some sort of scaffold structure into the patient, in order to either completely take over the function of (a specific part of) the affected bone organ, or in order to provide the substrate for the growth of new bone tissue. In the latter case, the production and functionalization of synthetic scaffolds has been one of the major goals in bone tissue engineering and hence advanced substantially over the past decades. Several textbooks and review papers are testament to related developments (Hutmacher, 2000; Hollister, 2005; Rezwan et al., 2006; Lanza et al., 2007; Williams, 2008; O'Brien, 2011; Geris, 2013).

In order to allow for adequate integration into the targeted physiological environment bone tissue engineering scaffolds must fulfill several requirements, the most important of which are introduced next:

- Biocompatibility: scaffold materials must not cause any harm to the targeted physiological environment.

**Advances in Ceramic Biomaterials.**
**DOI: http://dx.doi.org/10.1016/B978-0-08-100881-2.00013-0**

- Osteoconductivity: scaffolds must stimulate the regeneration of bone tissue. For that purpose, they must be suitable for hosting bone growth-promoting cells and growth factors, and they must be sufficiently porous, in order to provide enough physical space for substantial ingrowth of bone tissue.
- Biodegradability: once sufficient amounts of new bone tissue have been formed, degradation and eventual disappearance of the scaffold structure is desirable, as it has then fulfilled the purpose of providing temporary support and is no longer needed.
- Mechanical competence: since bone is often concerned with load-bearing tasks, bone tissue engineering scaffolds must exhibit suitable mechanical properties.

While each of these requirements (as well as additional requirements which have been disregarded in the above list) are equally important for the success of a specific bone tissue engineering material and structure, in this chapter the focus will be on the mechanical competence. Clearly, the scaffold material has to sustain the mechanical loading to which it is subjected, thus it must not be too soft. However, the biochemical processes related to bone regeneration are partly governed by the deformation characteristics of the scaffold (Simmons et al., 2001; Robling et al., 2006; Jacobs et al., 2010). This implies that for optimal integration of the scaffold into its bony vicinity, it must not be too stiff either, otherwise the biochemical processes involved cannot be initiated or maintained through the prevalent mechanobiological couplings. In the long run, the consequence would be potentially adverse, and phenomena such as stress shielding could occur, which may lead to bone degeneration in the proximity of the implant (Engh et al., 1987). For that reason, designing scaffold materials and structures with the just right stiffness (i.e., not too soft and not too stiff), which is the mechanical property determining the elastic deformation behavior, is a delicate task. In this respect, a nowadays much-stressed term comes into play, namely patient-specific design, meaning that a scaffold is implanted which fits as well as possible to the biological and mechanical environment which can be found in a specific patient.

Hence, patient-specificity implies that the all kinds of needs and circumstances of a specific patient are considered in the design of a clinical measure. In the particular context of the mechanical competence of bone tissue engineering scaffolds, patient-specific design is a challenging task in terms of both structural and material mechanics.

### 12.1.2 Measurements and observations are not enough

New scaffold materials and structures are usually tested experimentally, in order to investigate their suitability as bone replacement material. While creating in vitro an environment which adequately resembles the in vivo conditions is not necessarily straightforward, three of the four aforementioned required features, namely biocompatibility, osteoconductivity, and biodegradability, can be studied reasonably well. However, testing the mechanical properties of bone tissue engineering materials and structures is very challenging.

Firstly, realization of in vivo conditions for mechanical testing is very difficult, if not impossible. On the one hand, the specimen would have to be somehow integrated into a kind of artificial, yet physiologically representative bony environment, and, on the other hand, loading conditions would also have to be chosen according to the ones which are expected to occur in vivo. Secondly, once the scaffold has been implanted, bone regeneration starts and new bone tissue is added, while the scaffold may possibly dissolve concurrently. This dynamic behavior renders the definition of mechanical properties (which evolve accordingly) also a difficult task.

These intricacies are even worsened when aiming at patient-specific design of bone tissue engineering scaffolds, as patient-specific data should also be somehow integrated in the design and assessment strategy.

### 12.1.3 Integration of experimental, clinical, and computational approaches

Given the difficulties in studying the performance of materials and structures in bone tissue engineering applications based on a purely experimental approach, as briefly discussed in Section 12.1.2, following a "holistic" approach has been suggested as a remedy (Geris, 2013). In particular, utilizing the predictive capabilities of computational modeling, while also integrating data provided by experimental research and clinical studies, promises to provide a predictive assessment of materials and structures in terms of their performance when applied as bone replacement material.

Pointing out strategies how this task has been and is currently being attempted to be mastered is the focus of the remainder of this chapter.

## 12.2 Overview of mathematical models in bone tissue engineering

The starting point for most computational models in the field of bone tissue engineering is the acquisition of the exact shape and microstructure of the scaffold under investigation. To that end, the gold standard is scanning the scaffold by means of laboratory-based or clinical tomography. The resulting computed tomography (CT) or micro-computed tomography (micro-CT) data provides information concerning the three-dimensional distribution of attenuation coefficients, in terms of attenuation coefficient-proportional gray values. By employing suitable thresholding, the sought-after geometry of the scaffold structure can be deduced (Rüegsegger et al., 1996).

Mathematical models describing the mechanical behavior of a material across a spatial domain usually comprise sets of partial differential equations. Solution of such equations requires in most cases utilization of numerical methods – a brief (but certainly not complete) overview is presented next. If the exact geometry and microstructure of scaffold structures must be considered, large-scale simulations are typically employed. The majority of such simulations follow from solution of the underlying equations based on the Finite Element (FE) method. The complexity of the numerical models and the computational costs arising for the simulations depends on the morphology of the studied scaffold. If the latter exhibits some sort of periodicity, so-called unit cell models can be easily created (see e.g., Adachi et al., 2006; Lacroix et al., 2009; Melchels et al., 2010; Olivares et al., 2009; Sturm et al., 2010; Truscello et al., 2012; Dias et al., 2012; Hutmacher and Singh, 2008 and Fig. 12.1A for an exemplary model). For irregular microstructures, the aforementioned micro-CT data is often the basis for generation of a corresponding FE model (see e.g., Lacroix et al., 2006, 2009; Jaecques et al., 2004; Milan et al., 2009; Porter et al., 2005; Sandino et al., 2008; Sandino and Lacroix, 2011; Voronov et al., 2010; Williams et al., 2005; see also Fig. 12.1C). However, such micro-FE simulations are extremely costly in terms of computation time, because of which their application in a clinical environment is limited. As a remedy, so-called numerical multiscale models have been suggested, where the FE models are comparably coarse, and information from lower observation scales is integrated in a homogenized fashion. This strategy is particularly useful if certain domains within the numerical model are subjected to a dynamic evolution, as it is the case if bone tissue is formed in the pore spaces of a scaffold structure (Sanz-Herrera et al., 2008, 2009a,b); see e.g., Fig. 12.1B.

From a conceptual point of view, large-scale numerical modeling can be applied to study a wide range of different aspects relevant in bone tissue engineering, including the assessment of local effects occurring in response to physiological mechanical loading, the simulation of the pore fluid movement (see e.g., Fig. 12.1D), or the bone regeneration performance over time. The significance of these simulations is directly related to the reliability of the input parameters fed into the numerical model. This concerns in particular the mechanical properties. The simplest approach in this respect is to assume homogeneous material properties, thereby neglecting any material heterogeneities. Clearly, this approach is based on a quite strong simplification, and potentially entails inadequate simulation results, as demonstrated in Dejaco et al. (2012) and Luczynski et al. (2012). Furthermore, simplified empirical laws can be used for relating the distribution of gray values resulting from CT scanning to a corresponding distribution of material properties (Currey, 1986, 1988; Jacobs, 1994). Unarguably, this approach may work well for a certain material, whereas it may be completely wrong for another material.

In order to thoroughly process, based on a physically well substantiated theoretical framework, microstructural information in terms of corresponding macroscopic physical properties (such as mechanical properties), rigorous multiscale modeling approaches have been developed during the 20th century, and in the past 10 years adapted for application to bone tissue engineering scaffold materials and structures. The conceptual framework of these recent developments is continuum micromechanics, where a material is considered to be macrohomogeneous, but microheterogeneous. Granted that the so-called separation-of-scales-requirement is fulfilled (Hill, 1963, 1965a,b; Drugan and Willis, 1996; Zaoui, 2002; Dormieux et al., 2006), and upon introduction of material phases instead of taking into account all

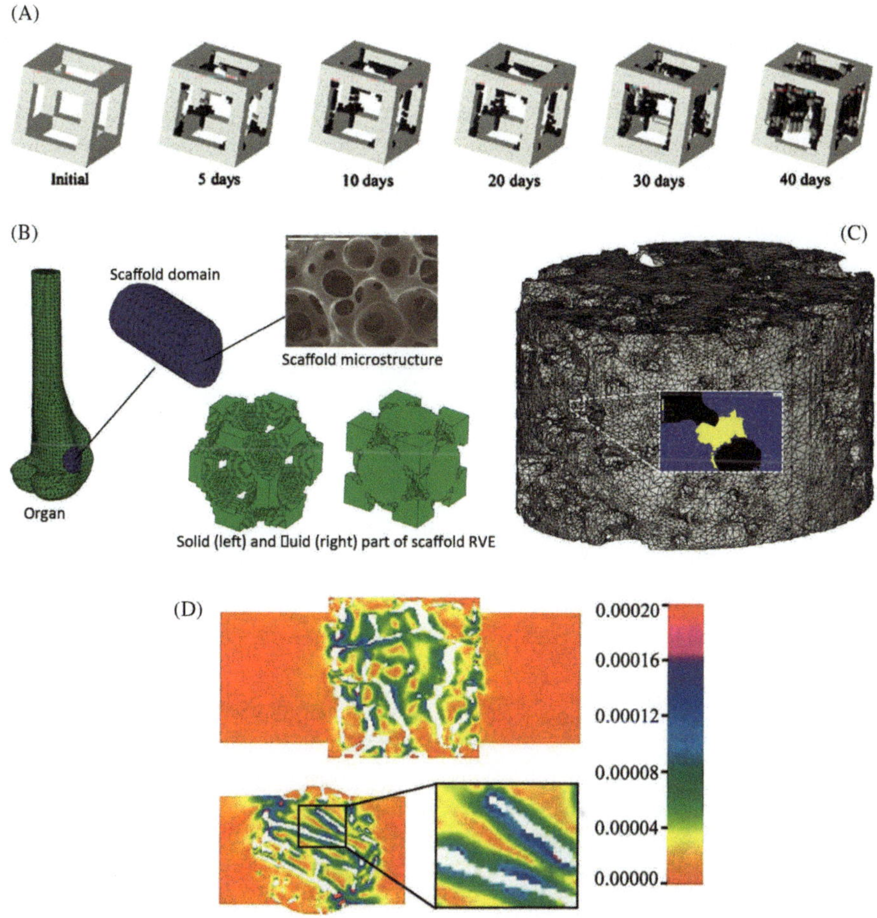


**Figure 12.1** Results of numerical simulations set up for assessing the performances of bone replacement materials. (A) Development of bone regeneration over 40 days, based on a unit cell model, reprinted from Adachi, T., Osako, Y., Tanaka, M., Hojo, M., and Hollister, S.J., 2006 Framework for optimal design of porous scaffold microstructure by computational simulation of bone regeneration. Biomaterials. 27(21):3964–3972, with permission from Elsevier. (B) Numerical multiscale model including a scaffold implanted in a rabbit distal femur, reprinted from Sanz-Herrera, J.A., García-Aznar, J.M., and Doblaré, M., 2008. Micro-macro numerical modelling of bone regeneration in tissue engineering. Comp. Methods Appl. Mech. Eng. 197(33–40):3092–3107, with permission from Elsevier. (C) Three-dimensional microfinite element model of a calcium phosphate-based tissue engineering material, with the magnified region showing the distribution of tensile and compressive stresses due to uniaxial compression, reprinted from Lacroix, D., Chateau, A., Ginebra, M.-P., and Planell, J.A., 2006. Micro-finite element models of bone tissue-engineering scaffolds. Biomaterials. 27(30):5326–5334, with permission from Elsevier. (D) The shear stresses caused by fluid flow in the pores of a scaffold sample, during a perfusion test, reprinted from Porter, B., Zauel, R., Stockman, H., Guldberg, R., and Fyhrie, D., 2005. 3-D computational modeling of media flow through scaffolds in a perfusion bioreactor. J. Biomech. 38(3):543–549, with permission from Elsevier.

microstructural features in minute detail, the mechanical properties of the elementary constituents of a (hierarchically organized) biomaterial can be upscaled through mathematical relations resulting from combination of Eshelby's matrix-inclusion problem (Eshelby, 1957), as well as stress and strain volume averaging. For example, this concept was successfully applied for estimating the strength of a hydroxyapatite-based biomaterial, by introducing a Coulomb-or Mohr-Coulomb-type failure criterion describing the brittle failure of the interfaces between the hydroxyapatite crystals and the surrounding material (Fritsch et al., 2007, 2009). Very recently, continuum micromechanics was also applied to a hydroxyapatite-based granular bone replacement material, for estimation of both macroscopic stiffness and strength (Scheiner et al., 2016a,b,c). Furthermore, it could be demonstrated how biomaterials can be modeled in a poromicromechanical framework, thereby allowing to study the influence of the respectively chosen poromechanical configuration on the macroscopic strength estimates (Fritsch et al., 2013).

What remains to be addressed is the link to patient-specific data, beyond using CT data as input for "only" creating FE models. The next section is devoted to shedding light on thoroughly exploiting the data available for specific patients in terms of computational assessment of bone tissue engineering scaffold materials and structures.

## 12.3 Utilization of mathematical models for patient-specific scaffold design

The focus of this section is the state-of-the art in patient-specific modeling of bone tissue engineering scaffolds. In particular, two computational strategies are discussed. On the one hand, "exhaustive" exploitation of CT data is reviewed, beyond plain thresholding for the sake of generating an FE model. On the other hand, an overview is presented regarding how the process of bone regeneration can be predicted.

### 12.3.1 X-ray physics-based analysis of CT data

During a CT scan, X-rays are sent through the studied object, and the reduction of the X-ray intensity upon passing through the object, referred to as attenuation, is measured. By varying the direction of the X-ray as well as the position of the source of the X-ray, a comprehensive set of attenuation data is gathered. The Radon transform (Radon, 1917) is then utilized, in order to process the attenuation behavior in terms of the three-dimensional distribution of attenuation coefficients. Usually, the attenuation coefficients are expressed in terms of gray values which are proportional to the attenuation coefficients. Depending on the setting of the tomograph, corresponding resolutions can be achieved, typically in the range of a few micrometers. Thus, the studied object is then reflected in the CT data as an assembly of voxels (which are cubic domains whose side length is defined via the resolution); and each voxel is characterized by a constant gray value, representing the average attenuation coefficient within this voxel.

For quantitative interpretation of the three-dimensional distribution of gray values, going beyond the establishment of the microgeometry of the studied object as well as gray value-based segmentation, some fundamental relations are recalled. Firstly, the relation between the gray value assigned to a specific voxel $i$, $GV^i$, and the corresponding attenuation coefficient, $\mu^i$, can be cast into mathematical form by means of a linear relation (Dejaco et al., 2012; Czenek et al., 2014; Hasslinger et al., 2016; Blanchard et al., 2013; Fritsch et al., 2011),

$$\mu^i(\epsilon) = a(\epsilon) \times GV^i + b(\epsilon), \tag{12.1}$$

where the voxel-specific attenuation coefficient $\mu^i$, as well as constants $a$ and $b$ are functions of the photon energy $\epsilon$ applied in the CT scanning. Secondly, considering the case that the material represented by one voxel is actually a composite material, volume averaging becomes relevant as well, thus

$$\mu^i(\epsilon) = \sum_j \mu_j(\epsilon) f_j^i, \tag{12.2}$$

where index $j$ represents the constituents found in voxel $i$. Hence, $\mu_j(\epsilon)$ is the energy-dependent attenuation coefficient of constituent $j$, and volume fraction $f_j^i$ quantifies the amount of constituent $j$ occurring in voxel $i$. Notably, the constituent-specific and energy-dependent attenuation coefficient follows from a comprehensive database provided by the National Institute of Standards and Technology (NIST) of the United States (Hubbel and Seitzer, 2004) if the chemical composition of the respective constituent is known. As demonstrated in a number of works (see e.g., Dejaco et al., 2012; Czenek et al., 2014; Hasslinger et al., 2016; Blanchard et al., 2013; Fritsch et al., 2011), the two laws given by Eqs. (12.1) and (12.2) suffice to interpret CT data in terms of the corresponding distribution of constituent volume fractions. For that purpose, assuming that the studied sample is actually a composite material, the following sequence of analysis steps has been shown to allow for extracting reliable compositional information from the CT data:

- CT scanning of the sample of interest is performed and, besides the sample, a phantom of one of the constituents making up the sample (in pure form) is also placed in the scanned domain.
- The resulting field of gray values is plotted in form of a frequency plot.
- Peaks within the frequency plots are identified; for a porous composite material which is supposed to be suitable as bone replacement material, peaks should be discernible relating to the air pores, to the phantom, and to the scaffold material.
- Applying Eq. (12.1) to both the air pore peak and to the phantom peak gives access to two equations:

$$\mu^{air}(\epsilon) = a(\epsilon) \times GV^{air} + b(\epsilon) \tag{12.3}$$

and

$$\mu^{\text{phantom}}(\epsilon) = a(\epsilon) \times \text{GV}^{\text{phantom}} + b(\epsilon). \tag{12.4}$$

These equations can be easily solved for the coefficients $a(\epsilon)$ and $b(\epsilon)$:

$$a(\epsilon) = \frac{\mu^{\text{air}}(\epsilon) - \mu^{\text{phantom}}(\epsilon)}{\text{GV}^{\text{air}} - \text{GV}^{\text{phantom}}} \tag{12.5}$$

and

$$b(\epsilon) = \frac{\mu^{\text{air}}(\epsilon)\text{GV}^{\text{phantom}} - \mu^{\text{phantom}}(\epsilon)\text{GV}^{\text{air}}}{\text{GV}^{\text{phantom}} - \text{GV}^{\text{air}}}. \tag{12.6}$$

- Considering that the average volume fractions of the constituents of the scaffold are known from the production of the material, evaluation of both Eqs. (12.1) and (12.2) for the scaffold peak, and equating the resulting two equations, allows us to back-calculate the photon energy used for the CT scanning.
- The volume averaging relation given by Eq. (12.2) then gives access to the volume fractions of the scaffold material constituents (if this is a binary composite) in any voxel.

The resulting field of material compositions can, in further consequence, be fed into micromechanical homogenization schemes, in order to obtain also a field of mechanical properties, discussed in Section 12.2 (see e.g., Dejaco et al., 2012; Czenek et al., 2014; Hasslinger et al., 2016; Blanchard et al., 2013; Fritsch et al., 2011; Scheiner et al., 2009). With regard to the stiffness properties, the theory of continuum micromechanics provides homogenization schemes for the macroscopic stiffness $\mathbb{C}^{\text{hom}}$, in the following format (Zaoui, 2002):

$$\mathbb{C}^{\text{hom}} = \sum_r f_r \mathbb{C}_r : [\mathbb{I} + \mathbb{P}_r^0 : (\mathbb{C}_r - \mathbb{C}^0)]^{-1} : \left\{ \sum_s f_s [\mathbb{I} + \mathbb{P}_s^0 : (\mathbb{C}_s - \mathbb{C}^0)]^{-1} \right\}^{-1}, \tag{12.7}$$

where $\mathbb{C}_r$ is the stiffness tensors of the single constituent (usually known from-experiments), $f_r$ is the constituent volume fraction (e.g., known from the analysis of CT images described above), $\mathbb{I}$ is the fourth-order unit tensor, $\mathbb{C}^0$ is the stiffness tensor of the matrix in which the constituents are embedded as inclusions, and $\mathbb{P}_r^0$ is the fourth-order Hill or inhomogeneity tensor relating to constituent $r$ embedded in a matrix which exhibits a stiffness $\mathbb{C}^0$. Different morphological situations can be considered based on the choice of stiffness tensor $\mathbb{C}^0$: if one of the material phases (i.e., constituents) acts as matrix in which all other material phases are embedded as inclusions, $\mathbb{C}^0$ is set to the stiffness of this matrix phase; this results in a so-called Mori–Tanaka-type homogenization scheme (Mori and Tanaka, 1973). If, however, no distinctive matrix phase can be identified, and all constituents are in mutual contact with each other, $\mathbb{C}^0$ is substituted by $\mathbb{C}^{hom}$—hence, the matrix in which all constituents are embedded is considered to be the homogenized material itself. Such an approach leads to a so-called self-consistent homogenization scheme (Hershey, 1954; Kröner, 1978). It should also be mentioned that such micromechanical homogenization schemes are not limited to the stiffness, but can be also used to estimate the macroscopic strength, poroelastic properties, viscoelastic behavior, as well as transport properties.

For the sake of demonstration, Fig. 12.2A shows the gray value distribution in a cross-section of a granular, hydroxyapatite-based biomaterial obtained by means of micro-CT scanning. Analyzing the distribution of gray values as described above gives access to the corresponding distribution of volume fractions of the constituents, i.e., of hydroxyapatite and of air pores. Considering the micromorphology of the studied material suggests employing Mori–Tanaka-type (Mori and Tanaka, 1973) stiffness homogenization. Feeding the resulting distribution of elastic constants into a structural model allows for simulation of the mechanical behavior of one of these granules when subjected to physiologically relevant mechanical loading, such as uniaxial compression, see Fig. 12.2B and C. Comparison of these two images clearly underpins the importance of taking into account the heterogeneous distribution of mechanical properties, as was done in the simulation behind Fig. 12.2B, instead of simply assuming, for simplicity, average mechanical properties which are constant for all voxels; see Fig. 12.2C.

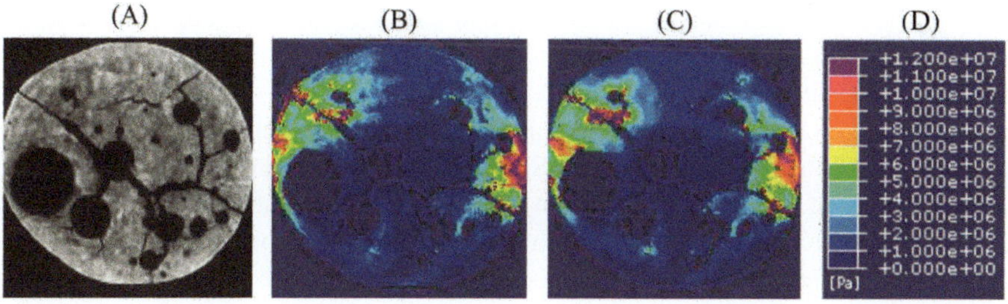


**Figure 12.2** (A) Gray value distribution in a cross-section of a granular, hydroxyapatite-based biomaterial, obtained by means of micro-CT scanning; distribution of the deviatoric stress norms resulting from finite element simulations considering uniaxial compression, with load initiation occurring on the lateral sides of the granule, for (B) heterogeneous and (C) homogeneous stiffness properties.
Source: Reprinted from Dejaco, A., Komlev, V.S., Jaroszewicz, J., Swieszkowski, W., and Hellmich, C., 2012. Micro CT-based multiscale elasticity of double-porous (pre-cracked) hydroxyapatite granules for regenerative medicine. J. Biomech. 45(6):1068–1075, with permission from Elsevier.

### 12.3.2 Prediction of bone regeneration based on mathematical modeling

Bone regeneration is a complicated biological process (Lieberman and Friedlaender, 2005; Petite et al., 2000). Essentially, the growth of new bone tissue in the pore spaces of bone tissue engineering scaffolds comprises numerous biochemically and mechanically stimulated mechanisms. First, they cause addition of bone tissue by mononuclear cells called osteoblasts, deriving from mesenchymal stem cells. In more detail, osteoblasts lay down osteoid to fill this cavity, a substance consisting mainly of collagen type I. Over time, osteoid gets mineralized, with the bone mineral mainly consisting of carbonated hydroxyapatite. Since the greater part of bone mineral is formed very fast (within a few days), osteoblasts are often, for simplicity, referred to as bone-forming cells, without explicitly mentioning the intermediate step of osteoid secretion. Hence, initiation of bone regeneration requires the attraction of such stem cells to the pore spaces of the implanted scaffold, and creation of a milieu which facilitates the required differentiation processes.

Once the scaffold is (at least partly) covered with bone tissue, remodeling events also take place, implying that the bone tissue is removed by multinuclear cells called osteoclasts, deriving from hematopoietic stem cells. More precisely, osteoclasts attach themselves to the bone surface, thereby creating an acidic environment in order to dissolve the bone matrix, thus leaving behind a resorption cavity. This cavity is subsequently filled with new bone tissue by osteoblasts. Moreover, osteocytes, a third cell type found in bone, have been identified as bone remodeling "conductors." In particular, osteocytes are former osteoblasts that have been "buried" in newly secreted osteoid. Osteocytes are the most abundant cell type in bone tissue, and they are considered to be capable of sensing changes in their environment, particularly concerning the mechanical loading. There is ample evidence that osteocytes transduce these changes into biochemical signals, which, in turn, lead to corresponding changes of cellular activities in the bone microenvironment.

As for the exact biochemical regulatory pathways, the discovery of the receptor activator of nuclear factor kappa $\beta$ (RANK) and its ligand (RANKL) allowed the understanding of the interplay between osteoblasts and osteoclasts. Namely, binding of RANKL, which is produced by both osteoblasts and osteocytes, to RANK, which is a transmembrane protein found on osteoclasts, is required for differentiation of osteoclasts. Furthermore, osteoprotegerin (OPG), a protein which is produced by osteoblasts, is a so-called decoy receptor, as it also binds to RANKL and thereby prevents osteoclastogenesis. Furthermore, parathyroid hormone (PTH) influences the RANK-RANKL-OPG pathway, through promoting the production of RANKL and inhibiting the production of OPG. Transforming growth factor beta (TGF-$\beta$), in turn, promotes the differentiation of osteoblast progenitor cells, inhibits the differentiation of osteoblast precursor cells, and promotes the apoptosis of osteoclasts. The list of factors contributing to the regulation of the bone cells could be easily extended to further proteins and hormones (such as nitric oxide, prostaglandins, vitamin D, corticosteroids, interleukins, calcitonin, the Wnt$\beta$-catenin pathway, just to mention a few) (see Robling et al., 2006; Jacobs et al., 2010; Bonewald, 2011 for respective review articles).

Mechanical excitation of bone cell activities is a heavily debated field, and several hypotheses have been brought forth over the years, including direct stretching of the cell-surrounding bone matrix, the hydrostatic pressure to which the cells are exposed, the fluid flow in the bone pore spaces, or microcracks emerging as result of local overloading (Robling et al., 2006; Jacobs et al., 2010). Also the exact consequences of changing mechanical loading, in terms of the mechanotransductive response, are not completely resolved. Experimentally confirmed hypotheses include the increase of osteoblast proliferation due to increased mechanical loading (with respect to "normal" loading conditions), and the increase of RANKL production due to decreased mechanical loading.

The above sketched regulatory mechanisms of bone formation and resorption have not yet been considered at all (to the best of the authors' knowledge) in the context of computational models of bone regeneration. The addition of bone tissue is usually considered based on simple laws, mostly involving scalar representatives of the location-dependent mechanical loading as functional argument, see e.g., Adachi et al. (2006), while biological details are completely neglected. The latter deficit could be eradicated by integrating into the structural simulations of bone tissue engineering scaffold systems biology-based bone models of the bone metabolism (see e.g., Lemaire et al., 2004; Pivonka et al., 2008, 2010; Scheiner et al., 2013; Graham et al., 2013). These models allow for consideration of cell populations, different developmental stages along the cell lineages, and regulation of cell differentiation, proliferation, and apoptosis processes by biochemical factors. In the work of Scheiner et al. (2013), bone systems biology models are furthermore coupled with a bone micromechanics model for estimating the local mechanical stimulus in the extravascular bone matrix, in order to include a physically meaningful argument for biomechanical regulation of the bone cell activities.

In the future, it seems desirable to include and study the effects of the suggested mechanical stimuli on the related, mechanically triggered bone cell activities. Continuum micromechanics is the conceptual tool which straight-forwardly allows related studies to be carried out: it could be shown that the hydrostatic pore pressures in the pore spaces of bone can be reliably predicted (Hellmich et al., 2009; Scheiner et al., 2016a,b,c); fluid flow in the canaliculi and lacunae, occurring in response to macroscopic mechanical loading, can be estimated by downscaling related pressure gradients to the relevant pore spaces, (see e.g., Abdalrahman et al., 2015); and microcracking can be introduced by taking into account suitable failure criteria defining the onset of cracking events in the bone matrix (Fritsch et al., 2009). Furthermore, an often disregarded aspect is related to the hierarchical organization of bone and scaffold materials implanted into a bony environment, spanning several orders of length scale magnitude (from cross-linked collagen molecules up to macroscopic bone tissue), and including different kinds of pore spaces (exhibiting respectively different characteristic dimensions). When aiming at the development of models related to bone regeneration characterized by maximum adequacy, the concentration change of the involved factors due to moving from one kind of pore space to another one must also be taken into account.

In this way, bone regeneration could be simulated specifically for a certain patient, based on considering the peculiarities of this patient through suitable parameter choices. While the endeavor of developing such models seems quite challenging, the potential benefits are certainly promising.

## 12.4 Conclusions and outlook

The mathematical modalities presented in Sections 12.3.1 and 12.3.2 show how the future of computer simulation-supported, patient-specific design of tissue engineering scaffolds could look. The initial situation of a scaffold can be digitalized based on physically substantiated analysis of CT data (yielding three-dimensional fields of composition data and mechanical properties), whereas the progress of bone regeneration can be predicted by means of systems biology-based modeling strategies.

While additional efforts are certainly necessary and will keep researchers busy for years to come, in order to actually introduce predictive computational simulations as tools regularly employed for the patient-specific design of tissue engineering scaffolds, the presented technologies are certainly promising and could be key in reaching this ambitious goal. Unarguably, *predictive* assessment strategies concerning the performance of bone tissue engineering materials and structures requires the development of capable mathematical models. However, it is of utmost importance to tackle the problem by means of an inter- and multidisciplinary approach, prioritizing that mathematical models are thoroughly informed by experimental and clinical data, and that practical requirements are taken into account, in order to maximize the significance of the model predictions.

## References

Abdalrahman, T., Scheiner, S., Hellmich, C., 2015. Is trabecular bone permeability governed by molecular ordering-induced fluid viscosity gain? Arguments from re-evaluation of experimental data in the framework of homogenization theory. J. Theor. Biol. 365, 433–444.

Adachi, T., Osako, Y., Tanaka, M., Hojo, M., Hollister, S.J., 2006. Framework for optimal design of porous scaffold microstructure by computational simulation of bone regeneration. Biomaterials. 27 (21), 3964–3972.

Blanchard, R., Dejaco, A., Bongaers, E., Hellmich, C., 2013. Intravoxel bone micromechanics for microCT-based finite element simulations. J. Biomech. 46 (15), 2710–2721.

Bonewald, L.F., 2011. The amazing osteocyte. J. Bone Mineral Res. 26 (2), 229–238.

Currey, J.D., 1986. Power law models for the mechanical properties of cancellous bone. Eng. Med. 15 (3), 153–154.

Currey, J.D., 1988. The effect of porosity and mineral content on the Young's modulus of elasticity of compact bone. J. Biomech. 21 (2), 131–139.

Czenek, A., Blanchard, R., Dejaco, A., Sigurjónsson, Ó.E., Örlygsson, G., Gargiulo, P., et al., 2014. Quantitative intravoxel analysis of microct-scanned resorbing ceramic biomaterials – perspectives for computer-aided biomaterial design. J. Mater. Res. 29 (23), 2757–2772.

Dejaco, A., Komlev, V.S., Jaroszewicz, J., Swieszkowski, W., Hellmich, C., 2012. Micro CT-based multiscale elasticity of double-porous (pre-cracked) hydroxyapatite granules for regenerative medicine. J. Biomech. 45 (6), 1068–1075.

Dias, M.R., Fernandes, P.R., Guedes, J.M., Hollister, S.J., 2012. Permeability analysis of scaffolds for bone tissue engineering. J. Biomech. 45 (6), 938–944.

Dormieux, L., Kondo, D., Ulm, F.-J., 2006. Microporomechanics. John Wiley & Sons, Chichester.

Drugan, W.R., Willis, J.R., 1996. A micromechanics-based nonlocal constitutive equation and estimates of representative volume element size for elastic composites. J. Mech. Phys. Solids. 44 (4), 497–524.

Engh, C.A., Bobyn, J.D., Glassman, A.H., 1987. Porous-coated hip replacement. The factors governing bone ingrowth, stress shielding, and clinical results. Bone Joint J. 69-B (1), 45–55.

Eshelby, J., 1957. The determination of the elastic field of an ellipsoidal inclusion, and related problems. Proc. Royal Soc. London, Series A. 241, 376–396.

Fritsch, A., Dejaco, A., Komlev, V.S., Swieszkowski, W., Jaroszewicz, J., Bongaers, E., et al., 2011. Translation of ct data into voxel-specific micromechanics-based elasticity tensors. SkyScan Micro-CT User Meeting. Bruker microCT, Kontich, Belgium.

Fritsch, A., Dormieux, L., Hellmich, C., Sanahuja, J., 2007. Micromechanics of crystal interfaces in polycrystalline solid phases of porous media: fundamentals and application to strength of hydroxyapatite biomaterials. J. Mater. Sci. 42 (21), 8824–8837.

Fritsch, A., Hellmich, C., Dormieux, L., 2009. Ductile sliding between mineral crystals followed by rupture of collagen crosslinks: experimentally supported micromechanical explanation of bone strength. J. Theor. Biol. 260 (2), 230–252.

Fritsch, A., Dormieux, L., Hellmich, C., Sanahuja, J., 2009. Mechanical behavior of hydroxyapatite biomaterials: An experimentally validated micromechanical model for elasticity and strength. J. Biomed. Mater. Res.-Part A. 88A (1), 149–161.

Fritsch, A., Hellmich, C., Young, P., 2013. Micromechanics-derived scaling relations for poroelasticity and strength of brittle porous polycrystals. J. Appl. Mech. (ASME). 80 (2), 020905.

Geris, L., 2013. Computational Modeling in Tissue Engineering, volume 10 of Studies in Mechanobiology, Tissue Engineering and Biomaterials. Springer-Verlag, Berlin Heidelberg.

Graham, J.M., Ayati, B.P., Holstein, S.A., Martin, J.A., 2013. The role of osteocytes in targeted bone remodeling: a mathematical model. PLoS One. 8 (5), e63884.

Hasslinger, P., Vass, V., Dejaco, A., Blanchard, R., Örlygsson, G., Gargiulo, P., et al., 2016. Coupling multiscale X-ray physics and micromechanics for bone tissue composition and elasticity determination from micro-ct data, by example of femora from ovx and sham rats. Int. J. Comp. Methods Eng. Sci. Mech. 17 (3), 222–244.

Hellmich, C., Celundova, D., Ulm, F.-J., 2009. Multiporoelasticity of hierarchically structured materials: micromechanical foundations and application to bone. J. Eng. Mech. (ASCE). 135 (5), 382–394.

Hershey, A.V., 1954. The elasticity of an isotropic aggregate of anisotropic cubic crystals. ASME J. Appl. Mech. 21, 236–240.

Hill, R., 1963. Elastic properties of reinforced solids: some theoretical principles. J. Mech. Phys. Solids. 11 (5), 357–372.

Hill, R., 1965a. Continuum micro-mechanics of elastoplastic polycrystals. J. Mech. Phys. Solids. 13 (2), 89–101.

Hill, R., 1965b. A self-consistent mechanics of composite materials. J. Mech. Phys. Solids. 13 (4), 213–222.

Hollister, S.J., 2005. Porous scaffold design for tissue engineering. Nat. Mater. 4 (7), 518–524.

Hubbel, J.H., and Seitzer, S.M. Tables of X-ray mass attenuation coefficients and mass energy-absorption coefficients from 1 kev to 20 mev for elements z 1 to 92 and 48 additional substances of dosimetric interest. Technical report, National Institute of Standards and Technology, U.S. Department of Commerce, 2004.

Hutmacher, D.W., Singh, H., 2008. Computational fluid dynamics for improved biore-actor design and 3d culture. Trends Biotechnol. 26 (4), 166–172.

Hutmacher, D.W., 2000. Scaffolds in tissue engineering bone and cartilage. Biomaterials. 21 (24), 2529–2543.

Jacobs, C.R., Temiyasathit, S., Castillo, A.B., 2010. Osteocyte mechanobiology and pericellular mechanics. Annu. Rev. Biomed. Eng. 12, 369–400.

Jacobs, C.R. *Numerical simulation of bone adaptation to mechanical loading*. PhD thesis, Stanford University, CA, USA, 1994.

Jaecques, S.V.N., Van Oosterwyck, H., Muraru, L., Van Cleynenbreugel, T., De Smet, E., Wevers, M., et al., 2004. Individualised, micro CT-based finite element modelling as a tool for biomechanical analysis related to tissue engineering of bone. Biomaterials. 25 (9), 1683–1696.

Kröner, E., 1978. Self-consistent scheme and graded disorder in polycrystal elasticity. J. Phys. F Metal Phys. 8, 2261–2267.

Lacroix, D., Chateau, A., Ginebra, M.-P., Planell, J.A., 2006. Micro-finite element models of bone tissue-engineering scaffolds. Biomaterials. 27 (30), 5326–5334.

Lacroix, D., Planell, J.A., Prendergast, P.J., 2009. Computer-aided design and finite-element modelling of biomaterial scaffolds for bone tissue engineering. Philos. Trans. Royal Soc. London A Mathemat. Phys. Eng. Sci. 367 (1895), 1993–2009.

Lanza, R., Langer, R., Vacanti, J.P., 2007. Principles of Tissue Engineering. Elsevier Academic Press, New York, NY.

Lemaire, V., Tobin, F.L., Greller, L.D., Cho, C.R., Suva, L.J., 2004. Modeling of the interactions between osteoblast and osteoclast activities in bone remodeling. J. Theor. Biol. 229 (3), 293–309.

Lieberman, J.R., Friedlaender, G.E., 2005. Bone Regeneration and Repair. Humana Press, Totowa, NJ.

Luczynski, K., Dejaco, A., Lahayne, O., Jaroszewicz, J., Swieszkowski, W., Hellmich, C., 2012. MicroCT/micromechanics-based Finite Element models and quasi-static unloading tests deliver consistent values for Young's modulus of rapid-prototyped polymer-ceramic tissue engineering scaffold. CMES – Comp. Model. Eng. Sci. 87 (6), 505–529.

Melchels, F.P.W., Bertoldi, K., Gabbrielli, R., Velders, A.H., Feijen, J., Grijpma, D.W., 2010. Mathematically defined tissue engineering scaffold architectures prepared by stereolithography. Biomaterials. 31 (27), 6909–6916.

Milan, J.-L., Planell, J.A., Lacroix, D., 2009. Computational modelling of the mechanical environment of osteogenesis within a polylactic acid–calcium phosphate glass scaffold. Biomaterials. 30 (25), 4219–4226.

Mori, T., Tanaka, K., 1973. Average stress in matrix and average elastic energy of materials with misfitting inclusions. Acta Metall. 21 (5), 571–574.

O'Brien, F.J., 2011. Biomaterials and scaffolds for tissue engineering. Mater. Today. 14 (3), 88–95.

Olivares, A.L., Marsal, È., Planell, J.A., Lacroix, D., 2009. Finite element study of scaffold architecture design and culture conditions for tissue engineering. Biomaterials. 30 (30), 6142–6149.

Petite, H., Viateau, V., Bensaid, W., Meunier, A., de Pollak, C., Bourguignon, M., et al., 2000. Tissue-engineered bone regeneration. Nat. Biotechnol. 18 (9), 959–963.

Pivonka, P., Zimak, J., Smith, D.W., Gardiner, B.S., Dunstan, C.R., Sims, N.A., et al., 2008. Model structure and control of bone remodeling: A theoretical study. Bone. 43 (2), 249–263.

Pivonka, P., Zimak, J., Smith, D.W., Gardiner, B.S., Dunstan, C.R., Sims, N.A., et al., 2010. Theoretical investigation of the role of the RANK-RANKL-OPG system in bone remodeling. J. Theor. Biol. 262 (2), 306–316.

Porter, B., Zauel, R., Stockman, H., Guldberg, R., Fyhrie, D., 2005. 3-D computational modeling of media flow through scaffolds in a perfusion bioreactor. J. Biomech. 38 (3), 543–549.

Radon, J., 1917. Über die Bestimmung von Funktionen durch ihre Integralwerte längs gewisser Mannigfaltigkeiten [On the determination of functions from their integrals along certain manifolds]. Berichte der Sächsischen Akademie der Wissenschaften. 29, 262–277, In German.

Rezwan, K., Chen, Q.Z., Blaker, J.J., Boccaccini, A.R., 2006. Biodegradable and bioactive porous polymer/inorganic composite scaffolds for bone tissue engineering. Biomaterials. 27 (18), 3413–3431.

Robling, A.G., Castillo, A., Turner, C.H., 2006. Biomechanical and molecular regulation of bone remodeling. Annu. Rev. Biomed. Eng. 8, 455–498.

Rüegsegger, P., Koller, B., Müller, R., 1996. A microtomographic system for the nondestructive evaluation of bone architecture. Calcif. Tissue Int. 58, 24–29.

Sandino, C., Lacroix, D., 2011. A dynamical study of the mechanical stimuli and tissue differentiation within a cap scaffold based on micro-ct finite element models. Biomech. Model. Mechanobiol. 10 (4), 565–576.

Sandino, C., Planell, J.A., Lacroix, D., 2008. A finite element study of mechanical stimuli in scaffolds for bone tissue engineering. J. Biomech. 41 (5), 1005–1014.

Sanz-Herrera, J.A., García-Aznar, J.M., Doblaré, M., 2008. Micro-macro numerical modelling of bone regeneration in tissue engineering. Comp. Methods Appl. Mech. Eng. 197 (33-40), 3092–3107.

Sanz-Herrera, J.A., García-Aznar, J.M., Doblaré, M., 2009a. On scaffold designing for bone regeneration: A computational multiscale approach. Acta. Biomater. 5 (1), 219–229.

Sanz-Herrera, J.A., García-Aznar, J.M., Doblaré, M., 2009b. A mathematical approach to bone tissue engineering. Philosop. Trans. Royal Soc. London A Math. Phys. Eng. Sci. 367 (1895), 2055–2078.

Scheiner, S., Pivonka, P., Hellmich, C., 2013. Coupling systems biology with multi-scale mechanics, for computer simulations of bone remodeling. Comp. Methods Appl. Mech. Eng. 254, 181–196.

Scheiner, S., Pivonka, P., Hellmich, C., 2016a. Poromicromechanics reveals that physiological bone strains induce osteocyte-stimulating lacunar pressure. Biomech. Model. Mechanobiol. 15 (1), 9–28.

Scheiner, S., Sinibaldi, R., Pichler, B., Komlev, V., Renghini, C., Vitale-Brovarone, C., et al., 2009. Micromechanics of bone tissue-engineering scaffolds, based on resolution error-cleared computer tomography. Biomaterials. 30 (12), 2411–2419.

Scheiner, S., Komlev, V.S., Gurin, A.N., Hellmich, C., 2016b. Multiscale mathematical modeling in dental tissue engineering: towards computer-aided design of a regenerative system based on hydroxyapatite granules, focusing on early and mid-term stiffness recovery. Front. Physiol. 7 (383), 1–18.

Scheiner, S., Komlev, V.S., Hellmich, C., 2016c. Strength increase during ceramic biomaterial-induced bone regeneration: a micromechanical study. Int. J. Fract. 202 (2), 217–235.

Simmons, C.A., Meguid, S.A., Pilliar, R.M., 2001. Differences in osseointegration rate due to implant surface geometry can be explained by local tissue strains. J. Orthop. Res. 19 (2), 187–194.

Sturm, S., Zhou, S., Mai, Y.-W., Li, Q., 2010. On stiffness of scaffolds for bone tissue engineering – a numerical study. J. Biomech. 43 (9), 1738–1744.

Truscello, S., Kerckhofs, G., Van Bael, S., Pyka, G., Schrooten, J., Van Oosterwyck, H., 2012. Prediction of permeability of regular scaffolds for skeletal tissue engineering: A combined computational and experimental study. Acta. Biomater. 8 (4), 1648–1658.

Voronov, R., VanGordon, S., Sikavitsas, V.I., Papavassiliou, D.V., 2010. Computational modeling of flow-induced shear stresses within 3d salt-leached porous scaffolds imaged via micro-ct. J. Biomech. 43 (7), 1279–1286.

Williams, D.F., 2008. On the mechanisms of biocompatibility. Biomaterials. 29 (20), 2941–2953.

Williams, J.M., Adewunmi, A., Schek, R.M., Flanagan, C.L., Krebsbach, P.H., Feinberg, S. E., et al., 2005. Bone tissue engineering using polycaprolactone scaffolds fabricated via selective laser sintering. Biomaterials. 26 (23), 4817–4827.

Zaoui, A., 2002. Continuum micromechanics: survey. J. Eng. Mech. (ASCE). 128 (8), 808–816.

# Tissue engineering and biomimetics with bioceramics

# 13

*Simone Sprio, Monica Sandri, Andrea Ruffini, Alessio Adamiano, Michele Iafisco, Massimiliano Dapporto, Silvia Panseri, Monica Montesi and Anna Tampieri*
National Research Council, Faenza, Italy

**Chapter Outline**

**13.1 Introduction 407**
**13.2 Multisubstituted apatites 408**
13.2.1 Superparamagnetic HA nanoparticles 411
**13.3 Apatitic, self-setting bone cements 412**
**13.4 Multifunctional, biohybrid scaffold obtained by bioinspired assembling/mineralization process 416**
**13.5 Porous bioceramics with hierarchical structure obtained by biomorphic transformation of natural structures 419**
**13.6 Conclusions and future perspectives 424**
**Acknowledgments 425**
**References 425**
**Further reading 432**

## 13.1 Introduction

The development of materials with high mimicry of target tissues is today a major research target for biomaterial scientists. Indeed, regenerative solutions for clinical needs of great societal impact such as those regarding the musculoskeletal system are increasingly urgent, also considering the steady aging of the population and the predictable increase in the number of bone diseases due to trauma or degenerative pathologies in the coming years. For decades, ceramic materials have been considered as elective materials for hard tissue regeneration; in particular, calcium phosphates (CaPs) are today the main research focus, as they strongly resemble the main inorganic component of mammalian hard tissues. However, bone scaffolds based on stoichiometric CaPs also demonstrated strong limitations in regenerating critical size defects. In fact, it is well accepted today that substantial tissue regeneration can occur only on the basis of intense exchange of signals between biomaterials and cells so that the attention of scientists is increasingly dedicated to the development of biomaterials with real mimicry of natural tissues. To this end, scientists are also investigating new approaches for biomaterial synthesis, particularly looking at natural processes and structures, as they are the nicest and smartest

**Advances in Ceramic Biomaterials.**
**DOI: http://dx.doi.org/10.1016/B978-0-08-100881-2.00014-2**

examples of nanotechnology, exhibiting still insuperable mechanical and functional properties.

The chapter illustrates recent developments in biomaterial development, also including new, nature-inspired synthesis methods by which bone scaffolds with enhanced bioactivity could be obtained, as reported by various in vitro and in vivo investigations. In particular, the chapter will describe the synthesis of biomimetic, ion-substituted apatite phases by various approaches to generate different bioactive devices in the form of nanopowders to solid porous ceramics, to new bioinspired hybrid and biomorphic scaffolds that, thanks to their high mimicry of host tissues, can enable regenerative applications in different diseased bony regions.

## 13.2 Multisubstituted apatites

Bone tissue possesses a unique ability to self-repair and reorganize its three-dimensional (3D) structure, on the basis of complex biochemical signaling continuously exchanged with cells. In this respect, the fine chemical features of the inorganic part of bone are a major source of information: bone mineral is represented by a nearly amorphous CaP with the structure of hydroxyapatite (HA) characterized by complex atomic composition, low crystallinity and nanosize. All these features play a pivotal role in activation of physiological processes related to new bone formation by osteoblasts and resorption by osteoclasts, for which bone is a living tissue with ability of self-repair and continuous remodeling (Olszta et al., 2007; Sprio et al., 2013). These unique characteristics are strictly related to the mineral bone composition which continuously evolve with its maturation, so that in spite of its inorganic nature, bone apatite can rightly be considered as a metabolically active phase.

HA is one of the most common biomaterial used for bone tissue engineering; however in most of the cases it is used in the form of a stoichiometric phase that generally has a reduced interaction with cells, due to its high thermodynamic stability at physiological pH that reduces ion exchange and bioresorption (Elliot, 1994). Indeed, incorporation of foreign ions in the apatite lattice yields crystal destabilization, thus preventing grain growth and enhancing ion release with higher solubility in physiological environment. All these features are typical of newly formed bone tissue, whereas mature bones assume a more stable composition that limit further tissue rearrangement (Rey et al., 2007a). The bone mineral is also characterized by highly active superficial layer, reported as nonapatitic environments, which extend for few nanometers in thickness and is characterized by a quite disordered structure, thus functioning as a buffer layer for ion exchanging with the physiological environment. (Rey et al., 2007b) Therefore, the use of nanocrystalline, doped apatite phases can be considered as the elective approach for bone tissue engineering to trigger and promote effective bone regeneration. Many different synthesis approaches have been developed in recent decades to synthesize CaPs and apatites to develop regenerative biomaterials (Wang and Shaw, 2007; Ben-Nissan and Choi, 2006; Lopez-Macipe et al., 1998; Manara et al., 2008; Iafisco et al., 2010; Ye et al.,

2008). In particular, wet methods based on acid–base neutralization and carried out at body temperature allowed the maintenance of a low crystalline ordering in the final product and the fine design of the atomic composition by introducing multiple foreign ions in the reaction vessel, mainly by dissolution of suitable soluble salts (Landi et al., 2008a; Sprio et al., 2008).

Among the various foreign ions, the partial replacement of phosphate with carbonate (B-carbonation) is considered as the most relevant, as it greatly increases the apatite solubility without penalizing the affinity with osteoblasts (Wang and Nancollas, 2008). When carbonate replaces the hydroxyl group (A-carbonation) the apatite lattice becomes more stable and insoluble; indeed such atomic configuration in the apatite phase is more typical of mature bone, for which a high resorbability is not required (Boskey, 2006; Bigi et al., 1992). Numerous studies were concerned with the development of carbonated apatites and their assessment as a biomaterial (Iafisco et al., 2010; Tadic et al., 2002; Landi et al., 2004; Tampieri et al., 2005).

Ionic substitutions in the apatite lattice can occur very easily, particularly in cationic sites where calcium can be partially replaced by a number of divalent ions, without impacting on the charge neutrality of the apatite crystal. From a biological perspective, magnesium has a major relevance because it increases the nucleation kinetics of HA on the assembling collagen matrix, but prevents grain growth, thus favoring the formation of mineral phase characterized by very small nuclei, that in turn enhance its bioavailability. Also, magnesium has a much higher affinity with water with respect to calcium, which strongly enhances hydrophilicity and the related process of protein binding which mediates focal adhesion of cells (Bertinetti et al., 2007, 2009). Similarly to carbonate, magnesium is particularly abundant in young bone (Bigi et al., 1992), thus being a major element stimulating the ossification process, for which the synthesis of magnesium-doped apatite has been widely investigated in previous studies (Landi et al., 2006, 2008a; Laurencin et al., 2011) also including several investigations in vivo (Crespi et al., 2009, 2012; Grigolato et al., 2015; Landi et al., 2008). In particular magnesium-doped apatite provided enhanced stimulation of new bone formation and osseointegration, with possible signs of bioresorption related to enhanced material fragmentation in vivo (Fig. 13.1). These properties were also assessed in recent clinical tests where Mg-doped nanocrystalline apatite particles were successfully used to augment alveolar bone when applied to fresh extraction sockets (Fig. 13.1: in vivo Mg-HA), thus showing excellent behavior in comparison with microcrystalline apatitic products (Checchi et al., 2011).

Strontium is a trace element in bone which has raised great interest in the last decade due to its proven ability to restore the bone turnover balance, especially when the treatment of bone fractures caused by degenerative diseases such as osteoporosis is demanded (Dahl et al., 2001; Marie et al., 2001). The beneficial effect of low doses of Sr in the treatment of osteoporosis is well known and growing evidence of positive results obtained in clinical studies on long-term Sr treatment (Reginster et al., 2009) has led to increased interest in the development of strontium-doped apatites (Landi et al., 2007, 2008b; Yıldız Yaralı Özbek et al., 2016; Sopyan et al., 2008). In particular the ability of Sr-doped apatite to be

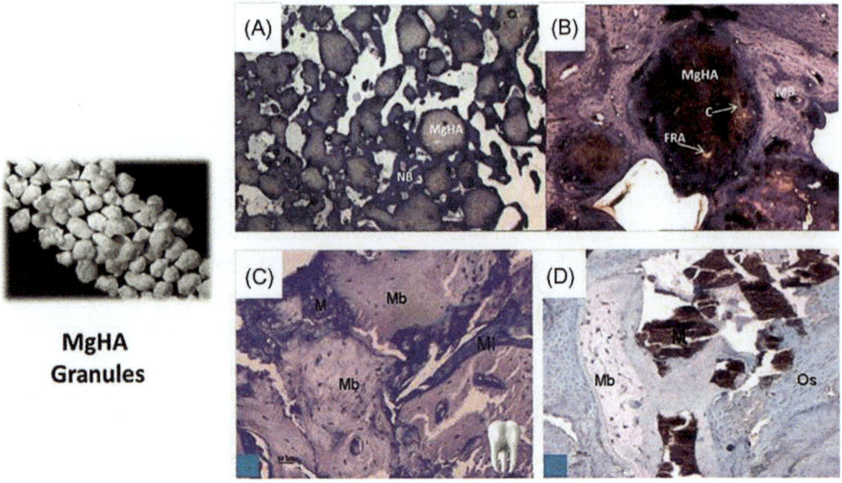


**Figure 13.1** In vivo assessment of Mg-doped hydrpxyapatite (Mg-HA) nanoparticles. (A, B) Preclinical study in rabbit femur. (A) Follow-up at 1 month, with complete filling with new woven, immature bone (NB); (B) follow-up at 3 months, showing remodeling into mature bone (MB) characterized by lamellar bone apposition in contact with the material, and focal resorptive areas (FRA) forming inside the Mg-HA appear, in conjunction with several cracks. (C, D) Clinical study in oral surgery. (C) Light micrographs of MgHA biopsies at the site of graft insertion, with marrow-like tissue (Ml) and mature bone (Mb) filling the defect; (D) active bone remodeling, mature bone (Mb), osteoid seams (Os).

released in situ as an active principle is an interesting perspective to avoid systemic administration by strontium-containing drugs which raised several concerns due to secondary adverse effects (Grynpas et al., 1996), and has been explored in previous studies (Andersen et al., 2013; Li et al., 2010).

Among the foreign ions of relevance in bone regeneration, silicon is known as an essential trace element for the activation of bone growth as also shown by various in vivo studies showing enhanced bone apposition and faster bone remodeling on the surface of Si-doped apatities. (Carlisle, 1981; Patel et al., 2002; Porter et al., 2003). Silicon ions enter as $SiO_4^{4-}$ replacing the phosphate group by nonisoelectronic substitution requiring charge compensation by elimination of a negative charge. In this respect, evidences were given on the elimination of hydroxyl ions following introduction of increasing amounts of silicon (Sprio et al., 2008; Gibson et al., 1999). Previous studies also confirmed the enhanced activity of Si-doped apatites with respect to stoichiometric phases (Botelho et al., 2006a,b).

The apatite doping with multiple ions has been proposed in previous studies to obtain biomaterials with very high mimicry of the bone mineral composition (Sprio et al., 2008; Iafisco et al., 2013). However, the simultaneous incorporation of foreign ions of different sizes, in replacement of calcium and phosphate, generates a complex scenario where a competition for the occupation of the apatite crystal sites is established, with lattice deformations related to cell volume modification and increased anisotropy (Sprio et al., 2008; Bigi et al., 2007; Donazzon et al., 1998). In this respect, the interaction between different foreign ions can reduce the extent of single ion substitutions; on the other hand it has been found that the presence of various ions can provide synergistic effects yielding enhanced stabilization, as was shown for cosubstitution with magnesium and carbonate (Landi et al., 2006), or silicon and magnesium (Sprio et al., 2008), where the two ions mutually stabilize against release in physiological media. These phenomena are intriguing as they confirm the possibility of design-specific ion substitutions in apatites, however this also opens up new queries on the fine mechanisms occurring in the bulk and the surface of nanocrystalline, bone-like apatites, particularly when in contact with physiological environment, to which deep investigation should still be dedicated.

### 13.2.1 Superparamagnetic HA nanoparticles

The possibility of introducing desired amounts of selected ionic species in substitutional lattice positions makes this an easy synthesis process as a multifunctional platform for the generation of biomaterials with properties designed for specific applications in medicine. Hence, codoping with divalent and trivalent ions was successfully carried out, thus obtaining a nanocrystalline superparamagnetic apatite (FeHA) characterized by high saturation magnetization value at room temperature (RT) (9.0 emu/g), associated with high specific surface area and large number of active adsorption sites with nonimmunogenicity, biocompatibility, and bioactivity. FeHA demonstrated excellent cytocompatibility and ability to enhance cell proliferation compared to iron-free apatite particles, particularly when a magnetic field was applied, associated with enhanced biodegradability in a pilot study in rabbit (Tampieri et al., 2014). The coexistence of these properties in a magnetic nanoparticle offers outstanding opportunities in some of the most innovative therapeutic approaches, such as stem-cell therapy for regenerative medicine (Panseri et al., 2016), and magnetic-controlled drug delivery for cancer treatment (Iafisco et al., 2016).

A full understanding of the mechanism underlying the unusual magnetic behavior of FeHA is still lacking and so far, the most common hypotheses implies (1) the hetero-epitaxial growth of magnetite on iron-doped HA crystallites (Wu et al., 2010), and (2) the occurrence of two distinct interacting structural domains or sublattices (Tampieri et al., 2012). Recently, it was proposed that the arising of FeHA outstanding magnetic properties is due to the oxidation induced by the synthesis process determining the arranging of $Fe^{2+/3+}$ ions that can adopt (1) the FeHA HA lattice as isolated ions, (2) the nonapatitic domain as interacting-paramagnetic ions, or (3) they can be segregated into external interacting-superparamagnetic maghemite nanoparticles having unusual A-site and B-site iron populations as conferred by the heterogeneous nucleation on the iron-doped HA nanoparticles (Iannotti et al., 2017).

This preliminary investigation shows that FeHA phase can open brilliant perspectives in the fields of tissue regeneration and nanomedicine, as they associate for the first time high physicochemical affinity with the human bone mineral (Tampieri et al., 2014; Panseri et al., 2012), and superparamagnetic properties

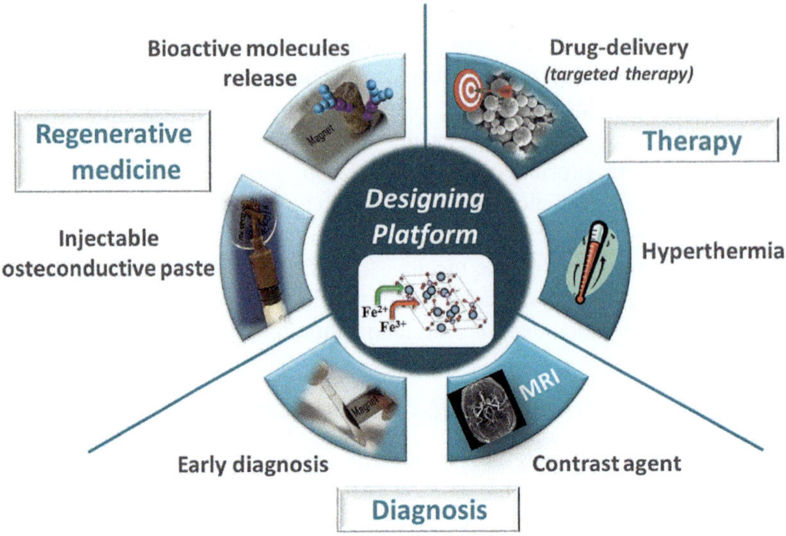


**Figure 13.2** Multifunctional platform in nanomedicine based on FeHA.

comparable to conventional magnetic nanoparticles. This can significantly enhance the perspective of circumventing critical toxicity-related effects deriving from the administration of superparamagnetic iron oxides nanoparticles to patients. Therefore, this new nanomaterial can be considered as the fulcrum of a new smart technological platform in theranostics that might open up improved therapies for a number of degenerative diseases (Fig. 13.2).

## 13.3 Apatitic, self-setting bone cements

Injectable self-hardening biomaterials directed at the treatment of bone diseases are a subject of major interest and intense investigation due to their capability of being implanted through minimal invasive surgery. Indeed, several bone disorders, such as osteonecrosis or osteopenia related to metabolic diseases such as osteoporosis, require mini-invasive surgery due to the difficulty of intervention and scaffold placement in anatomical regions such as vertebral bodies and femur heads. The treatment of damaged or partially collapsed vertebral bones is today among the most relevant clinical cases for which the use of injectable scaffolds is desired (Sprio et al., 2016a). In this respect, trauma and metabolic diseases such as osteoporosis are major causes of vertebral fractures, particularly affecting postmenopausal women (Stetzer, 2011), but also due to several interacting factors, including clinical, behavioral, nutritional, and genetic variables. The alteration of the physiological bone turnover due to osteoporosis results in depletion of bone mineral content with consequent weakening of the vertebra and increase in the fracture risk. Even after partial bone collapse, the patient has to be immediately stabilized to reduce pain and prevent detrimental nerve compression (Wilcox et al., 2003).

The treatment of vertebral compression fractures, also for the sake of prevention, has been addressed by drugs such as bisphosphonates, alendronates, and strontium-containing molecules (e.g., strontium ranelate). The use of strontium, in spite of its evident ability to reestablish the correct balance between osteoblast and osteoclast activity (Dahl et al., 2001; Marie et al., 2001), often resulted in adverse systemic effects. Minimally invasive surgery techniques offer fewer associated injuries, quicker recovery times and less pain, with a reduction in healthcare costs (Park et al., 2007). Balloon kyphoplasty and vertebroplasty are today well established techniques based on the injection of a bone cement in the vertebral body to provide immediate pain relief and physical stabilization.

The use of acrylic bone cements (mainly polymethylmetaacrylate, PMMA) leads to rapid strengthening of damaged vertebral bodies, with good recovery of mechanical capability after a few hours. These are the main reasons for the wide use of acrylic cements, together with the low cost, in most of the vertebroplasty procedures nowadays. However, acrylic cements exhibit several drawbacks associated with their use, particularly: (1) exothermic hardening reactions yielding strong local heating with potential damaging of surrounding tissues, (2) high stiffness, in comparison with natural bone, that can provoke secondary fractures at adjacent vertebrae (Bohner, 2000). Moreover, acrylic cements are completely bioinert and dense, thus hampering integration with surrounding bone. As these drawbacks can be acceptable for older patients, for which short immobilization times are mandatory, for young and physically active people the use of regenerative therapies would greatly help to prevent secondary effects and, above all, to recover full biomechanical functionality at the spine level.

With this in mind, biomimetic approaches have been investigated for many years, to develop bioactive cements with bone-like composition associated with open and interconnected porosity thus permitting cell colonization and proliferation of new mature bone inside the injected cement mass. CaP cements (CPCs) discovered and applied from the early 1980s (Brown and Chow, 1983; Friedman et al., 1998; Kamerer et al., 1994; Constantz et al., 1995; Horstmann et al., 2003; Welch et al., 2003; Maestretti et al., 2007; Takemasa et al., 2007).

CPCs are very interesting biomaterials as they do not show the typical drawbacks related to the use of acrylic cements; besides, due to their nanostructure and porosity, they offer the possibility of loading with biologics such as drugs, proteins, or growth factors (Vallet-Regi, 2014; Ginebra et al., 2006).

However, CPCs are characterized by lower mechanical strength and porosity insufficient to ensure substantial penetration of new bone (Khairoun et al., 1998). These features are the main weaknesses of CPCs for which material scientists are increasingly called to find a solution.

CPCs harden by means of dissolution-reprecipitation processes in aqueous media, involving one or more CaPs as metastable reactants that transform into nanocrystalline HA with elongated morphology ensuring physical entanglement and hardening. In this respect, the synthesis of CPCs based on transformation of

$\alpha$-$Ca_3(PO_4)_2$ ($\alpha$TCP) into ion-doped apatite is a recent trend, and is extremely promising due to the close similarity of nanocrystalline, ion-doped apatite to the bone mineral (Bohner, 2000).

In particular, the cement doping with strontium has been widely investigated in recent years by various synthesis approaches, due to its ability to reestablish the correct balance between osteoblast and osteoclast activity, altered by metabolic diseases such as osteoporosis (Schumacher and Gelinsky, 2015). In some cases, strontium has been added by means of soluble salts to be introduced in the initial formulation, together with commercial, stoichiometric $\alpha$TCP phase (Alkhraisat et al., 2008; Baier et al., 2013; Schumacher et al., 2013; Thormann et al., 2013). However, a major concern penalizing the development of CPCs for clinical use is related to the use of multiple inorganic components in CPC formulations, which can make the optimization of rheological properties related to flowability, injectability, cohesion extremely labor-consuming. The achievement of adequate rheological properties is a key aspect for CPC use, also with respect to achievement of suitable setting times, porosity, and mechanical performances. To this end, recent synthesis approaches were based on the synthesis of CPCs starting from a single inorganic component, appositely synthesized to host strontium ions in its structure (Saint-Jean et al., 2005; Sprio et al., 2016b).

The optimization of the cement formulation must also involve the adjustment of the composition of the setting solution. In fact, the simple use of water gave very slow reaction kinetics, so that setting accelerators are commonly used (Bohner, 2000), particularly based on acidic components (i.e., monocalcium phosphate or acid citric) or sodium phosphate solutions. However, the choice of the most adequate compound is made difficult by the prompt alteration of the rheological properties of the whole paste once modifying the formulation. In fact the simultaneous optimization of the key parameters related to the use and performance of CPCs is perhaps the most critical issue. Hence, in recent years researchers were pushed to investigate polymer-enriched formulations, with the aim of stabilizing rheological properties and improving physical stability of the paste (Perez et al., 2012; Maazouz et al., 2017). In this respect, recent investigations reported on the promising use of a thermoresponsive polymer (pluronic 127) with gelling ability at body temperature, so that the resulting ceramic paste, based on $\alpha$TCP phase, exhibited reversible temperature-dependent properties and improved rheological behavior, thus adequate for using in vivo (Maazouz et al., 2017).

Among polymeric additives tested in cement formulations, biopolymers are considered as elective materials, as they can undergo metabolic resorption and promote the formation of open porosity directly in vivo after hardening. (Zhang et al., 2014; Lee et al., 2011; Sprio et al., 2016b). Indeed, the use of natural polymers such as alginate was found to be promising as its use provided a clear increase in the cement strength, even after a long time aging in aqueous media, and also modulated the setting kinetics to times adequate for the clinical practice. The same cement was also tested in a small animal model, thus confirming good bioactivity and osteoconductivity, particularly related to higher porosity, in comparison with an Sr-doped bone cement used in clinics (Sprio et al., 2016b). The higher porosity and, possibly, the presence of alginate, could favor cement fragmentation in vivo and enhanced penetration. Besides, thanks to its compositional features, based on a single inorganic precursor, the cement showed enhanced ability to be remodeled in vivo thus suggesting that a bioresorption process could be active.

Sr-doped CPCs demonstrated enhanced bioactivity and degradability both under laboratory conditions and in vivo, even though a clear effect of strontium, also with respect to specific dosages, is still debated (Schumacher and Gelinsky, 2015). In this respect Sr-doped cements with different extents of ion doping were extensively tested in vitro (Montesi et al., 2017), thus giving some evidences on dose-dependent effects of strontium in inducing osteoblastic differentiation of mesenchymal stem cells, proliferation of osteoblasts, and inhibition of osteoclast activity. The study reported that low strontium doses such as 2% could give the better results.

In spite of all of the research discussed above, much more extensive investigation is required; the results obtained so far suggest that the use of ion-doped CPCs is a promising approach for tissue engineering in bony regions where injectable pastes are required. Besides, the use of small amounts of polymers as additives can greatly improve injectability, cohesion, mechanical strength and setting time, whilst maintaining high porosity. In this respect, as mechanical strength and porosity are inversely related, the use of cements with higher initial load-bearing properties, although very desirable, can be detrimental to the subsequent process of cement colonization by the newly formed bone. This would limit the whole regeneration process to the superficial layer of the injected cement, and might prevent the complete recovery of biomechanical ability. On the other hand, if sufficient strength is exhibited at the time of implantation, the early colonization by new bone could rapidly raise the biomechanical competence up to levels of healthy tissues (Fig. 13.3).

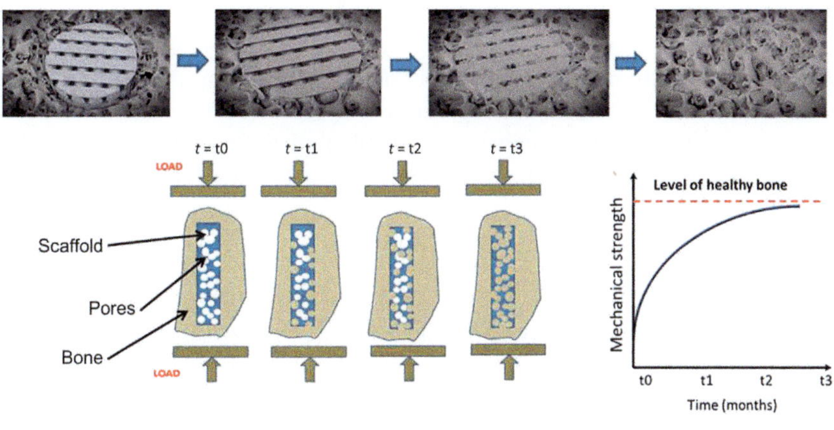


**Figure 13.3** Scheme of porous scaffold colonization progressively enhancing biomechanical competence.

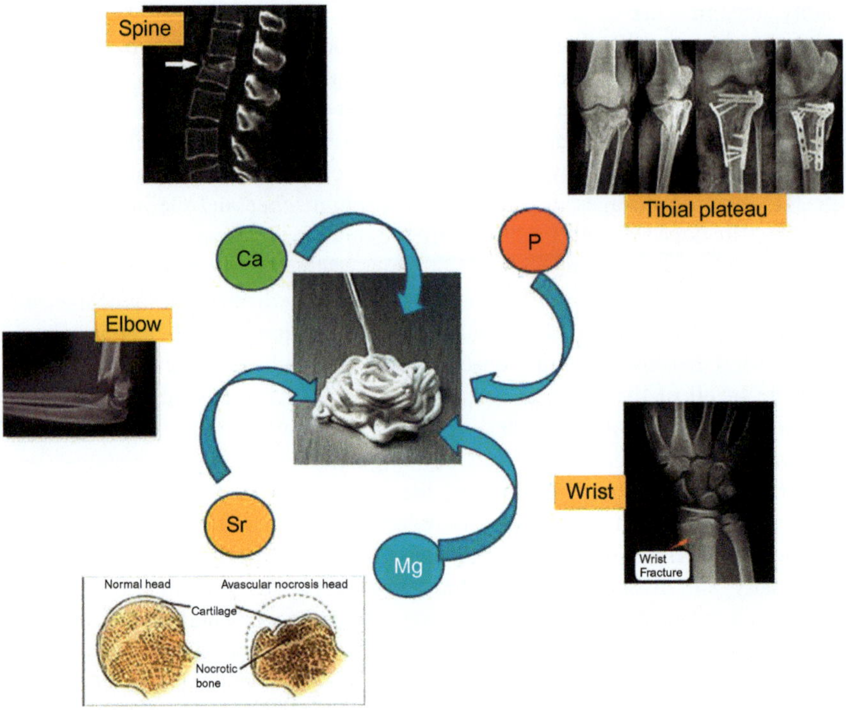


**Figure 13.4** Biomimetic apatitic bone cements and their potential uses in different bony regions.

Therefore, open questions still remain, and the future activity of scientists will certainly be dedicated to the optimization of these injectable biomaterials. However, thanks to the positive outcomes so far obtained, the development of ion-doped apatites as injectable bone cements can be considered as a promising pathway for the settling of new regenerative therapies in spinal surgery. Furthermore, thanks to the possibility of tailoring the viscosity and setting of the paste, new biomaterials could be developed, for regenerative applications also in bone diseases affecting different anatomical regions such as tibial plate or femur head, for which the use of injectable pastes rather than 3D scaffolds is preferred (Fig. 13.4).

## 13.4 Multifunctional, biohybrid scaffold obtained by bioinspired assembling/mineralization process

The bone mineral is a nearly amorphous apatitic phase presenting multiple ionic substitutions in cationic and anionic site. Its crystals are a few nanometers in size and present defined crystallographic arrangements thus favoring topotactic links of proteins relevant for focal adhesion of cells (Tampieri et al., 2011). All these features spontaneously establish during new bone formation, as directed by the physicochemical and ultrastructural information typical of the collagenous matrix on which the bone mineral heterogeneously nucleates. The process of bone formation is thus based on the progressive assembling of collagen molecules and simultaneous mineralization with apatitic crystals that evolve into a macroscopic, highly disordered construct that later organizes and remodels into mature bone tissue. This cascade of phenomena occurs in vivo under the influence of physicochemical conditions, namely the presence of ions such as calcium, phosphate, magnesium, and local variations of pH values, both of which combine to drive the self-assembling of collagen molecules and the simultaneous nucleation of the mineral phase (Weiner, 2008). Biopolymers involved in the formation of biologic tissues, such as collagen, contain complex information stored in chemical and ultrastructural features related to molecule organization and exposed functional groups. These characteristics enable spontaneous formation of hybrid materials with highly complex structure, which could not be obtained by classical additive techniques. Therefore, natural polymers are increasingly attracting the attention of materials scientists, as they could be the basis for new concepts of materials synthesis based on dynamic growing processes rather than on fabrication methods, based on prefixed and static design (Fratzl and Weinkamer, 2007). An example of this approach is given by the development of hybrid bone scaffold by application of a synthesis process reproducing the conditions of new bone formation (biomineralization). Hence, by controlled pH variations at body temperature, and in the presence of calcium, phosphate, and magnesium ions, collagen fibrils under aqueous suspensions could be induced to assemble into thicker fibers while heterogeneous nucleation of multi-substituted apatite nanocrystals took place, driven by linking of calcium ions to the free carboxylic groups exposed by collagen (Tampieri et al., 2003). The final construct, in the form of mineralized hydrogel, could be later processed by cross-linking and freeze drying to obtain a porous scaffold with outstanding mimicry of newly formed bone. The same process could be directed to obtain mineralized hydrogels with tailored amounts of mineral phase, to mimic different tissues of multifunctional regions such as osteochondral tissue and periodontium, all bony regions characterized by specific mineralization extent, porosity, and fiber organization (Cho and Garant, 2000; Nukavarapu and Dorcemus, 2013). Therefore, with a similar bioinspired approach, a graded scaffold could be obtained, made of thin layers mimicking subchondral bone, mineralized cartilage and hyaline cartilage, engineered in a monolithic construct (Tampieri et al., 2008). This scaffold demonstrated outstanding regenerative ability in a large animal model, without the use of any growth factor (Kon et al., 2010). This result demonstrated that biomimetic compositional and topological features inherent in scaffolds for tissue engineering are able to instruct cells to activate the regenerative cascade, as occurs with natural tissues. This result was also confirmed by further animal tests where hybrid scaffolds were implanted in ectopic sites in mice (Scaglione et al., 2012), thus revealing osteoinductive features (Fig. 13.5: mice).

The possibility of applying the above synthesis method in a flexible manner opens up the development of materials for wider applications. In fact, the

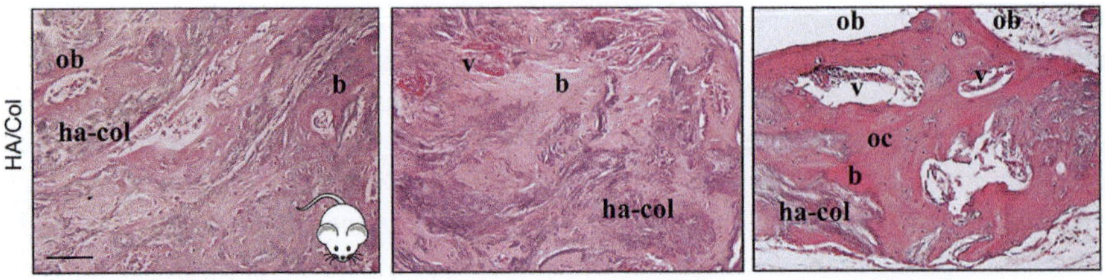


**Figure 13.5** Histology of new bone tissue formed in ectopic sites, and deposited by stromal cells within hydroxyapatite–collagen grafts. *b*, bone; *bm*, bone marrow; *ha-col*, hydroxyapatite-collagen composite; *ob*, osteoblasts; *oc*, osteocytes; *v*, blood vessels. Scale bar = 50 μm.

mineralization extent can be tailored over a wide range of values, and the type of mineral phase defined on the basis of the nature of the ions introduced in the reaction vessel. In a novel and recent study, the biomineralization process was modified by introducing also $Fe^{2+}/Fe^{3+}$ ions to induce heterogeneous nucleation of a superparamagnetic apatitic phase (Fe-HA) (Tampieri et al., 2014). Similar to that which was obtained with iron-free apatite, the biomineralization process method yielded biomimetic hybrid scaffolds mimicking bone and osteochondral tissues. In vitro studies revealed very good cytocompatibility and biodegradation profiles, with improved cell proliferation, in the presence of external magnetic fields. The use of biomimetic scaffolds with superparamagnetic ability enabling remote activation by magnetic signaling opens up new possible therapies boosting tissue regeneration in those patients with reduced endogenous regenerative potential (Higashi et al., 1993; Kotani et al., 2002; Xu and Gu, 2014). Magnetic scaffolds also offer the possibility of external, mini-invasive fixation methods (Tampieri et al., 2011) for which a preliminary proof of concept was provided by a previous study, where the fixating magnets were positioned in contact with the scaffolds (Panseri et al., 2013). Perhaps the most intriguing applications of hybrid bone scaffolds is the use of its magnetic properties to attract magnetized cells and force the scaffold colonization, to enhance the regenerative process, particularly in the case of large tissue defects for which scaffolds often fail in ensuring proper vascularization and cell penetration in the whole defect volume (Tampieri et al., 2014). This would greatly enhance the possibility of therapeutic intervention in the case of extensive bone deficiency, for which restorative interventions are still a major challenge.

The biomineralization process can be also formulated as a flexible process by means of using different macromolecular matrices enabling heterogeneous nucleation of nanoapatites, as in the case of a recent study, which developed a new hybrid scaffold where the organic template was a recombinant biopolymer (Ramírez-Rodríguez et al., 2016). Biomineralization is a process with interesting potential that still has to be investigated in depth; soft mineralized scaffolds obtained by this approach can be used in a variety of applications, thanks to the possibility of tailoring composition, mineralization extent, and microstructure, thus opening to a variety of applications, even outside the biomedical field (Fig. 13.6).

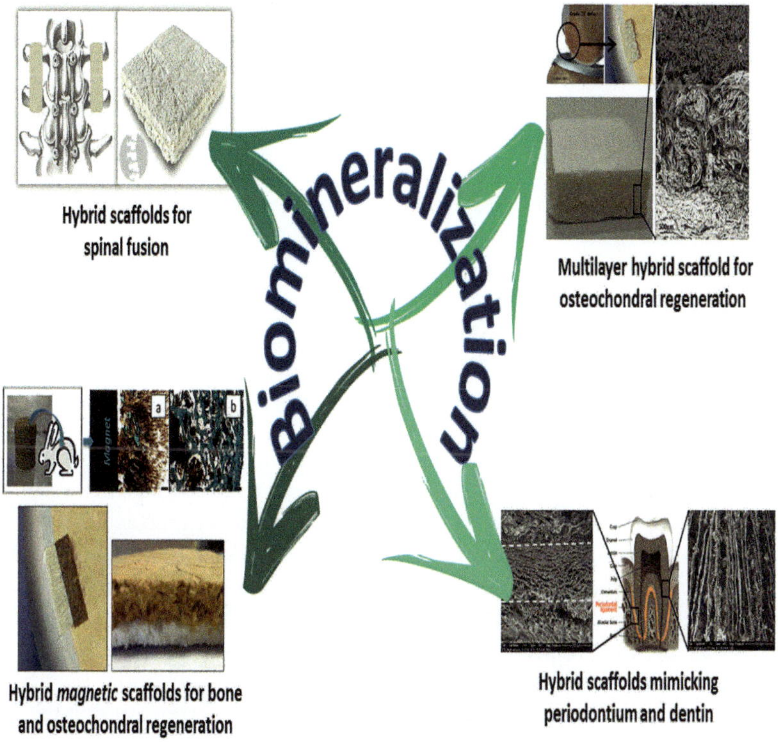


**Figure 13.6** Scheme of the multifunctional platform based on hybrid biomimetic constructs, having potential application in different mineralized anatomical regions.

The association with biocompatible, superparamagnetic phases further enhances the potential of smart applications, thus creating technological platforms with high potential impact in nanomedicine, and representing a remarkable leap forward in the current therapies against bone diseases (Fig. 13.2).

## 13.5 Porous bioceramics with hierarchical structure obtained by biomorphic transformation of natural structures

Porous scaffolds are elective materials for bone grafting, as they offer structural support for critical size bone defects, and open macroscopic voids where cells, blood vessels, and newly formed tissue can penetrate and form well-integrated bone/scaffold constructs with good physical stability (Sprio et al., 2014). This achievement is a key factor in improving the healing process and, in this respect, several fabrication technologies were developed in the last decades to produce porous ceramics (Studart et al., 2006). Additionally, compositional and ultrastructural aspects are extremely relevant, because they determine the extent of cell adhesion and hosting, with the ability of migration inside the scaffold pores. Therefore, as CaPs, and particularly HA, are elective materials for bone scaffolding, the effort of scientists was directed to the development of porous devices associating bioactive phase composition, wide open porosity. and bone-like mechanical properties. Basically, the existing manufacturing techniques can be addressed as template-based or template-free processes (Sprio et al., 2011). In the first approach manufacturers use porous organic constructs as 3D substrates to be infiltrated with ceramic slurries and then sintered to eliminate the matrix and leave a "positive" copy made of pure ceramic (Hsu et al., 2007; Zhao et al., 2008; Ji et al., 2011; Yunos et al., 2008; Jo et al., 2009; Tampieri et al., 2001). Alternative, template-based methods include the use of solid pore-forming agents, namely crystals of soluble salts or polymeric spheres (Le Ray et al., 2010; Chevalier et al., 2008). Template-free processes are rather based on the direct generation of pores into the ceramic slurry, which can be obtained either by the use of surfactants or during the application of directed drying processes (Deville et al., 2006; Deville, 2008; Moritz and Richter, 2007). Both approaches can give good results in terms of open porosity and mechanical strength; however, the presence of a sacrificial template requires the application of thermal processes dedicated to the elimination of the organic matrix, prior to the final sintering treatment. Such a debonding process requires slow heating, in order to prevent the occurrence of defects and to allow the coalescence of adjacent ceramic particles that yield ceramic consolidation. Failure, in this respect, significantly impacts on the final mechanical properties, so that the application of template-free methods is rapidly gaining ground. Among these, the direct foaming process can generate massive ceramics with highly homogeneous pore structure and high interconnectivity. Direct foaming is based on concentrated ceramic slurries containing dispersants and deflocculating agents which are processed by milling and then poured into molds for slow drying, prior to sintering (Sprio et al., 2011). During the foaming process, formation of interconnecting bubbles occurs through phenomena of nucleation, coalescence, and growth, that can be directed on the basis of the slurry concentration, and other process parameters related to the milling process (Fig. 13.7). Recently, an approach based on planetary ball milling allowed the homogeneity of the slurry and the solid/liquid ratio to be strongly improved, thus resulting in improved mechanical strength (Dapporto et al., 2016). Ceramic suspensions can also be processed by a freeze-drying process that, contrary to homogeneous drying at room temperature, is based on freezing/heating cycles. Here, the application of specific temperature gradients imparts designed porosity to the final ceramic body, in terms of pore size and orientation, due to specific arrangement of ice crystals formed during freezing (Deville et al., 2006; Lu et al., 1998).

Foamed apatite ceramics showed very good ability to induce fast colonization by cells (Fig. 13.7). Further studies showed that the process can be translated into different bioceramics thus representing a platform for the development of porous materials to be employed in wider application fields; in particular tricalcium phosphate and titania nanoparticles were engineered to obtain a precursor that, after

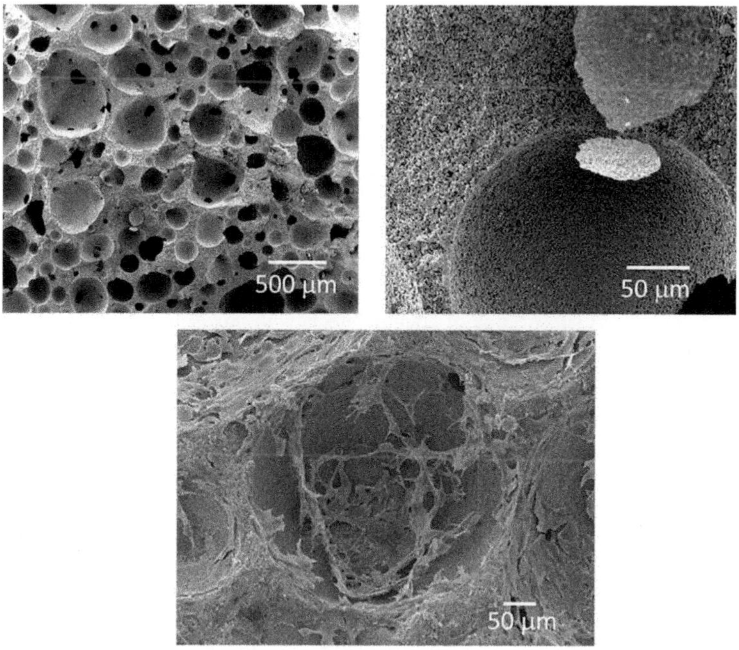


**Figure 13.7** Scanning electron micrograph images showing the typical porous structure of ceramic scaffolds obtained by direct foaming process (top) and extensive mesenchymal stem cell adhesion and spreading on its surface (bottom).

application of foaming and sintering processes, gave porous scaffolds with much higher mechanical strength than pure apatite and also exhibited enhanced osteogenic ability (Cunha et al., 2013).

Despite the fact that porous foamed ceramics usually exhibit open and percolating pathways for cells, their application in critical size defects was somewhat limited by the insufficient ability to derive the formation of blood vessels, particularly in the case of long bone defects where often the penetration extent of new tissue and vascular networks is limited to a few millimeters (Sprio et al., 2014). As an example, pilot clinical tests were carried out by implanting a porous apatite scaffold into a long segmental bone defect in lower limbs (Quarto et al., 2001). In these experiments, despite the fact that new bone formation at the interface yielded good stabilization of the defect, the random and tortuous porosity exhibited by the scaffolds did not allow extensive angiogenesis so that complete regeneration of the defect was not achieved. In the case of flat bones, conversely, the application of porous apatite scaffolds can be more satisfactory. In particular, in neurosurgery porous apatite scaffolds are today considered as the gold standard material for the regeneration of large bony regions of the skull, after a decade of clinical tests (Sprio et al., 2016c), also due to the possibility of obtaining personalized scaffolds by precise fitting of cranial defects (Fig. 13.8).

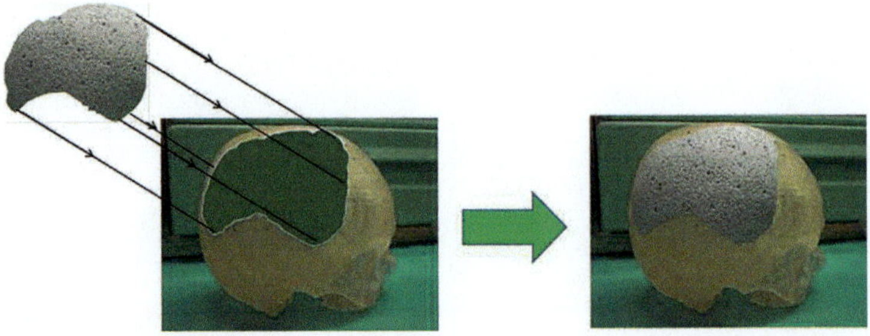

**Figure 13.8** Scheme of substitution of cranial defects with precisely fitting porous hydroxyapatite scaffolds.

The reduced thickness of cranial bones, in comparison with long bone of the limbs, allows extensive penetration of newly formed bone, with tight osteointegration and recovery of optimal physical stability. Furthermore, the close similarity of porous apatite with natural bone prevents the occurrence of physical discontinuities in the implanted area thus restoring biomechanical functions typical of the healthy bone. In comparison with the use of inert implants such as PMMA or titanium, the use of porous apatite is a new concept in neurosurgery, that further confirms the relevance of the use of biomimetic implants, able to closely reproduce compositional and morphological features of natural tissues. In fact the unique ability of macroporous apatite to rapidly host new bone tissue enables effective osteointegration even in the case of extended bony defects and can open up application in children, thanks to the self-adapting features of bone-like porous apatite (Sprio et al., 2016c).

Similar considerations can be made when attempting to reconstruct long segmental bones; in such cases, particularly with very serious bone defects or comminuted fractures, regenerative solutions are still missing. Indeed, these cases are considered to be among the most challenging for orthopedic surgeons, also due to the numerous complications typically associated with extensive bone damaging and compromised blood vessels in the area, such as infected pseudoarthrosis (Giannoudis and Atkins, 2007; Motsitsi, 2008; Calori et al., 2007; Lozada-Gallegos et al., 2013). Extensive vascularization of the treated bone defect is a serious concern; however, substantial reconstruction of new bone tissue with all its functions, a particularly critical requirement when treating load-bearing bones, requires scaffolds able to rapidly induce new bone formation with establishment of a tight callus and deep bone penetration in the inner region of the defect. These scaffolds must also exhibit adequate strength to withstand early biomechanical load, but must be compliant with the typical response of healthy bone. This ability is extremely relevant to activate and sustain mechano-transduction processes at the cell level, at the basis of the process of bone remodeling which gives biomechanical competence to the newly formed bone (Ingber, 1993; Pavalko et al., 2003; Sikavitsas, 2001; Bilezikian et al., 2002). The expression of all these properties in a bone scaffold, however, has never been obtained so far. Indeed, scaffolds exhibiting high compositional, morphological, and mechanical mimesis with natural bone have still not been achieved, because of intrinsic limitations in the current manufacturing technologies.

Therefore, nature-inspired processes are increasingly capturing the interest of materials scientists; natural structures exhibit unique morphologies and mechanical performances, still not surpassed by artificially produced materials. Among natural structures, wood can be taken as a model to realize bone scaffolds with hierarchically organized structure and superior performance (Fig. 13.9). In particular, a recent research developed a multistep transformation process, following a sequence of chemical reactions in highly controlled conditions of atmosphere, pressure, and temperature, to convert cylinders of Rattan wood (*Calamus rotang*) into scaffolds characterized by biomimetic composition, nanostructure and, from the macroscopic to the nanoscale, wide channeled porosity, interconnected with a number of hierarchically organized smaller canals (Tampieri et al., 2009). Rattan wood was selected on the basis of its 3D architecture very close to the Haversian structure with wide pores adequate for enhanced cell colonization and vascularization also throughout large volumes. Moreover, the channel-like structure of Rattan resulted in anisotropic mechanical properties with values in the range of the trabecular bone, that reflect the complex bone response to directional loading.

The biomorphic transformation process enabled controlled incorporation of carbonate ions in the apatite lattice and, also, tailoring of the final Ca/P ratio by varying the volume and ionic strength of the phosphate solution (Ruffini et al., 2013).

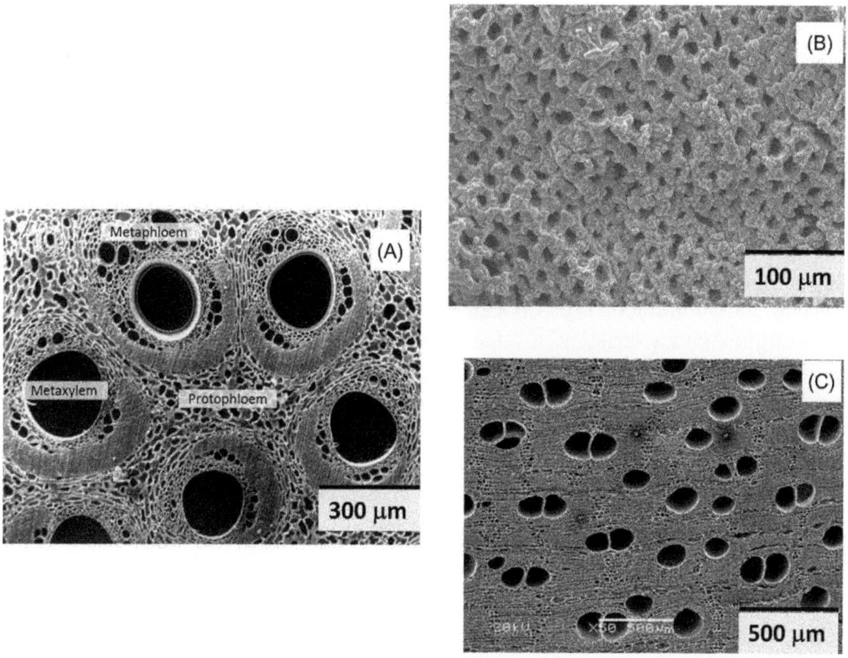


**Figure 13.9** Wood structures exhibiting high porosity, potentially suitable to inspire new hierarchically organized bone scaffolds. (A) Rattan wood; (B) pinewood; (C) Sipo wood.

Calcium-deficiency in apatites raises physiological solubility, thus increasing its potential bioactivity; moreover, the partial substitution with foreign ions that can be introduced in the last stage of the phosphatization reaction can make the final HA much closer to the natural bone tissue, thus potentially increasing its therapeutic effectivess. In particular, carbonate ions are known as major factors in the process of new bone formation and maturation (Dorozhkin, 2010), so that the new scaffolds have real potential for use in the treatment of long segmental bone defects. Preliminary tests in vitro and in vivo confirm that the biomorphic apatite scaffolds have very good ability to regenerate critical size bone defects (Sprio et al., 2016a).

The establishment of biomorphic transformations able to transform woods or other natural structures into functional materials is an emerging trend that can revolutionize material science and opens up a new generation of smart devices for wide applications. In the biomedical field, hierarchically organized porous scaffolds with biomimetic composition might represent a breakthrough in orthopedics and all surgery fields where load-bearing regenerative scaffolds are demanded.

## 13.6 Conclusions and future perspectives

Bioceramics designed for bone regeneration have been under thorough investigation for many decades, and a plethora of different materials and implantable devices have been developed so far. As the use of bioinert materials revealed severe limitations in determining substantial advances in regenerative bone therapies, particularly when it comes to treating critical size defects, the application of cell-instructive concepts by means of physicochemical and topological cues delivered by biomimetic synthetic scaffolds is, conversely, gaining ground and has been demonstrated to be a very promising approach for achieving substantial tissue regeneration. In this respect, several technological approaches have been developed in the past decade to generate highly porous scaffolds with bioactive composition and very good results have been obtained. However, to overcome critical limitations in conventional manufacturing processes, particularly when it comes to reproducing very complex characteristics of bone tissue, such as composition, porosity, and hierarchical organization, the adoption of nature-inspired approaches can result in a breakthrough in the biomedical field, as shown in several studies carried out in the past decade. In particular, it has been shown how the reproduction of natural assembling processes can be feasible, thanks to the huge information included in natural macromolecular compounds which can be delivered and exchanged with the surrounding environment by simple modulation of environmental conditions. On the other hand, nature exhibits innumerable nanocomposite structures that can be copied and transformed into inorganic materials, to exhibit outstanding and unpreceded performance, which can finally open up new solutions for highly critical and still unmet clinical needs, or at least to significantly improve the existing therapies.

From a broader perspective, the adoption of nature-inspired synthesis approaches, which today is still in the preliminary stages, could also guarantee potential repercussions for many other technological fields, particularly when materials with complex composition and 3D morphology activating smart and unusual properties are needed.

## Acknowledgments

The Authors wish to acknowledge the regional project NIPROGEN (POR-FESR Emilia Romagna 2014–2020: PG/2015/731448) and the project PNR-CNR 2012-2014, "Ageing" for funding the present research.

## References

Alkhraisat, M.H., Moseke, C., Blanco, L., Barralet, J.E., Lopez-Carbacos, E., Gbureck, U., 2008. Strontium modified biocements with zero order release kinetics. Biomaterials. 29, 4691–4697.

Andersen, O.Z., Offermanns, V., Sillassen, M., Almtoft, K.P., Andersen, I.H., Sorensen, S., et al., 2013. Accelerated bone ingrowth by local delivery of strontium from surface functionalized titanium implants. Biomaterials. 34 (24), 5883–5890.

Baier, M., Staudt, P., Klein, R., Sommer, U., Wenz, R., Grafe, I., et al., 2013. Strontium enhances osseointegration of calcium phosphate cement: a histomorphometric pilot study in ovariectomized rats. J. Orthop. Surg. 8, 16.

Ben-Nissan, B., Choi, A.H., 2006. Sol-gel production of bioactive nanocoatings for medical applications. Part 1: an introduction. Nanomedicine. 1, 311–319.

Bertinetti, L., Tampieri, A., Landi, E., Ducati, C., Midgley, P.A., Coluccia, S., et al., 2007. Surface structure, hydration, and cationic sites of nanohydroxyapatite: UHR-TEM, IR, and microgravimetric studies. J. Phys. Chem. C. 111 (10), 4027–4035.

Bertinetti, L., Drouet, C., Combes, C., Rey, C., Tampieri, A., Coluccia, S., et al., 2009. Surface characteristics of nanocrystalline apatites: effect of Mg surface enrichment on morphology, surface hydration species, and cationic environments. Langmuir. 25, 5647–5654.

Bigi, A., Foresti, E., Gregorini, R., Ripamonti, A., Roveri, N., Shah, J.S., 1992. The role of magnesium on the structure of biological apatite. Calcif. Tissue. Int. 50, 439–444.

Bigi, A., Boanini, E., Capuccini, C., Gazzano, M., 2007. Strontium-substituted hydroxyapatite nanocrystals. Inorganica. Chim. Acta. 360 (3), 1009–1016.

Bilezikian, J.P., Raisz, L.G., Rodan, G.A., 2002. Principles of Bone Biology, vol. 1. Academic Press, San Diego.

Bohner, M., 2000. Calcium orthophosphates in medicine: from ceramics to calcium phosphate cements. Injury. 31 (Suppl. 4), 37–47.

Boskey, A.L., 2006. Mineralization, structure and function of bone. In: Seibel, M.J., Robins, S.P., Bilezikian, J.P. (Eds.), Dynamics of Bone and Cartilage Metabolism. Academic Press, Toronto, pp. 201–212.

Botelho, C.M., Brooks, R.A., Best, S.M., Lopes, M.A., Santos, J.D., Rushton, N., et al., 2006a. Human osteoblast response to silicon-substituted hydroxyapatite. J. Biomed. Mater. Res. A. 79A, 723–730.

Botelho, C.M., Brooks, R.A., Spence, G., McFarlane, I., Lopes, M.A., Best, S.M., et al., 2006b. Differentiation of mononuclear precursors into osteoclasts on the surface of Si-substituted hydroxyapatite. J. Biomed. Mater. Res. A. 78A, 709–720.

Brown, W.E., Chow, L.C., 1983. A new calcium phosphate setting cement. J. Dent. Res. 62, 672–676.

Calori, G.M., Albisetti, W., Agus, A., Iori, S., Tagliabue, L., 2007. Risk factors contributing to fracture non-unions. Injury. 38, S11–S18.

Carlisle, E., 1981. Silicon: a requirement in bone formation independent of vitamin D. Calcif. Tissue. Int. 33, 27–34.

Checchi, V., Savarino, L., Montevecchi, M., Felice, P., Checchi, L., 2011. Clinical radiographic and histological evaluation of two hydroxyapatites in human extraction sockets: a pilot study. Int. J. Oral. Maxillofac. Surg. 40, 526–532.

Chevalier, E., Chulia, D., Pouget, C., Viana, M., 2008. Fabrication of porous substrates: a review of processes using pore forming agents in the biomaterial field. J. Pharm. Res. 97 (3), 1135–1154.

Cho, M.-I., Garant, P.R., 2000. Development and general structure of the periodontium. Periodontology. 2000 (24), 9–27.

Constantz, B.R., Ison, I.C., Fulmer, M.T., Poser, R.D., Smith, S.T., VanWagoner, M., et al., 1995. Skeletal repair by in situ formation of the mineral phase of bone. Science. 267, 1796–1799.

Crespi, R., Mariani, E., Benasciutti, E., Capparè, P., Cenci, S., Gherlone, E., 2009. Magnesium-enriched hydroxyapatite versus autologous bone in maxillary sinus grafting: combining histomorphometry with osteoblast gene expression profiles ex vivo. J. Periodontol. 80 (4), 586–593.

Crespi, R., Capparè, P., Addis, A., Gherlone, E., 2012. Injectable magnesium-enriched hydroxyapatite putty in peri-implant defects: a histomorphometric analysis in pigs. Int. J. Oral Maxillof. Impl. 27 (1), 95–101.

Cunha, C., Sprio, S., Panseri, S., Dapporto, M., Marcacci, M., Tampieri, A., 2013. High biocompatibility and improved osteogenic potential of novel Ca-P/titania composite scaffolds designed for regeneration of load-bearing segmental bone defects. J. Biomed. Mater. Res. Part A. 101A (6), 1612–1619.

Dahl, S.G., Allain, P., Marie, P.J., Mauras, Y., Boivin, G., Ammann, P., et al., 2001. Incorporation and distribution of strontium in bone. Bone. 28 (4), 446–453.

Dapporto, M., Sprio, S., Fabbi, C., Figallo, E., Tampieri, A., 2016. A novel route for the synthesis of macroporous ceramics for bone regeneration. J. Eur. Ceram. Soc. 36, 2383–2388.

Deville, S., Saiz, E., Tomsia, A.P., 2006. Freeze casting of hydroxyapatite scaffolds for bone tissue engineering. Biomaterials. 27, 5480–5489.

Deville, S., 2008. Freeze-casting of porous ceramics: a review of current achievements and issues. Adv. Eng. Mater. 10, 155–169.

Donazzon, B., Dechambre, G., Lacout, J.L., 1998. Calcium-strontium hydroxyapatite: hydrothermal preparation. Ann. Chim. Sci. Des Mater. 23 (1-2), 53–56.

Dorozhkin, S.V., 2010. Nanosized and nanocrystalline calcium orthophosphates. Acta. Biomater. 6, 715–734.

Elliot, J.C., 1994. Structure and Chemistry of the Apatites and Other Calcium Ortophosphates. Elsevier, Amsterdam.

Fratzl, P., Weinkamer, R., 2007. Nature's hierarchical materials. Prog. Mater. Sci. 52 (8), 1263–1334.

Friedman, C.D., Costantino, P.D., Takagi, S., Chow, L.C., 1998. BoneSource hydroxyapatite cement: a novel biomaterial for craniofacial skeletal tissue engineering and reconstruction. J. Biomed. Mater. Res. 43, 428–432.

Giannoudis, P.V., Atkins, R., 2007. Management of long-bone non-unions. Injury. 38 (Suppl 2), S1–S2.

Gibson, I.R., Best, S.M., Bonfield, W., 1999. Chemical characterization of silicon-substituted hydroxyapatite. J. Biomed. Mater. Res. 44, 422–428.

Ginebra, M.P., Traykova, T., Planell, J.A., 2006. Calcium phosphate cements as bone drug delivery systems: a review. J. Control. Release. 113, 102–110.

Grigolato, R., Pizzi, N., Brotto, M.C., Corrocher, G., Desando, G., Grigolo, B., 2015. Magnesium-enriched hydroxyapatite as bone filler in an ameloblastoma mandibular defect. Int. J. Clin. Exp. Med. 8 (1), 281–288.

Grynpas, M.D., Hamilton, E., Cheung, R., Tsouderos, Y., Deloffre, P., Hott, M., et al., 1996. Strontium increases vertebral bone volume in rats at a low dose that does not induce detectable mineralization defect. Bone. 18 (3), 253–259.

Higashi, T., Yamagishi, A., Takeuchi, T., Kawaguchi, N., Sagawa, S., Onishi, S., et al., 1993. Orientation of erythrocytes in a strong static magnetic field. Blood. 82, 1328–1334.

Horstmann, W.G., Verheyen, C.C.P.M., Leemans, R., 2003. An injectable calciumphosphate cement as a bone-graft substitute in the treatment of displaced lateral tibial plateau fractures. Injury. 34, 141–144.

Hsu, Y.H., Turner, I.G., Miles, A.W., 2007. Fabrication of porous bioceramics with porosity gradients similar to the bimodal structure of cortical and cancellous bone. J. Mater. Sci. Mater. Med. 18 (12), 2251–2256.

Iafisco, M., Morales, J.G., Hernandez-Hernandez, M.A., Garcia-Ruiz, J.M., Roveri, N., 2010. Biomimetic carbonate-hydroxyapatite nanocrystals prepared by vapor diffusion. Adv. Eng. Mater. 12, B218–B223.

Iafisco, M., Ruffini, A., Adamiano, A., Sprio, S., Tampieri, A., 2013. Biomimetic magnesium-carbonate-apatite nanocrystals endowed with strontium ions as anti-osteoporotic trigger. Mater. Sci. Eng. C. 35 (1), 212–219.

Iafisco, M., Drouet, C., Adamiano, A., Pascaud, P., Montesi, M., Panseri, S., et al., 2016. Superparamagnetic iron-doped nanocrystalline apatite as a delivery system for doxorubicin. J. Mater. Chem. B. 4, 57–70.

Iannotti, V., Adamiano, A., Ausanio, G., Lanotte, L., Coey, J.M.D., Aquilanti, G., et al., 2017. Fe Doping-induced magnetism in nano-hydroxyapatites. Inorg. Chem. (accepted manuscript).

Ingber, D.E., 1993. Cellular tensegrity: defining new rules of biological design that govern the cytoskeleton. J. Cell. Sci. 104, 613–627.

Ji, L., Jell, G., Dong, Y., Jones, J.R., Stevens, M.M., 2011. Template synthesis of ordered macroporous hydroxyapatite bioceramics. Chem. Commun. 47, 9048–9050.

Jo, I.-H., Shin, K.-H., Soon, Y.-M., Koh, Y.-H., Lee, J.-H., Kim, H.-E., 2009. Highly porous hydroxyapatite scaffolds with elongated pores using stretched polymeric sponges as novel template. Mater. Lett. 63 (20), 1702–1704.

Kamerer, D.B., Hirsch, B.E., Snyderman, C.H., Costantino, P., Friedman, C.D., 1994. Hydroxyapatite cement: a new method for achieving watertight closure in transtemporal surgery. Am. J. Otolaryngol. 15, 47–49.

Khairoun, I., Boltong, M., Driessens, F.C.M., Planell, J., 1998. Some factors controlling the injectability of calcium phosphate bone cements. J. Mater. Sci. Mater. Med. 9, 425–428.

Kon, E., Delcogliano, M., Filardo, G., Fini, M., Giavaresi, G., Francioli, S., et al., 2010. Orderly osteochondral regeneration in a sheep model using a novel nano-composite multilayered biomaterial. J. Orthop. Res. 28, 116–124.

Kotani, H., Kawaguchi, H., Shimoaka, T., Iwasaka, M., Ueno, S., Ozawa, H., et al., 2002. Strong static magnetic field stimulates bone formation to a definite orientation in vitro and in vivo. J. Bone Mineral Res. 17, 1814–1821.

Landi, E., Tampieri, A., Celotti, G., Vichi, L., Sandri, M., 2004. Influence of synthesis and sintering parameters on the characteristics of carbonate apatite. Biomaterials. 25, 1763–1770.

Landi, E., Tampieri, A., Mattioli-Belmonte, M., Celotti, G., Sandri, M., Gigante, A., et al., 2006. Biomimetic Mg- and Mg, $CO_3$-substituted hydroxyapatites: synthesis characterization and in vitro behaviour. J. Eur. Ceram. Soc. 26, 2593–2601.

Landi, E., Tampieri, A., Celotti, G., Sprio, S., Sandri, M., Logroscino, G., 2007. Sr-subtituted hydroxyapatites for osteoporotic bone replacement. Acta. Biomater. 3 (6), 961–969.

Landi, E., Logroscino, G., Proietti, L., Tampieri, A., Sandri, M., Sprio, S., 2008a. Biomimetic Mg-substituted hydroxyapatite: from synthesis to in vivo behaviour. J. Mater. Sci. Mater. Med. 19, 239–247.

Landi, E., Sprio, S., Sandri, M., Celotti, G., Tampieri, A., 2008b. Development of Sr and CO3 co-substituted hydroxyapatites for biomedical applications. Acta. Biomater. 4, 656–663.

Laurencin, D., Almora-Barrios, N., de Leeuw, N.H., Gervais, C., Bonhomme, C.,, Mauri, F., et al., 2011. Magnesium incorporation into hydroxyapatite. Biomaterials. 32 (7), 1826–1837.

Lee, G.S., Park, J.H., Won, J.E., Shin, U.S., Kim, H.W., 2011. Alginate combined calcium phosphate cements: mechanical properties and in vitro rat bone marrow stromal cell responses. J. Mater. Sci. Mater. Med. 22 (5), 1257–1268.

Le Ray, A.-M., Gautier, H., Bouler, J.-M., Weiss, P., Merle, C., 2010. A new technological procedure using sucrose as porogen compound to manufacture porous biphasic calcium phosphate ceramics of appropriate micro- and macrostructure. Ceram. Int. 36 (1), 93–101.

Li, Y.F., Li, Q., Zhu, S.S., Luo, E., Li, J.H., Feng, G., et al., 2010. The effect of strontium-substituted hydroxyapatite coating on implant fixation in ovariectomized rats. Biomaterials. 31 (34), 9006–9014.

Lopez-Macipe, A., Gomez-Morales, J., Rodriguez-Clemente, R., 1998. Nanosized hydroxyapatite precipitation from homogeneous calcium/citrate/phosphate solutions using microwave and conventional heating. Adv. Mater. 10, 49–53.

Lozada-Gallegos, A.R., Letechipia-Moreno, J., Palma-Lara, I., Montero, A.A., Rodríguez, G., Castro-Muñozledo, F., et al., 2013. Development of a bone nonunion in a noncritical segmental tibia defect model in sheep utilizing interlocking nail as an internal fixation system. J. Surg. Res. 183 (2), 620–628.

Lu, H., Qu, Z., Zhou, Y., 1998. Preparation and mechanical properties of dense polycrystalline hydroxyapatite through freeze-drying. J. Mater. Sci. Mater. Med. 9, 583–587.

Maazouz, Y., Montufar, E.B., Malbert, J., Espanol, M., Ginebra, M.P., 2017. Self-hardening and thermoresponsive alpha tricalcium phosphate/pluronic pastes. Acta. Biomater. 49, 563–574.

Maestretti, G., Cremer, C., Otten, P., Jakob, R.P., 2007. Prospective study of standalone balloon kyphoplasty with calcium phosphate cement augmentation in traumatic fractures. Eur. Spine J. 16, 601–610.

Manara, S., Paolucci, F., Palazzo, B., Marcaccio, M., Foresti, E., Tosi, G., et al., 2008. Electrochemically-assisted deposition of biomimetic hydroxyapatite-collagen coatings on titanium plate. Inorganica. Chim. Acta. 361, 1634–1645.

Marie, P.J., Ammann, P., Boivin, G., Rey, C., 2001. Mechanisms of action and therapeutic potential of strontium in bone. Calcif. Tissue. Int. 69 (3), 121–129.
Montesi, M., Panseri, S., Dapporto, M., Tampieri, A., Sprio, S., 2017. Strontium-substituted apatite nanophase direct mesenchymal stem cells, osteoblasts and osteoclasts fate. PLoS. One. 12 (2), e0172100.
Moritz, T., Richter, H.-J., 2007. Ice-mould freeze casting of porous ceramic components. J. Eur. Ceram. Soc. 27 (16), 4595–4601.
Motsitsi, N.S., 2008. Management of infected nonunion of long bones: the last decade (1996-2006). Injury. 39, 155–160.
Nukavarapu, S.P., Dorcemus, D.L., 2013. Osteochondral tissue engineering: current strategies and challenges. Biotechnol. Adv. 31, 706–721.
Olszta, M.J., Cheng, X.G., Jee, S.S., Kumar, R., Kim, Y.Y., Kaufman, M.J., et al., 2007. Bone structure and formation: a new perspective. Mater. Sci. Eng. R-Rep. 58, 77–116.
Panseri, S., Cunha, C., D'Alessandro, T., Sandri, M., Giavaresi, G., Marcacci, M., et al., 2012. Intrinsically superparamagnetic Fe-hydroxyapatite nanoparticles positively influence osteoblast-like cell behaviour. J. Nanobiotechnol. 10, 32.
Panseri, S., Russo, A., Sartori, M., Giavaresi, G., Sandri, M., Fini, M., et al., 2013. Modifying bone scaffold architecture in vivo with permanent magnets to facilitate fixation of magnetic scaffolds. Bone. 56, 432–439.
Panseri, S., Montesi, M., Sandri, M., Iafisco, M., Adamiano, A., Ghetti, M., et al., 2016. Magnetic labelling of mesenchymal stem cells with iron-doped hydroxyapatite nanoparticles as tool for cell therapy. J. Biomed. Nanotechnol. 12, 909–921.
Park, A., Kavic, S.M., Lee, T.H., Heniford, B.T., 2007. Minimally invasive surgery: the evolution of fellowship. Surgery. 142, 505–513.
Patel, N., Gibson, I.R., Hing, K.A., Best, S.M., Revell, P.A., Bonfield, W., 2002. A comparative study on the in vivo behavior of hydroxyapatite and silicon substituted hydroxyapatite granules. J. Mater. Sci. Mater. Med. 13, 1199–1206.
Pavalko, F.M., Norvell, S.M., Burr, D.B., Turner, C.H., Duncan, R.L., Bidwell, J.P., 2003. A model for mechanotransduction in bone cells: the load-bearing mechanosomes. J. Cell. Biochem. 88, 104–112.
Perez, R.A., Kim, H.W., Ginebra, M.P., 2012. Polymeric additives to enhance the functional properties of calcium phosphate cements. J. Tissue Eng. 3 (1), pp. 2041731412439555.
Porter, A.E., Patel, N., Skepper, J.N., Best, S.M., Bonfield, W., 2003. Comparison of in vivo dissolution processes in hydroxyapatite and silicon-substituted hydroxyapatite bioceramics. Biomaterials. 24, 4609–4620.
Quarto, R., Mastrogiacomo, M., Cancedda, R., Kutepov, S.M., Mukhachev, V., Lavroukov, A., et al., 2001. Repair of large bone defects with the use of autologous bone marrow stromal cells. New Engl. J. Med. 344 (5), 385–386.
Ramírez-Rodríguez, G.B., Delgado-López, J.M., Iafisco, M., Sandri, M., Sprio, S., Tampieri, A., 2016. Biomimetic mineralization of recombinant collagen type I derived protein to obtain hybrid matrices for bone regeneration. J. Struct. Biol. 196 (2), 138–146.
Reginster, J.Y., Bruyère, O., Sawicki, A., Roces-Varela, A., Fardellone, P., Roberts, A., et al., 2009. Long-term treatment of postmenopausal osteoporosis with strontium ranelate: results at 8 years. Bone. 45, 1059–1064.
Rey, C., Combes, C., Drouet, C., Sfihi, H., Barroug, A., 2007a. Physico-chemical properties of nanocrystalline apatites: implications for biominerals and biomaterials. Mater. Sci. Eng. C. 27, 198–205.
Rey, C., Combes, C., Drouet, C., Lebugle, A., Sfihi, H., Barroug, A., 2007b. Nanocrystalline apatites in biological systems: characterisation, structure and properties. Materwiss. Werksttech. 38, 996–1002.

Ruffini, A., Sprio, S., Tampieri, A., 2013. Study of the hydrothermal transformation of wood-derived calcium carbonate into 3D hierarchically organized hydroxyapatite. Chem. Eng. J. 217, 150–158.

Saint-Jean, S.J., Camire, C.L., Nevsten, P., Hansen, S., Ginebra, M.P., 2005. Study of the reactivity and in vitro bioactivity of Sr-substituted alpha-TCP cements. J. Mater. Sci. Mater. Med. 16, 993–1001.

Scaglione, S., Giannoni, P., Bianchini, P., Sandri, M., Marotta, R., Firpo, G., et al., 2012. Order versus disorder: in vivo bone formation within osteoconductive scaffolds. Sci. Rep. 2 (274), 1–6.

Schumacher, M., Henss, A., Rohnke, M., Gelinsky, M., 2013. A novel and easy-to-prepare strontium(II) modified calcium phosphate bone cement with enhanced mechanical properties. Acta. Biomater. 9, 7536–7544.

Schumacher, M., Gelinsky, M., 2015. Strontium modified calcium phosphate cements – approaches towards targeted stimulation of bone turnover. J. Mater. Chem. B. 3, 4626–4640.

Sikavitsas, V.I., 2001. Biomaterials and bone mechanotransduction. Biomaterials. 22, 2581–2593.

Sopyan, I., Mardziah, C.M., Toibah, A.R., Singh, R., 2008. Synthesis of strontium-doped hydroxyapatite powder via sol-gel method. Adv. Mater. Res. 47-50, 928–931.

Sprio, S., Tampieri, A., Landi, E., Sandri, M., Martorana, S., Celotti, G., et al., 2008. Physico-chemical properties and solubility behaviour of multi-substituted hydroxyapatite powders containing silicon. Mater. Sci. Eng. C. 28, 179–187.

Sprio, S., Ruffini, A., Valentini, F., D'Alessandro, T., Sandri, M., Panseri, S., et al., 2011. Biomimesis and biomorphic transformations: new concepts applied to bone regeneration. J. Biotechnol. 156 (4), 347–355.

Sprio, S., Sandri, M., Iafisco, M., Panseri, S., Cunha, C., Ruffini, A., et al., 2013. Biomimetic materials in regenerative medicine. In: Ruys, A.J. (Ed.), Biomimetic Biomaterials: Structure and Applications. Woodhead Publishing Limited, Cambridge, pp. 3–45.

Sprio, S., Sandri, M., Iafisco, M., Panseri, S., Filardo, G., Kon, E., et al., 2014. *Composite bio*medical foams for en*gineering bone tissue*. In: Netti, P.A. (Ed.), Biomedical Foams for Tissue Engineering Applications. Woodhead Publishing Limited, Cambridge, pp. 249–280.

Sprio, S., Ruffini, A., Dapporto, M., Tampieri, A., 2016a. New strategies for regeneration of load bearing bones. In: Tampieri, A., Sprio, S. (Eds.), Bio-inspired Regenerative Medicine: Materials, Processes and Clinical Applications. PAN Stanford Publishing, Singapore, pp. 85–117.

Sprio, S., Dapporto, M., Montesi, M., Panseri, S., Lattanzi, W., Pola, E., et al., 2016b. Novel osteointegrative Sr-substituted apatitic cements enriched with alginate. Materials. 9, 763–780.

Sprio, S., Fricia, M., Maddalena, G., Nataloni, A., Tampieri, A., 2016c. Osteointegration in cranial bone reconstruction: a goal to achieve. J. Appl. Biomater. Funct. Mater. 14 (4), e470–e476.

Stetzer, E., 2011. Identifying Risk Factors for Osteoporosis in Young Women. Int. J. Allied Health Sci. Practice. 9, Number 4.

Studart, A.R., Gonzenbach, U.T., Tervoort, E., Gauckler, L.J., 2006. Processing routes to macroporous ceramics: a review. J. Am. Ceram. So. 89 (6), 1771–1789.

Tadic, D., Peters, F., Epple, M., 2002. Continuous synthesis of amorphous carbonated apatites. Biomaterials. 23, 2553–2559.

Takemasa, R., Kiyasu, K., Tani, T., Inoue, S., 2007. Validity of calcium phosphate cement vertebroplasty for vertebral non-union after osteoporotic fracture with middle column involvement. Spine J. 7, 148S.

Tampieri, A., Celotti, G., Landi, E., Sandri, M., Roveri, N., Falini, G., 2003. Biologically inspired synthesis of bone-like composite: self-assembled collagen fibers/hydroxyapatite nanocrystals. J. Biomed. Mater. Res. Part A. 67, 618–625.

Tampieri, A., Celotti, G., Landi, E., 2005. From biomimetic apatites to biologically inspired composites. Anal. Bioanal. Chem. 381, 568–576.

Tampieri, A., Celotti, G., Sprio, S., Delcogliano, A., Franzese, S., 2001. Porosity-graded hydroxyapatite ceramics to replace natural bone. Biomaterials 22, 1365–1370.

Tampieri, A., Sandri, M., Landi, E., Pressato, D., Francioli, S., Quarto, R., et al., 2008. Design of graded biomimetic osteochondral composite scaffolds. Biomaterials. 29, 3539–3546.

Tampieri, A., Sprio, S., Ruffini, A., Celotti, G., Lesci, I.G., Roveri, N., 2009. From Wood to Bone: multi-step process to convert wood hierarchical structures into biomimetic hydroxyapatite scaffolds for bone tissue engineering. J. Mater. Chem. 19 (28), 4973–4980.

Tampieri, A., Sprio, S., Sandri, M., Valentini, F., 2011. Mimicking natural bio-mineralization processes: a new tool for osteochondral scaffold development. Trends. Biotechnol. 29, 526–535.

Tampieri, A., D'Alessandro, T., Sandri, M., Sprio, S., Landi, E., Bertinetti, L., et al., 2012. Intrinsic magnetism and hyperthermia in bioactive Fe-doped hydroxyapatite. Acta. Biomater. 8, 843–851.

Tampieri, A., Iafisco, M., Sandri, M., Panseri, S., Cunha, C., Sprio, S., et al., 2014. Magnetic bioinspired hybrid nanostructured collagen–hydroxyapatite scaffolds supporting cell proliferation and tuning regenerative process. ACS Appl. Mater. Interfaces. 6, 15697–15707.

Thormann, U., Ray, S., Sommer, U., ElKhassawna, T., Rehling, T., Hundgeburth, M., et al., 2013. Bone formation induced by strontium modified calcium phosphate cement in critical-size metaphyseal fracture defects in ovariectomized rats. Biomaterials. 34, 8589–8598.

Vallet-Regi, M., 2014. In: Vallet-Regi, Maria (Ed.), Bio-Ceramics with Clinical Applications, 2014. Wiley, ISBN: 978-1-118-40672-4.

Wang, J.W., Shaw, L.L., 2007. Morphology-enhanced low-temperature sintering of nanocrystalline hydroxyapatite. Adv. Mater. 19, 2364–2369.

Wang, J.W., Nancollas, G.H., 2008. Calcium orthophosphates: crystallization and dissolution. Chem. Rev. 108, 4628–4669.

Weiner, S., 2008. Biomineralization: a structural perspective. J. Struct. Biol. 163, 229–234.

Welch, R.D., Zhang, H., Bronson, D.G., 2003. Experimental tibial plateau fractures augmented with calcium phosphate cement or autologous bone graft. J. Bone. Joint. Surg. 85, 222–231.

Wilcox, R.K., Boerger, T.O., Allen, D.J., Barton, D.C., Limb, D., Dickson, R.A., et al., 2003. A dynamic study of thoracolumbar burst fractures. J. Bone. Joint. Surg. 85-A (11), 2184–2189.

Wu, H.C., Wang, T.-W., Bohn, M.C., Lin, F.H., Spector, M., 2010. Novel magnetic hydroxyapatite nanoparticles as non-viral vectors for the glial cell line-derived neurotrophic factor gene. Adv. Funct. Mater. 20, 67–77.

Xu, H.-Y., Gu, N., 2014. Magnetic responsive scaffolds and magnetic fields in bone repair and regeneration. Front. Mater. Sci. 8, 20–31.

Ye, F., Guo, H.F., Zhang, H.J., 2008. Biomimetic synthesis of oriented hydroxyapatite mediated by nonionic surfactants. Nanotechnology. 19 (24), 7–10.

Yıldız Yaralı Özbek, Y.Y., Baştan, F.E., Üstel, F., 2016. Synthesis and characterization of strontium-doped hydroxyapatite for biomedical applications. J. Therm. Anal. Calorim. 125 (2), 745–750.

Yunos, D.M., Bretcanu, O., Boccaccini, A.R., 2008. Polymer-bioceramic composites for tissue engineering scaffolds. J. Mater. Sci. 43, 4433–4442.
Zhang, J.T., Liu, W.Z., Schnitzler, V., Tancret, F., Bouler, J.M., 2014. Calcium phosphate cements for bone substitution: chemistry, handling and mechanical properties. Acta. Biomater. 10 (3), 1035–1049.
Zhao, J., Guo, L.Y., Yang, X.B., Weng, J., 2008. Preparation of bioactive porous HA/PCL composite scaffolds. Appl. Surf. Sci. 255 (5), 2942–2946, Part 2.

## Further reading

Bock, N., Riminucci, A., Dionigi, C., Russo, A., Tampieri, A., Landi, E., et al., 2010. A novel route in bone tissue engineering: magnetic biomimetic scaffolds. Acta. Biomater. 6, 786–796.
Guo, C., Kaufman, L.J., 2007. Flow and magnetic field induced collagen alignment. Biomaterials. 28, 1105–1114.
Hori, J., Deie, M., Kobayashi, T., Yasunaga, Y., Kawamata, S., Ochi, M., 2011. Articular cartilage repair using an intra-articular magnet and synovium-derived cells. J. Orthop. Res. 29, 531–538.
Jiang, M., Terra, J., Rossi, A.M., Morales, M.A., Baggio-Saitovitch, E.M., Ellis, D.E., 2002. $Fe\ 2+/Fe\ 3+$ substitution in hydroxyapatite: theory and experiment. Phys. Rev. B. 66, 2241071–22410715.
Laschke, M.W., Harder, Y., Amon, M., Martin, I., Farhadi, J., Ring, A., et al., 2006. Angiogenesis in tissue engineering: breathing life into constructed tissue substitutes. Tiss. Eng. 12, 2093–2104.
Patel, Z.S., Young, S., Tabata, Y., Jansen, J.A., Wong, M.E.K., Mikos, A.G., 2008. Dual delivery of an angiogenic and an osteogenic growth factor for bone regeneration in a critical size defect model. Bone. 43, 931–940.
Schicker, M., Seitz, H., Drosse, I., Seitz, S., Mutschler, W., 2006. Biomaterials as scaffold for bone tissue engineering. Eur. J. Trauma. 32, 114–124.
Simioni, A.R., Martins, O.P., Lacava, Z.G.M., Azevedo, R.B., Lima, E.C.D., Lacava, B.M., et al., 2006. Cell toxicity studies of albumin-based nanosized magnetic beads. J. Nanosci. Nanotechnol. 6, 2413–2415.
Tampieri, A., Sandri, M., Panseri, S., Adamiano, A., Montesi, M., Sprio, S., 2016. Biologically-inspired nanomaterials and nano-bio-magnetism: a synergy among new emerging concepts in Regenerative Medicine. In: Tampieri, A., Sprio, S. (Eds.), Bioinspired Regenerative Medicine: Materials, Processes and Clinical Applications. PAN Stanford Publishing, Singapore.

# Advanced processing techniques for customized ceramic medical devices

**14**

*Eric Champion, Amandine Magnaudeix, Patricia Pascaud-Mathieu and Thierry Chartier*
University of Limoges, Limoges, France

**Chapter Outline**

**14.1 Introduction 433**
**14.2 Additive manufacturing: towards automization of customized organ fabrication 434**
14.2.1 Overview of AM of ceramics 434
14.2.2 Powder-based technologies 435
14.2.3 Slurry extrusion-based techniques 439
14.2.4 SLA 440
14.2.5 Indirect additive manufacturing 441
14.2.6 Critical role of 3D geometrical features of pores in scaffolds 441
**14.3 Freeze-templating: towards biomimetic architectured ceramics 443**
**14.4 Bioreactors and 3D cell culture techniques 446**
14.4.1 3D dynamic cell cultures and bioreactors 450
14.4.2 Features to take into consideration: decisional chart and parameters to standardize 453
**14.5 Concluding remarks 458**
**References 459**

## 14.1 Introduction

The improvement of healthcare and well-being of populations results in a growing need for synthetic materials in order to repair diseased or damaged living bone tissues. Among the public health issues in the field of bone graft substitutes, there is a significant interest in synthetic materials to replace autografts or allografts. Though autograft remains the gold standard due to its osteogenic and osteoconductive properties, the demand for synthetic materials is an increasing trend as well as the need for individual solutions to treat various osseous pathologies (such as large bone defects resulting from osteoporosis, tumour removal, or injuries, etc.) for which there are currently no satisfying solutions. Thus, the development of customized ceramics is a challenge to provide new high-performance medical devices. Two great fields of applications can be targeted: personalized medicine, requiring personalized fabrication of synthetic implants and bone tissue engineering, requiring production of 3D

**Advances in Ceramic Biomaterials.**
**DOI: http://dx.doi.org/10.1016/B978-0-08-100881-2.00015-4**

scaffolds with complex tailored architecture. Conventional ceramic processing techniques suffer from limitation or inability to produce near-net-shape parts with highly complex design. Advanced tools for the production of such devices include two main trends. The first consists of implementing additive manufacturing technologies and the second consists of producing biomimetic architectures using freeze-templating (also called ice-templating). In association with customized processing, advanced techniques of characterization are also required. They are of prime importance for a better understanding of the biological behavior of implants, which is necessary in order to provide rational criteria for the design of high-performance devices. In this field, the classical approaches include mainly two-dimensional (2D) static in vitro assays using cell lines or in vivo evaluations using animal models. The current trend is to set up new in vitro methods, using bioreactors, allowing 3D dynamic cell culture. The aim is on the one hand to define more realistic conditions of culture mimic in vivo behavior, and on the other hand, to replace animal experiments as far as possible. This chapter will focus on these main approaches of advanced processing and characterization of ceramic medical devices.

## 14.2 Additive manufacturing: towards automization of customized organ fabrication

The development of computer applications in the industry led to computer aided design and computer aided manufacturing (CAD/CAM) and for some years to novel additive manufacturing (AM) technologies. AM technologies are considered as new frontiers by the economists, bringing customers' needs and suppliers' offers closer. AM technologies have become the most used methods of producing within a short time, via an automated process, an accurate low-cost prototype. These techniques are today developed to become a real production tool in various industrial fields. Depending on the nature of the final object, the versatile AM techniques can also be used to produce cost-effective single items or a low-volume manufacturing. Such a concept requires developing smart materials and real-time control of fabrication. Among the fields of interest, high-added-value components and systems, frequently associated with niche markets such as bioceramics for medical applications, are relevant targets (Chartier et al., 2015). Thus, AM technologies (ASTM F2792-10: Standard Terminology for Additive Manufacturing Technologies, ASTM Intern., USA.) for the on-demand fabrication of customized implants for bone repair or scaffolds for bone tissue engineering are of increasing interest due to the wide possibilities they offer. The principles and applications of the AM technologies currently used for the development of bioceramics are detailed hereafter.

### *14.2.1 Overview of AM of ceramics*

AM techniques enable the shaping of 3D ceramic scaffolds with good accuracy and complex geometry using a layer-by-layer manufacturing process. A 3D model can

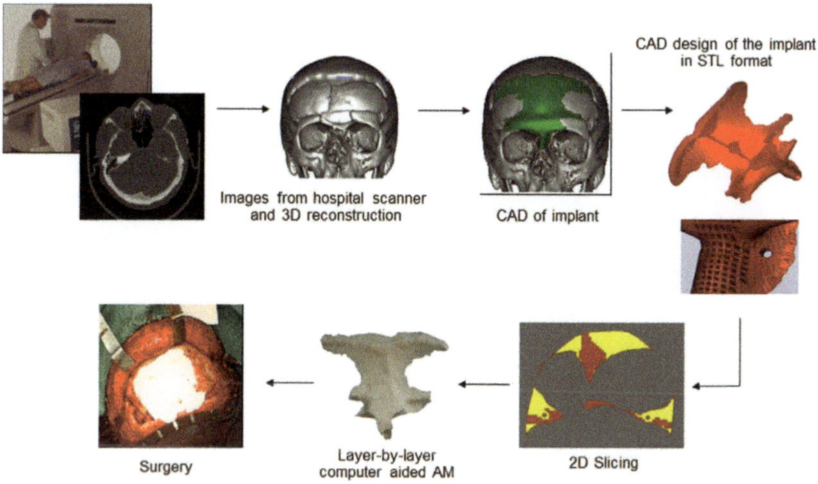


**Figure 14.1** Schematic representation of the main steps in the additive manufacturing (AM) approach. *CAD*, computer-aided design; *STL*, standard tessellation language. Courtesy of 3DCeram (Limoges, France, http://3dceram.com/) and University Hospital Centre of Limoges (France).

be designed from medical imaging techniques commonly used for diagnostic purposes or directly by CAD software treatment before being converted into a standard tessellation language (STL) file and then sliced into 2D layers in order to be loaded into the building machine (Fig. 14.1).

Depending on the fabrication principle, AM techniques set up for the fabrication of customized implants for bone repair or scaffolds for bone tissue engineering (Fig. 14.2) can be classified into four categories : selective laser sintering (SLS), 3D printing (3DP), slurry extrusion-based techniques, and stereolithography (SLA) (Brunello et al., 2016; Hutmacher, Sittinger and Risbud, 2004; Melchels, Feijen,and Grijpma, 2010; Mota et al., 2015; Zocca et al., 2015). These AM methods display different advantages and limitations in terms of accuracy, surface roughness and mechanical properties, as summarized in Table 14.1.

### 14.2.2 Powder-based technologies

#### 14.2.2.1 SLS

The SLS process is based on the selective sintering of ceramic powder bed, using a high-intensity laser beam (usually $CO_2$ laser) forming, layer-by-layer, solid 3D objects (Fig. 14.2A). The local densification of the powders can be obtained by directly sintering the ceramic powder or by mixing the powder with a binder phase which is then melted by the laser light. Unmelted powder serves as a support structure and this remaining powder is removed from the part after shaping.

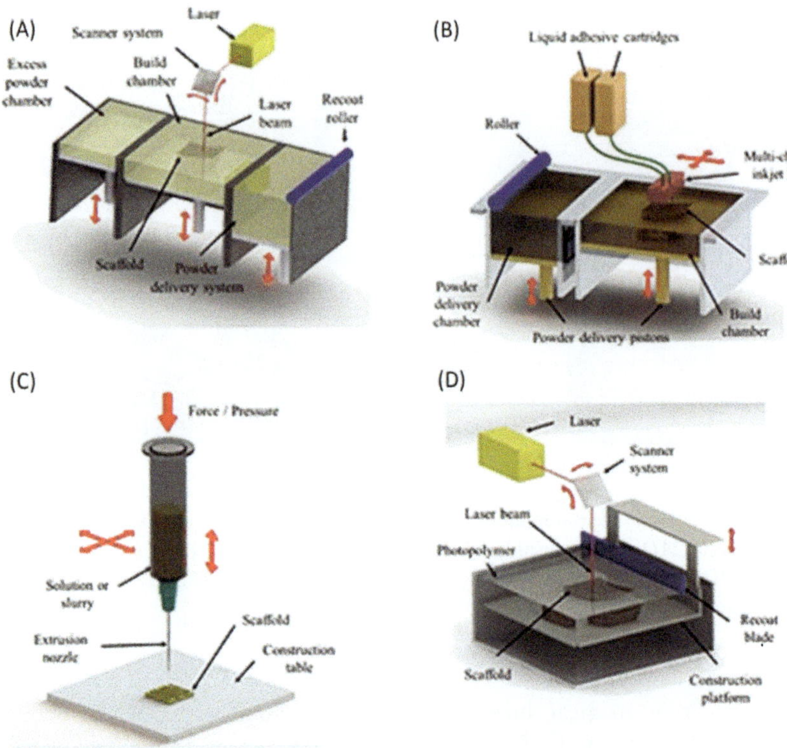


**Figure 14.2** Schematic representation of the most common additive manufacturing techniques employed in tissue engineering. (A) Selective laser sintering; (B) 3D printing; (C) slurry extrusion-based technique; and (D) stereolithography.
Reprinted from Mota, C., Puppi, D., Chiellini, F., Chiellini, E., 2015. Additive manufacturing techniques for the production of tissue engineering constructs. J. Tissue Eng. Regen. Med. 9, 174–190. doi:10.1002/term.1635, copyright © 2012, with permission from John Wiley & Sons.

Lee et al. were the first, in 1994, to use SLS to manufacture ceramic bone implants based on calcium phosphate powders (Lee and Barlow, 1994). More recently, Shuai et al. (2013) have reported the fabrication of biphasic calcium phosphate ceramic parts using the SLS process (Fig. 14.3(1)). However, SLS remains mainly limited in terms of mechanical properties and accuracy of the manufactured part (Table 14.1) even though some studies (Duan et al., 2010; Eosoly et al., 2012; Liu et al., 2013) have suggested the addition of a small amount of polymer to calcium phosphate powder in order to improve the mechanical properties of scaffolds fabricated via SLS (Fig. 14.3(2)).

**Table 14.1** **Tolerances, advantages and limitations of additive manufacturing methods used in tissue engineering**

| AM techniques | Type of feedstock (Zocca et al., 2015) | Tolerance | Advantages | Limitations |
|---|---|---|---|---|
| Selective laser sintering | Powder suspension | Smallest feature : 45–100 μm (Butscher et al., 2011) | High production rates, low cost<br>Complex designs | High roughness of the surface<br>Poor mechanical properties<br>Limited to materials which absorb IR light |
| Three-dimensional printing | Powder suspension | Smallest feature: 350–500 μm (Butscher et al., 2011) | Wide variety of materials<br>Simple technology | High roughness of the surface<br>Expensive technology<br>Poor mechanical properties |
| Slurry extrusion-based technique | Paste | Filament diameter: 50–1000 μm (Zocca et al., 2015) | Ease of support removal<br>Good mechanical properties<br>No material waste | Precision limited by the filament diameter |
| Stereolithography | Suspension | Layer thickness: 10–50 μm (Zocca et al., 2015) | Complex designs<br>Good surface finishing<br>Good mechanical properties<br>High accuracy | Expensive photosensitive resins<br>Cleaning step necessary<br>Debinding |

Adapted from (Chartier et al. 2015), copyright 2014, with permission from Göller Verlag.

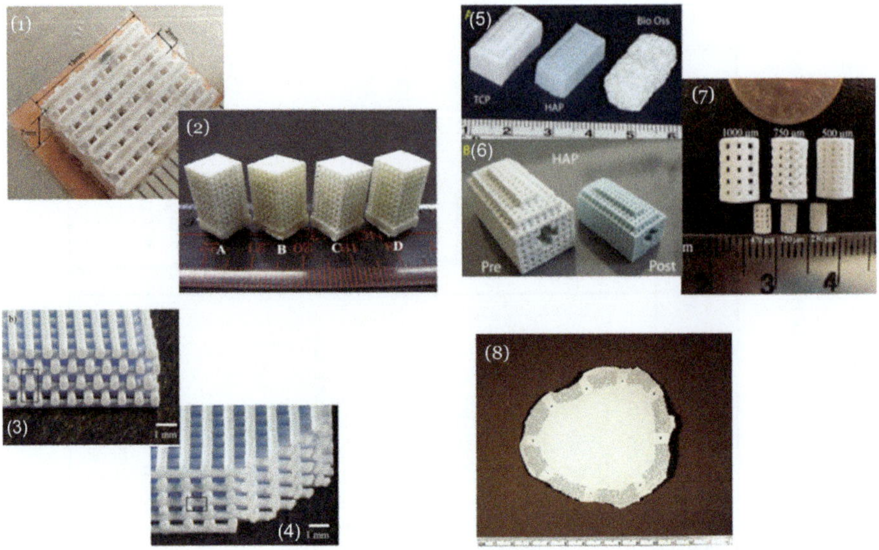


**Figure 14.3** Photographs of scaffolds produced through different additive manufacturing techniques. (1) Porous BCP scaffold fabricated by selective laser sintering, reprinted from Shuai, C., Li, P., Liu, J., Peng, S., 2013. Optimization of TCP/HAP ratio for better properties of calcium phosphate scaffold via selective laser sintering. Mater. Charact. 77, 23–31. doi:10.1016/j.matchar.2012.12.009, copyright © 2013, with permission from Elsevier. (2) Scaffolds produced by selective laser sintering: (A) PHBV; (B) Ca-P/PHBV; (C) PLLA; (D) CHAp/PLLA; reproduced from Duan, B., Wang, M., Zhou, W.Y., Cheung, W.L., Li, Z.Y., Lu, W.W., 2010. Three-dimensional nanocomposite scaffolds fabricated via selective laser sintering for bone tissue engineering. Acta Biomater. 6, 4495–4505. doi:10.1016/j.actbio.2010.06.024, copyright © 2010, with permission from Elsevier. (3) Periodic hydroxyapatite (HA)scaffolds built up by means of robocasting machine with three-dimensional (3D)interconnected porosity with simple tetragonal and (4) face-centered symmetries, reprinted from Dellinger, J.G., Cesarano, J., Jamison, R.D., 2007. Robotic deposition of model hydroxyapatite scaffolds with multiple architectures and multiscale porosity for bone tissue engineering. J. Biomed. Mater. Res. A 82, 383–394. doi:10.1002/jbm.a.31072, copyright © 2007, with permission from John Wiley & Sons. (5) Tricalcium phosphate (TCP) scaffolds – HA scaffolds produced by 3D printing and block of bone replacement material BioOss as a control and (6) HA block after printing (Pre) and after sintering (Post), reprinted from Warnke, P.H., Seitz, H., Warnke, F., Becker, S.T., Sivananthan, S., Sherry, E., et al., 2010. Ceramic scaffolds produced by computer-assisted 3D printing and sintering: characterization and biocompatibility investigations. J. Biomed. Mater. Res. B Appl. Biomater. 93, 212–217. doi:10.1002/jbm.b.31577, copyright © 2010, with permission from John Wiley & Sons. (7) Sintered β-TCP scaffolds manufactured using 3D printing, reprinted from Tarafder, S., Balla, V.K., Davies, N.M., Bandyopadhyay, A., Bose, S., 2013. Microwave-sintered 3D printed tricalcium phosphate scaffolds for bone tissue engineering. J. Tissue Eng. Regen. Med. 7, 631–641. doi:10.1002/term.555, copyright © 2013, with permission from John Wiley & Sons. (8) HA cranial prosthesis, reprinted from Brie, J., Chartier, T., Chaput, C., Delage, C., Pradeau, B., Caire, F., et al., 2013. A new custom made bioceramic implant for the repair of large and complex craniofacial bone defects. J. Craniomaxillofacial Surg. 41, 403–407. doi:10.1016/j.jcms.2012.11.005, copyright © 2013, with permission from Elsevier.

#### 14.2.2.2 3D printing

In powder-based 3D printing, ceramic scaffolds are built up by a liquid binder selectively sprayed by means of an inkjet head onto a powder bed (Fig. 14.2B), binding the particles together. The consolidated green part is subsequently sintered in order to obtain 3D ceramic scaffolds. The ease of use makes it one of the most implemented methods of producing a wide variety of ceramic parts (Table 14.1). In the field of ceramic medical devices, some specimens (Fig. 14.3(5–7)) have been built using powder-binder systems from hydroxyapatite (HA) and/or β-tricalcium phosphate (β-TCP) powders (Butscher et al., 2011; Fielding, Bandyopadhyay and Bose, 2012; Leukers et al., 2005; Tarafder et al., 2013; Warnke et al., 2010). For example, Tarafder et al. have manufactured 3D-printed TCP scaffolds containing multiscale porosity and investigated in vitro cell–materials interactions and behavior of scaffolds in vivo. Results showed that the presence of macro- and micropores improved osteoid-like new bone formation (Tarafder et al., 2013). Another team has evidenced that the addition of dopants (silica and zinc oxide) to the TCP increased mechanical strength of scaffolds and further cellular proliferation (Fielding, Bandyopadhyay and Bose, 2012) and highlighted the great potential of such bioresorbable scaffolds for bone tissue repair.

It should be noted that an extension of powder-based technology previously called "slurry-based 3D printing" (S-3DP) and "slurry-based SLS" (S-SLS) technologies exist. In this instance, a liquid suspension of ceramic particles, instead of dry powder, is spread as a thin layer in order to increase the powder packing density in the powder bed (Zocca et al., 2015).

### 14.2.3 Slurry extrusion-based techniques

Robocasting (RB) is an additive manufacturing technique, referred-to as a direct-write assembly (DWA) method based on robotic deposition of a viscous ceramic paste by means of continuous extrusion through a nozzle onto a construction platform (Fig. 14.2C). This technology, patented and developed by Cesarano for ceramic applications (Cesarano, 1999), requires complete control of the rheological properties of the paste filament. Indeed, the ceramic suspension must undergo a transformation from a pseudoplastic to a dilatant behavior during extrusion, to avoid deformation of the ceramic part after extrusion and sagging of the filaments, especially for the most porous scaffolds. Through RB, ceramic scaffolds can be built up with good mechanical characteristics (Table 14.1) but the accuracy remains conditioned by the diameter and the geometry of the nozzle, which are restrictive parameters.

Tailor-made calcium phosphate ceramic parts have lately been fabricated by extrusion techniques (Fig. 14.3(3–4)) based on HA and/or β-TCP slurries (Dellinger et al., 2007; Michna, Wu and Lewis, 2005; Miranda et al., 2006, 2008). Dellinger et al. have developed scaffolds based on HA powders with architecture including three varieties of porosities to promote bone ingrowth. Macropores (100–600 μm), micropores (1–30 μm), and submicron pores (<1 μm) were obtained, respectively, by controlling the design of raw scaffolds (arrangement and spacing between rods), by incorporating polymer microspheres as porogen agent in the HA paste, and by optimizing the sintering of raw scaffolds. Multiscale porosity, micropores, and submicron pores can serve as growth factor tank or drug reservoir for local release to induce vascularization and bone ingrowth (Dellinger et al., 2007). Besides, Miranda et al. have proved the excellent mechanical features of robocast calcium phosphate scaffolds even after immersion in simulated body fluid (SBF) pointing out their potential in load-bearing bone tissue engineering application (Miranda et al., 2008).

### 14.2.4 SLA

SLA is a process based on laser technology. A photosensitive ceramic-powder-loaded suspension is selectively polymerized by a laser beam or a ultraviolet (UV) light. The consolidated part, elaborated layer by layer, is subsequently cleaned to remove the excess of unpolymerized suspension, then debinded and sintered to obtain a dense ceramic part. Reactive slurry is composed of UV curable monomer, a photoinitiator and additives (diluent and dispersant) for the dispersion of the ceramic powder.

The use of stereolithographic fabrication methods, commercially available for more than 20 years, to custom ceramics medical devices is flourishing. Indeed scaffolds produced by SLA present a good surface finishing, good mechanical properties, and high accuracy. Yet, the main limitations of SLA remain the cleaning and the debinding steps.

Different calcium phosphate scaffolds designed by SLA for bone replacement have been currently marketed[1]. Besides, this technique has recently revealed its efficiency to produce large customized patient-specific implants for bone repair, from a suspension of hydroxyapatite, marketed and successfully implanted on complex craniofacial bone defects (Fig. 14.3(8–9)) by the Neurosurgery and Maxillofacial surgery Departments of Limoges University Hospital Centre (Brie et al., 2013).

In parallel to the traditional SLA technique, the microstereolithography (μSLA) process has been developed and recently implemented to produce scaffolds with higher accuracy by increasing the dimensional resolution up to approximately 10-times greater than SLA. The principle is based on the illumination by a UV light of the suspension layer to be polymerized, through a dynamic mask generated by a digital micromirror device (Chartier et al., 2015). The use of such an accurate technique requires an optimal formulation of UV curable suspension combined with full control of μSLA processing parameters. The processability of silicon-substituted hydroxyapatite scaffolds by μSLA has been subjected to a specific study (Lasgorceix, Champion and Chartier, 2016) in which authors propose an empiric

[1] http://www.lithoz.com/en/products/materials/
http://blog.sirris.be/fr/blog/ladditive-manufacturing-pour-favoriser-la-reconstruction-osseuse
http://www.osseomatrix.com/
http://3dceram.com/category/biomedical/applications/

dimensioning model taking into account the overcure phenomena, which occur because of light scattering on ceramic particles, during the photopolymerization step and the shrinkage during sintering, for the reliable production of porous ceramic parts. μSLA allows good control of pore shape, a parameter of prime importance in scaffold design for cell colonization (see Section 14.2.6), which is hardly achievable by any other direct methods of ceramic parts shaping using AM.

### 14.2.5 Indirect additive manufacturing

Additive manufacturing can be used to shape ceramic scaffolds directly, as described above, or indirectly by the initial AM of a polymer mould, which will serve as a negative sacrificial organic template of the ceramic part to be produced. Then, a ceramic suspension is cast in the mold before heat treatments of debinding, to burn the mold, and sintering of the ceramic part (Fig. 14.4). The mold can be fabricated either by 3D printing of stereolithography (Skoog, Goering and Narayan 2014, Charbonnier, Laurent and Marchat 2016). In fact, indirect AM to shape ceramic parts is considered to be much easier than direct AM because of the use of polymers instead of ceramic powder-loaded suspensions, for which formulation is difficult to optimize. Indeed, direct AM requires highly loaded suspensions with specific rheological behavior for the AM step. Polymers would also permit finer features because there is no scattering of the laser beam on ceramic particles as well as a much easier cleaning step to remove unpolymerized liquid in the case of SLA and to overcome the lack of architectural control at local and global scales especially for 3D printing. Indirect SLA for the production of porous HA implants and calcium phosphate scaffolds with designed external architecture has been developed by Chu et al. (2001) and indirect 3D priting by Charbonnier et al. (2016).

### 14.2.6 Critical role of 3D geometrical features of pores in scaffolds

Several studies have investigated the effects of porosity and pore size of biomaterial scaffolds produced by AM on new tissue ingrowth. Several requirements have been identified as essential for the production of scaffolds. An interconnected porous network, with interconnections of around 50–100 μm and pores with a size in the range 300–600 μm, is recommended to allow cell migration and transport and to promote vascularization (Karageorgiou and Kaplan, 2005; Marques et al., 2017; Sachlos and Czernuszka, 2003).

The impact of the macroscopic geometry of the substrate on the kinetics of tissue deposition has been recently revealed through a model of curvature-driven growth (Rumpler et al., 2008, Bidan et al., 2013). Results highlight that the significant parameters of influence are the radius of curvature, the convexity, and the presence and size of angles. The effects of pore shape on blood vessel guidance and angio-conductive potential have been shown using an ex ovo model (Magnaudeix et al., 2016). Therefore, the optimization of pore shapes is a relevant approach for improving the rate of ingrowth of bone tissue into ceramic scaffolds. This accurate control of pore shape

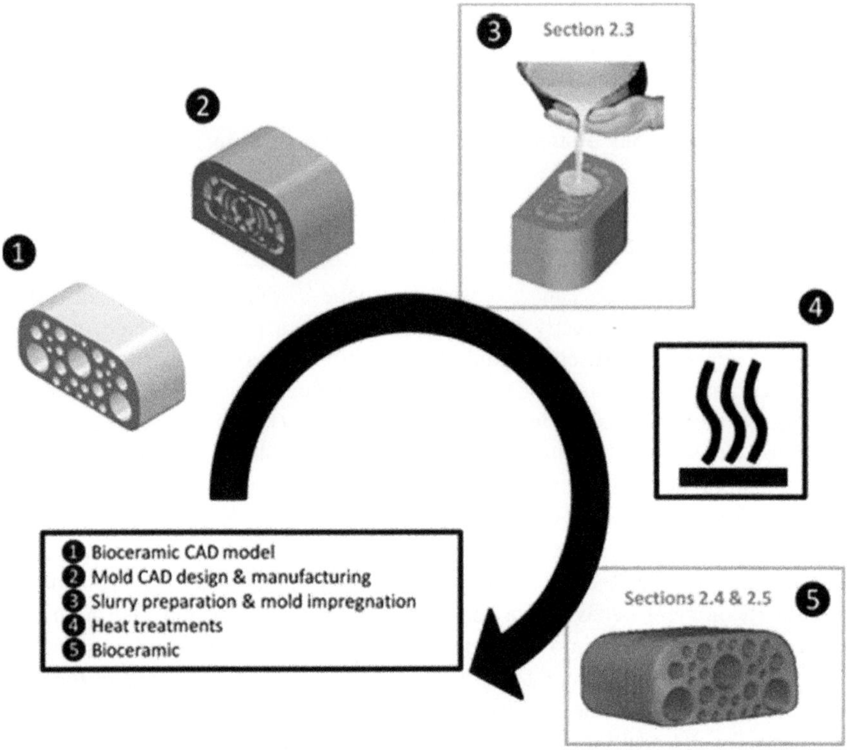


**Figure 14.4** Representation of the developed manufacturing process including : (1) the bioceramic computer-aided design (CAD) model, (2) the mold CAD model, which is a negative of the bioceramic structure, and its production using a 3D printer, (3) mold impregnation by a ceramic suspension, (4) heat-treatments of debinding and sintering to obtain, and (5) the bioceramic.
Reprinted from Charbonnier, B., Laurent, C., Marchat, D., 2016. Porous hydroxyapatite bioceramics produced by impregnation of 3D-printed wax mold: Slurry feature optimization. J. Eur. Ceram. Soc. 36, 4269-4279., copyright © 2016, with permission from Elsevier.

and more generally of the architectural design of the porous network of ceramic scaffolds is now possible thanks to AM techniques. Several authors have investigated specific architectures from the 3D periodic reproduction of unit cells (Fig. 14.5). Numerical approaches using such models have been developed with the aim to optimize the scaffold architectures (Hollister, Maddox and Taboas, 2002; Rajagopalan and Robb, 2006; Hollister and Lin, 2007; Yoo, 2011). They focus mainly on the optimization of the mechanical properties of scaffolds and on their permeability.

Finally, AM technologies are efficient for generating bioceramic scaffolds with controlled architectural design, either at the macroscopic scale to produce customized ceramic implants or at the microscopic scale to control the internal porous architecture of ceramic scaffolds. They open a new way of thinking and fabricating scaffolds more selectively designed to display the specificity of bone

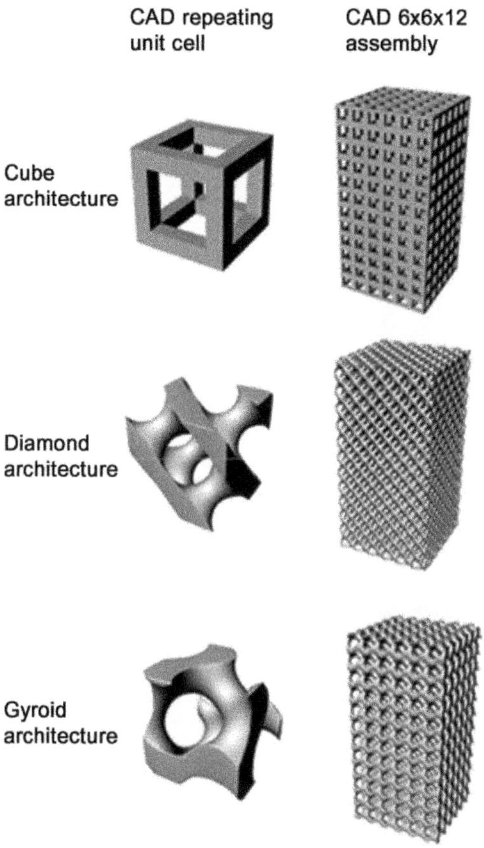


**Figure 14.5** Visualizations of the different porous architectures. Left: CAD-designs of the repeating unit cells. Right: CAD-designs of assemblies of 6 × 6 × 12 unit cells. Reprinted from Melchels, F.P., Bertoldi, K., Gabbrielli, R., Velders, A.H., Feijen, J., & Grijpma, D.W. (2010). Mathematically defined tissue engineering scaffold architectures prepared by stereolithography. Biomaterials, 31(27), 6909-6916, copyright © 2010, with permission from Elsevier.

repair needs (see Chapter 8: Ceramic devices for bone regeneration: mechanical and clinical issues and new perspectives, for more details on this point). In the field of scaffolds for applications in bone tissue engineering, as reviewed by Giannitelli et al., the current trend is to combine several AM technologies, and further developments should combine AM with biofabrication methods (Giannitelli et al., 2015).

## 14.3 Freeze-templating: towards biomimetic architectured ceramics

Freeze-templating is a direct foaming method to create a porous network in ceramic materials. Its principle (Fig. 14.6) consists of freezing a ceramic suspension in order

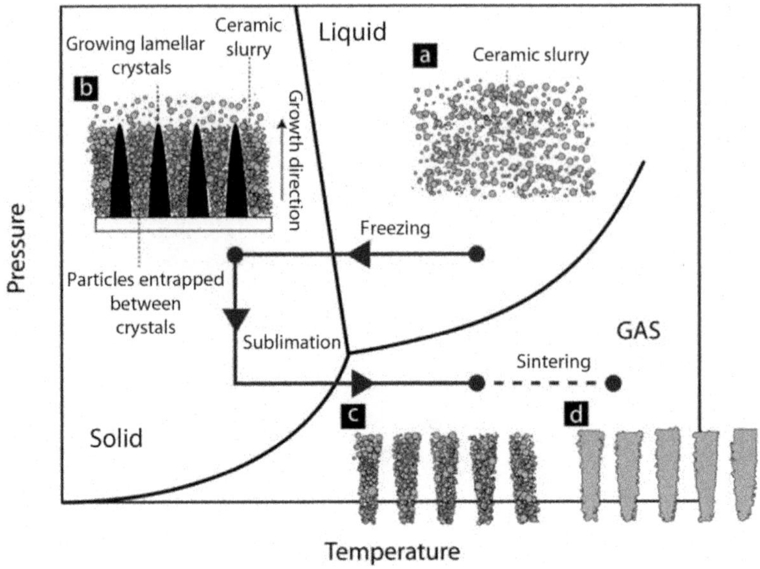


**Figure 14.6** The four processing steps of freeze-casting: slurry preparation, solidification, sublimation, and sintering.
Reprinted from Deville, S., 2008. Freeze-casting of porous ceramics: a review of current achievements and issues. Adv. Engng Mat. 10, 155-169, copyright © 2008, with permission from Wiley-VCH Verlag.

to form crystals of solvent entrapping the ceramic particles. The solvent is then sublimated to form pores and the remaining green ceramic sintered.

Schematic of freezing process is given in Fig. 14.7A (see Meurice et al., 2016 for example of equipment). A suspension is poured in a container placed on a metallic plate whose temperature is controlled by a refrigerant (e.g., nitrogen, ethanol). The key point of the process is the step of freezing that must induce solidification and crystal growth of solvent. This stage will construct the porous network by growth of crystal solvent (Deville, 2008), whose direction is guided by the temperature gradients imposed on the mould. The solvent is usually water or camphene ($C_6H_{16}$). The latter, with a melting point of 51°C, allows freezing at ambient temperature. Crystallization of these solvents produces typical dendritic-like crystals (Fig. 14.7B) whose growth results in the formation of aligned lamellar pores crossing the ceramic after solvent sublimation and sintering (Fig. 14.8A). Such a porous microstructure is expected to be of interest in the biomedical field for the development of porous biomaterials with improved properties (for a review, see Deville, 2010; Pawelec et al., 2014). For instance, due to this specific lamellar porosity, enhanced mechanical properties were found compared to porous hydroxyapatite ceramics produced by other methods (Deville, Saiz and Tomsia, 2006; see Fig. 8.4).

The control of pore morphology, size and 3D organization of porous networks is the main issue to overcome to obtain scaffolds that promote effective bone tissue ingrowth.

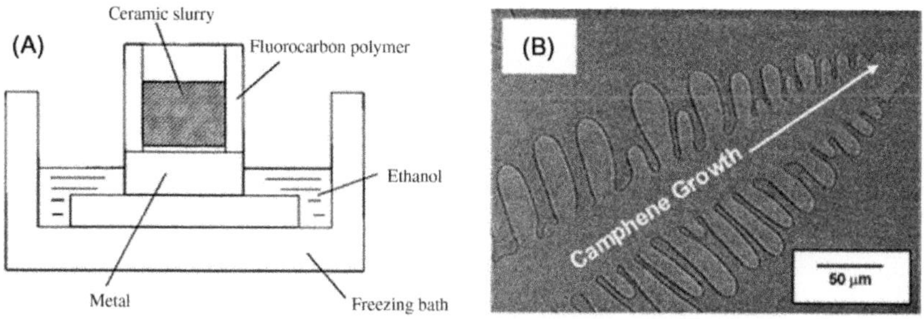


**Figure 14.7** (A) Schematic of freezing process. The container was composed of two parts: the container bottom made of metal with high thermal conductivity and the side of fluorocarbon polymer. Only the container bottom face was immersed in a refrigerant in a freezing bath, reprinted from Fukasawa, T., Z.-Y. Deng, Ando, M., Ohji, T., Goto, Y., 2001. Pore structure of porous ceramics synthesized from water-based slurry by freeze-dry process. J. Mat. Sci. 36, 2523–2527 (Fukasawa et al., 2001), copyright © 2001, with permission from Springer Science. (B) Solidified camphene dendrites leading to the formation of a dendritic porous structure, reprinted from Yoon, B.-H., Lee, E.-J., Kim, H.-E., Koh, Y.-H., 2007. Highly aligned porous silicon carbide ceramics by freezing polycarbosilane/camphene solution, J. Am. Ceram. Soc. 90, 1753–1759, copyright © 2007, with permission from John Wiley & Sons.

Numerous parameters may influence the porosity design; the main ones (listed in (i)) relate to the formulation of suspensions and the others (listed in (ii)) to the equipment settings and freeze conditions.

**i.** Different solvents (e.g., water, camphene, tert-butyl alcohol) (Deville, Saiz and Tomsia, 2006; Lee et al., 2007; Zhang et al., 2013, Yoon et al., 2007; Macchetta, Turner and Bowen, 2009) or mixtures of solvents (e.g., mixtures of water and dioxane or glycerol to form binary pro- or hyper-eutectic liquids) have been investigated (Rahaman and Fu, 2008). Depending on the formulation, various crystal morphologies can be obtained during freezing (for a review, see Pawelec et al., 2014). This results in different microstructures of freeze-cast scaffolds with lamellar or prismatic pores (Fig. 14.8A–D). The addition of $H_2O_2$ in water was also investigated with the aim of produce both lamellar and spherical pores (Cheng, Zhao and Wu, 2015). Besides the solvent formulation, ceramic particle size and distribution will also affect the behavior during freezing and may influence the final microstructure (Deville, 2008). And more generally, the whole formulation of suspensions (i.e., ceramic/liquid ratio, amount of dispersants, binders) must also be taken into account (Fu et al., 2007, Zhang et al., 2013).

**ii.** Conditions of freezing will also influence the porous network design. Various equipments were set up to control the direction of freezing. Different thermal gradients can be applied to orient the crystal growth and therefore the pore direction within the scaffold: from bottom to top using setup similar to the schematic of Fig. 14.7 or radial from inner to outer surface of scaffolds using a rod located in the center of the mould (Moon et al., 2003) or using a controlled temperature gradient, as illustrated in Fig. 14.8E and F (Macchetta et al., 2009).

As described above, attempts have been made to control of porous design of freeze-templating scaffolds for further application in bone surgery, but up until

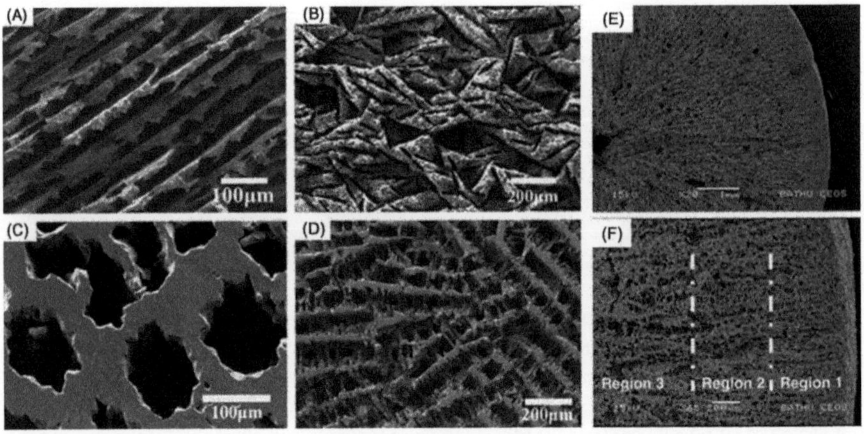


**Figure 14.8** Scanning electron microscopic images of hydroxyapatite constructs prepared from aqueous suspensions (A), and suspensions with 8 mol% (30 wt%) dioxane (B), 23 mol% (60 wt%) dioxane (C), and 1.25 mol% (5 wt%) glycerol (D), reprinted from Rahaman, M.N., Fu, Q., 2008. Manipulation of porous bioceramic microstructures by freezing of suspensions containing binary mixtures of solvents, J. Am. Ceram. Soc. 91[12], 4137-4140, copyright ©2008, with permission from John Wiley and Sons. (E, F) Graded porosity with three distinct regions, from Macchetta, A., Turner, I.G., Bowen, C.R., 2009. Fabrication of HA/TCP scaffolds with a graded and porous structure using a camphene-based freeze-casting method. Acta Biomater. 5, 1319–1327, copyright ©2009, with permission from Elsevier.

now, very few works have investigated the biological behavior of scaffolds (Fu et al., 2009, Meurice et al., 2016). Observation of scaffolds after in vitro culture using MG63 (Meurice et al., 2016) or MC3T3-E1 cell lines (Fu et al., 2009) showed that lamellar pores were not favorable to cell colonization, cellular (spherical) pores being much more colonized (Fig. 14.9). These observations result probably from the size of lamellar pores whose widths appear too small, leading to a fast closure of pores near the outer surface of scaffolds. The in vitro set up used in these studies, i.e., 2D static cell culture, may also account for such behavior of cells. This latter point is also crucial to better understanding the influence of porous architecture (i.e., size, shape and 3D network) on tissue ingrowth and further validate scaffold designs; this will be discussed in the following Section 14.4.

Finally, freeze-templating appears of particular interest to produce porous bioceramics but efforts are still needed in the control of processing parameters and setup to achieve the manufacture of high-performance scaffolds with adjusted design to the target applications in bone tissue engineering.

## 14.4 Bioreactors and 3D cell culture techniques

Efforts are being made to develop a new generation of bioceramic scaffolds for the repair of large bone defects using tissue engineering strategies (see Chapter 8:

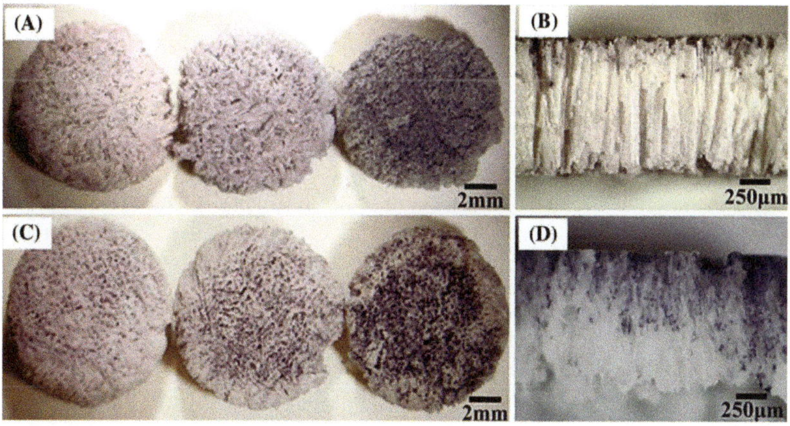


**Figure 14.9** Cell-seeded hydroxyapatite constructs treated with tetrazolium dye (MTT): (left) surface of constructs with (A) lamellar-type and (C) cellular type microstructure after culture intervals of 2, 4, and 6 days (left to right, respectively); (right) freeze-fracture section of scaffold cultured for 6 days, showing considerably greater infiltration of MTT-labeled cells into the interior of the cellular microstructure (D) than in the lamellar microstructure (B). Reprinted from Fu, Q., Rahaman, M.N., Sonny Bal, B., Brown, R.F., 2009. Proliferation and function of MC3T3-E1 cells on freeze-cast hydroxyapatite scaffolds with oriented pore architectures. J. Mater. Sci: Mater. Med. 20, 1159–1165, copyright © 2009, with permission from Springer Science.

Ceramic devices for bone regeneration: mechanical and clinical issues and new perspectives, for more details). Ideally, the scaffold should be bioactive (i.e., able to actively induce a desired biological response) and possibly resorbing, so that the implanted devices would be totally replaced by de novo functional and vascularized bone tissue. While, per se rather artefactual, by allowing strict control of cell environment parameters, in vitro methods are the minimum prerequisite to all procedures of evaluation and characterization of the biological behavior of a given biomaterial (Grayson et al., 2009). Advanced methods are necessary to evaluate the biological properties of scaffolds supporting cellular activities and new tissue ingrowth at a long distance from the native host tissues. First of all, it is fundamental to keep in mind and to understand how the targeted healthy tissue is organized and structured, in order to optimize and make as pertinent as possible the experimental set ups. Overall, these tissues are complex, involving interactions between several different cell types constituting them with intrinsic specificities (Cazzaniga et al., 2014) that can be evidenced in vitro using 3D coculture settings (Grellier et al., 2009; Penolazzi et al., 2016). In an obvious tri-dimensional configuration (Griffith and Swartz, 2006; Liu et al., 2015), and immersed in interstitial fluid, most cells are sensitive and responsive to mechanical cues, especially flow shear (Barbee et al., 1995; Klein-Nulend et al., 2005; Skerry, 2008; Missirlis, 2016; Ren et al., 2015; Rosa et al., 2015). Mechanical stimulation is essential for tissue homeostasis maintenance, and in numerous healing and regenerative processes

(Chatzizisis et al., 2007; Chien, 2006). Hence, at the cellular level, mechanical forces affect cell behaviors such as proliferation, migration, or differentiation (Gjorevski et al., 2015; Griffith and Swartz, 2006; Paluch et al., 2015; Viswanathan et al., 2015). Cellular morphology in 2D settings is very different (flattened cells in cell monolayer) from morphology adopted in a 3D configuration (Cukierman, 2001; Harunaga and Yamada, 2011). Depending on the size of voids in the scaffold, cells emit extensions and span through them with a totally different sensitivity and behavior toward physical stress (McCoy and O'Brien, 2012, 2010; Morris et al., 2010). Some cell types present even only physiological responses when cultured in three dimensions. This is the case for the very specialized bone mechanosensitive osteocytes (Boukhechba et al., 2009) whose communication with other cells is of importance for bone homeostasis maintenance (Nakashima et al., 2011). In 2D culture, seeded scaffolds are transferred to a fresh culture plate after cell attachment but cells can migrate to the culture plastic and induce artefactual effects on the surface and inside the scaffold (Bjerre et al., 2008) (Fig. 14.10(1)). Moreover, cells grow in a monolayer at the surface of a biomaterial, becoming rapidly confluent, and produce an impermeable extracellular matrix (ECM) resulting in an encapsulation effect (Campos et al., 2014). This distorts the ECM role to support and constitute tri-dimensional environment sustaining tissue growth and the differentiation behavior of the cells (Datta et al., 2006; Bjerre et al., 2008; Campos et al., 2014). Additionally, the absence of flow, one of drawbacks of static culture, results in a poor diffusion and availability of gas and nutrients and makes the evacuation of metabolic wastes impossible (Martin et al., 2004). Consequently, an inhomogeneity of cell distribution over the scaffolds forms with cells mainly found in peripheral zones and a decrease in cell viability in the center (absence of nutrient, hypoxia) associated with necrosis.

For these reasons, usual 2D static in vitro cell culture should be considered as a strong oversimplification (Grayson et al., 2009). Accordingly, numerous works have evidenced that 3D dynamic cell culture in bioreactors is essential to mimic cell microenvironment with controlled parameters (nutrient availability, pH, oxygenation, etc.) and to obtain physiological and realistic responses (Bouet et al., 2015; Boukhechba et al., 2009; Braccini et al., 2005; Grayson et al., 2009). Cell functions and activities are enhanced in dynamic 3D culture when compared to static 2D settings (Almela et al., 2016; Grellier et al., 2009; Silva et al., 2014; Yu et al., 2004; Bancroft et al., 2003; Bjerre et al., 2008; Holtorf et al., 2005; Katayama et al., 2013; Sailon et al., 2009). Despite providing supplemental cellular responses owing to mechanical strain input using a plate-flow chamber, dynamic 2D culture remains very simplified because of the absence of a third dimension (McCoy and O'Brien, 2010 ; Morris et al., 2010). By improving mass transfer of oxygen and nutrients as well as metabolic waste, on the one hand and, on the other through the third dimension increasing the surface for cell culture and modifying cell responses features, bioreactors allow longer culture duration providing thus more comprehensive data on cell differentiation processes (Penolazzi et al., 2016; Sikavitsas et al., 2003). Consequently, they are ideally suitable for the assessment of biological properties of scaffolds.

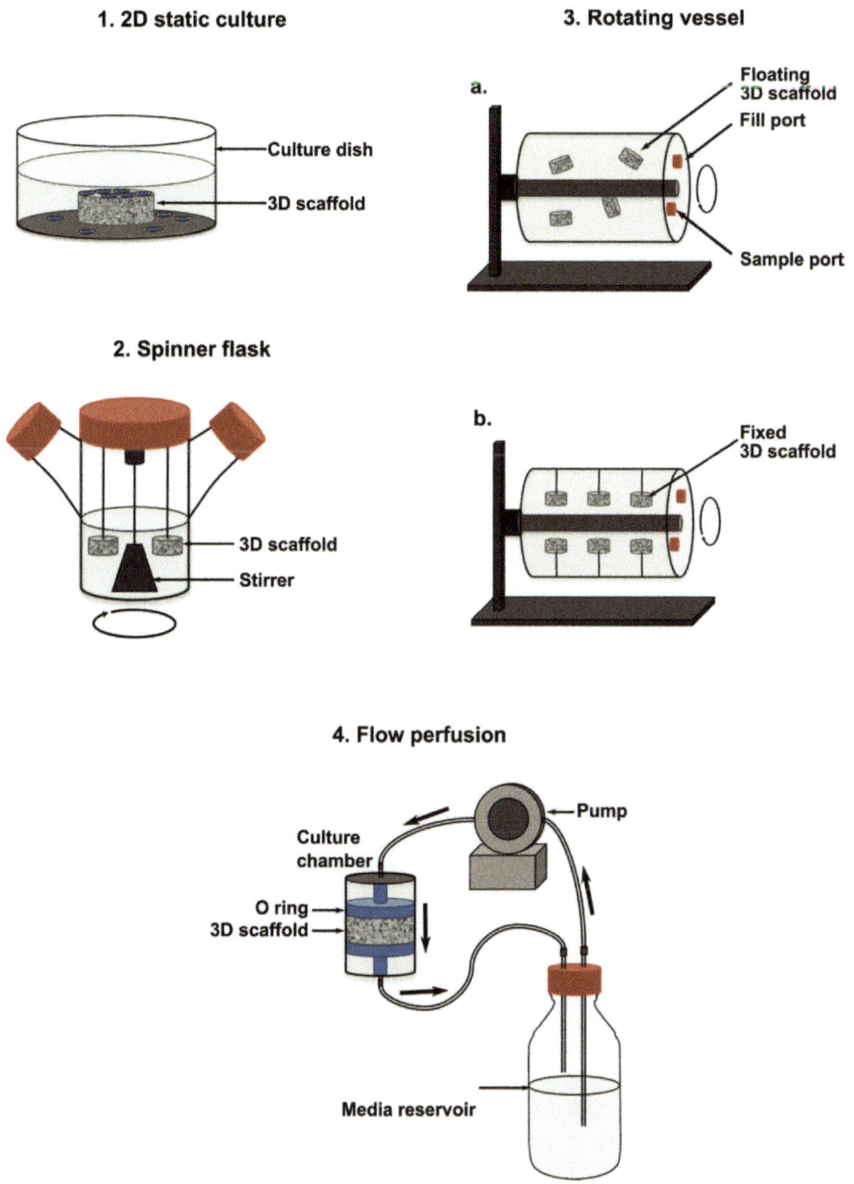


**Figure 14.10** Cell culture methods used in bone engineering studies. (1) 2D static culture. (2–4) Bioreactors for dynamic 3D cell culture: (2) spinner flask; (3a) rotating wall vessel with floating 3D scaffolds and (3b) with fixed scaffolds. An outer vessel rotates at a defined velocity while the inner vessel remains stationary or rotates at a different velocity inducing thus the rotation of culture medium in a laminar flux. The inner cylinder allows gas exchanges. (4) Common principles of flow perfusion-based reactor with a continuous (or oscillating or waving) flow of culture media, throughout a culture chamber containing the 3D scaffold (often custom-made), by a controllable pump allowing tuning of the flow rate. Between devices, the medium can be continuously recycled as presented here or thrown away in a "waste" bottle.

### 14.4.1 3D dynamic cell cultures and bioreactors

Among the growing number of studies using bioreactors, three main system families dominate: spinner flasks, rotating wall vessels, and flow-perfusion based bioreactors (Fig. 14.10) providing different hydrodynamic environments (Meinel et al., 2004). Some bioreactor designs allow also application of fully controlled physical constrains such as compression, mechanical load, stretch, electromagnetic fields, etc. (Barron et al., 2003; Dermenoudis and Missirlis, 2010; Hoffmann, 2015; Zong Ming et al., 2013). Most of the studies comparing static conditions and 3D dynamic cultures showed a global improvement in cellular functions in bioreactors (for a review, see Rauh et al., 2011; Vetsch et al., 2015; Yeatts and Fisher, 2011a). Moreover, constant efforts are made in order to improve the efficiency and accuracy of these devices (e.g., see Leferink et al., 2015; Sailon et al., 2009; Song et al., 2013; Teixeira et al., 2014). Table 14.2 summarizes the main features, advantages, and drawbacks of 3D bioreactors and 2D static culture systems, whose brief overview is presented in the following subsections.

#### 14.4.1.1 Spinner flasks

Spinner flasks are commercially available devices consisting of a glass flask with a main aperture and two arms (T-flasks) closed by filter caps allowing gas exchanges (Fig. 14.10(2)). A stirring system allows culture medium homogenization and the formation of a convective flux. The bioreactor is placed in a temperature- and atmosphere- controlled incubator similar to that for 2D static culture. Scaffolds are attached and the distance between scaffolds and stirring can be set. Culture medium is added in sufficient quantity to totally immerse scaffolds (Bancroft et al., 2003; Gaspar et al., 2012; Rauh et al., 2011; Vetsch et al., 2015). Because of poor internal diffusion of medium inside the scaffold, cells grow preferentially on its outer surface resulting in the formation of the ECM only at the surface (Meinel et al., 2004). Moreover, the flow forces inside the culture flask are not homogeneous creating a convective force gradient from the bottom to the top. Consequently, flow shear is not uniform around the scaffold and cells growing on the scaffold periphery are subjected to a turbulent flow that can be detrimental (Meinel et al., 2004 ; Gardel et al., 2014 ; Gaspar et al., 2012).

Despite these limitations, numerous studies showed an enhanced cell dispersion (homogeneity at the construct surface), viability, and proliferative activity compared to static culture (Grellier et al., 2009). Almela et al. successfully engineered a bony part on hydroxyapatite disks, with the aim of establishing a model of tissue-engineered bone/oral mucosa composite (Almela et al., 2016).

#### 14.4.1.2 Rotating vessels

Rotating wall bioreactors (or rotating wall vessels) constitute two imbricated cylinders (Fig. 14.10(3)). The inner cylinder is fixed or may rotate (Gaspar et al., 2012; Rauh et al., 2011), and the second cylinder is always in rotation. The rotation of the outer cylinder at a controlled speed creates a laminar flux inside the system together

Table 14.2 **Comparison of 3D bioreactor and 2D static culture features**

| | 2D static culture | Spinner flasks | Rotating vessels | Flow perfusion |
|---|---|---|---|---|
| **Flow** | None | Convective | Laminar | Laminar |
| **Nutrient diffusion** | Poor (< ~100 μm depth) | Homogeneous mixing but poor diffusion inside the scaffold | | Perfusion throughout the scaffold. Suppression of diffusion limitations |
| **Cell distribution** | Inhomogeneous, denser in periphery | Possible superficial cell growth, cells and matrix encapsulating scaffold | | Homogeneous throughout all the scaffold (outside and inside) |
| **Scaffold requirements** | Small volume | | If not fixed, a lower bulk density than the culture medium is required | Interconnectivity from one side to the other by channels or high porosity rates (>75%) |
| **Shear forces tuning and values** | Not applicable | Stirring rate (rpm) | Rotating velocity (rpm) | Flow rate (mL/min or μm/s) |
| **Advantages** | | Low cost<br>Commercially available in different sizes | | The medium passes directly through the scaffolds: homogeneous distribution of nutrient and oxygen throughout the scaffold |
| **Drawbacks** | Culture limited in time, poor colonisation of the scaffold (only close to the surface)<br>Cells migration and adhesion at the bottom of culture dishes<br>No mechanical strain<br>Cell death at the interior of scaffolds (hypoxia)<br>Artefactual late differentiation phenotype of osteoblastic cells due to 2D confluence (contact inhibition which stops proliferation) | Nonuniform medium flow around the scaffolds (gradient of convective forces)<br>Limited mass transfer to the interior of the scaffold | Nonuniform medium flow around the scaffolds<br>Limited mass transfer to the interior of the scaffold | Require customized parts adapted to the scaffold architecture |

with microgravity conditions leading to free-floating scaffolds (Katayama et al., 2013; Rauh et al., 2011, Freed and Vunjak-Novakovic, 1997; Schwarz et al., 1992; Hammond and Hammond, 2001). Besides these conditions of free floating scaffolds, it is noteworthy to consider the bulk density of the used biomaterials. When their density is higher than that of the culture medium, centrifugal forces push the scaffolds to collude with the outer vessel wall. This phenomenon is detrimental for the cell and the production and preservation of ECM (Braccini et al., 2005; Yeatts and Fisher, 2011b; Wang et al., 2014; Yu et al., 2004). Microgravity may also modify the expression of osteogenesis-related markers (Cazzaniga et al., 2014; Inanç et al., 2007) since it was proved that weightlessness affects bone homeostasis (loss of bone density) by decoupling osteoblasts and osteoclasts actions (Cancedda et al., 2012; Canciani et al., 2015; Cazzaniga et al., 2014; Goyden et al., 2015; Lloyd et al., 2015). Microgravity and scaffold bulk density problematics can be reduced with the use of rotating vessel systems allowing the scaffold fixation by pinning to the vessel wall or to the lid (Fig. 14.10(3b)) (Rauh et al., 2011; Leferink et al., 2015; Katayama et al., 2013; Song et al., 2013). But, for a given scaffold, depending on its location in the outer cylinder and the flow velocity, hydrodynamic forces intensity and distribution are modulated (Song et al., 2013). With the aim of improving medium circulation and flow dynamics, models with perpendicular bi-axial vessel rotation were set up and combined to a system of flow medium replacement (additional medium reservoir) (Leferink et al., 2015).

Cell cultures onto scaffolds were successfully conducted in order to produce tissue-engineered construct with endothelial cells (Dermenoudis and Missirlis, 2010), and as well as culture performed with spinner flask systems, an improvement of osteoblast viability and matrix production was demonstrated using this system (Yu et al., 2004).

#### *14.4.1.3 Flow perfusion*

The flow perfusion-based bioreactors principle lies on a closed-loop or open circuit circulation of the culture medium (Fig. 14.10(4)) (Bancroft et al., 2003, Campos et al., 2014). The culture medium is pumped, with a controlled flow rate, from a reservoir to a flow chamber where the 3D scaffold is tightly enclosed between perforated covers (O-rings on the figure) in a such way that the culture medium passes throughout all the scaffold volume. By changing the perforation pattern, hydrodynamic forces throughout the scaffold can be modified. The medium is pumped from a medium reservoir and after crossing the flow chamber is evacuated into a collection reservoir (Bancroft et al., 2003, Holtorf et al., 2005). In the literature, an important number of flow systems are composed of customized parts (e.g., Bancroft et al., 2003; Grayson et al., 2009; Leferink et al., 2015; Wang et al., 2014; Yeatts and Fisher, 2011b). Gas exchanges can be possible through gas-permeable silicone tubing (Bancroft et al., 2003; Li et al., 2008; Meinel et al., 2004) or sometimes by adding an oxygenator on the circuit (Chen and Lin, 2006; Chen et al., 2016; Janssen et al., 2006; Miyoshi et al., 2010).

Flow perfusion systems overcome the internal diffusion limitations described for the two previous systems, since nutrients and gases are perfused inside the scaffold making this system the most common for biomaterial-related biological studies. Moreover, the passage of the flow throughout the construct distributes physical strains into the whole volume of the scaffold. Flow direction through the scaffold is often unilateral (from the top to the bottom) but some oscillatory or bidirectional systems were described where medium flow passes alternatively from top-to-bottom to bottom-to-top (Braccini et al., 2005; Tseng et al., 2014). While generally steady-state, a pulsatile medium flow was described in several studies without clear improvement in terms of cell density (Jaasma et al., 2008) but inducing enhanced contractile properties of cardiac cells (Brown et al., 2008). Perfusion in the chamber can be direct, but in this case, the flow must be adapted to the scaffold (Bancroft et al., 2003). A nontight sealing of scaffold inside the bioreactor results in different hydrodynamic features with an indirect perfusion modifying cell distribution and attachment/migration. For instance, Katayama et al. described a radial flow-perfusion bioreactor in which the flow is allowed to pass around the construct (Katayama et al., 2013). Whatever the flow features, some works highlighted a direct relation between shear stress intensity and cellular behavior (Bancroft et al., 2003; Meinel et al., 2004; McCoy and O'Brien, 2012; Campos et al., 2014).

### 14.4.2 Features to take into consideration: decisional chart and parameters to standardize

Several works have been devoted to the biological evaluation of 3D scaffolds but the variety of experimental settings (e.g., design of customized bioreactor, architecture of scaffold, etc.) makes it difficult to compare results. Examples for calcium phosphate ceramics tested in a flow perfusion bioreactor are given in Table 14.3. For instance, cell density at seeding is given either as cell number per medium unit volume or per scaffold. Consequently, it is crucial to harmonize terminology and units. Concerning flow dynamic settings, values should be given in terms of common features such as flow shear stress intensity in addition to device-specific parameters (usually given in rpm, ml/min, etc.), which are strictly dependent on the bioreactor design.

Numerous scaffold parameters must also be taken into account. They have been arranged in a decision chart (Fig. 14.11). Porosity amount, pore size and shape, and pore interconnectivity will influence construct permeability as well as global porous architecture and tested volume of scaffold (Uebersax et al., 2006; Bouet et al., 2015). All of them will condition hydrodynamic features around and inside the construct (flow direction, shear strain, etc.). Applied shear force is of high importance since the cell will behave differently according to mechanical forces (Campos et al., 2014; Datta et al., 2006; McCoy and O'Brien, 2010; Song et al., 2013). Geometry regularity (e.g., symmetric and straight channels vs random pore distribution) will strongly affect flow shear outside and inside the scaffolds (McCoy and O'Brien, 2012). Regular channels in a scaffold will not induce the same fluid

**Table 14.3 Calcium phosphate ceramic scaffolds used in flow perfusion bioreactors and main results**

| Authors | Study | Scaffold features | Bioreactor/ hydrodynamic regime | Cells/seeding | Main results (3D vs 2D culture) |
|---|---|---|---|---|---|
| Holtorf et al. (2005) | Comparison of static condition vs flow perfusion bioreactor (culture of MSCs) | Cylinder: $\phi$=8 mm, $h$ = 8 mm<br>BCP scaffolds: 60% HA/40% β -TCP<br>Porosity: 90% pores size ~500 μm | Flow perfusion system (Bancroft et al., 2003)<br>0.3 mL/min for 1 day then 1 mL/min | Rat MSCs<br>Static seeding: 500,000 cells/scaffold, dropwise in 3 × 100 μL (2 h adhesion and 4 h attachment)<br>Osteogenic medium ~2–3 days<br>Duration: 4, 8, and 16 days | ↑ scaffold cellularity with more homogeneous distribution of cells throughout the scaffold<br>↑ proliferation<br>↑Alkaline phosphatase (ALP) activity and osteopontin (OPN) secretion<br>↑ ECM production and mineralization |
| Bjerre et al. (2008) | Comparison of static versus dynamic culture conditions | Cylcinder: $\phi$=11 mm, $h$ = 2 mm<br>Si-TCP<br>Porosity: 74%<br>Pore size: 200 μm < $\phi$ <500 μm | Flow perfusion system (Bancroft et al., 2003)<br><0.1 mL/min | Human MSC-TERT (immortalized)<br>Static seeding (2 h attachment)<br>Growth medium supplemented with vitamin D<br>Duration: 7, 14, and 21 days | ↑ proliferation<br>↑ differentiation<br>↑ cell/ECM deposition |
| Wang et al. (2014) | Comparison of seeding and/or culture using 2D static versus 3D dynamic culture | Scaffold: 6 × 6 × 16 mm$^3$<br>β-TCP<br>Pores: interconnected channel (~300 μm) | Customized flow perfusion system<br>1 mL/min, 0.5 mL/min then 2 mL/min | Primary rabbit osteoblasts<br>Osteogenic medium<br>30 days of cultuture then *in vivo* study in a rabbit bone defect for 3 months. | Better performance of scaffolds seeded and cultured in flow perfusion bioreactor. Better cell distribution<br>Accelerated osteogenesis differentiation |

| | | | | | |
|---|---|---|---|---|---|
| | | | | | Allograft was superior overall |
| Chen et al. (2016) | Effect of scaffold design on cell behavior (porosity and pore size gradients vs homogeneous scaffold) | Amorphous calcium polyphosphate<br>Cylinder:<br>$\phi = 10$ mm, $h=8$ mm<br>Gradient porosity (average 32%)<br>Pores: average size 210 μm, variable along the gradient | Customized flow perfusion<br>1 mL/s (2 Pa) | Mouse MC3T3-E1 preosteoblastic cell line Static seeding: 900,000 cells/scaffold , dropwise in 30 × 10 μL (attachment overnight) Growth medium supplemented with β-glycerophosphate Duration: 4 and 14 days | Improvement of scaffold biological behavior by creating a gradient of porosity |
| Mygind et al. (2007) | Comparison of static versus dynamic cell culture: influence of scaffold pore size | Cylinder: $\phi = 10$ mm, h = 2 mm<br>Commercial coralline HA ($CaCO_3$ core and thin external layer of HA)<br>Porosity : 75% and 88%<br>Pore size: 200 μm or 500 μm | Commercial spinner flasks (4 needles, 2 scaffolds/needle) 30 rpm | Human MSC-TERT (immortalized)<br>Static seeding: 2,000,000 cells/scaffold, dropwise in 50 μl (attachment: 2 h, adhesion: overnight) Growth medium supplemented with vitamin D<br>Duration: 1, 7, 14, and 21 days | ↑ proliferation, influence of pore size<br>Cells found in the center of the scaffold<br>↑ECM production<br>↑expression of ALP Overall superiority of dynamic conditions |

HE, hydroxyapatite; MSCs, mesenchymal stem cells; TCP, tricalcium phosphate

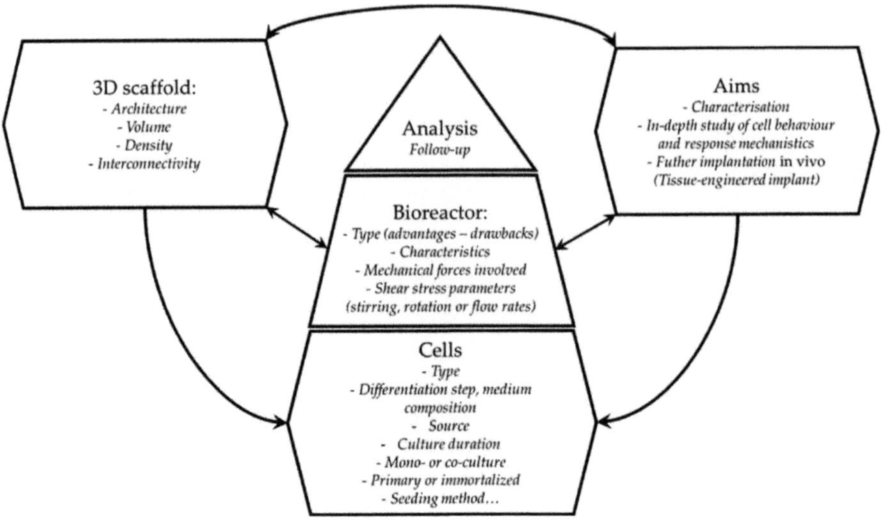


**Figure 14.11** Decisional chart for *in vitro* biological evaluation of bioceramic devices. Aims and context are at the origin of scaffold design, which defines specific features to take into account in the choice of the bioreactor (e.g., suitable for rotating vessel or spinner flask, usable or not in flow-perfusion devices). Target objective will also restrain the choice of *in vitro* settings, especially cell source and type choice. When tissue-engineered scaffold is intended to be implanted *in vivo*, this choice is crucial for the compatibility between cells and further animal models (animal species and immune status) or human. It is important to note that different scaffold/cell/bioreactor combinations may lead to result variation since each parameter may influence another one (e.g., local flow shear may change depending on scaffold pore size and morphology and consequently affect cell response).

dynamic forces as scaffold with random interconnected porosity (Bouet et al., 2015; Guyot et al., 2016; Vetsch et al., 2015). Several models highlighted these differences which depends also on both bioreactor device and flow rate (Guyot et al., 2014; Ismadi et al., 2014; Jones et al., 2007; Jungreuthmayer et al., 2008; Lacroix et al., 2006; McCoy and O'Brien, 2012; Vetsch et al., 2015). Surface properties and microstructure (e.g., roughness, topography, microporosity amount, etc.) are also known to affect cell behavior (e.g., adhesion/attachment, lineage commitment and differentiation) (Samavedi et al., 2013; Gariboldi and Best, 2015). Pursued objectives, characterization of biological properties, such as depth of cell migration, cell response (activity, signalling, behavior, etc.), or tissue-engineered scaffold evaluation for further implantation will also influence choice regarding bioreactor and cell culture settings.

Numerous cell types can be used for *in vitro* experiments (stem cells, precursors, predifferentiated). The choice is closely linked to the study context. For instance, a further animal study using a specific animal model (immuneincompetent, syngeneic, etc.) requires autologous source and/or the use of nonimmunogenic cells such as mesenchymal stem cells (MSCs) (Baldwin et al., 2017). The nature of the cell line is also important: primary cells, more physiological but with a lot of constraints (low number of passages, behavior highly dependent on donor status), immortalized primary (e.g., MSC-TERT) or immortalized cell lines (more reproducible but potentially different response). Due to their responsive abilities, MSCs of adults are the most common cell type of interest for biomaterial characterization (Jaiswal et al., 1997; Pittenger, 1999). Fetal MSCs presenting improved plastic and functional properties should be considered with a large amount of caution (Zhang et al., 2010, 2012; Leferink et al., 2015).

Some studies have also tested the feasibility of coculture to reproduce more accurately bone tissue but also to introduce more complexity. Considering the crucial role of vascularization in regenerative medicine, endothelial cells are the cell type of choice for coculture experiments (Baldwin et al., 2017; Grellier et al., 2009; Hofmann et al., 2008; Liu et al., 2015). MSCs as sampled from donor (bone marrow aspirate, adipose stromal vascular fraction, SVF) contain mesenchymal and vascular precursors and can constitute a potent base for coculture settings. For instance, Papadimitropoulos et al. have mimicked the bone tissue behavior by a coculture system in a flow-perfusion bioreactor to construct engineered tissue containing human MSCs and monocytes further engrafted in a murine animal model (Papadimitropoulos et al., 2011).

Because seeding is very crucial and will condition the culture success, this parameter should not be neglected (Gaspar et al., 2012). Scaffolds are commonly preseeded dropwise with a defined cell number that are allowed to attach for an initial duration before the sample is placed in the bioreactor (see examples in Bancroft et al., 2003; Chen et al., 2016; Mygind et al., 2007; Strobel et al., 2014). Alternatively, cells can be encapsulated together with scaffold in a hydrated polymer before incorporation in dynamic culture (Grellier et al., 2009; Inanç et al., 2007; Yeatts and Fisher, 2011b). The positive influence of dynamic culturing through higher mass transfer and application of shear stress allows a better distribution of cells throughout scaffolds (Alvarez-Barreto et al., 2007; Bancroft et al., 2003; Katayama et al., 2013; Li et al., 2014), but depends on applied shears, too-high flow forces leading to low cell attachment (Campos et al., 2014). Dynamic seeding methods were also used (cells added as a suspension in the bioreactor) (Alvarez-Barreto et al., 2007; Braccini et al., 2005; Janssen et al., 2006; Wang et al., 2014). The comparison with static seeding highlights a better viability because attachment is thus active, selecting only viable cells (Wang et al., 2014). The benefit is high when seeding bone marrow aspirates or adipose SVF (with the objective of coculture experiments), because it allows the insertion in the system of nonadherent precursors which are eliminated by conventional plating methods (Braccini et al., 2005; Papadimitropoulos et al., 2011, 2014). Culture medium viscosity can be modified by supplementing with molecules such as dextran allowing the increase of shear forces (Rauh et al., 2011; Sikavitsas et al., 2003). Again, according to the experimental settings, results can differ and are not easy to compare. These results confirm the reality of scaffold/bioreactor/cell combination in modulation of cell response.

Analysis of biological response obtained in a 3D environment may also need some adaptations compared to monolayer culture at the scaffold surface. For example, several studies showed an improvement of ECM production associated with the hydrodynamic conditions (Holtorf et al., 2005; Li et al., 2008). As a result, DNA extraction and quantification to characterize cellularity is difficult to perform with sometimes underestimated results or discrepancies due to the cell entrapment (Bjerre et al., 2011; Holtorf et al., 2005). Consequently, complementary assays and methods suited to experiment settings should be adapted or developed. Thus, Janssen et al. used oxygen consumption monitoring to estimate cell growth (Janssen et al., 2006). Recent studies used nondestructive imaging methods allowing a time-monitoring of construct changes and parallel modeling of the events (Chen et al., 2016; Yue et al., 2011).

In conclusion, bioreactors, by providing a better physiological model of the tissue microenvironment with tightly controlled parameters, are promising and already crucial tools in the tissue-engineering field. The transposition of 2D models to the third dimension is not obvious from various aspects. For instance, a pore configuration suitable for cell growth in a 2D configuration will not necessarily lead to the same results in a dynamic 3D bioreactor because of additional parameters such as hydrodynamic behavior. While the flow perfusion bioreactor appears to be the most suitable device for ceramic scaffold characterization, the strategy needs to consider the scaffold/cells/bioreactor system as a whole. Because each experimental setting will not necessarily provide the same aspects of the phenomena occurring at the cellular–biomaterial interface, special attention should be given to versatile tools allowing more accurate analysis.

## 14.5 Concluding remarks

Issues remain in the clinical treatment of large osseous defects for which there are still no satisfying solutions. Advanced ceramic processes have been widely investigated for some years to produce high-performance medical devices for applications in bone surgery and to provide answers for these issues. Additive manufacturing opens a new way of thinking and fabricating systems, which is of particular interest for the development of a new generation of ceramic-based devices. Though these versatile technologies appear effective, few (e.g., stereolithography, 3D printing) have already proved clinically the efficiency of manufactured devices and led to commercially available customized implants or scaffolds. For some other processes, such as freeze-templating, a better knowledge and improvements are necessary to control the architecture and porous network in large scaffolds. The current trends focus on combined approaches, especially with biofabrication methods to manufacture hybrid devices.

However, achievements in the development of complex devices cannot reasonably be made without a better knowledge of the biological behavior of scaffolds. In this field, the use of 3D bioreactors appears of prime importance to provide rational criteria allowing production of tunable scaffold designs. But to be efficient, such an approach needs some standardization depending on the target objective: characterization or tissue-engineered scaffold. The latter combined with AM of customized scaffolds gets into personalized medicine. Such a personalized medicine will also require the capacity of our society to produce not only high-performance but also cost-effective devices.

# References

Almela, T., Brook, I.M., Moharamzadeh, K., 2016. Development of three-dimensional tissue engineered bone-oral mucosal composite models. J. Mater. Sci. Mater. Med. 27, 65. Available from: http://dx.doi.org/10.1007/s10856-016-5676-7.

Alvarez-Barreto, J.F., Linehan, S.M., Shambaugh, R.L., Sikavitsas, V.I., 2007. Flow perfusion improves seeding of tissue engineering scaffolds with different architectures. Ann. Biomed. Eng. 35, 429–442. Available from: http://dx.doi.org/10.1007/s10439-006-9244-z.

Baldwin, J.G., Wagner, F., Martine, L.C., Holzapfel, B.M., Theodoropoulos, C., Bas, O., et al., 2017. Periosteum tissue engineering in an orthotopic in vivo platform. Biomaterials. 121, 193–204. Available from: http://dx.doi.org/10.1016/j.biomaterials.2016.11.016.

Bancroft, G.N., Sikavitsas, V.I., Mikos, A.G., 2003. Design of a flow perfusion bioreactor system for bone tissue-engineering applications. Tissue Eng. 9, 549–554. Available from: http://dx.doi.org/10.1089/107632703322066723.

Barbee, K.A., Mundel, T., Lal, R., Davies, P.F., 1995. Subcellular distribution of shear stress at the surface of flow-aligned and nonaligned endothelial monolayers. Am. J. Physiol. Heart Circ. Physiol. 268, H1765–H1772.

Barron, V., Lyons, E., Stenson-Cox, C., McHugh, P.E., Pandit, A., 2003. Bioreactors for cardiovascular cell and tissue growth: a review. Ann. Biomed. Eng. 31, 1017–1030. Available from: http://dx.doi.org/10.1114/1.1603260.

Bidan, C.M., Kommareddy, K.P., Rumpler, M., Kollmannsberger, P., Fratzl, P., Dunlop, J.W.C., 2013. Geometry as a factor for tissue growth: towards shape optimization of tissue engineering scaffolds. Adv. Healthc. Mater. 2, 186–194. Available from: http://dx.doi.org/10.1002/adhm.201200159.

Bjerre, L., Bünger, C., Baatrup, A., Kassem, M., Mygind, T., 2011. Flow perfusion culture of human mesenchymal stem cells on coralline hydroxyapatite scaffolds with various pore sizes. J. Biomed. Mater. Res. A. 97A, 251–263. Available from: http://dx.doi.org/10.1002/jbm.a.33051.

Bjerre, L., Bünger, C.E., Kassem, M., Mygind, T., 2008. Flow perfusion culture of human mesenchymal stem cells on silicate-substituted tricalcium phosphate scaffolds. Biomaterials. 29, 2616–2627. Available from: http://dx.doi.org/10.1016/j.biomaterials.2008.03.003.

Bouet, G., Marchat, D., Cruel, M., Malaval, L., Vico, L., 2015. *In vitro* three-dimensional bone tissue models: from cells to controlled and dynamic environment. Tissue Eng. Part B Rev. 21, 133–156. Available from: http://dx.doi.org/10.1089/ten.TEB.2013.0682.

Boukhechba, F., Balaguer, T., Michiels, J.-F., Ackermann, K., Quincey, D., Bouler, J.-M., et al., 2009. Human primary osteocyte differentiation in a 3D culture system. J. Bone Miner. Res. 24, 1927–1935. Available from: http://dx.doi.org/10.1359/jbmr.090517.

Braccini, A., Wendt, D., Jaquiery, C., Jakob, M., Heberer, M., Kenins, L., et al., 2005. Three-dimensional perfusion culture of human bone marrow cells and generation of osteoinductive grafts. STEM CELLS. 23, 1066–1072. Available from: http://dx.doi.org/10.1634/stemcells.2005-0002.

Brie, J., Chartier, T., Chaput, C., Delage, C., Pradeau, B., Caire, F., et al., 2013. A new custom made bioceramic implant for the repair of large and complex craniofacial bone defects. J. Craniomaxillofacial Surg. 41, 403–407. Available from: http://dx.doi.org/10.1016/j.jcms.2012.11.005.

Brown, M.A., Iyer, R.K., Radisic, M., 2008. Pulsatile perfusion bioreactor for cardiac tissue engineering. Biotechnol. Prog. 24, 907–920.

Brunello, G., Sivolella, S., Meneghello, R., Ferroni, L., Gardin, C., Piattelli, A., et al., 2016. Powder-based 3D printing for bone tissue engineering. Biotechnol. Adv. 34, 740–753. Available from: http://dx.doi.org/10.1016/j.biotechadv.2016.03.009.

Butscher, A., Bohner, M., Hofmann, S., Gauckler, L., Müller, R., 2011. Structural and material approaches to bone tissue engineering in powder-based three-dimensional printing. Acta Biomater. 7, 907–920. Available from: http://dx.doi.org/10.1016/j.actbio.2010.09.039.

Campos, D.M., Soares, G.A., Anselme, K., 2014. Role of culture conditions on in vitro transformation and cellular colonization of biomimetic HA-Col scaffolds. Biomatter. 3, e24922. Available from: http://dx.doi.org/10.1359/jbmr.1999.14.3.351.

Cancedda, R., Liu, Y., Ruggiu, A., Tavella, S., Biticchi, R., Santucci, D., et al., 2012. The Mice Drawer System (MDS) Experiment and the Space Endurance Record-Breaking Mice. PLoS ONE. 7, e32243. Available from: http://dx.doi.org/10.1371/journal.pone.0032243.

Canciani, B., Ruggiu, A., Giuliani, A., Panetta, D., Marozzi, K., Tripodi, M., et al., 2015. Effects of long time exposure to simulated micro- and hypergravity on skeletal architecture. J. Mech. Behav. Biomed. Mater. 51, 1–12. Available from: http://dx.doi.org/10.1016/j.jmbbm.2015.06.014.

Cazzaniga, A., Castiglioni, S., Maier, J.A.M., 2014. Conditioned media from microvascular endothelial cells cultured in simulated microgravity inhibit osteoblast activity. BioMed Res. Int. 2014, 857934. Available from: http://dx.doi.org/10.1155/2014/857934.

Cesarano III, J., 1999. A Review of robocasting technology. Mat. Res. Soc. Symp. Proc. 542, 133–139.

Charbonnier, B., Laurent, C., Marchat, D., 2016. Porous hydroxyapatite bioceramics produced by impregnation of 3D-printed wax mold: Slurry feature optimization. J. Eur. Ceram. Soc. 36, 4269–4279.

Chartier, T., Dupas, C., Lasgorceix, M., Brie, J., Delhote, N., Chaput, C., 2015. Additive manufacturing to produce complex 3D ceramic parts. J. Ceram. Sci. Technol. 6, 95–104.

Chatzizisis, Y.S., Coskun, A.U., Jonas, M., Edelman, E.R., Feldman, C.L., Stone, P.H., 2007. Role of endothelial shear stress in the natural history of coronary atherosclerosis and vascular remodeling. J. Am. Coll. Cardiol. 49, 2379–2393. Available from: http://dx.doi.org/10.1016/j.jacc.2007.02.059.

Chen, J.-P., Lin, C.-T., 2006. Dynamic seeding and perfusion culture of hepatocytes with galactosylated vegetable sponge in packed-bed bioreactor. J. Biosci. Bioeng. 102, 41–45. Available from: http://dx.doi.org/10.1263/jbb.102.41.

Chen, L., Song, W., Markel, D.C., Shi, T., Muzik, O., Matthew, H., et al., 2016. Flow perfusion culture of MC3T3-E1 osteogenic cells on gradient calcium polyphosphate scaffolds with different pore sizes. J. Biomater. Appl. 30, 908–918. Available from: http://dx.doi.org/10.1177/0885328215608335.

Cheng, Z., Zhao, K., Wu, Z.P., 2015. Structure control of hydroxyapatite ceramics via an electric field assisted freeze casting method. Ceram. Int. 41, 8599–8604.

Chien, S., 2006. Mechanotransduction and endothelial cell homeostasis: the wisdom of the cell. AJP Heart Circ. Physiol. 292, H1209–H1224. Available from: http://dx.doi.org/10.1152/ajpheart.01047.2006.

Chu, T.-M.G., Halloran, J.W., Hollister, S.J., Feinberg, S.E., 2001. Hydroxyapatite implants with designed internal architecture. J. Mat. Sci. Mater Med. 12, 471–478.
Cukierman, E., 2001. Taking cell–matrix adhesions to the third dimension. Science. 294, 1708–1712. Available from: http://dx.doi.org/10.1126/science.1064829.
Datta, N., Pham, Q.P., Sharma, U., Sikavitsas, V.I., Jansen, J.A., Mikos, A.G., 2006. *In vitro* generated extracellular matrix and fluid shear stress synergistically enhance 3D osteoblastic differentiation. Proc. Natl. Acad. Sci. U. S. A. 103, 2488–2493.
Dellinger, J.G., Cesarano, J., Jamison, R.D., 2007. Robotic deposition of model hydroxyapatite scaffolds with multiple architectures and multiscale porosity for bone tissue engineering. J. Biomed. Mater. Res. A. 82, 383–394. Available from: http://dx.doi.org/10.1002/jbm.a.31072.
Dermenoudis, S., Missirlis, Y., 2010. Design of a novel rotating wall bioreactor for the *in vitro* simulation of the mechanical environment of the endothelial function. J. Biomech. 43, 1426–1431. Available from: http://dx.doi.org/10.1016/j.jbiomech.2010.01.012.
Deville, S., 2008. Freeze-casting of porous ceramics: a review of current achievements and issues. Adv. Engng Mat. 10, 155–169.
Deville, S., 2010. Freeze-casting of porous biomaterials: struture, properties and opportunities. Materials. 3, 1913–1927.
Deville, S., Saiz, E., Tomsia, A.P., 2006. Freeze casting of hydroxyapatite scaffolds for bone tissue engineering. Biomaterials. 27, 5480–5489.
Duan, B., Wang, M., Zhou, W.Y., Cheung, W.L., Li, Z.Y., Lu, W.W., 2010. Three-dimensional nanocomposite scaffolds fabricated via selective laser sintering for bone tissue engineering. Acta Biomater. 6, 4495–4505. Available from: http://dx.doi.org/10.1016/j.actbio.2010.06.024.
Eosoly, S., Vrana, N.E., Lohfeld, S., Hindie, M., Looney, L., 2012. Interaction of cell culture with composition effects on the mechanical properties of polycaprolactone-hydroxyapatite scaffolds fabricated via selective laser sintering (SLS). Mater. Sci. Eng. C32. Available from: http://dx.doi.org/10.1016/j.msec.2012.06.011.
Fielding, G.A., Bandyopadhyay, A., Bose, S., 2012. Effects of silica and zinc oxide doping on mechanical and biological properties of 3D printed tricalcium phosphate tissue engineering scaffolds. Dent. Mater. Off. Publ. Acad. Dent. Mater. 28, 113–122. Available from: http://dx.doi.org/10.1016/j.dental.2011.09.010.
Freed, L.E., Vunjak-Novakovic, G., 1997. Microgravity tissue engineering. Vitro Cell. Dev. Biol.-Anim. 33, 381–385.
Fu, Q., Rahaman, M.N., Dogan, F., Sonny Bal, B., 2007. Freeze casting of porous hydroxyapatite scaffolds. I. Processing and general microstructure. J. Biomed. Mater. Res. Part B: Appl Biomater. 86B, 125–137.
Fu, Q., Rahaman, M.N., Sonny Bal, B., Brown, R.F., 2009. Proliferation and function of MC3T3-E1 cells on freeze-cast hydroxyapatite scaffolds with oriented pore architectures. J. Mater. Sci: Mater. Med. 20, 1159–1165.
Fukasawa, T., Deng, Z.-Y., Ando, M., Ohji, T., Goto, Y., 2001. Pore structure of porous ceramics synthesized from water-based slurry by freeze-dry process. J. Mat. Sci. 36, 2523–2527.
Gardel, L.S., Serra, L.A., Reis, R.L., Gomes, M.E., 2014. Use of Perfusion Bioreactors and Large Animal Models for Long Bone Tissue Engineering. Tissue Eng. Part B Rev. 20, 126–146. Available from: http://dx.doi.org/10.1089/ten.teb.2013.0010.
Gariboldi, M.I., Best, S.M., 2015. Effect of Ceramic Scaffold Architectural Parameters on Biological Response. Front. Bioeng. Biotechnol. 3, 151. Available from: http://dx.doi.org/10.3389/fbioe.2015.00151.

Gaspar, D.A., Gomide, V., Monteiro, F.J., 2012. The role of perfusion bioreactors in bone tissue engineering. Biomatter. 2, 167. Available from: http://dx.doi.org/10.4161/biom.22170.

Giannitelli, S.M., Mozetic, P., Trombetta, M., Rainer, A., 2015. Combined additive manufacturing approaches in tissue engineering. Acta Biomater. 24, 1–11.

Gjorevski, N.S., Piotrowski, A., Varner, V.D., Nelson, C.M., 2015. Dynamic tensile forces drive collective cell migration through three-dimensional extracellular matrices. Sci. Rep. 5, 11458. Available from: http://dx.doi.org/10.1038/srep11458.

Goyden, J., Tawara, K., Hedeen, D., Willey, J.S., Oxford, J.T., Jorcyk, C.L., 2015. The effect of OSM on MC3T3-E1 osteoblastic cells in simulated microgravity with radiation. PLoS ONE. 10, e0127230. Available from: http://dx.doi.org/10.1371/journal.pone.0127230.

Grayson, W.L., Martens, T.P., Eng, G.M., Radisic, M., Vunjak-Novakovic, G., 2009. Biomimetic approach to tissue engineering. Semin. Cell Dev. Biol. 20, 665–673. Available from: http://dx.doi.org/10.1016/j.semcdb.2008.12.008.

Grellier, M., Granja, P.L., Fricain, J.-C., Bidarra, S.J., Renard, M., Bareille, R., et al., 2009. The effect of the co-immobilization of human osteoprogenitors and endothelial cells within alginate microspheres on mineralization in a bone defect. Biomaterials. 30, 3271–3278. Available from: http://dx.doi.org/10.1016/j.biomaterials.2009.02.033.

Griffith, L.G., Swartz, M.A., 2006. Capturing complex 3D tissue physiology in vitro. Nat. Rev. Mol. Cell Biol. 7, 211–224. Available from: http://dx.doi.org/10.1038/nrm1858.

Guyot, Y., Papantoniou, I., Chai, Y.C., Van Bael, S., Schrooten, J., Geris, L., 2014. A computational model for cell/ECM growth on 3D surfaces using the level set method: a bone tissue engineering case study. Biomech. Model. Mechanobiol. 13, 1361–1371. Available from: http://dx.doi.org/10.1007/s10237-014-0577-5.

Guyot, Y., Papantoniou, I., Luyten, F.P., Geris, L., 2016. Coupling curvature-dependent and shear stress-stimulated neotissue growth in dynamic bioreactor cultures: a 3D computational model of a complete scaffold. Biomech. Model. Mechanobiol. 15, 169–180. Available from: http://dx.doi.org/10.1007/s10237-015-0753-2.

Hammond, T.G., Hammond, J.M., 2001. Optimized suspension culture: the rotating-wall vessel. Am. J. Physiol.-Ren. Physiol. 281, F12–F25.

Harunaga, J.S., Yamada, K.M., 2011. Cell-matrix adhesions in 3D. Matrix Biol. 30, 363–368. Available from: http://dx.doi.org/10.1016/j.matbio.2011.06.001.

Hoffmann, W., 2015. Novel perfused compression bioreactor system as an in vitro model to investigate fracture healing. Front. Bioeng. Biotechnol.3. Available from: http://dx.doi.org/10.3389/fbioe.2015.00010.

Hofmann, A., Ritz, U., Verrier, S., Eglin, D., Alini, M., Fuchs, S., et al., 2008. The effect of human osteoblasts on proliferation and neo-vessel formation of human umbilical vein endothelial cells in a long-term 3D co-culture on polyurethane scaffolds. Biomaterials. 29, 4217–4226. Available from: http://dx.doi.org/10.1016/j.biomaterials.2008.07.024.

Hollister, S.J., Lin, C.Y., 2007. Computational design of tissue engineering scaffolds. Comput. Methods Appl. Mech. Engng. 196, 2991–2998.

Hollister, S.J., Maddox, R.D., Taboas, J.M., 2002. Optimal design and fabrication of scaffolds to mimic tissue properties and satisfy biological constraints. Biomaterials. 23, 4095–4103.

Holtorf, H.L., Sheffield, T.L., Ambrose, C.G., Jansen, J.A., Mikos, A.G., 2005. Flow perfusion culture of marrow stromal cells seeded on porous biphasic calcium phosphate ceramics. Ann. Biomed. Eng. 33, 1238–1248. Available from: http://dx.doi.org/10.1007/s10439-005-5536-y.

Hutmacher, D.W., Sittinger, M., Risbud, M.V., 2004. Scaffold-based tissue engineering: rationale for computer-aided design and solid free-form fabrication systems. Trends Biotechnol. 22, 354–362. Available from: http://dx.doi.org/10.1016/j.tibtech.2004.05.005.

Inanç, B., Eser Elçin, A., Koç, A., Baloş, K., Parlar, A., Murat Elçin, Y., 2007. Encapsulation and osteoinduction of human periodontal ligament fibroblasts in chitosan-hydroxyapatite microspheres. J. Biomed. Mater. Res. A. 82, 917–926. Available from: http://dx.doi.org/10.1002/jbm.a.31213.

Ismadi, M.-Z., Gupta, P., Fouras, A., Verma, P., Jadhav, S., Bellare, J., et al., 2014. Flow Characterization of a Spinner Flask for Induced Pluripotent Stem Cell Culture Application. PLoS ONE. 9, e106493. Available from: http://dx.doi.org/10.1371/journal.pone.0106493.

Jaasma, M.J., Plunkett, N.A., O'Brien, F.J., 2008. Design and validation of a dynamic flow perfusion bioreactor for use with compliant tissue engineering scaffolds. J. Biotechnol. 133, 490–496. Available from: http://dx.doi.org/10.1016/j.jbiotec.2007.11.010.

Jaiswal, N., Haynesworth, S.E., Caplan, A.I., Bruder, S.P., 1997. Osteogenic differentiation of purified, culture-expanded human mesenchymal stem cells in vitro. J Cell Biochem. 64, 295–312.

Janssen, F.W., Hofland, I., van Oorschot, A., Oostra, J., Peters, H., van Blitterswijk, C.A., 2006. Online measurement of oxygen consumption by goat bone marrow stromal cells in a combined cell-seeding and proliferation perfusion bioreactor. J. Biomed. Mater. Res. A. 79A, 338–348. Available from: http://dx.doi.org/10.1002/jbm.a.30794.

Jones, J.R., Poologasundarampillai, G., Atwood, R.C., Bernard, D., Lee, P.D., 2007. Non-destructive quantitative 3D analysis for the optimisation of tissue scaffolds. Biomaterials. 28, 1404–1413. Available from: http://dx.doi.org/10.1016/j.biomaterials.2006.11.014.

Jungreuthmayer, C., Donahue, S.W., Jaasma, M.J., Al-Munajjed, A.A., Zanghellini, J., Kelly, D.J., et al., 2008. A comparative study of shear stresses in collagen-glycosaminoglycan and calcium phosphate scaffolds in bone tissue-engineering bioreactors. Tissue Eng. Part A. 15, 1141–1149.

Karageorgiou, V., Kaplan, D., 2005. Porosity of 3D biomaterial scaffolds and osteogenesis. Biomaterials. 26, 5474–5491. Available from: http://dx.doi.org/10.1016/j.biomaterials.2005.02.002.

Katayama, A., Arano, T., Sato, T., Ikada, Y., Yoshinari, M., 2013. Radial-flow bioreactor enables uniform proliferation of human mesenchymal stem cells throughout a three-dimensional scaffold. Tissue Eng. Part C Methods. 19, 109–116. Available from: http://dx.doi.org/10.1089/ten.TEC.2011.0722.

Klein-Nulend, J., Bacabac, R.G., Mullender, M.G., 2005. Mechanobiology of bone tissue. Pathol. Biol. 53, 576–580. Available from: http://dx.doi.org/10.1016/j.patbio.2004.12.005.

Lacroix, D., Chateau, A., Ginebra, M.-P., Planell, J.A., 2006. Micro-finite element models of bone tissue-engineering scaffolds. Biomaterials. 27, 5326–5334. Available from: http://dx.doi.org/10.1016/j.biomaterials.2006.06.009.

Lasgorceix, M., Champion, E., Chartier, T., 2016. Shaping by microstereolithography and sintering of macro–micro-porous silicon substituted hydroxyapatite. J. Eur. Ceram. Soc. 36, 1091–1101.

Lee, E.J., Koh, Y.H., Yoon, B.H., Kim, H.E., Kim, H.W., 2007. Highly porous hydroxyapatite bioceramics with interconnected pore channels using camphene-based freeze casting. Mat. Let. 61, 2270–2273.

Lee, G., Barlow, J., 1994. Selective laser sintering of calcium phosphate powders. Proc. Solid Free. Fabr. Symp.191−197.

Leferink, A.M., Chng, Y.-C., van Blitterswijk, C.A., Moroni, L., 2015. Distribution and viability of fetal and adult human bone marrow stromal cells in a biaxial rotating vessel bioreactor after seeding on polymeric 3D additive manufactured scaffolds. Front. Bioeng. Biotechnol. 3, 169. Available from: http://dx.doi.org/10.3389/fbioe.2015.00169.

Leukers, B., Gülkan, H., Irsen, S.H., Milz, S., Tille, C., Schieker, M., et al., 2005. Hydroxyapatite scaffolds for bone tissue engineering made by 3D printing. J. Mater. Sci. Mater. Med. 16, 1121−1124. Available from: http://dx.doi.org/10.1007/s10856-005-4716-5.

Li, D., Li, M., Liu, P., Zhang, Y., Lu, J., Li, J., 2014. Tissue-engineered bone constructed in a bioreactor for repairing critical-sized bone defects in sheep. Int. Orthop. 38, 2399−2406. Available from: http://dx.doi.org/10.1007/s00264-014-2389-8.

Li, X., Li, D., Wang, L., Lu, B., Wang, Z., 2008. Osteoblast cell response to beta-tricalcium phosphate scaffolds with controlled architecture in flow perfusion culture system. J. Mater. Sci. Mater. Med. 19, 2691−2697. Available from: http://dx.doi.org/10.1007/s10856-008-3391-8.

Liu, D., Zhuang, J., Shuai, C., Peng, S., 2013. Mechanical properties' improvement of a tricalcium phosphate scaffold with poly-l-lactic acid in selective laser sintering. Biofabrication. 5, 025005. Available from: http://dx.doi.org/10.1088/1758-5082/5/2/025005.

Liu, Y., Chan, J.K.Y., Teoh, S.-H., 2015. Review of vascularised bone tissue-engineering strategies with a focus on co-culture systems. J. Tissue Eng. Regen. Med. 9, 85−105. Available from: http://dx.doi.org/10.1002/term.1617.

Lloyd, S.A., Morony, S.E., Ferguson, V.L., Simske, S.J., Stodieck, L.S., Warmington, K.S., et al., 2015. Osteoprotegerin is an effective countermeasure for spaceflight-induced bone loss in mice. Bone. 81, 562−572. Available from: http://dx.doi.org/10.1016/j.bone.2015.08.021.

Macchetta, A., Turner, I.G., Bowen, C.R., 2009. Fabrication of HA/TCP scaffolds with a graded and porous structure using a camphene-based freeze-casting method. Acta Biomater. 5, 1319−1327.

Magnaudeix, A., Usseglio, J., Lasgorceix, M., Lalloue, F., Damia, C., Brie, J., et al., 2016. Quantitative analysis of vascular colonisation and angio-conduction in porous silicon-substituted hydroxyapatite with various pore shapes in a chick chorioallantoic membrane (CAM) model. Acta Biomater. 38, 179−189. Available from: http://dx.doi.org/10.1016/j.actbio.2016.04.039.

Marques, C.F., Perera, F.H., Marote, A., Ferreira, S., Vieira, S.I., Olhero, S., et al., 2017. Biphasic calcium phosphate scaffolds fabricated by direct write assembly: Mechanical, anti-microbial and osteoblastic properties. J. Eur. Ceram. Soc. 37, 359−368. Available from: http://dx.doi.org/10.1016/j.jeurceramsoc.2016.08.018.

Martin, I., Wendt, D., Heberer, M., 2004. The role of bioreactors in tissue engineering. Trends Biotechnol. 22, 80−86. Available from: http://dx.doi.org/10.1016/j.tibtech.2003.12.001.

McCoy, R.J., O'Brien, F.J., 2010. Influence of shear stress in perfusion bioreactor cultures for the development of three-dimensional bone tissue constructs: a review. Tissue Eng. Part B Rev. 16, 587−601. Available from: http://dx.doi.org/10.1089/ten.teb.2010.0370.

McCoy, R.J., O'Brien, F.J., 2012. Visualizing feasible operating ranges within tissue engineering systems using a "windows of operation" approach: A perfusion-scaffold bioreactor case study. Biotechnol. Bioeng. 109, 3161−3171.

Meinel, L., Karageorgiou, V., Fajardo, R., Snyder, B., Shinde-Patil, V., Zichner, L., et al., 2004. Bone tissue engineering using human mesenchymal stem cells: effects of scaffold material and medium flow. Ann. Biomed. Eng. 32, 112–122.

Melchels, F.P., Bertoldi, K., Gabbrielli, R., Velders, A.H., Feijen, J., Grijpma, D.W., 2010. Mathematically defined tissue engineering scaffold architectures prepared by stereolithography. Biomaterials. 31 (27), 6909–6916.

Melchels, F.P.W., Feijen, J., Grijpma, D.W., 2010. A review on stereolithography and its applications in biomedical engineering. Biomaterials. 31, 6121–6130. Available from: http://dx.doi.org/10.1016/j.biomaterials.2010.04.050.

Meurice, E., Bouchart, F., Hornez, J.C., Leriche, A., Hautcoeur, D., Lardot, V., et al., 2016. Osteoblastic cells colonization inside beta-TCP macroporousstructures obtained by ice--templating. J. Eur. Ceram. Soc. 36, 2895–2901.

Michna, S., Wu, W., Lewis, J.A., 2005. Concentrated hydroxyapatite inks for direct-write assembly of 3-D periodic scaffolds. Biomaterials. 26, 5632–5639. Available from: http://dx.doi.org/10.1016/j.biomaterials.2005.02.040.

Miranda, P., Saiz, E., Gryn, K., Tomsia, A.P., 2006. Sintering and robocasting of beta-tricalcium phosphate scaffolds for orthopaedic applications. Acta Biomater. 2, 457–466. Available from: http://dx.doi.org/10.1016/j.actbio.2006.02.004.

Miranda, P., Pajares, A., Saiz, E., Tomsia, A.P., Guiberteau, F., 2008. Mechanical properties of calcium phosphate scaffolds fabricated by robocasting. J. Biomed. Mater. Res. A. 85, 218–227. Available from: http://dx.doi.org/10.1002/jbm.a.31587.

Missirlis, Y.F., 2016. Mechanoepigenetics. Front. Cell Dev. Biol.4. Available from: http://dx.doi.org/10.3389/fcell.2016.00113.

Miyoshi, H., Ehashi, T., Kawai, H., Ohshima, N., Suzuki, S., 2010. Three-dimensional perfusion cultures of mouse and pig fetal liver cells in a packed-bed reactor: Effect of medium flow rate on cell numbers and hepatic functions. J. Biotechnol. 148, 226–232. Available from: http://dx.doi.org/10.1016/j.jbiotec.2010.06.002.

Moon, J.-W., Hwang, H.-J., Awano, M., Maeda, K., 2003. Preparation of NiO–YSZ tubular support with radially aligned pore channels. Mat. Letters. 57, 1428–1434.

Morris, H.L., Reed, C.I., Haycock, J.W., Reilly, G.C., 2010. Mechanisms of fluid-flow-induced matrix production in bone tissue engineering. Proc. Inst. Mech. Eng. [H]. 224, 1509–1521. Available from: http://dx.doi.org/10.1243/09544119JEIM751.

Mota, C., Puppi, D., Chiellini, F., Chiellini, E., 2015. Additive manufacturing techniques for the production of tissue engineering constructs. J. Tissue Eng. Regen. Med. 9, 174–190. Available from: http://dx.doi.org/10.1002/term.1635.

Mygind, T., Stiehler, M., Baatrup, A., Li, H., Zou, X., Flyvbjerg, A., et al., 2007. Mesenchymal stem cell ingrowth and differentiation on coralline hydroxyapatite scaffolds. Biomaterials. 28, 1036–1047. Available from: http://dx.doi.org/10.1016/j.biomaterials.2006.10.003.

Nakashima, T., Hayashi, M., Fukunaga, T., Kurata, K., Oh-hora, M., Feng, J.Q., et al., 2011. Evidence for osteocyte regulation of bone homeostasis through RANKL expression. Nat. Med. 17, 1231–1234. Available from: http://dx.doi.org/10.1038/nm.2452.

Paluch, E.K., Nelson, C.M., Biais, N., Fabry, B., Moeller, J., Pruitt, B.L., et al., 2015. Mechanotransduction: use the force(s). BMC Biol.13. Available from: http://dx.doi.org/10.1186/s12915-015-0150-4.

Papadimitropoulos, A., Piccinini, E., Brachat, S., Braccini, A., Wendt, D., Barbero, A., et al., 2014. Expansion of human mesenchymal stromal cells from fresh bone marrow in a 3D scaffold-based system under direct perfusion. PLoS ONE. 9, e102359. Available from: http://dx.doi.org/10.1371/journal.pone.0102359.

Papadimitropoulos, A., Scherberich, A., Guven, S., Theilgaard, N., Crooijmans, H.J., Santini, F., et al., 2011. A 3D *in vitro* bone organ model using human progenitor cells. Eur Cell Mater. 21, 445–558.

Pawelec, K.M., Husmann, A., Best, S.M., Cameron, R.E., 2014. Ice-templating structures for biomedical tissue repair: From physics to final scaffolds. Appl. Phys. Rev. 1, 021301.

Penolazzi, L., Lolli, A., Sardelli, L., Angelozzi, M., Lambertini, E., Trombelli, L., et al., 2016. Establishment of a 3D-dynamic osteoblasts-osteoclasts co-culture model to simulate the jawbone microenvironment in vitro. Life Sci. 152, 82–93. Available from: http://dx.doi.org/10.1016/j.lfs.2016.03.035.

Pittenger, M.F., 1999. Multilineage potential of adult human mesenchymal stem cells. Science. 284, 143–147. Available from: http://dx.doi.org/10.1126/science.284.5411.143.

Rahaman, M.N., Fu, Q., 2008. Manipulation of porous bioceramic microstructures by freezing of suspensions containing binary mixtures of solvents. J. Am. Ceram. Soc. 91 (12), 4137–4140.

Rajagopalan, S., Robb, R.A., 2006. Schwarz meets Schwann: Design and fabrication of biomorphic and durataxic tissue engineering scaffolds. Med. Im. Analysis. 10, 693–712.

Rauh, J., Milan, F., Günther, K.-P., Stiehler, M., 2011. Bioreactor systems for bone tissue engineering. Tissue Eng. Part B Rev. 17, 263–280. Available from: http://dx.doi.org/10.1089/ten.TEB.2010.0612.

Ren, L., Yang, P., Wang, Z., Zhang, J., Ding, C., Shang, P., 2015. Biomechanical and biophysical environment of bone from the macroscopic to the pericellular and molecular level. J. Mech. Behav. Biomed. Mater. 50, 104–122. Available from: http://dx.doi.org/10.1016/j.jmbbm.2015.04.021.

Rosa, N., Simoes, R., Magalhães, F.D., Marques, A.T., 2015. From mechanical stimulus to bone formation: A review. Med. Eng. Phys. 37, 719–728. Available from: http://dx.doi.org/10.1016/j.medengphy.2015.05.015.

Rumpler, M., Woesz, A., Dunlop, J.W., van Dongen, J.T., Fratzl, P., 2008. The effect of geometry on three-dimensional tissue growth. J. R. Soc. Interface. 5, 1173–1180. Available from: http://dx.doi.org/10.1098/rsif.2008.0064.

Sachlos, E., Czernuszka, J.T., 2003. Making tissue engineering scaffolds work. Review: the application of solid freeform fabrication technology to the production of tissue engineering scaffolds. Eur. Cell. Mater. 5, 29–39-40.

Sailon, A.M., Allori, A.C., Davidson, E.H., Reformat, D.D., Allen, R.J., Warren, S.M., 2009. A novel flow-perfusion bioreactor supports 3D dynamic cell culture. J. Biomed. Biotechnol. 2009, 873816. Available from: http://dx.doi.org/10.1155/2009/873816.

Samavedi, S., Whittington, A.R., Goldstein, A.S., 2013. Calcium phosphate ceramics in bone tissue engineering: a review of properties and their influence on cell behavior. Acta Biomater. 9, 8037–8045. Available from: http://dx.doi.org/10.1016/j.actbio.2013.06.014.

Schwarz, R.P., Goodwin, T.J., Wolf, D.A., 1992. Cell culture for three-dimensional modeling in rotating-wall vessels: an application of simulated microgravity. J. Tissue Cult. Methods. 14, 51–57.

Shuai, C., Li, P., Liu, J., Peng, S., 2013. Optimization of TCP/HAP ratio for better properties of calcium phosphate scaffold via selective laser sintering. Mater. Charact. 77, 23–31. Available from: http://dx.doi.org/10.1016/j.matchar.2012.12.009.

Sikavitsas, V.I., Bancroft, G.N., Holtorf, H.L., Jansen, J.A., Mikos, A.G., 2003. Mineralized matrix deposition by marrow stromal osteoblasts in 3D perfusion culture increases with increasing fluid shear forces. Proc. Natl. Acad. Sci. 100, 14683–14688.

Silva, A.R.P., Paula, A.C.C., Martins, T.M.M., Goes, A.M., Pereria, M.M., 2014. Synergistic effect between bioactive glass foam and a perfusion bioreactor on osteogenic differentiation of human adipose stem cells. J. Biomed. Mater. Res. A. 102, 818–827. Available from: http://dx.doi.org/10.1002/jbm.a.34758.

Skerry, T.M., 2008. The response of bone to mechanical loading and disuse: Fundamental principles and influences on osteoblast/osteocyte homeostasis. Arch. Biochem. Biophys. 473, 117–123. Available from: http://dx.doi.org/10.1016/j.abb.2008.02.028.

Skoog, S.A., Goering, P.L., Narayan, R.J., 2014. Stereolithography in tissue engineering. J. Mater. Sci. Mater. Med. 25, 845–856. Available from: http://dx.doi.org/10.1007/s10856-013-5107-y.

Song, K., Wang, H., Zhang, B., Lim, M., Liu, Y.C., 2013. Numerical simulation of fluid field and in vitro three-dimensional fabrication of tissue-engineered bones in a rotating bioreactor and in vivo implantation for repairing segmental bone defects. Cell Stress Chap. 18, 193–201.

Strobel, L., Rath, S., Maier, A., Beier, J., Arkudas, A., Greil, P., et al., 2014. Induction of bone formation in biphasic calcium phosphate scaffolds by bone morphogenetic protein-2 and primary osteoblasts: Induction of bone formation in biphasic calcium phosphate scaffolds. J. Tissue Eng. Regen. Med. 8, 176–185. Available from: http://dx.doi.org/10.1002/term.1511.

Tarafder, S., Balla, V.K., Davies, N.M., Bandyopadhyay, A., Bose, S., 2013. Microwave-sintered 3D printed tricalcium phosphate scaffolds for bone tissue engineering. J. Tissue Eng. Regen. Med. 7, 631–641. Available from: http://dx.doi.org/10.1002/term.555.

Teixeira, G.Q., Barrias, C.C., Lourenço, A.H., Gonçalves, R.M., 2014. a multicompartment holder for spinner flasks improves expansion and osteogenic differentiation of mesenchymal stem cells in three-dimensional scaffolds. Tissue Eng. Part C Methods. 20, 984–993. Available from: http://dx.doi.org/10.1089/ten.tec.2014.0067.

Tseng, C.L., Chang, K.M., Wu, C.C., Wang, Y.K., 2014. Rabbit mesenchymal stem cells cultured in a dynamic culture system displayed superior cell proliferation and osteogenetic induction. J. Exp. Clin. Med. 6, 10–15.

Uebersax, L., Hagenmüller, H., Hofmann, S., Gruenblatt, E., Müller, R., Vunjaknovakovic, G., et al., 2006. Effect of scaffold design on bone morphology *in vitro*. Tissue Eng. 12, 3417–3429.

Vetsch, J.R., Müller, R., Hofmann, S., 2015. The evolution of simulation techniques for dynamic bone tissue engineering in bioreactors. J. Tissue Eng. Regen. Med. 9, 903–917. Available from: http://dx.doi.org/10.1002/term.1733.

Viswanathan, P., Ondeck, M.G., Chirasatitsin, S., Ngamkham, K., Reilly, G.C., Engler, A.J., et al., 2015. 3D surface topology guides stem cell adhesion and differentiation. Biomaterials. 52, 140–147. Available from: http://dx.doi.org/10.1016/j.biomaterials.2015.01.034.

Wang, L., Ma, X.-Y., Zhang, Y., Feng, Y.-F., Li, X., Hu, Y.-Y., et al., 2014. Repair of segmental bone defect using Totally Vitalized tissue engineered bone graft by a combined perfusion seeding and culture system. PLoS ONE. 9, e94276. Available from: http://dx.doi.org/10.1371/journal.pone.0094276.

Warnke, P.H., Seitz, H., Warnke, F., Becker, S.T., Sivananthan, S., Sherry, E., et al., 2010. Ceramic scaffolds produced by computer-assisted 3D printing and sintering: characterization and biocompatibility investigations. J. Biomed. Mater. Res. B Appl. Biomater. 93, 212–217. Available from: http://dx.doi.org/10.1002/jbm.b.31577.

Yeatts, A.B., Fisher, J.P., 2011a. Bone tissue engineering bioreactors: dynamic culture and the influence of shear stress. Bone. 48, 171–181. Available from: http://dx.doi.org/10.1016/j.bone.2010.09.138.

Yeatts, A.B., Fisher, J.P., 2011b. Tubular perfusion system for the long-term dynamic culture of human mesenchymal stem cells. Tissue Eng. Part C Methods. 17, 337–348. Available from: http://dx.doi.org/10.1089/ten.TEC.2010.0172.

Yoo, D.J., 2011. Porous scaffold design using the distance field and triply periodic minimal surface models. Biomaterials. 32, 7741–7754.

Yoon, B.-H., Lee, E.-J., Kim, H.-E., Koh, Y.-H., 2007. Highly aligned porous silicon carbide ceramics by freezing polycarbosilane/camphene solution. J. Am. Ceram. Soc. 90, 1753–1759.

Yu, X., Botchwey, E.A., Levine, E.M., Pollack, S.R., Laurencin, C.T., 2004. Bioreactor-based bone tissue engineering: the influence of dynamic flow on osteoblast phenotypic expression and matrix mineralization. Proc. Natl. Acad. Sci. U.S.A. 101, 11203–11208. Available from: http://dx.doi.org/10.1073/pnas.0402532101.

Yue, S., Lee, P.D., Poologasundarampillai, G., Jones, J.R., 2011. Evaluation of 3-D bioactive glass scaffolds dissolution in a perfusion flow system with X-ray microtomography. Acta Biomater. 7, 2637–2643. Available from: http://dx.doi.org/10.1016/j.actbio.2011.02.009.

Zhang, Y., Zhou, K., Bao, Y., Zhang, 2013. Effects of rheological properties on ice templated porous hydroxyapatite ceramics. Mat. Sci. Engng. C. 33, 340–346.

Zhang, Z.-Y., Teoh, S.-H., Teo, E.Y., Khoon Chong, M.S., Shin, C.W., Tien, F.T., et al., 2010. A comparison of bioreactors for culture of fetal mesenchymal stem cells for bone tissue engineering. Biomaterials. 31, 8684–8695. Available from: http://dx.doi.org/10.1016/j.biomaterials.2010.07.097.

Zhang, Z.-Y., Teoh, S.-H., Hui, J.H.P., Fisk, N.M., Choolani, M., Chan, J.K.Y., 2012. The potential of human fetal mesenchymal stem cells for off-the-shelf bone tissue engineering application. Biomaterials. 33, 2656–2672. Available from: http://dx.doi.org/10.1016/j.biomaterials.2011.12.025.

Zocca, A., Colombo, P., Gomes, C.M., Günster, J., 2015. Additive manufacturing of ceramics: issues, potentialities, and opportunities. J. Am. Ceram. Soc. 98, 1983–2001. Available from: http://dx.doi.org/10.1111/jace.13700.

Zong Ming, W., Jian, Yu, L., Rui Xin, L., Hao, L., Yong, G., Lu, L., et al., 2013. Bone formation in rabbit cancellous bone explant culture model is enhanced by mechanical load. Biomed. Eng. Online. 12, 35. Available from: http://dx.doi.org/10.1186/1475-925X-12-35.

# Index

*Note*: Page numbers followed by "*f*" and "*t*" refer to figures and tables, respectively.


**A**

A-carbonation, 409
Acid washing, 58
Acrylic bone cements, 413
Active oxides, 22–34
calcium carbonates, 33
calcium phosphates (CaPs)-based systems, 22–33, 23*t*
biphasic HA/β-TCP and related mixtures, 28–29
for drug delivery systems, 31–33
inorganic cement formulations, 29–30
organic/inorganic composites, 30–31
pure and substituted HA and related apatitc compounds, 24–28
calcium sulfates, 33–34
Acute systemic toxicity, 117
Additive manufacturing (AM), 15, 434–443, 435*f*, 436*f*
critical role of 3D geometrical features of pores in scaffolds, 441–443
indirect additive manufacturing, 441
powder-based technologies, 435–439
scaffolds produced through, 438*f*
slurry extrusion-based techniques, 439–440
stereolithography (SLA), 440–441
tolerances, advantages and limitations of, 437*t*
$Al_2O_3/SiO_2$ ratio in the glass, 55–56
All-ceramic implants, 365
All-ceramic restorations, 217, 358
Alumina ceramics, 9–10, 34–35, 132–136, 314–315, 331–332
Alumina/zirconia ceramic composites, characteristics of, 143*t*
Alumina-toughened zirconia (ATZ), 10–11, 38, 141–143, 143*f*, 184–185, 333
Alumina–zirconia composites, 38–39, 140–143
Aluminoborate glasses, 55
Aluminosilicate glasses, 54–55
Aluminosilicate polyacrylate-I (ASPA-I), 51
Aluminum-polyacrylate gels, 8–9
Amedica Corp, 166
Ames test, 114, 115*f*
Amorphous calcium phosphate (ACP), 25
Animal Welfare Act, 115–116
Ankle joints, application of load-bearing ceramics in, 157
Antimicrobial effectiveness, 59–60
Apatites, multisubstituted, 408–412
Apatitic bone cements, 416*f*
Apatitic tricalcium phosphate, 24
Arteriovenous (AV) loop, 291
Artificial pulp chamber (APC), 359–360, 360*f*
Attenuation, 396–397
Attenuation coefficients, 393, 396–397
Autologous transplantation methods, 380, 381*f*

**B**

Bacterial adherence and response of the tissues, 212–216
Balloon kyphoplasty and vertebroplasty, 413
B-carbonation, 409
Bioactive ceramics, 83–84, 111
Bioactive glass plates, use of, 260*f*
Bioactive glasses, 44–49
commercial, 96*t*, 258*t*
and glass ceramics, 14–15, 93–95, 256–262
Bioactive oxides, 22, 28

Biocompatibility
assessing, 359–360
*in vivo* evaluation of, 117–120
of zirconia implants, 187–188
Biocompatible ceramics, coatings with, 341–344
Bioglass 45S5 particles, 45, 48
Bioinert ceramics, 63
structural, 102–105
Bio-inspired composites
design and fabrication of, 378*f*
Biological assessment of bioceramics, 111
*in vitro* models, advanced preclinical, 120–123
co-culture *in vitro* models, 121–122
three-dimensional models, 122–123
*in vitro* tests, 113–115
Ames test, 114, 115*f*
micronucleus assay (MN), 114–115
*in vivo* evaluation of biocompatibility, 117–120
*in vivo* tests, 115–116
pathological models, 120
regulations and international standard organization rules, 112
Biolox delta ceramic, 103, 104*f*, 316–317, 323, 332–333
BIOLOXdelta components, 155–156, 161–162
BIOLOXOption, 162, 164*f*
Biomimetic apatitic bone cements, 416*f*
Biomimetic architectured ceramics, 443–446
Biomimetic nanocrystalline apatite, 26
Biomimetics with bioceramics
tissue engineering and. *See* Tissue engineering and biomimetics with bioceramics
Biomineralization, 417–418
Biomorphic SiC, 44
Biomorphic transformations, 424
Biopolymers, 414–417
Bioreactors, for 3D culture, 450–453, 451*t*
flow perfusion, 452–453
rotating vessels, 450–452
spinner flasks, 450
Biphasic calcium phosphates (BCPs), 12–13, 282
Biphasic HA/β-TCP and related mixtures, 28–29
Bis-GMA (bisphenol A glycidyl dimethacrylate), 376–377
Bisphenol A glycidyl methacrylate (bis-GMA)-based composite, 207
Bisphosphonates, 32–33
Bisurface Knee replacement, 155
BonAlive S53P4, 48
Bone cements, 13–14
Bone fracture healing interactions, diamond model of, 281*f*
Bone fracture model, 123
Bone mineral, 83, 408–409, 416–417
Bone regeneration, ceramic devices for, 279, 408–409, 424
biology of bone healing, 280–281
calcium phosphates (CaP) ceramics, 282–288
mechanical properties of new forming bone, 287–288
mechanical properties of scaffolds, 284–287
current biomaterials, osteogenic substances, and surgical procedures, 281–282
implant-based tissue engineering strategies, rationale for development of, 288–297
BTE strategies, 290–291
CaP bioceramics, 291–297
from research to clinic: issues, 289
Bone regeneration, prediction of
based on mathematical modeling, 400–402
Bone replacement, ceramics for, 249
assessing the performances of, 395*f*
bioactive glasses and glass ceramics, 256–262
calcium orthophosphates of synthetic origin, 254–256
composites, 262–264
human and animal origin, bone substitutes of, 250–252
moldable and injectable ceramic-based cements, 264–269
nonanimal biological origin, bone substitutes of, 252–254

Bone Source, 266–267
Bone tissue engineering (BTE), 288–289
  BTE scaffolds, 391–392
Bone tissue engineering
  mathematical models in, 393–396
BoneAlive, 261
Bone-forming cells, 400
BPH-S total knee replacement, 156*f*
BPO (benzoyl peroxide), 376–377
Bridging stresses, 93
Bulk ceramics, 331–341
  new developments
    nonoxides, 340–341
    oxides, 334–340
  from a retrospect to the current state-of-the-art, 331–333

C
Calcium carbonates, 33
Calcium orthophosphates of synthetic origin, 254–256
Calcium oxide (CaO), 54
Calcium phosphate cements (CPCs), 13, 100–102, 413–414
Calcium phosphate ceramic scaffolds
  in flow perfusion bioreactors, 454*t*
Calcium phosphate scaffolds, 440
Calcium phosphates (CaP) and CaP composites, 95–100
Calcium phosphates (CaP) bioceramics, 279–280, 291–297
  architectural features of the scaffold, 294–297
  composition of, 292–294
Calcium phosphates (CaP) ceramics, 256, 282–288, 407
  mechanical properties of new forming bone, 287–288
  mechanical properties of scaffolds, 284–287
Calcium phosphates (CaPs)-based systems, 22–33, 23*t*
  biphasic HA/β-TCP and related mixtures, 28–29
  CaPs for drug delivery systems, 31–33
  inorganic cement formulations, 29–30
  organic/inorganic composites, 30–31
  pure and substituted HA and related apatite compounds, 24–28
  nanocrystalline apatites, 26–28
  well-crystallized apatites, 24–26
Calcium sulfate, 33–34, 264–265
Calcium-deficiency in apatites, 423–424
Calcium-fluoroalumino-silicate glass particles, 8–9
Canine bioengineered tooth, 380
Carbide and nitride thin films and surfaces, 345–346
  oxidized titanium, 346
  surface oxidized zirconium, 346
Carbon based coatings, 344–345
  diamond-like carbon films, 344–345
  nano-crystalline diamond (NCD), 345
  pyrolytic carbon (PyC), 345
Carbon nanotubes (CNT), 323–324
Carboxyl-containing molecules, 31
Caries filling, materials for, 8–9
CBS (Crystalline Bone Screw), 133–134
Cell culture methods, in bone engineering studies, 449*f*
Cell-seeded hydroxyapatite, 447*f*
Ceramic bearings, 320
  design of, 147–151
Ceramic coatings in joint replacements, 159–161
  diamond-like carbon coatings, 160–161
  nitride coatings, 159–160
  zirconium dioxide coatings, 160
Ceramic crown material, Young's modulus of, 374–375
Ceramic fracture, 318, 318*t*, 319*f*, 320
Ceramic posts, 201–202
Ceramic suspensions, 419–420
Ceramic-on-ceramic (CoC), 317–318, 321–322
  CoC bearings, 130–131, 322
  CoC implants, 321
Ceramic-on-polyethylene (CoP), 131
Ceramic-on-polymer (CoP) implants, 321
Ceramic–polymer composites, 15, 98
Ceramics for bone repair, 12–15
  bioactive glasses and glass ceramics, 14–15
  bone cements, 13–14
  ceramic-polymer composites, 15
  sintered calcium orthophosphates, 12–13

CeramTec, 38–39, 161–162
Cerasmart (GC America, Alsip, IL, USA), 231
Cerasorb, 255
Ceraver, 165
CEREC system, 183
Ceria-doped zirconia ceramics (Ce-TZP) composites, 362–363, 365, 368–370
  Ce-TZP-alumina, 372*t*
  Ce-TZP-alumina-Sr aluminate, 372*t*
  Ce-TZP-Mg spinel, 372*t*
  fracture toughness, 367*f*
Chlorapatite, 25
Chondrocytes, 187
Coatings, 341–346
  with biocompatible ceramics, 341–344
  carbide and nitride thin films and surfaces, 345–346
    oxidized titanium, 346
    surface oxidized zirconium, 346
  carbon based coatings, 344–345
    diamond-like carbon films, 344–345
    nano-crystalline diamond (NCD), 345
    pyrolytic carbon (PyC), 345
Cobalt–chromium alloys, 8
CoC hip resurfacing (CoCHR) design, 322–323
Cojet treatment, 227
Commercial ceramics for joint replacements bearings, 161–167, 162*f*
  Amedica Corp, 166
  CeramTec, 161–162
  Ceraver, 165
  CoorsTek medical, 166
  Groupe Lépine, 167
  Kyocera, 165–166
  Mathys, 162–165
  Morgan advanced ceramics, 167
  Signal Medical Corporation, 167
Commercial load-bearing ceramics, 217–231
  glass ceramics, 227–231
    glass-infiltrated ceramics, 229–231
    reinforced, 227–229
  load-bearing polymer–ceramic composites, 231
    Cerasmart (GC America, Alsip, IL, USA), 231
    Lava Ultimate CAD/CAM Restorative, 231
    Paradigm MZ100, 231
    PICN-Vita Enamic, Vita Zahnfabrik, 231
  toughened ceramics, 217–227
    fully sintered polycrystalline alumina ceramics, 217
    fully sintered polycrystalline zirconia ceramics, 217–227
Commercially available ceramic-based/ ceramic-containing cements, 266*t*
Commission Internationale de l'Eclairage (CIE), 360–361
CoMplete Acetabular Hip System, 152
Composites, 262–264
Computational models, 393
Computed tomography (CT), 393
Computer-aided design and computer-aided manufacturing (CAD/CAM), 140, 284–285, 434
Computer-assisted design–computer-assisted machining (CAD-CAM) methods, 7
Continuum micromechanics, 394–396, 401–402
Conventional glass-ionomer cements (C-GIC), 51
CoorsTek medical, 166
Coral-based bioceramics, commercial, 253*t*
Coralline bioceramics, 252
Coralline calcium carbonate, 252
Corals, ceramics from, 252–254
Crack–surface interactions, 93
Cross-linked polyethylene (XLPE), 131
Cross-linked polyethylene (XPE), 321–322
Crowns and structures, materials for, 6–8
Customized ceramic medical devices, advanced processing techniques for, 433
  additive manufacturing (AM), 434–443
    critical role of 3D geometrical features of pores in scaffolds, 441–443
    indirect additive manufacturing, 441
    powder-based technologies, 435–439
    slurry extrusion-based techniques, 439–440
    stereolithography (SLA), 440–441

bioreactors and 3D cell culture techniques, 446–458
3D dynamic cell cultures and bioreactors, 450–453
decisional chart and parameters to standardize, 453–458
freeze-templating, 443–446
Customized ceramics, 433–434

**D**
Decoy receptor, 400–401
Dense polycrystalline ceramics, 184
Dental applications, 4–9
caries filling, materials for, 8–9
crowns and structures, materials for, 6–8
dental implants, materials for, 5–6
esthetics, materials for, 8
of load-bearing ceramics, 182–216
Dental ceramics, 181
commercial load-bearing ceramics: a comparative analysis, 217–231
glass ceramics, 227–231
load-bearing polymer–ceramic composites, 231
toughened ceramics, 217–227
design of, 355
bio-inspired design, 374–379
dental tissue regeneration, 379–383
indirect restoration, 357–358
minimum flexural strength for, 359*t*
requirements for, 357–361
zirconia as a dental material, 361–365
$ZrO_2$-based dental materials, 365–374
load-bearing ceramics, dental applications of, 182–216
biocompatibility of zirconia implants, 187–188
biomechanical properties of zirconia implants, 187
CAD/CAM systems, 183–185
ceramic implant abutments, 210–216
endodontic post, 201–210
*in vivo* behavior of the main zirconia implant systems, 188–200
marginal fit, 185
Dental restoration, 8, 63
Dental tissue regeneration, 379–383
Dental zirconia ceramics, mechanical properties of, 372*t*
Dentin, 356–357
Dentin–enamel junction (DEJ), 355–356
Diamond-like carbon (DLC) coatings, 143, 160–161, 344–345
Direct foaming, 419–420, 421*f*
Direct write assembly (DWA) method, 439
Doxorubicin (DOX), 32–33
Drug delivery devices, 63
Drug delivery systems, CaPs for, 31–33

**E**
Enamel, 355–356, 356*f*
Endosseous Ridge Maintenance Implant (ERMI), 46, 259
Eshelby's matrix-inclusion problem, 394–396
Esthetic requirements, 360–361
Esthetics, 4, 363–364
materials for, 8
Expanded polytetrafluoroethylene (e-PTFE), 381–382
Extracellular matrix (ECM), 446–448

**F**
Failure analysis, 321–323
FeHA, 411–412
multifunctional platform in nanomedicine based on, 412*f*
Fiber-reinforced composite (FRC) posts, 201
Fiber-reinforced CPCs (FRCPCs), 100–102
Fibroblasts, 187
Finger joints, application of load-bearing ceramics in, 157–158
Finite element (FE) method, 393–394, 396
Finite-element simulation, 375
First-generation ceramic materials, 3–4
Fixed partial dentures (FPDs), 184
Flexural test methods, 358–359
Flow perfusion-based bioreactors, 452–453, 454*t*
Fluoride, 52, 56–57, 59
Fluoride release and recharge ability, 58–59
Fluorohydroxyapatite (FHA), 25
Foamed apatite ceramics, 420–421
45S5 Bioglass, 256–262
Fracture of ceramics, 84–85
Fracture toughness, mechanisms of increase in, 90–93
Freeze-casting technique, 377

Freeze-templating, 443–446, 444*f*, 445*f*
Fully sintered polycrystalline alumina ceramics, 217
Fully sintered polycrystalline zirconia ceramics, 217–227
auto-catalytic transformation, 225
occlusal function, 221
thermal expansion/contraction and residual stress, 225
unsupported porcelain, 221–225
weaker porcelain, 225
zirconia cementation, 226–227
Cojet treatment, 227
hydrofluoric acid etching, 227
Rocatec treatment, 226
sandblasting, 226
silica coating process, 227
tribochemical treatment, 226
Functionally graded materials (FGM), 364–365, 375

**G**
Genotoxicity, 114
Glass ceramics, 111, 227–231
and bioactive glass ceramics, 49–50
bioactive glasses and, 93–95, 256–262
glass-infiltrated ceramics, 7, 229–231
1993 Vita-CAD/CAM InCeram-Alumina -Single anterior and posterior crowns, 230
1994-CEREC inLab-inlay, crown-anterior restorations, vital teeth, 230
In-Ceram Alumina-Slip-cast or milled, 229–230
In-Ceram Spinell, 230
In-Ceram Zirconia, 230–231
synthoceram, 230
reinforced, 227–229
leucite reinforced glass ceramics, 227–228
lithium disilicate glass ceramics, 228–229
Glass reactivity, 57–58
acid washing, 58
heat treatment, 57
Glass-ionomer cements (GICs), 8–9, 50–60, 63
antimicrobial effectiveness, 59–60
chemistry of, 53–54
fluoride release and recharge ability, 58–59
glass compositions to form, 54–55
aluminoborate glasses, 55
aluminosilicate glasses, 54–55
zinc silicate glasses, 55
key factors affecting the properties of, 55–58
$Al_2O_3/SiO_2$ ratio in the glass, 55–56
$F^-$ content in the glass, 56–57
glass reactivity, 57–58
$Na^+$ content in the glass, 57
particle size, 58
phosphorus content in the glass, 56
Groupe Lépine, 167
Guided bone regeneration (GBR), 380–382
$ZrO_2$ membranes for, 383

**H**
HAPEX, 262–264
Hard tissue applications, materials for, 1
ceramics for bone repair, 12–15
bioactive glasses and glass ceramics, 14–15
bone cements, 13–14
ceramic-polymer composites, 15
sintered calcium orthophosphates, 12–13
dental applications, 4–9
materials for caries filling, 8–9
materials for crowns and structures, 6–8
materials for dental implants, 5–6
materials for esthetics, 8
orthopedic applications, 9–12
alumina, 9–10
composites, 10–11
materials in development, 11–12
zirconia, 10
replacement of damaged hard tissues, 3–4
Hard-on-hard bearings, 151–152
Hard-on-soft bearings with ceramic heads, 152–154
Hierarchically organized scaffolds, 423, 423*f*
High velocity oxyfuel spraying (HVOF), 342–343
High-density PTFE (d-PTFE), 381–382
High-velocity suspension flame spraying (HVSFS), 342–343

Hip- and knee implants, 334
Hip- and knee-replacement bearings, 42
Hip replacements, application of ceramics in, 133*f*, 145–154
ceramic bearings, design of, 147–151
hard-on-hard bearings, 151–152
hard-on-soft bearings with ceramic heads, 152–154
Hip resurfacing (HR), 322–323
Hot isostatic pressing (HIP), 136, 314–315
Human and animal origin, bone substitutes of, 250–252
Hybrid scaffold, 416–419
Hydrofluoric acid etching, 227
Hydrogen fluoride, 59
Hydrothermal degradation/aging, 102–103
Hydroxyapatite (HA), 83, 120, 292–293, 408–409
Hydroxyapatite (HA) ceramic, 342
Hydroxycarbonated apatite (HCA) layer, 45, 95
Hypoxia-induced cell death, 290

## I

Ice-templating. *See* Freeze-templating
Ilizarov device, 282
Implant abutments, ceramic, 210–216
bacterial adherence and response of tissues, 212–216
implant/abutment fitting, 211
zirconia abutments strength, 212
Implant-based tissue engineering strategies, rationale for development of, 288–297
BTE strategies, 290–291
calcium phosphates bioceramics, 291–297
architectural features of the scaffold, 294–297
composition of, 292–294
from research to clinic, 289
*In vitro* models, advanced preclinical, 120–123
co-culture *in vitro* models, 121–122
osteoblasts/chondrocytes differentiated from mesenchymal stem cells, 122
osteoblasts/osteoclasts, 121
osteoblasts/osteoclasts/endothelial cells, 121–122
three-dimensional models, 122–123
*In vitro* tests, 113–115, 120–121
Ames test, 114, 115*f*
micronucleus assay (MN), 114–115
*In vivo* tests, 113*t*, 115–116, 359–360
Indirect additive manufacturing, 441, 442*f*
Indirect restoration, 183, 357–358
Inert high-strength ceramics, 382
Inert oxides and composites, 34–39
alumina ceramics, 34–35
alumina–zirconia composites, 38–39
further developments, 39
zirconia ceramics, 37–38
Ion-doped apatites, 413–414
Ion-doped CPCs, 415
ISO 7405:2009, 359–360

## J

Joint replacement, ceramics for, 127
ceramic coatings, 159–161
diamond-like carbon coatings, 160–161
nitride coatings, 159–160
zirconium dioxide coatings, 160
commercial ceramics, 161–167, 162*f*
Amedica Corp, 166
CeramTec, 161–162
Ceraver, 165
CoorsTek medical, 166
Groupe Lépine, 167
Kyocera, 165–166
Mathys, 162–165
Morgan advanced ceramics, 167
Signal Medical Corporation, 167
development, 132–145
nonoxide bioceramics, 143–145
oxide biomaterials, 132–143
hip replacements, application of ceramics in, 133*f*, 145–154
design of ceramic bearings, 147–151
hard-on-hard bearings, 151–152
hard-on-soft bearings with ceramic heads, 152–154
knee replacements, applications of ceramic in, 154–156
load-bearing ceramics, application of, 157–159
in ankle joints, 157
in finger joints, 157–158
in shoulder joints, 157
in spine joints, 158–159

Joint replacement, ceramics for (*Continued*)
requirements, 145–159

**K**

Keramische Werk Hermsdorf (KWH), 135
$K_{IC}$ and curve R-behavior of ceramics, 90
Knee replacements, 130
applications of ceramic in, 154–156
Bisurface Knee replacement, 155
BPH-S total knee replacement, 156*f*
Multigen Plus Total Knee Replacement, 155–156, 156*f*
total knee replacements (TKRs), 131
Kyocera, 140, 142, 154–155, 157, 165–166

**L**

Lava Ultimate CAD/CAM Restorative, 231
Leucite reinforced glass ceramics, 227–228
1986-IPS-Empress (Ivoclar)-heat pressed, 228
1998-IPS ProCAD-milled, 228
2006-IPS-Empress CAD, 228
Liquid-phase sintered silicon nitride, 333, 340–341
Lithium disilicate glass ceramics, 228–229
1998-IPS Empress2-IPS e.max (Ivoclar), 228–229
2006-IPS e.max CAD (Ivoclar-Vivadent), 229
Lithium-disilicate-based glass ceramics, 6–8
Load-bearing ceramics, application of, 157–159
in ankle joints, 157
in finger joints, 157–158
in shoulder joints, 157
in spine joints, 158–159
Load-bearing ceramics, dental applications of, 182–216
biocompatibility of zirconia implants, 187–188
biomechanical properties of zirconia implants, 187
CAD/CAM systems, 183–185
ceramic implant abutments, 210–216
bacterial adherence and response of the tissues, 212–216
implant/abutment fitting, 211
zirconia abutments strength, 212
*in vivo* behavior of main zirconia implant systems, 188–200
Axis Biodental, 197, 198*f*
BIO-HIP Metoxit AG, Thayngen, Switzerland, 195–196
Bredent (Senden Germany), 196
CeraRoot-Oral Iceberg Barcelona, Spain, 196, 197*f*
Goei implants (Goei Industry, Akitsu-Hiroshima, Japan), 194
Incermed SA, Losanna, 188–193
Konus Dental, 197
ReImplant; Hagen Germany, 197
Straumann, 199–200, 200*f*
ZERAMEX T Implants system (Dentalpoint AG, Zurich, Switzerland), 200
Ziterion, 197
ZiUnite; Nobel Biocare, 198–199, 199*f*
Z-systems AG, Konstanz, Germany, 194–195
marginal fit, 185
zirconia endodonic posts
bond strength of, 207–208
clinical studies of, 209–210
fracture strength of, 201–202
retentive strength of, 202–206
Load-bearing polymer–ceramic composites, 231
Cerasmart (GC America, Alsip, IL, USA), 231
Lava Ultimate CAD/CAM Restorative, 231
Paradigm MZ100, 231
PICN-Vita Enamic, Vita Zahnfabrik, 231
Low Friction Anatomical (LFA-1), 155
Low-temperature degradation (LTD), 102–103, 138–139, 332, 361–362
Low-temperature hydrothermal degradation (LTD), 37–38
Lymphocytes, 187

**M**

Macrophage, 187–188
Macroporous biphasic calcium phosphate ceramics, 256
Macroscopic porous network, 294–295
Macroscopic stiffness, 394–396, 398–399

Magnesia partially stabilized zirconia (Mg-PSZ), 11, 138*f*, 315–316
Magnesium-doped apatite, 409
Magnetic ceramic materials in medicine, 60–62
Magnetic scaffolds, 417–418
Masquelet technique, 282
Mathematical models
  in bone tissue engineering, 393–396
  for patient-specific scaffold design, 396–402
    prediction of bone regeneration based on mathematical modeling, 400–402
    X-ray physics-based analysis of CT data, 396–399
Mathys, 135, 162–165, 333
Mechanical properties of ceramic materials, 83
  bioactive glasses and glass ceramics, 93–95
  bioceramics, 83–84
  calcium phosphate cements (CPCs), 100–102
  calcium phosphates (CaP) and CaP composites, 95–100
  fracture of ceramics, 84–85
  fracture toughness, mechanisms of increase in, 90–93
  $K_{IC}$ and curve R-behavior of ceramics, 90
  structural bioinert ceramics, 102–105
  subcritical crack growth (SCCG), 88–90
  Weibull statistics of the strength, 85–88, 87*f*
Mesenchymal stem cells (MSCs), 122, 290, 456–457
  osteoblasts/chondrocytes differentiated from, 122
Metal-on-polymers (MoPs) couples, 321
Mg-doped hydrpxyapatite (Mg-HA) nanoparticles
  *in vivo* assessment of, 410*f*
Micro-computed tomography (micro-CT), 393
Microcracking phenomenon, 37–38
Micro-FE simulations, 393–394
Micronucleus assay (MN), 114–115, 115*f*
Microstereolithography (μSLA), 440–441
Microtomography, 119–120
Mimix Bone Void Filler, 267
Mixed stabilizer systems, 339
Moldable and injectable ceramic-based cements, 264–269
Molding, 6–7
Morgan advanced ceramics, 167
Mori–Tanaka-type homogenization scheme, 398–399
Multigen Plus TKR, 155–156
Multigen total knee replacement, 156*f*

**N**

$Na^+$ content in the glass, 57
Nanocrystalline, 408–409
Nanocrystalline apatites, 26–28
Nano-crystalline diamond (NCD), 345
Nanocrystalline superparamagnetic apatite, 411
NANOZR, 39, 337–338, 368, 372*t*
National Institute of Standards and Technology (NIST), 397–398
Neutral Red dye, 113, 114*f*
Nitride coatings, 159–160
Nitrides, 143
Noise production, 319–320
Nonanimal biological origin, bone substitutes of, 252–254
Nonbridging oxygens (NBOs), 54
Nonoxide bioceramics, 143–145
Nonoxide ceramics, 40–44
  silicon carbide, 43–44
  silicon nitride, 40–43
    emergence of silicon nitride as a biomedical material, 41–43
Nonoxides, 333, 340–341
NovaBone, 46, 259–262, 260*f*
Numerical multiscale models, 393–394

**O**

Odontogenesis, 379–380
Orthopedic applications, 4, 9–12, 42, 142–143, 340–341
  alumina, 9–10
  composites, 10–11
  materials in development, 11–12
  zirconia, 10
Orthopedic devices, design of ceramic materials for, 329
  bulk ceramics, 331–341
    nonoxides, 340–341

Orthopedic devices, design of ceramic materials for (*Continued*)
oxides, 334–340
from a retrospect to the current state-of-the-art, 331–333
coatings, 341–346
carbide and nitride thin films and surfaces, 345–346
carbon based coatings, 344–345
coatings with biocompatible ceramics, 341–344
compositional design, 347
microstructural design, 347
Orthopedic medical devices, ceramics as
advantages and disadvantages, 317–320
challenges and future trends, 323–324
*in vitro* performance and *in vivo* failure analysis, 321–323
technical issues and surgical aspects, 320–321
Osteoblasts, 187, 400
Osteoblasts/chondrocytes differentiated from mesenchymal stem cells, 122
Osteoblasts/osteoclasts, 121
Osteoblasts/osteoclasts/endothelial cells, 121–122
Osteochondral model, 122–123
Osteoconductivity, 392
Osteocytes, 400
Osteoporosis, 120, 409–410, 414
Osteoprotegerin (OPG), 400–401
Oxide and fluoride glasses, 54
Oxide biomaterials, 132–143
alumina, 132–136
alumina–zirconia composites, 140–143
zirconia, 136–140
Oxide ceramics bearings, 131
Oxides, 54, 334–340
Oxidized titanium, 199, 346
OXINIUM-Oxidized Zirconium, 346
Oxygen plasma irradiation, 364

**P**

Paradigm MZ100, 231
Parathyroid hormone (PTH), 400–401
Parfitt formulae, 119
Partially stabilized zirconia (PSZ), 365–366
Patient-specific design
definition and implied requirements, 391–392
integration of experimental, clinical, and computational approaches, 393
realization of *in vivo* conditions, 392–393
utilization of mathematical models for, 396–402
PerioGlas, 46, 259
Phosphate-buffered saline (PBS), 42
Phosphate-free bioactive $Na_2O$–$CaO$–$SiO_2$ glass particles, 49
Phosphorus content in the glass, 56
Physical vapor deposition (PVD), 342
PICN-Vita Enamic, Vita Zahnfabrik, 231
Polyacrylic acid (PAA), 51, 53–54
Polycrystalline ceramics, 182, 184
Polymer–ceramic composites, 377
Polymer-infiltrated-ceramic-network materials (PICNs), 7–8, 376–377
Polymethylmetaacrylate (PMMA), 29, 413, 422
Porcelain, 8, 181, 218–221, 376
Porous architectures, visualizations of, 443*f*
Porous bioceramics, 419–424
Porous scaffolds, 25, 48, 415*f*, 419–420
Powder-based technologies, 435–439
Powder-binder systems, 439
Preclinical models, 120
Predictive assessment strategies, 402
Primary Irritation Index (PII), 117
Procera AllCeram system, 217
Prosthetic hip- and knee-replacement bearings, 42
Pyrolytic carbon (PyC), 158, 345

**R**

RANK-RANKL-OPG pathway, 400–401
Rattan wood, 423, 423*f*
R-curve behavior, 90–93, 94*f*
Reaction-bonded silicon nitride (RBSN), 40
Reamer–Irrigator–Aspirator (RIA) System, 282
Receptor activator of nuclear factor kappa β (RANK), 400–401
Regenerative cascade, 416–417
Reinforced glass ceramics, 227–229
leucite, 227–228
lithium disilicate glass ceramics, 228–229

Reinforced glassy materials, 182
Resin-modified glass-ionomer cement (RM-GIC), 51–52
Revision surgery, 320–321
Robocasting (RB), 439
Rocatec treatment, 226
Rosenthal Technik, 135
Rotating wall bioreactors, 450–452

**S**
Sandblasting, 195, 226
Sandhaus dental implant, 186, 186*f*
Scaffolds, 84, 286–287, 438*f*
  critical role of 3D geometrical features of pores in, 441–443
  design, 296, 298
  magnetic scaffolds, 417–418
  mechanical properties of, 284–287
  porous scaffolds, 419–420
Second-generation ceramic materials, 3–4
Selective laser sintering (SLS), 435–438, 436*f*, 437*t*
Self-consistent homogenization scheme, 398–399
Semi-quantitative grading scores, 119
Separation-of-scales-requirement, 394–396
SEVNB method, 370–371
Shoulder joints, application of load-bearing ceramics in, 157
Signal Medical Corporation, 140, 167
Silica coating process, 208, 227
Silicon carbide, 43–44
Silicon nitride, 11–12, 40–43, 144, 341
  emergence of, as a biomedical material, 41–43
Silicon-doped apatites, 410
Sintered calcium orthophosphates, 12–13
Sintering window, 48, 261
Slip casting techniques, 140, 230–231
Slip-casting technology, 377–379, 378*f*
Slow crack growth, 97, 185, 337–338
Slurry extrusion-based techniques, 436*f*, 437*t*, 439–440
Slurry-based 3D printing (S-3DP) technologies, 439
Slurry-based SLS (S-SLS) technologies, 439
Soda–lime–silica ($Na_2O$–CaO–$SiO_2$) glass, 44
Sol-gel processing, 49
Sol-gel synthesis, 140
Spine joints, application of load-bearing ceramics in, 158–159
Squeaking, 318–319, 324
Sr-doped CPCs, 415
Stereolithography (SLA), 436*f*, 437*t*, 440–441
Stoichiometric HA, 24
*Streptococcus mutans*, 59–60
Stress-induced transformation phenomenon, 37–38
Strontium ranelate, 413
Strontium-doped apatites, 409–410
Subchronic systemic toxicity, 117
Subcritical crack growth (SCCG), 88–90
Superparamagnetic HA nanoparticles, 411–412
Superparamagnetic iron oxide nanoparticles (SPIONs), 62
Superparamagnetism, 62
Surface oxidized zirconium, 346
Surface-coating elaboration method, 370
Surgical-grade calcium sulfate cements, 265
Synovial fluid analysis, 320
Synthetic origin, calcium orthophosphates of, 254–256
Systemic toxicity test, 117

**T**
Tartaric acid (TA) accelerators, 51
TEGDMA (tri(ethyl-englycol) dimethacrylate), 376–377
Template-based methods, 419–420
Template-free processes, 419–420
Tetragonal zirconia polycrystal (TZP), 130, 217
Third-body metallic particles, 319–320
Third-generation ceramic materials, 3–4
3D dynamic cell cultures, 449*f*, 450–453
Three-dimensional models, 122–123
  bone fracture model, 123
  osteochondral model, 122–123
3D printing, 436*f*, 437*t*, 439
3Y-TZP, 372*t*
Tissue engineering and biomimetics with bioceramics, 407
  future perspectives, 424–425

Tissue engineering and biomimetics with bioceramics (*Continued*)
multifunctional, biohybrid scaffold obtained by bioinspired assembling/ mineralization process, 416–419
multisubstituted apatites, 408–412
superparamagnetic HA nanoparticles, 411–412
porous bioceramics with hierarchical structure obtained by biomorphic transformation of natural structures, 419–424
Tissue engineering in dentistry, 384
Titanium, 5–6, 185–186, 211, 422
Titanium alloys, 8
Titanium mesh, 381–382
Titanium nitride (TiN), 159, 345–346
Titanium oxide, 346
Titanium-reinforced PTFE, 381–382
Tooth development, stages in, 379–380
Total hip arthroplasty (THA)
of ceramics for, 317*f*
noise, 321
THA ceramic bearings, failure of, 320
Total hip replacements (THR), 131, 314
Total knee replacements (TKRs), 131, 133*f*
Total shoulder replacement (TSR) systems, 157
Toughened ceramics, 217–227
fully sintered polycrystalline alumina ceramics, 217
fully sintered polycrystalline zirconia ceramics, 217–227
auto-catalytic transformation, 225
occlusal function, 221
thermal expansion/contraction and residual stress, 225
unsupported porcelain, 221–225
weaker porcelain, 225
zirconia cementation, 226–227
Toughness/strength relationship for Mg PSZ and Y-PSZ materials, 366–367, 366*f*
Transformation toughening, in ceramics, 361, 365–366
Transforming growth factor beta (TGF-β), 400–401
Tribochemical treatment, 226
Tricalcium phosphate (TCP), 120
Tri-culture model, 121–122, 122*f*
Triethyleneglycoldimetacrylate (TEGMA), 7–8
Tubingen (Frialit) implants, 186
Types of ceramics, 21
active oxides, 22–34
calcium carbonates, 33
calcium phosphates (CaPs)-based systems, 22–33, 23*t*
calcium sulfates, 33–34
bioactive glasses, 44–49
glass ceramics and bioactive glass ceramics, 49–50
glass-ionomer cements (GICs), 50–60, 63
antimicrobial effectiveness, 59–60
chemistry of, 53–54
fluoride release and recharge ability, 58–59
glass compositions to form, 54–55
key factors affecting the properties of, 55–58
inert oxides and composites, 34–39
alumina ceramics, 34–35
alumina–zirconia composites, 38–39
further developments, 39
zirconia ceramics, 37–38
magnetic ceramic materials in medicine, 60–62
nonoxide ceramics, 40–44
silicon carbide, 43–44
silicon nitride, 40–43
TZ-3YB-E, 372*t*

**U**

Ultra-high-molecular-weight polyethylene (UHMWPE), 131, 149, 315
Urethane dimetacrylate (UDMA), 7–8

**V**

Vertebral compression fractures, treatment of, 413
Vita Enamic, 7–8, 376–377
Voxel-specific attenuation coefficient, 397–398

**W**

Weibull statistics of the strength, 85–88, 87*f*
Well-crystallized apatites, 24–26
White-Sky implants, 196, 196*f*
Whole-tooth complex, 379, 384

**X**

Xenografts, 251–252
X-ray physics-based analysis of CT data, 396–399

**Y**

Yokohama Medical Ceramic Knee (YMCK), 155
Yttria partially stabilized zirconia implants (Y-PSZ), 187
Yttria-stabilized tetragonal zirconia polycrystals (Y-TZP), 315–316, 358–359, 361, 365
Yttria-stabilized zirconia (Y-TZP), 131–132, 138, 331, 339

**Z**

ZA8Sr8, 370
ZA8Sr8-Ce10.5, 372*t*
Zinc silicate glasses, 55
Zirconia, 5, 10, 103, 136–140, 332–333
  as a dental material, 361–365
    $ZrO_2$-based dental materials, 365–374
Zirconia abutments, 211
  strength, 212
Zirconia- and platelets-toughened alumina, 142*f*
Zirconia cementation, 226–227
  Cojet treatment, 227
  hydrofluoric acid etching, 227
  Rocatec treatment, 226
  sandblasting, 226
  silica coating process, 227
  tribochemical treatment, 226
Zirconia ceramics, 8, 37–38, 315–316
Zirconia endodonic posts
  bond strength of, 207–208
  clinical studies of, 209–210
  fracture strength of, 201–202
  retentive strength of, 202–206
Zirconia implant systems, *in vivo* behavior of, 188–200
  Axis Biodental, 197, 198*f*
  BIO-HIP Metoxit AG, Thayngen, Switzerland, 195–196
  Bredent (Senden Germany), 196
  CeraRoot-Oral Iceberg Barcelona, Spain, 196, 197*f*
  Goei implants (Goei Industry, Akitsu-Hiroshima, Japan), 194
  Incermed SA, Losanna, 188–193
  Konus Dental, 197
  ReImplant; Hagen Germany, 197
  Straumann, 199–200, 200*f*
  ZERAMEX T Implants system (Dentalpoint AG, Zurich, Switzerland), 200
  Ziterion, 197
  ZiUnite; Nobel Biocare, 198–199, 199*f*
  Z-systems AG, Konstanz, Germany, 194–195
Zirconia implants
  biocompatibility of, 187–188
  biomechanical properties of, 187
Zirconia sheet, customized, 382*f*
Zirconia-based materials
  development of strong, tough, and stable zirconia-based materials, 369*f*
Zirconia-toughened alumina (ZTA), 10–11, 38, 141, 184–185, 316–317, 331, 333*f*, 335, 336*f*
Zirconium dioxide coatings, 160

CPI Antony Rowe
Chippenham, UK
2017-10-31 21:07